Consultation Skills

for Mental Health Professionals

Consultation Skills
for Mental Health Professionals

Richard W. Sears

John R. Rudisill

Carrie Mason-Sears

WILEY

JOHN WILEY & SONS, INC.

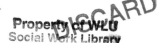

To Ashlyn and Jeremy,
from whom we have learned so much.

Contents ———————————————

Preface ———————————————————————————————

This book is based on the class notes for the core course on consultation for doctoral clinical psychologists created by John R. Rudisill, dean of the Wright State University School of Professional Psychology. Our intent is to educate mental health professionals on the practical aspects of consultation. This material covers traditional mental health consultation models, but also focuses on consulting with organizations, which is a rapidly growing area of the field. Regardless of which area you find most attractive (or even if you believe you may never actively engage in formal consultation work), the diverse array of knowledge covered in this book will prove useful to all mental health clinicians. The book is organized into four parts: (1) Individual-Level Consulting Issues, (2) Consulting to Small Systems, (3) Consulting to Large Systems, and (4) Special Topics.

The chapters in this book cover a broad variety of consulting topics and make ample use of disguised case examples taken from actual practice as well as fictional scenarios to illustrate and enliven the concepts discussed.

Chapter 1 provides an overview of consultation, discussing definitions, different types of consultation, and the fields that have contributed to the research and knowledge base. It reviews the settings in which consultants work and highlights the basic skills and competencies needed by consultants. Basic problem-solving skills are also outlined.

Part One covers issues related to consulting at the individual level. Chapter 2 covers career counseling. Assessment and other issues are discussed for individuals who are seeking employment, changing fields, being promoted, or simply are not happy with their current jobs. Chapter 3 covers concepts concerning a variety of organizational contexts, including job stress, burnout, and how jobs are structured. Theories of human and work motivation are explored, as well as basic legal issues regarding employment. Chapter 4 deals with leadership, management, and supervision. Beginning with historical models of leadership, the evolution of ideas about how to manage others in the workplace is traced, culminating in a multidimensional approach to conceptualizing leadership. Important leadership skills are taught, including supportive communication, dealing with difficult employees, networking, negotiation skills, organizational politics, and how to deal with conflict. Chapter 5 investigates the tools and skills needed for executive assessment, employment selection, effective interviewing, and professional development. Chapter 6 covers executive coaching and performance enhancement, a rapidly growing field in which the consultant or "coach" works to improve the executive's job performance. This chapter presents a variety of strategies, including how to apply psychotherapeutic theories to a coaching situation.

Part Two focuses on issues involved in working with small systems, such as groups and teams. Chapter 7 explores the nature of teams and groups (using systems theory, role theory, and group theory), how to effectively conduct a meeting, and how to facilitate a group (which involves feedback, basic skills, methods and tools, and designing effective facilitation). Chapter 8 discusses how to plan and conduct training and team-building sessions. Though important diversity issues are highlighted throughout the book, Chapter 9 focuses specifically on the many diversity issues that are important in workplace and consultation settings, including how to educate managers and how to make the workplace more inclusive.

Part Three investigates consultation as it applies to large systems. Chapter 10 discusses the nature of organizations, and covers organizational structure, terms, concepts, culture, change, and resistance. Chapter 11 explores assessment issues, including the characteristics of healthy and dysfunctional workplaces, targets and goals of assessment activities, and how to perform effective assessment interviews. Chapter 12 looks at intervention issues and outlines the steps in process consultation, discusses organizational change and development, considerations in the use of differing consulting styles, and strategic planning.

Part Four introduces special consulting topics. Chapter 13 covers the practical issues of running a consulting practice, including charting, billing, and the development of a marketing strategy. Ethical issues are also discussed. Chapter 14 provides information on clinical consultation and explores Caplan's mental health consultation model, behavioral and ecological models of consultation, as well as general knowledge and skills required for successful clinical consulting. Chapter 15 covers consultation services for special populations, including school and pediatric consultation. Annotated bibliographies are included for those who would like to know more about these settings. Chapter 16 covers crisis consultation and outlines strategies for intervening when organizations experience traumatic events, including critical incident stress management (CISM), psychological first aid, phases of disaster recovery, how to communicate with the media, and crisis response in school settings.

The field of mental health is changing. With nationwide budget cuts, community mental health centers and other agencies are cutting back on the number of high-level mental health providers they employ. Aside from the positive aspects of doing consultation work, consulting may become a necessity for many clinicians to provide the means to make a decent living.

Recently, there has been a rapid expansion of research into the field of consulting. Although it is important to have an understanding of the research base, this book focuses more on the practical aspects of consulting. References provided at the end of the book show readers where to find more details about the empirical research.

As a final caution, remember not to "consult" in areas for which you are not competent to practice. Just as you would not work with a deaf client (even through an interpreter) without specific training in deaf culture and issues unique to that population, you should not begin to do work in large organizational strategic planning without specialized knowledge, training, and supervision. In mental health work, the client's mental health is at stake. In organizational consulting, the organizational health and the financial health of the institution and all of its employees are at stake.

Acknowledgments ───────────────────

We would like to thank the many students who have stimulated our thinking and pressed for increasingly helpful ways to impart this material, especially Erika Driver and LaToya Gregory.

Also, we appreciate the support of the generous and welcoming psychologists of the American Psychological Association, Division 13.

Many thanks to our diligent research team, who are doctoral students at the School of Professional Psychology at Wright State University: Shelley Leiphart and Brandon Kozar, for their background research and painstaking indexing work, and Tricia Giessler, Lindsey Slaughter, and Jayme Arose for finding difficult to find citations. Thanks also to Susan Foskuhl, for all of her administrative support.

Thanks also to Elfriede and Charles Sears for all of their support over the years, and to Ashlyn and Jeremy, for all those times we told them we did not have time to play. The mentorship of Joseph Petrick in business consulting and ethics is also greatly appreciated. The inspiration of ninjutsu teacher Stephen K. Hayes has also had a profound impact.

We would also like to thank Tracey Belmont, senior editor at Wiley, Ester Mallach, editorial assistant, and all of the Wiley staff for their encouragement and support of this project. Special thanks also to Charlotte Saikia for her diligent editing work, and to Pam Blackmon and Nancy Land of Publications Development Company of Texas.

This material was gathered from many sources over a number of years, and although every effort was made to appropriately cite material, errors are possible. The authors apologize in advance for any such oversights, and request that we be made known of such instances so that proper credit can be given in future editions of this book.

Consultation Skills

for Mental Health Professionals

Chapter 1

INTRODUCTION

What exactly is consultation? Even very experienced practitioners in this field have a difficult time answering this question with precision. However, one way to define consultation is through consideration of the activities involved. Although the variety of activities makes it difficult to say what a "typical day" might be like, Box 1.1 shows a sampling of a day in the life of a consultant in private practice.

As mental health clinicians, most of us are not particularly interested in consultation during the early years of our career. We usually want to do therapy, most often individual therapy, and are enlivened by the opportunity to intimately connect with individuals in a safe, structured environment. Consultation is sometimes neglected in mental health professions because students conclude that clinical practice is the only legitimate professional expression of clinical skills. As we progress (and sometimes "burn out"), we

---

Box 1.1

A Typical Day for a Full-Time Consultant

7:30 A.M.	Have breakfast at the Racquet Club with the managing partner of a law firm to discuss her business and personal concerns.
9:30 A.M.	Work with an executive who is the victim of downsizing on career assessment.
11:00 A.M.	Consult with a company concerned about a potentially violent employee.
12:00 P.M.	Put on a team-building and planning workshop with a small financial firm around the organization's future.
4:00 P.M.	Meet with an owner and company president who are having difficulty getting along.
5:00 P.M.	Analyze a test battery from a selection candidate for an executive position.
6:00 P.M.	Coach a supervisor who was demoted by his company because of his poor people skills.

On the way home, think about the survey requested by a large social service agency and a consultation request by a medical practice.

---

often begin to feel some comfort with individual therapy, and want to add increased complexity by seeing couples or families. From family or group therapy, the next step in our developmental mastery of complexity may be supervision or organizational consultation.

All the lessons we learn and the experience we gain from individual and group therapy are useful when doing consulting work. Therefore, this book begins with individual interventions, moves into considerations for group interventions, and progresses into principles for organizational consultation. Consultation is one of the most complex and challenging interventions a mental health provider can perform, but with that challenge comes great potential for service. We can often create major impact through our consultation efforts by using the important principle of leverage. As individual service providers, we are limited in the number of individuals we can help. By providing group therapy, we can further increase the number of individuals we help. Through consultation, however, we can ultimately help many more individuals, especially when viewed from a systems perspective. Assisting a work supervisor not only improves the quality of work and life for the supervisor, it can foster a healthier work environment for all the employees at that worksite. Consulting with other mental health providers about specific clinical skills (e.g., systems perspectives and diversity issues) can positively affect every client seen by each provider. Consulting with CEOs of large corporations can help improve the mental health of every employee in that organization.

Once we become more aware of the suffering in the world, we feel compelled to do more about the systems in which the suffering is perpetuated. You may feel that you have little to offer, but what seems like common sense to you may be enlightening to the consultee. As clinicians, we often experience this with psychotherapy clients. When asked later what was most helpful in therapy, clients often point out incidents that we did not recognize as meaningful at the time and discover that the client has no recollection of what we felt was the most meaningful therapeutic event. Whatever the perceptions of either person, the end result is life-altering change.

Consultation has several unique features that may appeal to mental health professionals, depending on their vocational and avocational interests. Often our clinical client base consists of individuals with severe psychopathology with whom it can be extremely challenging to work. Consultation clients are often highly skilled and accomplished "normal" individuals who are extremely grateful for the consultant's services. Consultants typically earn a relatively high fee, which is received promptly, avoiding the hassle of insurance companies and managed care forms and oversight. On the downside, consultation can be anxiety-provoking, tapping into our deep-seated fears and worries about our competence. There is also a large degree of ambiguity in consulting situations—you may find yourself staring at the client with neither of you knowing what the other one really wants or needs. The knowledge that we have learned and relied on in clinical situations, such as the importance of avoiding dual relationships, often becomes less applicable. Consultants must rely on a broad knowledge base, including fields such as business, education, and health. It also typically requires either an ability to market yourself well or a strong personal "face validity," or presence.

We can use our past training and experiences to overcome most of these challenges (Bellman, 1990). We frequently face ambiguous moments or awkward silences in therapy, and ask questions or reflect the conversation to the client when in doubt (or we develop a comfort in using the silence therapeutically). We continuously face ethical issues and devise a systematic framework for thinking about them. We are accustomed to being seen as an authority figure, with all the advantages and disadvantages entailed in such a perception. And those of us who have invested so much time and effort in our educations are likely to enjoy learning new things.

Martin (1996) also encourages mental health professionals to remember the valuable qualities we possess, which will give us confidence to do consulting work. He does this by reminding us about the unique skills we have developed from our psychotherapy experiences:

1. *You are an expert at forming and building a trusting relationship.* The most significant element of the consulting process is the client relationship. Skills that you take for granted, like bonding, empathizing, confronting and disciplining, provide a competitive advantage in the consulting industry.
2. *You have multidimensional training and experience.* Organizational life is complex; and you will find your deeper analysis of the issues useful. The corporate client may not see a problem as intrapsychic, as well as interpersonal, structural or systemic. As a result, he/she will appreciate your broader perspective.
3. *You are hypervigilant and tuned in to people.* This makes you keenly aware of the symbolic aspects of what you observe. Clients, particularly when recruiting executives, find this ability extraordinary in preventing bad hiring decisions that literally cost millions.
4. *You have conducted psychotherapy with extremely challenging cases, including borderlines and multiple personalities.* As such, you have experienced firsthand the commitment required for healing and change. Your ability to stay in close proximity with organizations undergoing the turbulence and pain of change will reap rewards from your grateful clients. Particularly artful transformation of negative transference is admired. (p. 16)

DEFINITIONS OF CONSULTATION

The practice of consultation probably dates back to prehistoric humankind. Even before the emergence of spoken language, someone more skilled at hunting could have assisted someone less skilled on becoming a more efficient hunter. As a serious and formal area of systematic study, however, the complex field of psychological consultation based on scientific principles began in the late twentieth century.

The National Council of Schools and Programs of Professional Psychology (NCSPP) considers consultation to be a core competency in the training of psychologists. Consultation is defined as "A planned, collaborative interaction that is an explicit intervention process based on principles and procedures found within psychology and related disciplines in which the psychologist does not have direct control of the change process" (Bent, 1992, p. 77). For systemic competency, the NCSPP expects psychologists to develop the capacity to use a systemic epistemology, systemic assessment processes, interpersonal relationship skills, and systemic intervention to assist larger social systems and organizations.

Another definition might be that mental health consultation, especially when working with organizations, is the act of applying psychological principles and understanding to promote the accomplishment of organizational goals. The accomplishment of these goals always depends on being able to mobilize the energies, dedication, teamwork and synergy of its workforce. Organizations with the desire to achieve sustainable, long-term growth and prosperity should have the development and fulfillment of individual growth as a part of their mission. The most precious resource of an organization is its people, and understanding and being able to work with people is the most

---

Box 1.2

Definitions of Consultant

"A consultant is a person with special knowledge, skills, and talent, who makes needed expertise available to a client for a fee." This is perhaps the broadest definition of a consultant, and is applicable to any consultant in any field of knowledge.

"A consultant is someone who helps people deal with their organizational issues and opportunities, in order to accomplish strategic directions" (Widdis, 2005). This is a general business definition of consultant, perhaps best capturing the function of the management consultant: someone who works directly with the management and leadership teams in an organization to improve performance.

"A consultant is an expert who charges you for looking at your watch and telling you what time it is." Though this is said tongue-in-cheek, sometimes a consultant may feel that he or she is receiving a lot of money for seemingly commonsense information. However, some clients are happy to pay someone with more expertise to oversee new projects, if only for the emotional comfort of knowing that help is close at hand should the need arise.

---

important quality in skillful management and leadership. The task of the mental health professional when consulting with organizations is to offer ways to accomplish goals that heighten productivity through the effective management of people. Box 1.2 provides additional definitions of consultant.

THE TRIPARTITE NATURE OF CONSULTATION

Consultation generally involves three parties: the consultant, the consultee, and the client. The consultee is the individual with whom the consultant works directly. The client is the individual or group with whom the consultee works. For consultation in clinical settings, the consultee may be a mental health provider who has little experience with a particular type of client. The consultant is called in to discuss the client's unique case factors with the consultee. In an organizational setting, a company (the client) may hire a consultant to work with the CEO (the consultee) to enhance that person's managerial style.

The consultant, consultee, and client system are involved in a problem-solving process that includes relationship development, data gathering, problem identification, goal setting, strategy selection and implementation, evaluation, and often a recycling of the process. This sequence is not necessarily linear (e.g., evaluation of how things are going can occur at any point during the course of consultation).

Caplan (1970), the founder of mental health consultation, originally restricted consultation to two professionals and their agreed-on work and firmly believed that therapy should never occur in a consulting relationship. This stance is generally accepted, but most mental health consultants would likely agree that the boundary between therapy and consultation is sometimes blurred and that it is difficult to avoid therapeutic issues when working closely with a consultee. However, it must be stressed that consultation is *not* the same as psychotherapy. In psychotherapy, the therapist works with the client's personal issues. In consultation, the consultant works with the consultee to enhance the consultee's effectiveness in a job situation or some other specific capacity. Although in practice, this distinction has many shades of gray, the consultant should refer the consultee to another mental health provider should it become apparent that psychotherapy is indicated.

The goal of consultation is to improve the consultee or client system in some way. Helping the consultee with the client system enhances the consultee's knowledge, skills, and attitudes, leading to improved handling of the client system.

Another definition of consultation is tailored specifically to the field of human service (Goodstein, 1978). Dougherty (1995) characterized consultation as a process in which a human services professional assists a consultee with a specific work-related or caretaking-related problem within a client system. This process helps both the consultee and the client system. Box 1.3 lists the core characteristics of consultation.

Unlike clinical, counseling, school, and industrial/organizational psychology, consulting psychology has only recently become a formally recognized area of training. Many mental health provider educational programs provide only some basic coursework, and quite a few programs do not offer any explicit consultation training. Because there is a growing interest in the field, many programs are now offering special tracks in consulting, sometimes in collaboration with business schools. Still, at the present time, no specific credentials or licenses are necessary to do consulting work. Only in the last few years has there been postdoctoral recognition of consultation expertise, such as the American Board of Professional Psychology's Diplomate in Consulting Psychology, which was first offered in 2003. The Society of Consulting Psychology, Division 13 of the American Psychology Association, produces a publication called *Consulting Psychology Journal: Practice and Research*. Clinical psychologists make up the largest percentage of the Division's membership. The career path for becoming a consulting psychologist has not yet been clearly defined but typically has started from clinical, counseling, industrial/organizational psychology, or social psychology, with predictable differences in emphasis and skills. Industrial/organizational psychologists tend to be more measurement oriented; counseling psychologists tend to be more career oriented and coaching oriented; clinical psychologists tend to be more involved with employee assistance programs and with troubled employees; and social psychologists tend to focus on an interpersonal and systems orientation with strong quantitative skills.

Even less clear are the roles and boundaries of competence for mental health providers such as counselors, social workers and psychiatric nurses, who have not been traditionally as involved in organizational consulting. The unique training and strengths of each discipline are likely to translate into valuable consulting niches. Practitioners from each field are advised to discuss these issues with their mentors.

CONSULTATION AS AN INTERDISCIPLINARY FIELD

Approximately 30 years ago, consulting psychology began to emerge from the shadow of clinical psychology. It became a truly interdisciplinary field, borrowing and integrating concepts, models, and research from business, organizational behavior, general systems theory, group dynamics, action research, community mental health, family systems, and social psychology, in addition to the "godparent" fields of clinical psychology, counseling psychology, social psychology, and industrial/organizational psychology.

═══ Box 1.3 ═══

Core Characteristics of Consultation

1. Either the consultee or the client system may be given priority over the other at a given time, depending on the approach to consultation that is taken.
2. The consultant provides indirect service to the client system by providing direct service to the consultee.
3. A consultant can be either separate from or part of the system in which consultation is to occur. Consultants who are not part of the system in which consultation is to occur are termed external consultants, while those who are part of the system are called internal consultants.
4. Participation in consultation is voluntary for all parties involved.
5. Consultees are free to do whatever they wish with the consultant's suggestions and recommendations. They are under no obligation to follow the consultant's recommendations.
6. The relationship between the consultee and consultant is one of peers— two equals. Although the consultation relationship is equal in terms of the power of the consultant and consultee, it is unequal in terms of need; that is, the consultee needs help with a problem and the consultant does not, at least as far as the consultation relationship is concerned.
7. The consultation relationship is temporary. Depending on the type, consultation may range from a single session to weekly sessions for years. Whatever its length, however, the relationship is always temporary—the consultant does not replace the consultee.
8. Consultation deals exclusively with the consultee's work-related or caretaking-related problems (Herlihy & Corey, 1997). Consultation, by definition, only deals with the personal concerns of the consultee when they impact work performance. Sometimes, major personal concerns are better addressed in psychotherapy.
9. The consultant can take on a variety of roles in consultation, depending on the nature of the problem, the skills of the consultee, the purpose and desired outcomes of consultation, and the skills of the consultant.
10. Consultation tends to be collaborative in nature; that is, consultants and consultees work together to complement each other in solving the problems defined in consultation. Typically, consultants do not do for consultees what consultees can do for themselves. One exception is when consultees have the skills but not the time to do a given task. For example, a consultee might ask a consultant to lead an in-service workshop on substance-abuse counseling for the consultee's organization, even though the consultee is skilled in that area (Bennett & Lehman, 2003).

The mental health consultant can benefit from knowledge related to a broad array of disciplines. Following are brief descriptions of the many fields that contribute to the knowledge base of consultation.

Business: Research in the areas of business gives the consultant a background into the processes that take place in organizations, including how organizations are structured, managed, and how they survive. Such information can be important to consultants so that they may freely work in organizational environments, and better understand the reciprocal effects between organizations and individuals.

- *Organizational behavior:* The study of individuals and groups in organizations (Schermerhorn, Hunt, & Osborn, 2000). This field draws heavily from both business and psychology research (Kolb, Rubin, & Osland, 1995; Matteson & Ivancevich, 1993).
- *Human resource management:* The design of formal systems in an organization to ensure effective and efficient use of human talent to accomplish organizational goals (Mathis & Jackson, 2003).
- *Management:* The use of organizational resources to achieve objectives through planning, staffing, leading, and controlling (DuBrin, 2000).
- *Marketing:* The conception, pricing, promotion, and distribution of ideas, goods, and services to create exchanges that satisfy individual and organizational goals (American Marketing Association, 2005; Lamb, Hair, & McDaniel, 2003).

Sociology: The structure and functioning of societies. Knowledge of human behavior in groups is crucial to consultants who must find interventions for individuals and groups within a larger organizational and societal context.

- *Structural sociology:* A sociological theory based on the premise that society comes before individuals (Wordreference.com, 2005). It is the study of the various effects of structure on collective behavior.
- *Social psychology:* The study of the influences that people have on the beliefs or behavior of others (Aronson, 1999). Social psychology can be considered as a subfield of both sociology and psychology.

Psychology: The study of human behavior. The science of psychology gives the consultant a strong background in the functioning of individuals and groups.

- *Clinical:* The evaluation, diagnosis, and treatment of individuals with psychological disorders, as well as treatment of less severe behavioral and emotional problems. Clinical psychologists typically perform psychological testing, interview clients, and provide group or individual psychotherapy (Weiten, Stalling, & Wasden, 1998).
- *Counseling:* Overlaps with clinical psychology. Specialists in both areas engage in similar activities—interviewing, testing, and providing therapy. Counseling psychologists tend to focus more on enhancing normal functioning or providing assistance with everyday problems of moderate severity, often specializing in family, marital, or career counseling (Weiten et al., 1998).
- *Industrial-organizational (IO):* The development and application of psychological theory and methodology to problems of organizations and individuals and groups in organizational settings (American Psychological Association, 1981; Jewell, 1998).
- *Organizational health:* The application of the principles of health psychology in organizational settings (Klarreich, 1998). Health psychology is the scientific study of behaviors that relate to health enhancement, disease prevention, and rehabilitation (Brannon & Feist, 1997).
- *Community:* The branch of applied psychology that is concerned with modifying both the individual and the structure of the social system to produce optimal benefits for both society and the individual. Community psychologists are primarily interested in preventing maladaptive behavior (Gladding & Newsome, 2004;

Goodspeed, 1998; J. A. Lewis, Lewis, Daniels, & D'Andrea, 1998; Sarason & Sarason, 1996).

Psychiatry: A branch of medicine that recognizes the impact of physiological functioning and health on an individual's performance in group and organizational settings.

- *Administrative:* Deals with the challenge of delivery system configuration and integrated service delivery in the behavioral health system. Areas of study include organizational theories, leadership requirements, planning models, information system solutions, models of program evaluation, quality management, and training and human resource development (Talbott & Hales, 2001).

- *Consultation-liaison (C-L):* The subspecialty of psychiatry concerned with medically and surgically ill patients (Academy of Psychosomatic Medicine, 1992). The C-L consultant has an extensive clinical understanding of physical/neurological disorders and their relation to abnormal illness behavior. The C-L consultant is a diagnostician, who teases apart and formulates the patient's multiaxial disorders, and develops treatment plans. The C-L consultant also knows psychotherapeutic and psychopharmacological interventions as well as the wide-ranging medicolegal aspects of psychiatric and medical illness and hospitalization. The psychiatric physician, by virtue of professional stature and knowledge, can supervise a multidisciplinary team (Academy of Psychosomatic Medicine, 1998). Viewed separately, liaison work involves developing the skills of other staff in assessment and management of psychological problems, whereas consultation work assumes that the other staff already possess these skills and need a greater depth of expertise (Gelder, Gath, Mayou, & Cowen, 1996; Stoudemire & Fogel, 1993).

WHY CONSULTATION IS IMPORTANT FOR MENTAL HEALTH PRACTITIONERS

Private practitioners have felt increasingly squeezed financially after the growth of the managed care industry. To find out how practitioners were dealing with this, Steven Walfish (2001) surveyed psychologists and asked them to identify activities in their independent practice that fall outside the purview of managed care. A total of 180 specific activities were identified and were rationally grouped into 10 categories: (1) business psychology, (2) consultation to organizations, (3) fee-for-service, (4) forensic psychology, (5) group therapy, (6) health psychology, (7) psychoeducational services, (8) services to government, (9) teaching and supervision, and (10) miscellaneous. Several of these options are related to the core competency of consultation.

Although consultation can be considered a separate practice specialty, it encompasses an important set of skills that support a clinical practice, such as the ability to work more effectively with parents, agencies, colleagues, and community groups.

Consultation skills are important for every mental health practitioner in performing the following activities:

- Addressing community needs and fostering social betterment
- Advocating for underserved populations
- Programming interventions, especially primary prevention interventions
- Working with multidisciplinary teams

All mental health professionals need to understand systems and organizations because their work is done and their time is spent in a systems context (family, office, hospital, clinic, university). The mental health provider and the clients that are served do not operate in a vacuum.

As the managed care model, the industrialization, and the commoditization of mental health services continue, clinical providers will need more markets and new services to ensure their financial survival and a medium for the creative application and growth of their skills (Ackley, 1997). They may also work directly with organizations to provide capitation and other traditional services. *Capitation* is an agreement with an organization to provide mental health services to a set number of employees for a set fee for a set period of time. Organizations are increasingly looking to mental health providers for improvements in their operating efficiency (and therefore, bottom-line profits). According to an article from the *Journal of Management* (Danna & Griffin, 1999), "U.S. industry loses approximately 550 million working days annually to absenteeism, with an estimated 54% of these absences being stress-related. Estimates place the annual cost at more than $43 billion" (p. 377). As experts in stress management, mental health clinicians can directly help the performance of organizations and improve the work environments of individuals, thus contributing to the prevention of mental illnesses.

Another important reason for learning about organizational factors is that many mental health professionals eventually become supervisors and managers, usually without adequate training. Knowledge of consultation skills will help prepare practitioners for potential leadership and management roles.

HOW DOES CONSULTATION DIFFER FROM OTHER COMPETENCIES?

Consultation is a complex competency that overlaps with all the other aspects of mental health practice: management, supervision, therapy, assessment, diversity/relationship, research/basic science. The development of consultation skills involves integrating these various specialty areas. However, one must keep in mind important differences in how these areas of competency are applied in consultation:

- *Management:* A manager is directly responsible for the work of subordinates. A consultant is not directly responsible for the work results, but works indirectly through others.
- *Supervision:* A supervisor exercises authority over the supervisee and holds evaluation power. Consultants typically have a peer relationship with the client— though the client pays the consultant for his or her time, the relationship is ideally one of colleagues mutually working to solve a problem.
- *Therapy:* In psychotherapy, the clinician helps clients directly. In consultation, clients are helped indirectly, through the medium of the consultee. The consultant is not contracted to do therapy, although therapeutic skills are important in the consulting relationship. Consultants may also find themselves doing "therapy" for the organization as a whole through systems intervention.
- *Assessment:* When performing psychological assessments, the clinician must often make diagnoses based on limited information, usually provided only by the

individual being assessed and any empirical data in the individual's record. In consultation, it becomes much more crucial to assess the broader influences on a complex system of many interacting variables. This usually involves gathering data from a variety of sources through interviews, questionnaires, and other techniques.

- *Diversity/relationship:* Diversity issues, neglected in the mental health field until recently, are becoming increasingly recognized as crucial to efficacious therapeutic interventions. These are also important considerations for consultants. Consulting builds on this competency in designing accurate assessments and effective interventions that consider diversity issues within an organization.
- *Research/basic science:* Research skills and the basic ideas of the scientific method are important for the clinician to understand in order to develop and use the most effective assessment and intervention tools. Likewise, these skills are important to accurately assess and intervene in an organization without being swayed by potential biases. However, these skills constitute only a subset of the background knowledge needed for effective consultation.

CHARACTERISTICS OF THE PLAYERS IN AN ORGANIZATIONAL SETTING

Only in the past 25 years or so have social scientists done much detailed, systematic study on how organizations work. Special areas of study such as *organizational behavior,* which combines the fields of business and the social sciences, are becoming very popular. Consulting psychologists working with businesses are known as *corporate, business,* or *organizational psychologists.* Community psychology involves working with nonprofit agencies.

Though mental health professionals possess many skills that they can leverage in an organizational setting or consulting situation, it is important to understand the major differences between clients in the business world and in the helping professions.

Executives

Business executives, whether in a corporate or nonprofit setting, are responsible for the survival of the organization. Hence, their primary attitude toward people in their organization involves seeing them as tools to meet organizational goals. Executives work to develop the skills of visioning (leading), motivating (selling), monitoring, and rewarding (management), as well as their individualized specialty technical skills (e.g., accounting, finance, human resources, information systems, operations management, project management, or strategic planning; Applegate, Austin, & McFarlan, 2003; Baker & Baker, 1998; Brigham & Ehrhardt, 2002; Chase, Aquilano, & Jacobs, 2001; F. David, 2001; Mathis & Jackson, 2003; Meredith & Mantel, 2003; Stickney & Weil, 2000). The performance of most executives is measured (either by their bosses or by the company stockholders) in terms of their bottom-line outcomes, and hence their main emphasis is on monetary profit.

Mental Health Providers

Most clinicians' primary attitude involves helping people maximize their human potential. Clinicians work to develop the skills of conceptualizing, listening with the third ear (empathy), understanding, accepting, and intervening. Hence, the clinician's main emphasis is on helping people (Corey, 1991).

Organizational Psychologists and Counselors

For organizational psychologists and counselors, the primary attitude toward people involves maximizing human potential to meet organizational goals, by helping organizations deal effectively with their employees. This requires rapport building, problem solving, analyzing systems, and influencing others to implement interventions. Hence, they emphasize both process and people (Gallessich, 1982; Harrison, 2004; Rothwell, Sullivan, & McLean, 1995).

The inherent role conflicts among these differing attitudes and emphases suggest several implications for consultation:

- As clinicians, we tend to treat individuals within the system as clients or patients.
- As consultants, we tend to accept individual pathology and focus on the system and its structure, which involves the organization's norms, rules, policies, culture, and climate.
- Businesses exist to provide a return on investment to shareholders. Nonprofit and government agencies exist to accomplish a nonmonetary mission, such as helping people. These purposes can sometimes conflict. What is being recognized more and more today, however, is that most of the time, what is good for the individual is also good for the organization. The relationship between process and people and profit is complementary. When employees are treated fairly and work in an environment wherein they feel respected and valued, they will treat customers fairly, and the customers will continue to do business with that company.

CONSULTATION SETTINGS

Consultation can take place in any organizational or work setting. What follows are some of the most common settings where mental health professionals engage in consultation work.

Community Agencies

Because community agencies operate through government funding or on a nonprofit basis, they usually cannot afford to hire a full-time advanced-level mental health professional. Such agencies include child welfare departments, social service agencies, and mental health centers. Consultants may be called on to help staff therapists deal with problems they are having with one or more clients in their caseload, provide training for work with diverse clients, or perform psychological assessments.

Educational Institutions

School systems may have special needs that their guidance counselors or school psychologists cannot meet. A consultant may perform such services as working with a schoolteacher to improve classroom management techniques, consulting with a special-education teacher about a student who has Asperger's syndrome, or providing didactic sessions for school counselors in family systems theory.

Legal System

Courts and prisons frequently ask mental health professionals to provide diagnostic assessments, therapeutic interventions, and program evaluations. For example, a clinician may be called on to diagnose the reasons for high turnover in a prison staff.

Health Care Systems

Mental health consultants are increasingly playing varied roles in medical settings. A consultant may assist the staff of a multispecialty medical practice in identifying its major work concerns and then assist in designing a strategic plan for overcoming those concerns.

Organizations

Consultants can be useful in both for-profit and nonprofit organizations. Properly trained mental health professionals can assist an organization with long-range strategic planning, short-range business planning, and executive selection and development. As an example, a consultant may help a human resources director develop and evaluate an employee satisfaction survey.

Government

The number and variety of government agencies that can profitably use a mental health consultant is continually growing. A consultant can perform evaluations and interventions at the local, state, and federal level. A consultant could assist a job corps center staff in increasing its morale, or could assist a Head Start program in evaluating its parent training program.

Private Practice

Mental health providers who work alone or in a small group in private practice settings may feel isolated from their colleagues and from the frontiers of the mental health fields. These clinicians may need outside consultants to provide training in specific interventions for special populations or may provide in-service training for doing consultation work.

TYPES OF CONSULTATION

There are many types of consultation, depending on the setting and the desired goals. These types are not mutually exclusive. Consultants may choose to specialize in a specific type, may work in some or all of the following areas, or may creatively develop unique practice niches.

Clinical Consultation

Clinical consultation is the area that is most familiar to mental health professionals. It might include an initial session with a client to determine suitability for working with the therapist, a referral from another department for an assessment of someone else's therapy client, a session with a colleague to share special expertise, or a session with parents when treating a child.

Mental Health Consultation

Mental health consultation involves the prevention of mental health problems. The Community Mental Health Centers Act of 1963 required mental health centers that received federal monies to implement programs of consultation with other agencies and professionals in their communities. Mental health professionals were generally not trained in this capacity, and the community often resented their advice (Brown, Pryzwansky, & Schulte, 2001).

Caplan (1970) was a pioneer in the field of mental health consultation. He conceptualized the role of the mental health consultant as one who helps other professionals work more effectively with their clients around four key areas:

1. *Lack of knowledge:* The consultee may simply not have the knowledge base to understand the problem at hand. The consultant serves the role of teacher, providing education and information resources to the consultee.
2. *Lack of skill:* The consultee may not have the therapeutic skills to deal with the client's presenting issues. The consultant serves the role of teacher, enhancing the consultee's skills through discussing "what-if" scenarios, demonstrations, and role-play.
3. *Lack of confidence:* Often, the consultee may be performing very well, but is dealing with a complicated case or has little experience with the interventions being used. The consultant may simply need to provide support and reassurance that the consultee is doing well, and may offer some minor suggestions for improvement.
4. *Lack of objectivity:* When working with clients on material of an intimate and personal nature, it may be difficult for the therapist to remain objective, particularly if the topics are bringing up unresolved issues for the therapist. The consultant can provide a fresh perspective for the consultee, relatively free of the complications of transference and countertransference.

Behavioral Consultation

Bergan (1977) developed a consultation model based on the principles of behavioral psychology. Harrison (2004, pp. 189–190) nicely summarizes the characteristics of behavioral consultation approaches:

- Behavioral consultation approaches are indirect services and usually are focused on cases and clients even when conducted in organizational settings (Dougherty, 1995; Gallessich, 1982; Keller, 1981).
- Behavioral consultation approaches are most often used to problem-solve as well as enhance consultee competence (Bergan & Kratochwill, 1990; Mannino, Trickett, Shore, Kidder, & Levin, 1986; Vernberg & Reppucci, 1986).

- The goals of most behavioral approaches are to alter the client's behaviors, to change the consultee's behaviors, and to produce changes in organizations (Brown, Pryzwansky, & Schulte, 2001).
- The length of the consulting relationship varies from minutes to months (Bergan & Kratochwill, 1990; Brown, Pryzwansky, & Schulte, 2001; Myrick, 1987).
- In all cases, consultants should have a degree of expert knowledge in learning principles and utilize social learning theory and behavioral technology principles to design, implement, and assess interventions (Bergan & Kratochwill, 1990; Gallessich, 1982; Vernberg & Reppucci, 1986).
- The consultant/consultee relationship ranges from collegial to the consultant having some control in the relationship (Bergan & Kratochwill, 1990; Myrick, 1977).
- The consultant's major role ranges from facilitator (Myrick, 1977) to expert who imparts psychological information and principles to consultees (Bergan, 1977; Bergan & Kratochwill, 1990).
- A primary task of the consultant ranges from helping the consultee problem solve (Myrick, 1977) to enhancing the probability that the consultee will accept the consultant's recommendations (Bergan, 1977; Bergan & Kratochwill, 1990).
- In behavioral consultation approaches, the client or consultee "goals" or both need to be defined in behavioral terms (Bergan, 1977; Bergan & Kratochwill, 1990; Dougherty, 1990; Gallessich, 1982; Myrick, 1977).
- Most approaches emphasize direct observation techniques (Keller, 1981) and focus on present, current influences on overt behavior (Bergan, 1977; Doughterty, 1990; Myrick, 1977).
- In most cases, the interventions and evaluations lend themselves to empirical testing (Bergan, 1977; Bergan & Kratochwill, 1990; Mannino et al., 1986; Vernberg & Reppucci, 1986).

Consultation-Liaison

Consultation-liaison work refers to a mental health professional in a hospital setting who consults with medical professionals on psychological matters. The liaison works with other disciplines (e.g., medicine, nursing, and social work) to detect, treat, refer, or some combination of these three, those patients who have mental health or stress-related issues, especially those that affect their medical treatment. The liaison may also work with the patient's family or support system for such things as emotional support. The liaison also works on improving the overall medical care system, and may conduct research on the interaction of medical and psychiatric comorbidity (Rundell & Wise, 1999).

Program Consultation

In program consultation, a mental health professional provides services to a key figure in an agency or organization for the purposes of assisting in the planning of a new program, evaluating and revising an existing program, or in dealing with the factors that affect a current program (e.g., a community mental health center may wish to begin an adolescent substance abuse program, but not have any experience with starting or running such a program). The primary goal is to provide an organization with the technical assistance it requires to have successful programs and to accomplish its mission (Dougherty, 1995; Harrison, 2004).

Community Consultation or Organizing (Advocacy)

Advocacy for the community entails getting involved in the community to create positive change for everyone, especially for the underserved. Advocacy is for those who want to change the world from what it is to what they believe it should be (Alinsky, 1969, 1971). Mental health professionals are especially well-suited to understand the psychological consequences of oppression and low socioeconomic status.

Organizational Consultation or Development

Organizational development (OD) is the application of behavioral science knowledge in a long-range effort to improve an organization's ability to cope with change in its external environment and increase its problem-solving capabilities (Cummings & Worley, 1993; Golembiewski, 1993).

Massarik and Pei-Carpenter (2002) offer the following working definition of OD:

> In the context of continuing natural change at all interrelated levels of environment, society, organization, group, and individual, with focus on specified client systems, OD engages people within and among human systems (organizations) in activities (interventions) intended to bring about positive change for specifiable clients and stakeholders and directed toward improvement of the human condition—guided by humane values—by means of significant application of knowledge rooted in the social and behavioral sciences. (p. 2)

The National Center for Organizational Development, which is an internal consultation branch for the entire Veterans Health Administration (VHA), describes its services as including executive coaching, leadership development and assessment, team building, strategic planning, large and small group facilitation, work redesign, survey design and analysis, and psychoeducational interventions. Schein (1969) first introduced the idea of Process Consultation, which he defines as "a 'set of activities' on the consultant's part that are aimed at helping clients understand their internal and external environments better so that they can act on the process events that occur" (p. 34).

THE ROLE OF THE CONSULTANT

The roles taken on by consultants are unlike those of most clinicians, though there may be some similarities to therapists' traditional roles. Consultants focus on the *empowerment* of others. Just as in therapy, consultants do not want their clients to become dependent on them, but seek to replace themselves so that clients can continue to grow when their consultant is not around. Hence, the consultant is really a servant, helping others to achieve their goals. The consultant is not a manager or an employee, but uses lateral relationships to accomplish goals. This requires a tolerance for ambiguity, and requires negotiation skills (since it is easier to terminate a consultant than it is to terminate a subordinate). The consultant must respect the organization's culture and must learn to work within that framework to effect lasting change.

SKILLS OF THE CONSULTANT

There are three major skills areas for consultants: technical skills, interpersonal skills, and consulting skills. Technical skills comprise an area of expertise. If you have 30 years of experience in managing inpatient hospital units, then you can probably consult with developing inpatient programs on how to run their units efficiently. If you are a newly licensed mental health professional, you may be considered an expert on group dynamics, stress management, or mental health issues (assuming you have had the necessary training to work with organizations in these areas).

Interpersonal skills are also important for consultants. These are skills that most clinicians work on diligently in the course of their training, and they are accustomed to working to improve these skills in their clients. As a consultant, it is especially important to understand the client context and to be able to make and sustain relationships by joining with the client and building rapport. Important areas of knowledge include an in-depth understanding of assertiveness, supportiveness, confrontation, listening, management style, and group process.

Finally, consultants must possess skills specific to consulting, which is the major focus of this book. There are five basic phases of consulting: entry and contracting; discovery and dialogue; feedback and the decision to act; engagement and implementation; and extension, recycle, or termination (Block, 2000; Block & Markowitz, 2001). Entry involves making a connection with the client or organization, and contracting involves negotiating wants, coping with mixed motivations, dealing with concerns about exposure and the loss of control, as well as contracting for the work to be done. Discovery and dialogue are analogous to assessment and diagnosis. They involve surfacing layers of analysis, dealing with political climate, resisting the urge for complete data, and seeing the interview as an intervention. Feedback and decision making involve funneling data, identifying and working with different forms of resistance, presenting personal and organizational data, running group meetings, focusing on here-and-now choices, and not taking things personally. At this point, the consultant must decide if the work needs to be continued, reconceptualized, or terminated.

One of the best compliments a consultant can receive is to be thought of as "a person who asks good questions." Asking questions allows consultees to think out loud, to solve their own problems, and to become invested in potential solutions. It is a key skill for consultants. Caplan (1970; Caplan & Caplan, 1993) maintains that the consultees' problem-solving capabilities can be influenced by the consultant's questions. As mental health clinicians, we work to become comfortable avoiding direct suggestions about how clients should handle their problems. We know that advice-giving (except in such instances as crisis intervention) is a lose-lose proposition: If we give good advice, the client becomes dependent on us; and if we give bad advice, the client is harmed and terminates therapy.

Box 1.4 contains a checklist of the diverse competencies necessary for consultation work.

CONSULTING CORE COMPETENCY DOMAINS

The American Psychological Association's Division of Consulting Psychology (2002) has suggested incorporating the following consulting core competency areas into training programs for consultants. The areas are divided into three levels:

1. Primarily Individual-Level Core Competencies:
   • Individual assessment for purposes of career and vocational assessment
   • Individual assessment for purposes of employee selection or development
   • Job analysis for purposes of individual assessment

Box 1.4

Checklist of Consultant Competencies

Personal and Interpersonal Effectiveness

1. *Self-knowledge:* Awareness of the values and beliefs that influence the way one works.
2. *Self-awareness:* Awareness of one's own emotional responses to situations and people, especially patterns.
3. *Active listening:* Attending to the content and process level in communication.
4. *Self-expression:* Ability to express one's own thoughts, ideas, and feelings clearly.
5. *Relationship-building:* Building open, collaborative relationships. Exchanging feedback in constructive ways.
6. *Conflict-handling:* Valuing and exploring differences. Ability to challenge without alienating.
7. *Personal and professional limits:* Awareness of the limit of one's own competencies. Willingness to ask for help.

Qualities of a Change Agent

1. *Tolerance of ambiguity:* Ability to live with uncertainty and complexity without stress. Tolerate incompleteness.
2. *Maintaining a long-term perspective:* Helping clients identify and articulate desired futures.
3. *Maintaining a wide perspective:* Not drawing boundaries tightly.
4. *Understanding the nature of change:* Developing an intellectual and experiential understanding of how and why people change.
5. *Facilitating change:* Encouraging widespread participation in the design and implementation of change.

Consulting Skills

1. *Contracting:* Clarifying mutual expectations and responsibilities.
2. *Data collection:* Choosing appropriate methods of gathering information that will help to address the issues and concerns of the client.
3. *Diagnosis:* Having a range of frameworks and models for understanding individuals, groups, and organizations. Encouraging joint diagnosis with clients.
4. *Design:* Being creative and purposeful in designing interventions. Being willing to redesign on the spot.
5. *Closure:* Disengaging well from the project. Avoiding mutual dependency.

- Executive and individual coaching
- Individual-level intervention for job- and career-related problems
2. Primarily Group-Level Core Competencies:
    - Assessment of functional and dysfunctional group behavior
    - Assessment and development of teams
    - Creating group-level teams in organizations (e.g., self-directed work groups)
    - Intergroup assessment and intervention

- Group boundary assessment and intervention
- Identity group (racial, gender, ethnic) management in the organizational context
3. Primarily Organizational/Systemic-Level Core Competencies:
  - Organizational diagnosis including systemic assessment of the entire organization or large component parts of the organization
  - Attitude, climate, and satisfaction surveys
  - Evaluation of corporate management philosophy, organizational culture and nature of systemic stressors
  - Work flow and project planning activities
  - Identification of aggregate performance measures
  - Assessment of organizational values and management practices
  - Organizational-level interventions
  - Change management of organizational systems (p. 776)

INTERNAL VERSUS EXTERNAL CONSULTANTS

As evidenced by the foregoing, there are many types of consulting work, and many kinds of professionals who may call themselves consultants. We can divide consultants into two broad categories: internal and external.

An *internal consultant* provides consulting services within the organization. An internal consultant is a direct employee of the organization, and usually works within or in collaboration with the human resources department.

An *external consultant* provides consulting services on a contractual basis and is brought into the organization for a specific purpose. As a person with presumed objectivity and special expertise, a consultant does not have direct responsibility for goal achievement. External consultants are used when sufficient time, people power, objectivity, or competence is lacking within the organization to solve the problem or concern at hand. Because of this, external consultants hold a marginal role for the long-term operations of the organization and are generally under contract for a specific, time-limited purpose. Table 1.1 shows the advantages and disadvantages of internal and external consultants.

ELEMENTS OF THE CONSULTANT-CONSULTEE INTERACTION

The quality of the interactions with consultees is crucial to the success of consultation, just as the quality of interactions with clients is crucial to success in therapy.

Gallup (1998) listed several qualities that characterize a good consulting relationship: a workable rapport, compatible problem-solving style, integrity, open communications, clear goals, and reasonable outcome measures. Successful consultants have the following four characteristics:

1. *Responsibility:* Consultants should assume all the responsibility in their own thinking, but must also work to build a sense of responsibility in the consultee to resolve the challenges being faced.
2. *Feelings:* As mental health providers, consultants know the power of emotions, and the importance of managing the consultee's feelings as well as the consultant's own reactions.
3. *Trust:* To build trust, consultants must always deliver on what they promise. This means being careful about what they promise, and being quick to admit when

Table 1.1   Internal versus External Consultants

Internal Consultants

Advantages	Disadvantages
Knows the system (formally and informally) and how to use it.	May have difficulty establishing visibility and credibility.
Knows the language and how to express ideas in an acceptable way.	Has a history, such as past failures, old allegiances, that may get in the way of success.
May know key people and how to influence them.	May be too much a part of the system—not sufficiently detached.
May have a well-established network of contacts.	May be part of the problem.
May already have a lot of information about the problem.	May be perceived to be too much a part of the system, thus limiting trust.
Can work unobtrusively at times.	May feel wary of confronting superiors, especially senior managers.
Is well placed to seize opportunities.	May be subject to political/hierarchical pressures.
Is less likely to be expected to provide instant solutions than the external consultant.	May have limited room to maneuver because of tight role definitions.
Can keep in close touch with the long-term consequences of a project.	May not be able to refuse.

External Consultants

Advantages	Disadvantages
Is more likely to be seen as outside the politics of the organization.	May be "put on a pedestal," leading to deference/resentment/disillusionment.
People more likely to be open.	May need a lot of time to discover how the system really works.
People more willing to listen to and hear an "outsider."	May only see part of the problem.
Can bring new perspectives and fresh insights.	Leaves at the end of a project and may not see the long-term results.
Can more easily provide contacts with other organizations.	May use ideas that are too different from the organization's current way of thinking.
Can become an important communication channel, especially upward.	
Likely to have high visibility because of heightened expectations.	
Can more easily be direct and confronting.	
Has freedom to turn down an assignment.	

Source: A Consultancy Approach for Trainers and Developers, second edition, by K. Phillips and P. Shaw, 1998, Brookfield, VT: Gower.

trouble develops in delivering those promises. Sometimes the difference between success and failure is strong follow-through.

4. *The right of consultants to their own needs:* Consultants must be aware of their own desires and needs for acceptance, inclusion, validation, access to the company, and support from management, and must recognize how these desires will influence their work.

THE CLASSICAL PROBLEM-SOLVING SEQUENCE

As a consultant, you will frequently be called on to solve problems. Some may argue that consultation can be defined as problem solving. In many instances, your clients will have repeatedly attempted and failed to solve the problems they are currently facing. Bringing in an outside, objective perspective can be helpful in re-conceptualizing the situation. A simple device, the classical problem-solving sequence, can assist clients in systematically dealing with the problems at hand, and will give them the tools to more effectively work with future challenges.

How thoroughly the problem-solving sequence is conducted depends on the complexity of the problem, the seriousness of the issues involved, the amount of time available, and the potential consequences of any decisions made. However, the same six problem-solving steps are useful whether the consultant is assisting in the development of a treatment plan for a consultee's deaf client or helping to manage the merger of two giant corporations.

The first step is to *define the problem.* Although at first this appears to be the easiest step, in practice, the presenting problems often are fuzzy and ill-defined. Consultees may know that something is not right, but may not know precisely what is going on within the organization or client system. In addition, even if they know they are dissatisfied with the current state of affairs, they may not have identified what the end goal should be. Just as in individual psychotherapy, a thorough assessment of current functioning and clarification of how things would be different if the consultee could "wave a magic wand" can often be a major intervention in and of itself. The formulation of a succinct goal statement will guide the rest of the problem-solving process.

The second step is to *identify alternative solutions.* The consultee and the consultant can brainstorm various possible solutions to the identified problem; they also can conduct research and discuss the situation with others to develop a list of possibilities. At this stage, it is important not to prematurely filter out ideas, but to generate as many ideas as possible. Even if an idea initially sounds untenable, it may spark other, more plausible ideas.

The third step is to *weigh the consequences of alternative solutions.* The implications of each solution should now be examined. What are the short-term and long-term costs? Who else will this affect? How feasible is each solution? What time factors are involved?

The fourth step is to *implement the decision.* As clinicians know, this step can be difficult. Making a choice involves many factors, and there is often a great deal of ambiguity. The most difficult decisions are those that preclude other possibilities. People sometimes procrastinate in making choices so that they will not have to face the consequences of the decision, even if they know it is the best decision in the long run. The consultant should be supportive during this stage, but must always allow the consultee

---

Box 1.5

The Classical Problem-Solving Sequence

1. Define the problem.
2. Identify alternative solutions.
3. Weigh the consequences of alternative solutions.
4. Implement the decision.
5. Evaluate the consequences of the decision.
6. Redefine the problem and restart the problem-solving sequence.

---

to make the final decision, since the consultee must feel invested in the decision and is the one who bears the burden of the consequences.

The fifth step is to *evaluate the consequences of the decision.* Once the decision has been implemented, the results should be monitored and evaluated. Are the desired results being achieved? Quantitative results are best if possible. Instead of asking if morale has improved, the consultant could determine if employee absences have decreased. Instead of asking if the mental health client has improved, the consultant could determine if the client has had fewer return visits to the emergency room. Subjective measures are also important, but results that can be measured (e.g., by using a standardized or individualized survey instrument) provide justification for charging a fee for services.

The final step is to *redefine the problem and restart the problem-solving sequence.* Complex problems are seldom fully resolved with a single perfect solution. Even if you were to arrive at a perfect solution, environments that are internal and external to the organization or client may change with time. You must monitor the situation to see if new problems have arisen, or if the old problem still exists in other forms. Then you can move once again through the entire problem-solving sequence. This general sequence, which is used frequently in consulting, is shown in Box 1.5.

Consulting can be thought of as helping people solve their own problems, and psychological consulting can be thought of as solving people problems. Eventually, this process becomes internalized, just as experienced clinicians no longer need to meticulously follow a rigid list of assessment steps for every diagnosis. Although this sequence serves as a guide, many influences affect a person's problem-solving ability (DuBrin, 2000), and mental health professionals should be well suited to deal with the effects of psychological and contextual factors.

PART ONE

INDIVIDUAL-LEVEL CONSULTING ISSUES

Chapter 2

CLINICAL CAREER ASSESSMENT AND COUNSELING

We begin our exploration of consulting techniques by looking at interventions at the individual level. This chapter investigates individual personality variables and how they relate to the differing demands of the workplace. This information is valuable to young men and women who approach the consultant seeking advice about suitable careers. It is also valuable for people who are interested in changing careers or who are having difficulties with their current careers but are not sure why. The topics in this chapter will be useful to mental health professionals whether they are engaged in formal consultation in organizational settings or are simply assisting their therapy clients with career counseling (Savickas & Walsh, 1996).

The information in this chapter is also valuable for consultants who enter organizations for what may ostensibly be a systems-level change. Consultants who can identify personality and work styles will be able to design interventions that are more likely to be well received and implemented. They are also more likely to detect mismatches between individual styles and performance expectations. Knowing the workers' strengths and weaknesses, the consultant can make recommendations that optimize the functioning and satisfaction of the employees within a given system.

Career counseling should involve several interviews with the client. Sperry (1996) describes five phases for this process:

1. An intake interview in which the career counselor or consultant and worker establishes a working relationship such that some working hypotheses about the worker's needs and well-being can be formulated.
2. A phase involving what might be called "problem definition" in which the worker's major concerns are made more explicit than in the initial interview, and a priority order of these concerns is established.
3. An assessment phase that involves some more or less systematic appraisal of the worker's attributes that seem to be most closely related to the defined problem or problems. This assessment can be done using interview methods or might involve a rather extensive variety of psychological tests and inventories (Lowman, 1991). Furthermore, the assessment phase can include work simulation or job sample tasks and techniques.
4. The feedback phase in which the consultant reports back to the worker the results and the potential meaning of the previous phases, particularly the assessment phase.
5. Finally, an implementation phase in which the worker's main responsibility is to make decisions pertinent to putting into action, in appropriate ways, some of the major information and attitudes gleaned from the previous four phases. (p. 106)

The consultant should encourage individuals to try out new careers before investing a lot of time in preparing for them. This may be best achieved through interviews, shadowing, internships, or even part-time work in the career field (Boldt, 1999).

When helping individuals with career choices, it is important to assess and integrate three domains: occupational interests, abilities, and work-related personality characteristics (Lowman, 1991). When a client comes to you and asks for help with career choices, exploration of the client's interests is a good place to begin (Watkins & Campbell, 2000).

HOLLAND'S HEXAGONAL MODEL OF INTERESTS

Psychologist John L. Holland used factor analysis with the empirical findings on vocational interests to create a theory of six basic occupational personality types: Realistic, Investigative, Artistic, Social, Enterprising, and Conventional, as shown in Figure 2.1 (Gottfredson & Holland, 1996; Holland, 1966; Lowman, 1991).

Those types closest to each other are more similar, whereas dissimilar types are most distant from each other. That is, adjacent types share more commonalities than do those that are opposite one another.

For career assessments, an individual takes a written test that produces a classification based on the initial letters of the top three type scores. The Holland Vocational Types are commonly measured by several existing assessment instruments: the Self-Directed Search (Holland, 1994; Spokane & Catalano, 2000), the Vocational Preference Inventory (Holland, 1985; Lowman, 1991), the Career Assessment Inventory (Johansson, 2002), and the Strong Interest Inventory (Hansen, 2000; Harmon, Hansen, Borgen, & Hammer, 1994). Most occupations have associated code types that characterize the typical worker in that position. The prototypical manager would be ESC (Enterprising, Social, and Conventional, with the highest score listed first). Engineers might typically be IRC, IRE, RIC, or RIE. Small differences in code types can make big differences in interests. People with consistent codes (codes with types that are

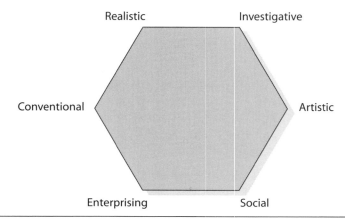

Figure 2.1   Holland's six occupational personality types.

next to each other on the diagram, which means they are somewhat similar) will have an easier time finding a career match because doing any one job effectively usually requires similar qualities. If their occupational type code does not match that which is traditional for individuals in their chosen career, they will tend to approach job tasks in a discrepant manner, leading to career frustration, both personally and professionally. People tend to do a good job in selecting their own careers, which is probably related to genetics (their predispositions) and reinforcement (if they don't enjoy a particular job, they seek out another one). Values are an implicit part of interests. To make the best career decisions, people need exposure to a variety of careers that match their interests.

Needless to say, these classification codes are to be used as tools. No one particular client will neatly fit into any one category. As always, be careful to avoid pigeon-holing clients.

Though not as accurate as a full written assessment, you can do a quick self-assessment by writing down the six types on a piece of paper (especially after reading more about them in this chapter). Mark your primary interest, second strongest interest, and third strongest interest. You can then mark the area in which you have the least interest.

Here are the typical occupational types for mental health professionals:

SAI or SIA	Counselor, clinical or counseling psychologist, clinician
SAE	Social worker, counselor
ISA	Research psychologist
SEC	Teacher
S versus I	"The scientist/practitioner dilemma"

What occupational code type best describes you? You can work in the mental health field with any code type, but if your occupational code type is very different from the typical ones, you may find yourself doing things in a different way from many of your colleagues, perhaps feeling as though you are swimming upstream from time to time.

When assessing clients, have them explain what their typical interests and activities are, instead of simply having them choose from the list of six. Ask them what kinds of things they most enjoyed in the past, and what they most long for in the present and future. Ask them to recall occasions when they felt most alive, most content, and which of their work activities cause time to "fly by."

If you get a flat profile (the client doesn't really have any interests that stand out above the others) or a high profile (all or most interests are rated highly), the clinician should consider the possibility of psychopathology. People with serious mental health concerns should prioritize psychological treatment over career assessment, as it will be difficult for them to truly reflect on interests when they are overwhelmed with daily stressors. This is especially true if they have low profiles suggesting depression and/or burnout. Work must first be done in psychotherapy to build motivation and hope within the client.

Some people have not had enough experience to define their interests. In this case, mutual exploration between the consultant and consultee may be helpful. Although you should avoid overt dissuasion of the consultee's thoughts about career possibilities (it is fortunate that the Wright brothers did not seek career consultation before inventing a means for practical flight), you should encourage people to do things that make sense in terms of their abilities and talents.

HOLLAND THEMES

Following are brief descriptions of the six Holland types (Harmon et al., 1994; Lowman, 1991; Prince & Heiser, 2000).

Realistic

People who score high in this area exhibit an emphasis on doing and things (e.g., building, repairing, working outdoors, mechanical interests).

Realistic individuals tend to be employed in occupations such as the military, engineering (some types), skilled trades, and work with mechanical objects. Jobs could range from simple blue-collar work to highly skilled work as an airline pilot. Typically, individuals who score high in the Realistic category graduate from high school and get jobs instead of long-term careers.

Realistic people often have superior physical abilities and express a preference for the concrete, for tangible things, and for the real world. They take what is given and have difficulty when the job isn't there (when unemployed). Realistic types exhibit direct, simplistic coping abilities and may be less adept at coping with others. Typically they are hardheaded, tough, practical, and asocial. When problems occur, they are at risk for substance abuse and acting out.

More men are of this type, most likely due to cultural conditioning and the perpetuation of stereotypes. This does not seem to be changing very much yet.

Interests include machines, tools, and the outdoors. Work activities include operating equipment, using tools, building, and repairing. Potential skills include mechanical ingenuity, dexterity, and physical coordination. Values include tradition, practicality, and common sense.

Occupational Fields of Realistic Types

Machine trades

Skilled trades

Protective service

Outdoor occupations

Construction work

Common Leisure Interests of Realistic Types

Sports

Woodworking

Repairing automobiles

Investigative

People who score high in this area emphasize thinking and ideas (e.g., researching, analyzing, inquiring). Typical descriptors include "analytical," "achievement-oriented," and "independent."

These individuals tend to be found in occupations involved with science (e.g., engineering and medicine), though they are not usually involved in pure science (such as chemistry). They enjoy working with their brains and are data-oriented.

Investigative types typically have good reasoning, analytical, and conceptual skills. They are often bright, with a high IQ and a high achievement orientation. They tend to be introverted, and are often cool, distant, and unemotional. They like a rational and analytic approach to things and will challenge the status quo. They tend to be asocial and do not gravitate toward people, preferring to work alone. They believe in an external reality that can be discovered and are also field independent (less influenced by the environment). These people theorize about what is given within the rules. They tend to be focused, detail-oriented, and narrow. They are adept at conceptualizing ideas and using inductive and deductive reasoning, but tend not to be creative. More men tend to hold these occupational positions, but this is changing rapidly.

Interests include science, theories, ideas, and analysis of data. Work activities include performing lab procedures, solving abstract problems, and researching. Potential skills include math, writing, and analysis. Values include independence, curiosity, and learning.

Occupational Fields of Investigative Types

Physical or natural science

Mathematics

Research

Medicine and health

Computer science

Common Leisure Interests of Investigative Types

Computers

Sailing

Math games

Astronomy

Artistic

People who score high in this area emphasize creating ideas or things (e.g., creating and enjoying art, drama, music, and writing). Typical descriptors for Artistic types include "expressive," "unstructured," and "independent."

Occupations for the Artistic type include the visual arts, writing, acting, dancing, and architecture. Of course, only a small percentage of such individuals do very well in these professions. Artistic success requires interest, talent, and enormous persistence against the odds, along with the unflappable belief that you will make it.

These individuals tend to be creative and self-expressive. They enjoy self-exploration, and also derive pleasure from creating something that hasn't existed before. Unstructured, flexible environments are best suited for the Artistic type. They enjoy novelty. They are hard on themselves as well as society; an elitist (defensive) attitude is typically apparent. Artistic types are more likely to work with others in a personal, emotional, and nontraditional manner. They have high aspirations and often experience discrepancies in life (never completely fulfilling their idealistic dreams). To earn a living, they often end up doing something other than what they want to be doing.

Keeping the real world in mind is a difficult task for the Artistic type. They are often odd, oppositional, and narcissistically self-focused. Substance abuse and marital problems are not uncommon. They also must often deal with age-limiting restrictions (e.g., professional dancers typically only perform regularly until their mid-20s).

Interests include self-expression and art appreciation. Work activities include composing music, writing, and creating visual art. Potential skills include creativity, musical talent, and artistic expression. Values include beauty, originality, independence, and imagination.

Occupational Fields of Artistic Types

Art

Music

Design

Theater

Writing

Entertainment

Commercial or fine arts

Common Leisure Interests of Artistic Types

Attending plays/concerts

Visiting museums

Painting

Playing music

Social

Individuals who score high in this area exhibit an emphasis on people (e.g., helping, instructing, and caregiving). Typical descriptors include "outgoing," "concerned for others," "humanistic," "verbal," and "generous."

People-oriented occupations such as teaching, nursing, some types of psychology, counseling, or social work are often suitable for Social types. To these individuals, the helping process is key, with focus on other people as an end product. Jobs usually require at least a BA degree, and often involve highly responsible positions but little pay.

These people attempt to please. They are nurturing, assisting, and dependent. Social types are agreeable, cooperative, and enjoyable to work with. Their social skills include being patient, generous, friendly, and tactful. Problem solving is typically handled through verbal interactions (including discussion of feelings) with others. They tend to be group-oriented.

Typically, more women than men exhibit characteristics of this vocational type, likely as a result of cultural conditioning (men tend to not be frequently reinforced for proactive social behaviors).

Interests include people, teamwork, human welfare, and community service. Work activities include teaching, explaining, and helping. Potential skills include people skills, verbal ability, listening, and showing understanding. Values include cooperation, generosity, and service to others.

Occupational Fields of Social Types

Teaching

Counseling

Psychology

Social work

Health services

Religious vocations

Common Leisure Interests of Social Types

Entertaining

Volunteer work

Family gatherings

Enterprising

Individuals who score high in this area place emphasis on managing and people (e.g., selling, managing, and persuading).

These people tend to hold occupations such as managers (rather than leaders), salespersons, directors, politicians, and attorneys. They tend to focus on people, but the emphasis is on people as a means to an end. They use people to get a job done. They are often well paid (depending on their performance). Persons of this type are seen as counterdependent and will often struggle over who is in charge. They are achievement-oriented and competitive and use their understanding of people in a goal-oriented way (instrumentally oriented). Enterprising types are more likely to deal with others in enterprising ways such as by asserting dominance. IQ is a factor in predicting how high they will rise.

Interests include business, politics, leadership, and influence. Work activities include selling, managing, and persuading. Potential assets include verbal skills and the ability to motivate and direct others. Values include risk taking, status, and competition.

Occupational Fields of Enterprising Types

Business

Sales

Political activity

Management

Law

Common Leisure Interests

Social involvement in local clubs and community organizations

Sports that involve a social component

Conventional

Individuals who score high in this area emphasize confirmation and data (e.g., accounting, organizing, and processing data).

Conventional types are found in occupations such as accountants, computer programmers, secretaries, and clerical support staff.

Conventional and conforming, these individuals are rule-oriented, enforcers of rules. They work because they need to, not because it is desirable. They are "orderly," open, attentive to detail, rigid and conforming, and good enforcers; suffer routine gladly; enjoy predictability; and are good at occupations and tasks requiring perceptual speed and accuracy. Conventional types are more likely to deal with others in a conventional manner (by being controlling and practical).

Statistically, women more frequently hold these occupations, particularly at the lower end, perhaps because continuing subtle discrimination in the workforce makes it more difficult for women to achieve leadership roles.

Interests include organization, data, and finance. Work activities include setting up procedures, organizing, and operating computers. Potential skills include math, data analysis, record keeping, and attention to detail. Values include accuracy, stability, and efficiency.

Occupational Fields

Accounting

Administrative occupations

Clerical occupations

Banking

Finance

Common Leisure Interests

Involvement in civic organizations

Home improvement projects

Collecting

DUAL TYPE EXPLANATIONS

Commonly, individuals score highly on two adjacent domains, making it difficult to choose a predominant set of interests. The following are examples of dual-type explanations, adapted from the Strong Vocational Inventory (Harmon et al., 1994).

Enterprising-Social People

People with Enterprising and Social interests may enjoy managing a service business or a for-profit organization. They like work environments that allow them to have a lot of contact with other people inside and outside the organization. Optimistic and enthusiastic, they are often skilled at motivating others or convincing them of the personal value of a product or service. These people may work as human resources directors, fund-raisers, or sales managers.

Artistic-Social People

Because the Artistic and Social Themes are next to each other on the hexagon, they share many similar interests. People with interests in the Artistic-Social Themes enjoy intense, personal relationships with others, creative work environments where they feel they are making a difference in people's lives, using creativity to facilitate personal growth, or empowering others to be better.

Examples of career fields that connect the Artistic and Social Themes are art, dance, or journal therapy; art or music teaching; written and oral communication; counseling and psychotherapy.

For someone whose interest is highest in the Artistic Theme, his or her strongest motivator is expressing creativity. If he or she also expresses high interest in the Social Theme, helping others will be a strong motivator as well. The work that would bring such individuals the most career satisfaction would most likely involve expressing creativity in friendly, helpful, and service-oriented ways.

CAMPBELL INTEREST AND SKILL SURVEY

Another popular career interest assessment is the Campbell Interest and Skill Survey (Campbell, Hyne, & Nilson, 1992). Though not as popular as the Strong Vocational Inventory, it remains a commonly used instrument. This instrument looks at seven orientations (compared with the six Holland themes): Influencing, Organizing, Helping, Creating, aNalyzing (using N as the abbreviation to avoid confusion with Adventuring), Producing, and Adventuring.

Prince and Heiser (2000) provide a succinct overview of the seven orientations:

1. *Influencing:* Covers the general area of leading and influencing others. People who score high are interested in making things happen. They want to take charge and are willing to accept responsibility for results. Influencers are generally confident of their ability to persuade others to their viewpoints. They typically work in organizations and often want to take charge of the specific activities that particularly interest them. They enjoy public speaking and like to be visible in public. Occupations include company presidents, corporate managers, and school superintendents.
2. *Organizing:* Includes activities that bring orderliness and planfulness to the working environment, such as managing projects, planning procedures, and directly supervising the work of others. Generally emphasize efficiency and productivity. Organizers are good with details, and usually enjoy solving the day-to-day problems that inevitably appear in organizations. They understand budgets and cash flow and are often good with investments. Occupations include accountants, financial planners, office managers, and administrative assistants.
3. *Helping:* Involves helping and developing others through activities usually related to personal services, such as teaching, counseling, or healing. Compassionate and deeply concerned about the well-being of others. Helpers enjoy having close, personal contact with others and are genuinely concerned with helping their students or clients live full, satisfying lives. They readily understand the feelings of others and can provide emotional support. Occupations include counselors, teachers, and religious leaders.
4. *Creating:* Includes artistic, literary, and musical activities, such as writing, painting, dancing, and working in the theater, and also various design activities such as interior design and fashion design. Interested in, and confident of, their ability to create new products, new visions, and new concepts within these artistic areas. Creators see the world through innovative eyes and are frequently uncomfortable with traditional organizational constraints. They see themselves as free spirits and are often fluent and expressive. Occupations include artists, musicians, designers, and writers.
5. *Analyzing:* Involves scientific, mathematical, and statistical activities. Comfortable with data and numbers and have a strong need to understand the world in a scientific sense. They usually prefer to work alone or in small groups in laboratory or academic settings. Analyzers have a strong need to be autonomous and like to work through problems for themselves. Occupations include scientists, medical researchers, and statisticians.

6. *Producing:* Covers practical, hands-on, productive activities, such as construction, farming, and mechanical activities. Like to work with their hands, generally enjoy being outdoors, and like to be able to see the visible results of their labors. Producers are usually good with tools, and they enjoy taking on new construction projects or repairing mechanical breakdowns. Occupations include mechanics, veterinarians, and landscape architects.

7. *Adventuring:* Covers athletic, police, and military activities involving physical endurance, risk-taking, and competing with others. Enjoy physical activities, and they like to confront competitive situations. They are confident of their physical skills and often seek out excitement. Adventurers enjoy winning, but they also are resilient in defeat. They often like working closely with others in teams. Occupations include military officers, police officers, and athletic coaches. (pp. 97–98)

ABILITIES ASSESSMENT

After ascertaining an individual's interests, it is important to assess the person's abilities: what a person can and is able to do. There is no assurance that a person's abilities and interests will match. People are not created equal—each individual has unique strengths. Statistically, there is a normal distribution of abilities in a given population, but in various career fields, these abilities may not be distributed equally. Some areas require higher levels of abilities to be effective and competitive. To become a physician requires the ability to memorize a great deal of information for rapid recall. Individuals who are lacking in this ability will have a difficult time succeeding in medical school.

There are two dimensions to the measurement of abilities: general cognitive ability and career-relevant primary abilities. General cognitive ability is considered to be a person's overall intelligence and is usually measured by IQ tests. Career-relevant primary abilities measure the specific abilities that will be needed for specific career

---

Box 2.1

Career-Relevant Primary Abilities

1. Physical abilities
2. Mechanical reasoning
3. Spatial reasoning ability
4. Verbal reasoning
5. Nonverbal reasoning
6. Aesthetic ability
   a. Reproductive drawing ability
   b. Musical abilities
7. Verbal fluency
8. Social intelligence
9. Emotional intelligence
10. Managerial intelligence
11. Computational ability
12. Perceptual speed and accuracy

fields (e.g., a litigator will need good verbal reasoning abilities). Box 2.1 lists some of the major career-relevant primary abilities. Although formal assessment instruments measure some of these abilities (such as the subtests of the Wechsler scales), others are more difficult to quantify (Lowman, 1991; Prince & Heiser, 2000; Watkins & Campbell, 2000).

PERSONALITY ASSESSMENT

An individual's personality is also important when matching up interests and abilities. Although it is important not to stereotype (e.g., to assume that an introverted person would make a good accountant), it is helpful to at least discuss how an individual's personality traits may affect that person's choice of careers, and how these traits may present an advantage or a disadvantage for any given job (H. W. Roberts & Hogan, 2001).

One of the most popular ways to conceive personality is to look at five dimensions (known as the "Big Five"): Neuroticism, Extroversion, Openness to Experience, Agreeableness, and Conscientiousness (Costa & Widiger, 2002). The NEO Personality Inventory, Revised Edition (NEO-PI-R; Costa & McCrae, 1992) is one such instrument that measures these traits. Following are brief descriptions of the Big Five. For more details, see Costa and McCrae (1992), Costa and Widiger (2002), De Raad and Perugini (2002), and Piedmont (1998).

1. *Neuroticism:* Refers to a person's chronic emotional adjustment and instability. Individuals who are high in neuroticism are prone to distress, have difficulty tolerating frustration, and generally have maladaptive coping responses. For career counseling, it is important to note that such individuals tend to have high levels of job dissatisfaction (as a long-term personality trait more than as a situational state). This factor has a relationship with overall performance across occupations (individuals high in this trait tend to have difficulty feeling satisfied with their job, and individuals low in this trait tend to feel satisfied with a variety of jobs).

2. *Extraversion:* Refers to the need for social interactions, lots of activity and stimulation, and to the capacity for joy. For career counseling, whether an individual who is high or low in extroversion would be suited for a particular type of work depends on the demands of that occupation. This factor predicts some criteria for some occupations.

3. *Openness to experience:* Relates to an individual's desire to seek out new experiences, as displayed in curiosity, imagination, and ability to see things unconventionally. This quality is especially important in some occupations (e.g., artistic ones). This factor also predicts criteria for some occupations.

4. *Agreeableness:* Refers to an individual's interpersonal style. Those with high levels of agreeableness tend to be helpful, trusting, forgiving, and soft-hearted. This trait may be helpful in customer service occupations. Again, this factor is useful for predicting criteria for some occupations.

5. *Conscientiousness:* This factor refers to how motivated, persistent, and organized a person is to achieve goals. A high level of conscientiousness is important for most occupations that require reliability. This factor is consistently related to performance in all occupations.

Other multifaceted personality traits can be thought of as "compound traits":

Integrity

Service orientation

Managerial potential

Proactive personality

Social competence

Emotional intelligence

Clinicians are generally well trained in personality assessment and may use a wide variety of methods in working with clients to help them with an ideal career choice. Keep in mind, however, that normal personality traits (like the Big Five) are most often important for career counseling; therefore, consultants should not use personality assessment instruments that measure psychopathology (e.g., the MMPI-2).

The Myers-Briggs Type Indicator

An instrument that remains popular within organizations is the Myers-Briggs Type Indicator (MBTI; Myers, McCaulley, Quenk, & Hammer, 1998) which is now in its third edition. This instrument is designed to assess aspects of healthy personality along four dimensions: extraversion versus introversion; sensing versus intuition; thinking versus feeling; and judging versus perceiving. Combinations of these dimensions produce 16 different personality types. For example, an ISTJ personality type would score higher on the Introversion, Sensing, Thinking, and Judging scales than on the Extraversion, Intuition, Feeling, and Perceiving scales. Each of the 16 types has a distinct personality description for the test taker. The newer version also has an option for viewing how test takers score on subscales of each of the four dimensions.

Quenk (2000) notes a number of strengths and weaknesses of the MBTI:

Strengths

The comprehensive theory provides a context for understanding individual complexity.

Clients recognize the types as real and the typology as a useful way of describing themselves and others.

Nonnormative basis of preferences and types identifies and affirms client individual differences as normal.

Questions about simple surface behaviors adequately identify the complex constructs that interact, as specified in the theory.

Test yields four large psychometrically independent scales that are relatively unambiguous in what they measure.

The test is parsimonious: It requires only four measured constructs to yield rich personality descriptions with broad applicability.

Weaknesses

Adequate understanding of the theory is needed to administer and interpret the instrument.

Clients and professionals ascribe trait qualities to type preferences, leading to inappropriate interpretations of type.

From a normative perspective, positive type descriptions too easily gloss over real psychological problems.

Simplicity of questions encourages the idea that the typology itself is simple and static rather than complex and dynamic.

The scales look like familiar trait measures, and can easily be interpreted as four independent traits.

The 16 types are not measured directly; knowledge of theoretical assumptions regarding how the four scales interact dynamically is needed to identify types. (pp. 90–91)

Despite its weaknesses, the Myers-Briggs remains a popular instrument among executives (Baron, 1998; Kroeger & Thuesen, 1992), probably because it is easy to administer and interpret, and emphasizes healthy personality traits. Baron (1998) divides the 16 types into four categories, based on the combination of two of the four factors:

1. *Sensing Judging Types (SJ): Duty Seekers:* SJs are motivated by a need to be useful and of service. They like to stick to the standard ways of doing things and value the traditions, customs, and laws of society.
2. *Sensing Perceiving Types (SP): Action Seekers:* SPs are motivated by a need for freedom and action. They value and enjoy living in the here and now.
3. *Intuiting Thinking Types (NT): Knowledge Seekers:* NTs are motivated by a need to understand the world around them. They value competency and the powers of the mind.
4. *Intuiting Feeling Types (NF): Ideal Seekers:* NFs are motivated by a need to understand themselves and others. They value authenticity and integrity and strive for an ideal world. (pp. 44–47)

Kroeger and Thuesen (1992) developed succinct descriptions that can serve as a quick guide to each of the types:

ESTJ   "Life's natural administrators"
ESFJ   "Everyone's trusted friend"
ISTJ   "Life's natural organizers"
ISFJ   "Committed to getting the job done"
ESTP   "Making the most of the moment"
ESFP   "Let's make work fun"
ISTP   "Just do it"
ISFP   "Action speaks louder than words"
ENTJ   "Life's natural leaders"
ENTP   "Progress is the product"
INTJ   "Life's independent thinkers"
INTP   "Life's problem solvers"
ENFJ   "Smooth-talking persuaders"
ENFP   "People are the product"
INFJ   "An inspiring leader and follower"
INFP   "Making life kinder and gentler"

Table 2.1 contains brief descriptions of each of the 16 types (Baron, 1998). Note the focus on positive personality traits.

Table 2.1   The 16 Myers-Briggs Types

ESTJ: Outgoing, energetic, and dependable. Efficient, organized, and decisive. Likes administrating and being in charge. Excellent at organizing and deciding policies and procedures. Assertive, outspoken, and direct. Focuses on solving problems. Responsible, hard-working, and goal-oriented.

ESFJ: Enthusiastic, sociable, and engaging. Likes to be needed and appreciated. Personable, sympathetic, and cooperative. Likes being helpful, active in service organizations. Trustworthy, loyal, and responsible.

ISTJ: Reserved, persevering, loyal, and careful. Systematic, organized, and focused on the facts. Hardworking, thorough, and good at follow-through. Down-to-earth, pragmatic, and trustworthy. Honor their commitments.

ISFJ: Conscientious, trustworthy, and cooperative. Loyal, dependable, and self-disciplined. Strong work ethic, completes tasks on time. Excellent memory for details. Quietly friendly, thoughtful, and reserved. Often works behind the scenes helping others. Modest and unassuming.

ESTP: Likes risk, challenge, and adventure. Energetic and constantly on the go. Lives life to the fullest. Alert, confident, and persuasive. Can be outrageous, direct, and impulsive. Competent, resourceful, and responds well to crises. Realistic, pragmatic, and matter-of-fact.

ESFP: Caring, generous, cooperative, and enjoys helping others. Friendly, gregarious, energetic, vivacious, and charming. Often the life of the party. Tolerant and accepting of self and others. Has practical common sense. Accentuates the positive.

ISTP: Prefers action to conversation. Likes adventure and challenge. Does well in crisis. Enjoys working with tools, machines, and anything requiring hands-on skills. Resourceful, independent, and self-determined. Logical, realistic, and practical. Reserved, detached, curious observer.

ISFP: Gentle, loyal, and compassionate. Appears reserved and unassuming. Quietly does things for others. Patient, accepting, and nonjudgmental. Has a live-and-let-live attitude. Sensitive to conflicts and disagreement.

ENTJ: Confident leader who likes to be in charge. Decisive and ambitious. Likes intellectual exchange. Ingenious and resourceful in solving complex problems. Innovative, analytical, and logical. Self-determined and independent.

ENTP: Outspoken and thrives on challenge and debate. Enthusiastic, charming, gregarious, and witty. Values freedom and independence. Innovative, enterprising, and resourceful. Spontaneous and impulsive. Risk-taker who is alert to all possibilities.

INTJ: Independent and individualistic. Has great insight and vision. Skilled in creating theories and systems. Drives self and others toward goals and self-improvement. Ingenious and creative problem-solver. Organized, determined, and good at follow-through.

INTP: Analytical and brilliant. Conceptual problem-solver and original thinker. Idiosyncratic and nonconforming. Values precision in thought and language. Notices inconsistencies, contradictions, and logical flaws in others' thinking. Independent, curious, and insightful.

ENFJ: Friendly, charming, enthusiastic, and socially active. Persuasive speaker and inspiring, charismatic leader who motivates others. Empathic, warm, helpful, and supportive. Can idealize people and relationships. Responsible, conscientious, and goal-oriented.

ENFP: Warm-spirited, helpful, accepting, and compassionate. Full of enthusiasm and new ideas. Values freedom and autonomy. Good at communicating and inspiring action.

Table 2.1 *Continued*

INFJ: Sensitive, deep, and sometimes mystical. Single-minded regarding personal values and convictions. Has a rich inner life, and values personal integrity. Creative, original, and idealistic. Reserved, gentle, and compassionate.

INFP: Devoted, compassionate, open-minded, and gentle. Dislikes rules, orders, schedules, and deadlines. Likes learning and being absorbed in own projects. Has passionate convictions, and drive for ideals. Sets high standards for self.

Source: From *What Type Am I? Discover Who You Really Are* (pp. 44–47), by R. Baron, 1998, New York: Penguin Putnam.

Sixteen Personality Factor Questionnaire

The Sixteen Personality Factor Questionnaire (16PF; Russell & Karol, 1994), though not as widely used as the Myers-Briggs Type Indicator among those in the business world, is still popular due to its better research and validity support (H. B. Cattell, 1989; Golden, 1990; M. Karson, Karson, & O'Dell, 1997; Krug, 1977; Meyer, 1993). The 16PF gives a broad picture of an individual's personality. Though experienced clinicians can sometimes detect signs of psychopathology in test scores, it is designed to measure normal variations in human personality, and reveals an individual's strengths as well as weaknesses.

The 16PF is based on the work of Raymond Cattell (1943), who used factor analyses on the 18,000 adjectives that Allport and Odbert (1936) found as they searched the dictionary for descriptors of human personality. Cattell was able to reduce the descriptors to 16 factors. M. Karson et al. (1997) give an excellent overview of the 16PF and its interpretation.

The score yielded on each of the scales ranges from 1 to 10 (a "sten" score). A sten of 4, 5, 6, or 7 indicates that the respondent scored in the average range on that scale; and scores of 1 to 3 (– pole) or 8 to 10 (+ pole) indicate extreme scores.

Validity Scales

The validity or "response set" scales attempt to measure the test taker's attitude and approach toward the test. The Impression Management (IM) scale attempts to determine if the test taker's responses are defensive or exaggerated. The Acquiescence scale monitors a test taker's tendency to choose the "true" item (which always comes first on the test) regardless of whether the item truly applies to the person. Infrequency (INF), like the F scale on the MMPI-2, measures the number of items that were not chosen by the normative sample very often, which can indicate random responding, poor comprehension, and general deviance (M. Karson et al., 1997).

After confirming the validity of the test, the consultant can interpret the main scales. Following are brief descriptions of the 16 personality factors measured by the 16PF.

Factor A: Warmth measures a person's desire for interpersonal warmth, sociability, and emotional connections with others. A high score suggests that the individual is warm, outgoing, and attentive to others. Low scores indicate that the person is reserved, impersonal, and distant.

Factor B: Reasoning measures the test taker's thinking style. A low score indicates that the individual tends to think in concrete terms, and a high score indicates that the individual tends to think in more abstract ways.

Factor C: Emotional Stability, also called "Ego Strength," measures an individual's ability to deal with both internal and external challenges and stresses without being thrown off balance. Low scores suggest that the individual is reactive and emotionally changeable, whereas high scores suggest that the individual is emotionally stable, adaptive, and mature.

Factor E: Dominance measures one's desire to express oneself to others (rather than a desire to control others). M. Karson et al. (1997) prefer the term "assertiveness" for this factor. Low scores suggest a tendency to be deferential, cooperative, avoidant of conflict, whereas high scores indicate a tendency to be dominant, forceful, and assertive.

Factor F: Liveliness refers to a person's outlook on and enthusiasm regarding life. People who score low on this factor tend to be serious, restrained, and careful. Those who score high tend to be lively, animated, and spontaneous.

Factor G: Rule-Consciousness is a measure of how well an individual conforms to the rules of the social game and the ideals of one's identified group (S. Karson and O'Dell, 1976). Low scores indicate that an individual tends to be expedient and nonconforming. High scores suggest that the individual tends to be rule-conscious and dutiful.

Factor H: Social Boldness is a measure of an individual's degree of inhibition in social situations. Low scores indicate shyness, timidity, and sensitivity to threats. People with high scores on this factor tend to be socially bold, venturesome, and thick-skinned.

Factor I: Sensitivity factor ostensibly measures an individual's sensitivity to feelings, though it is heavily influenced by cultural ideas of gender (which should be kept in mind when interpreting this scale). Low scores suggest a tendency to be utilitarian, objective, and unsentimental. People with high scores tend to be sensitive, aesthetic, and sentimental.

Factor L: Vigilance refers to how strongly the test taker monitors the external environment. Low scores suggest that a person is trusting, unsuspecting, and accepting, whereas high scores suggest a tendency to be vigilant, suspicious, skeptical, and wary. Clinicians should be cautious of very high scores, which can suggest pathological paranoia.

Factor M: Abstractedness, also known as "impracticality," measures how practical an individual is. Individuals with low scores tend to be grounded, practical, and solution-oriented. High scorers tend to be abstracted, imaginative, and idea-oriented.

Factor N: Privateness measures a person's tendency to be private or forthright in interactions with others. Low scorers tend to be forthright, genuine, and artless, whereas high scorers tend to be private, discreet, and nondisclosing.

Factor O: Apprehension represents, in psychodynamic terms, the struggle between one's conscience and one's identified sense of self. Individuals with low scores tend to be self-assured, unworried, and complacent. Individuals with high scores are often apprehensive, self-doubting, and worried.

The "Q" factors are based solely on internal states as measured by the questionnaire, as opposed to the previous factors, which were based on observational data (M. Karson et al., 1997).

Factor Q1: Openness to Change is a relatively straightforward measure of an individual's attitude toward change. Low scores suggest a tendency to be traditional and attached to the familiar, whereas high scores indicate that the person is open to change and likes to experiment.

Factor Q2: Self-Reliance attempts to measure a preference for being alone versus doing things with others. Low scores are indicative of someone who prefers to be group-oriented and affiliative. High scores suggest a tendency to be self-reliant, solitary, and individualistic.

Factor Q3: Perfectionism, also known as "compulsivity," measures an individual's tendency to develop and live up to ideals of behavior. Low scorers tend to be tolerant of disorder and are unexacting and flexible; whereas high scorers tend to be perfectionistic, organized, and self-disciplined.

Factor Q4: Tension is a measure of free-floating anxiety and general level of frustration. Due to the face validity of the test items that load on this factor, it is susceptible to manipulation by the test taker. Low scores are indicative of someone who is relaxed, placid, and patient, and high scores suggest a tendency to be tense, highly energized, impatient, and driven.

The 16PF also contains five *global factors,* derived from a factor analysis of the 16 scales. They resemble the "Big Five" personality factors:

Extraversion (EX) measures an individual's desire to participate in social activities. Low scorers tend to be introverted and socially inhibited, and high scorers tend to be extraverted and socially participative.

Anxiety (AX) measures what R. B. Cattell, Eber, and Tatsuoka (1970) called "Anxiety versus Dynamic Integration." Low scores indicate someone with low anxiety who is unperturbed, and high scores suggest a person with high anxiety who is perturbable. Low scores could indicate a denial of problems, and high scores could indicate that a person is feeling overwhelmed. This factor is correlated with the Neuroticism scale of the NEO-PI-R.

Tough-Mindedness (TM) measures emotionality that stems from comfort and conversance with feelings (M. Karson et al., 1997). People with low scores tend to be receptive, open-minded, and intuitive. High scores suggest a tendency to be tough-minded, resolute, and unempathic. This factor is correlated with the Openness to Experience scale of the NEO-PI-R.

Independence (IN) measures an individual's degree of independence. People with low scores tend to be accommodating, agreeable, and selfless; high scores suggest a tendency to be independent, willful, and persuasive. This factor is correlated with the Agreeableness scale of the NEO-PI-R.

Self-Control (SC) measures people's tendency to respect rules, maintain order, and consider the practical consequences of their actions. Low scorers tend to be unrestrained and follow their urges, whereas high scorers tend to be self-controlled and capable of inhibiting their urges. This factor is correlated with the Conscientiousness scale of the NEO-PI-R.

CAREER STAGES

Consultants should also consider the career stage of the individuals with whom they are working. There are likely to be different emphases and different considerations for individuals based on their age and career stage. Lussier (2002) breaks these stages into the 20s, the 30s, the 40s and 50s, and the 60s and 70s. Following are descriptions of the important aspects of each career stage for managers.

The 20s

Managers have just graduated college and are entering the workforce in their 20s. The challenge at this stage is to prove to employers that the manager can do the job effectively (*Journal of Accountancy,* 2000). There is a lot of pressure and competition to do well. Women and minorities who seek advancement in a world dominated by White men tend to feel additional personal pressure to try harder. At this stage, people are working to develop their skill level and professional identity. They need initiative and foresight to prepare for future advancement. Young people tend to work long, hard hours to get ahead, often postponing family plans.

Today's young managers have higher expectations for having a good life and a prestigious position, though they are operating in an environment with fewer organizational levels than in times past. Because there are relatively fewer management positions available, it takes more time to progress, and lateral promotions are frequent. Most professionals don't stay at their first job for more than 3 years (Tejada, 2000).

The 30s

Once they have had some seasoning, managers have begun to develop an expertise and have an opportunity to display their strengths as bosses. They continually strive to prove their worth to members of top management. This decade is also when people begin to question their career path. Where am I going? Is this where I should be? How much job security do I really have right now? This time of doubt is especially tough for individuals who must decide whether and how to combine having children and pursuing a career. Even if they are not satisfied with their current jobs or careers, people often feel trapped by financial demands and are frightened of changing careers, which may require a cut in pay or a change in benefits or retirement packages. However, it is now rare for an individual to work 20 to 30 years for the same organization. Career changes are more common, and managers typically work for two to four organizations in the course of their career years (Karr, 2000).

The 40s and 50s

By their mid-40s, managers have usually experienced numerous successes and failures and have a sense of their capabilities. Not everyone has the capacity to become a top-level manager, and the majority of individuals come to accept that they must abandon the race they began in their 20s. However, as middle-management jobs are being reduced in many organizations, people may be forced to find a new career, or may be pressured to take an early retirement (along with a cut in pay and lifestyle). Individuals may begin to mourn the loss of their youth and their dreams of big financial success.

The 60s and 70s

People begin to prepare for retirement at this stage. If they pass along what they have learned, they provide continuity to the next generation and can feel a sense of accomplishment from taking on the role of mentor to junior managers. Mentors can boost young careers, but are not available to most younger managers (*Wall Street Journal,* 1996).

INTEGRATING DATA

Mental health professionals understand the challenge of integrating data and strive to do this on a regular basis when working with clients. A psychological assessment may include a personality assessment, a cognitive assessment, and a clinical interview. The clinician then looks for themes among these responses. One of the great skills of the mental health consultant is the ability to integrate and analyze data, which can help the client to see the "big picture" and to consider multiple alternatives.

Lowman (1991) described six important considerations when integrating data:

1. *Separately evaluate the data in each domain (interests, abilities, and personality) as if other data did not exist.* It is important to remain unbiased when looking at each domain, so that unique pieces of data are not overlooked.

2. *After hypotheses have been independently generated in each domain, cross-domain comparisons can be made.* Once each domain has been analyzed, the consultant looks for connections and themes between the domains.

3. *Each tentative conclusion ideally should be supported by at least two sources of data.* Although unique pieces of data from one domain should not be ignored, more weight should be given to information that is found to be consistent across domains.

4. *Inconsistent hypotheses may not need to be fully resolved.* It is perfectly acceptable to present multiple hypotheses, even if they do not appear to fit together. For example, a given individual may be well suited for both office management and lion-taming.

5. *Major conclusions should be summarized in a point-by-point fashion.* This facilitates communication with the client, and allows him or her to easily grasp the results.

6. *Conclusions should be tentative and hypothetical rather than definitive and dogmatic.* When dealing with people's lives and futures, it is important to acknowledge the fallibility of the assessment instruments. There will always be individuals who go on to accomplish great things despite not having the "ability" to do so. As in therapy, the consultant must be aware of the power of suggestion created by his or her role as authority figure.

Regardless of the results of the interest, abilities, and personality assessments, the client is likely to come away from the process having learned something, and having become a bit more self-aware. As in individual psychotherapy, just being able to freely explore issues can be very helpful to clients. It is difficult to know the long-term effects of your interventions—even if you feel that you did not discover the perfect career for the client, you may have set into motion a series of life-altering events (assuming you performed your services competently!).

CASE EXAMPLE: THE DISCONTENTED AUTO SALESPERSON

An auto salesperson came in complaining of being miserable at work. He was running the family business with his father and brother. He felt trapped by the high salary and financial needs of his wife and three children, and he was tired of customers treating him like the stereotypical car salesperson, who is perceived to be a crook. He always tried to deal fairly with people, but people would haggle with him over price and assume that he was being dishonest. This hurt him very much. He was also in constant conflict with his father and brother about how best to run the business. He personally emphasized customer service and fairness, whereas he felt his family was most concerned about profit margin. Clinical career assessment revealed the various sources of the mismatch between his job and his personality and interests. Although the prospect of changing careers appealed to him (perhaps returning to school and doing graduate training in a profession such as optometry), he felt that he could not justify the disruption to his family. After several months of indecision and deepening vocational despair, he made a unique decision that was later to help ease his distress. He developed one of the first auto sales companies in the United States to adopt a fixed price with no negotiation or haggling on price. The price assured a reasonable profit margin but avoided many of the discomforts that plagued him on the job. Since he couldn't change jobs, he changed the job itself to better suit him.

Chapter 3

ORGANIZATIONAL CONTEXT

Before entering the organizational setting, consultants should be familiar with the ways that organizations motivate their employees, the problems faced by employees, legal issues involved in employment, and other contextual issues. Once consultants feel comfortable in organizational settings, they can focus more energy on designing and implementing effective interventions.

MULTILEVEL ORGANIZATION OF WORK

People spend a large percentage of their lives working. The work environment has a profound influence on an organization's employees and on the mental health of clients in psychotherapy. Before mental health professionals can suggest interventions for individuals in a work context, they must first explore the theoretical background of work.

When considering work, it is necessary to look at multiple levels (Quick & Tetrick, 2003; Sauter et al., 2002). First, there is the external context (factors that affect the economy as a whole); next, the organizational context (factors that affect the specific organization under consideration); and finally, the job context (the employee's specific job). In this chapter, we explore how these contexts might affect a therapist in a group practice.

External Context

The external context includes the economic, legal, political, technological, and demographic forces that operate at the national and international level:

- Economic developments (e.g., globalization of the economy)
- Regulatory, trade, and economic policies (e.g., deregulation)
- Technological innovations (e.g., computer technology)
- Changing worker demographics and labor supply (e.g., aging populations)

Thus, therapists must be aware of the latest developments in the external environment. Although the demand for psychotherapy for serious psychopathology may remain fairly robust despite changes in the economy, people may be less likely to pay out-of-pocket for growth-oriented therapy during recessions. Therapists also need to be aware of changes in policies by the state board and professional organizations that may affect their practice. Technological innovations such as multimedia therapy and computerized data management may help them become more competitive (or may needlessly distract them from more important activities). Demographic changes, such as the aging of the baby boomers, may inspire a therapist to seek more specialized training in working with geriatric populations.

Organizational Context

The organizational context includes the management structures, supervisory practices, production methods, and human resource policies of the organization:

- Organizational restructuring (e.g., downsizing)
- New quality and process management initiatives (e.g., high performance work systems)
- Alternative employment arrangements (e.g., contingent labor)
- Work/life/family programs and flexible work arrangements (e.g., telecommuting)
- Changes in benefits and compensation systems (e.g., gainsharing)

Therapists need to be aware of the policies of the organization for which they are working. Who will cover the client load for after-hours emergencies, or while the therapist is on vacation? What is included in the compensation and benefits package? Is there a procedure for handling suicidal or homicidal clients? Is the therapist expected to be in the office at set times, or is a flexible schedule permitted? How will client scheduling and billing be handled?

Job Context

The job context includes the specific characteristics of a job or task:

- Task attributes: temporal aspects, complexity, autonomy, physical and psychological demands
- Social-relational aspects of work
- Worker roles
- Working hours and schedule
- Employee development and job security
- Safety climate

Therapists need to be aware of the demands of their job, and how it might affect their stress level. If the job is demanding (as therapy can be), what buffers are in place? Is it a safe environment? Can downtime be scheduled between clients? How much autonomy and how much supervision will the therapist receive?

Although a consultant may be called in to work on only one level, any of these variables can be important to the consultee's work situation. A consultee may be doing wonderful work at the job context level, but may be encountering barriers at the organizational or external environment level.

THE POSITIVE ASPECTS OF WORK

Although it is sometimes fashionable in our society to grumble about working and to long for retirement, clinicians who have worked with unemployed or retired people understand that work provides many benefits to a person's life. Work provides structure (a reason to get up in the morning); social contact (friends, involvement with others); group identity ("our company is the best at what we do"); a sense of meaning or purpose; money and benefits to help workers acquire the resources they need to live; intrinsic value (if the work is inherently fulfilling); enforcement of activity (physical exercise, exercise of thought, and exercise of a person's capabilities)—and it often leads to the development of goals transcending the simple desire for a paycheck. Losing these benefits can be devastating to those who are unable to work.

The *manifest benefits* of work, which include pay and benefits, are what most people bring to mind. The secondary benefits, such as having a time structure and a sense of purpose, are known as *latent benefits* (Manning, Curtis, & McMillen, 1996).

Consultants are not usually called upon because an individual or an organization is experiencing too many positive work experiences. The negative consequences of work, such as work-related stress, are being increasingly recognized as a significant problem in the workplace.

WORK MOTIVATION

Why do people do the jobs that they do? Most people immediately think of money, but in reality there are many motivations. Blais, Briere, Lachance, Riddle, and Vallerand (1993) created the Blais Work Motivation Inventory (BWMI) to help clinicians assess the various types of motivation. To implement an effective intervention, the consultant should listen carefully to clients to gauge the source of their motivation and how it is regulated. Consider the following examples:

Intrinsic motivation: "Because I frequently learn interesting things doing this job."

Extrinsic motivation, identified regulation: "Because it is the job I chose to work toward fulfilling my career plans."

Extrinsic motivation, internal regulation: "Because my work is my life and I don't want to fail."

Extrinsic motivation, external regulation: "Because I get a paycheck."

Amorphous motivation, external regulation: "I don't know; our work conditions are too different."

Amorphous motivation, internal regulation: "I don't know; I just can't manage to do the important tasks of this work well."

Intrinsic motivation for work, or doing something you enjoy, is key for long-term life satisfaction (Csikszentmihalyi, 2003). Despite any superficial claims that money is all-important, clients would like consultants to help them develop goals that transcend their biweekly paychecks (the test is: would you continue to do your job if you were not paid to do so?). Seligman (2002) distinguishes three kinds of "work orientation":

1. A job
2. A career
3. A calling:

You do a *job* for the paycheck at the end of the week. It is just a means to another end, and when the wage stops, you quit. A *career* entails a deeper personal investment in work. You mark your achievements through money, but also through advancement. Each promotion brings you higher prestige and more power, as well as a raise. When the promotions stop—when you "top out"—alienation starts, and you begin to look elsewhere for gratification and meaning. A *calling* (or vocation) is a passionate commitment to work for its own sake. Individuals with a calling see their work as contributing to the greater good, to something larger than they are, and hence the religious connotation is entirely appropriate. The work is fulfilling in its own right, without regard for money or for advancement. When the money stops and the promotions end, the work goes on. Traditionally, callings were reserved to very prestigious and rarified work—clergy, Supreme Court justices, physicians, and scientists. But there has been an important discovery in this field: any job can become a calling, and any calling can become a job. (p. 168)

The importance of this background information to the topic of workplace stress is that a deep understanding and sense of the importance of work will tend to support clients in their job and buttress them from experiencing workplace stress. Clients can accept a lot more stress on the job if they view the work as a calling rather than a job. Work stress and conflict rise significantly in times of cutbacks and reduced profits, when uncertainty prevails and the "big picture" of where the organization is headed and the employee's future role is fuzzy. However, workers can endure the most difficult conditions if they find meaning in what they do. An example is the morale of soldiers who served in World War II versus those who fought in Vietnam.

Job satisfaction is more of a trait than a response to a work setting. People can find great satisfaction in many job settings. Consider the following quotes, taken from Terkel (1972):

Hots Michaels, piano player in a New York bar—". . . because I enjoy the action. I enjoy people. If I were suddenly to inherit four million dollars, I guarantee you I'd be playin' piano, either here or at some other place. I can't explain why. I would miss the flow of people in and out." (p. 336)

Cathleen Moran, nurse's aide—"I really don't know if I mind the work as much as you always have to work with people, and that drives me nuts. I don't mind emptying the bedpan, what's in it, blood, none of that bothers me at all. Dealing with people is what I don't like. It just makes everything else blah." (p. 613)

Nora Watson, newspaper editor—"Jobs are not big enough for people. It's not just the assembly line worker whose job is too small for his spirit, you know. A job like mine, if you really put your spirit into it, you would sabotage immediately. You don't dare. So you absent your spirit from it. My mind has been divorced from my job, except as a source of income, it's really absurd." (p. 675)

Elmer Ruiz, gravedigger—"Not anybody can be a gravedigger. You can dig a hole any way they come. A gravedigger, you have to make a neat job. I had this fella once; he wanted to see a grave. He was a fella that digged sewers. He was impressed when he seen me diggin' this grave—how square and perfect it was. A human body is goin' into this grave. That's why you need skill when you're gonna dig a grave. . . . I start early, about seven o'clock in the morning, and I have the part cleaned before the funeral. We have two funerals tomorrow, eleven and one o'clock. That's my life.

"I enjoy it very much, especially in summer. I don't think any job inside a factory or an office is so nice. You have the air all day and it's just beautiful. The smell of the grass when it's cut, it's just fantastic. Winter goes so fast sometimes you just don't feel it." (p. 658)

Research has found a relatively low correlation between workers' levels of job satisfaction and their performance on the job. Employees may be very happy, but not producing much for the company. Many of us may have had the experience in our youth of excitedly starting on a new job, eager to perform well, only to be looked down on by senior workers. These senior workers may have subtly (or not-so-subtly) encouraged us to lower our productivity so that we would not make everyone else look bad. Organizations may sometimes need to work creatively to foster an environment where employees experience high job satisfaction and high productivity.

For most people, job satisfaction is significantly tied to life satisfaction in general. Workers perhaps feel this most poignantly after losing a job.

UNEMPLOYMENT

Exploring the importance of work helps in understanding the importance of unemployment and job transitions resulting from mergers, downsizings, and reductions in force. Job transitions are increasing in our society, and unemployment represents the loss of all the rewards that people receive from working. To illustrate the importance of work, deterioration in both mental and physical health typically follows unemployment. Although a small minority of the recently unemployed (about 10%) report an improvement in health following job loss, the majority show signs of increased stress, anxiety, and depression, with decreased self-esteem and self-efficacy. Frequently, there is also an increase in somatic complaints, physical illnesses, and injuries. Rapid improvements in health usually occur after a return to paid employment, which suggests that the decline in mental and physical health is the result of unemployment rather than its cause.

When planning interventions, mental health consultants should bear in mind that there are two categories of unemployed individuals: the "Hard-Core Unemployed" and the "Soft-Core Unemployed." The Hard-Core Unemployed refers to people who have been unemployed for at least 6 months, have few marketable skills, are living at or below the poverty level, and have less than a high school education. The Soft-Core Unemployed includes people who find themselves unexpectedly without a job, often after having worked most of their adult lives.

The Age Discrimination in Employment Act protects older employees (those between the ages of 40 and 70) against unfair discrimination. Performance of older employees has been found to be comparable to that of younger employees, and any deficits tend to be compensated for by greater dependability, less absenteeism, and increased effort. Declines in performance are more likely to be due to decrements in psychomotor skills (e.g., slower reaction time) than to changes in intellectual functioning.

CASE EXAMPLE

A 25-year-old African American man presented in crisis seeking counseling and career assessment. Delray had been an outstanding college basketball player and for the past several years had been playing basketball in Europe. He came home because of an injury and discovered that his wife of 4 years had an affair during his last absence. He sought therapy for help in changing careers and getting over his wife's affair.

The clinician would need to consider many things in working with this client. How was Delray's work a factor in his psychological difficulties? How might his career progression and wife's affair affect his self-esteem? What adjustment issues will Delray have to overcome?

This case also illustrates the concept of *spillover,* which refers to the common experience of work-related issues affecting one's personal life. Spillover can include both positive and negative effects. An example of a negative effect would be a busy executive's tendency to continually think about work challenges when interacting with her family, which would weaken the emotional connection she once had with them. A positive effect would be bringing home a sense of purpose and fulfillment from a job, and treating other people with greater kindness.

THE PROBLEM OF JOB STRESS

Work-related stress is dynamic and multidimensional—the causes are multiple, interacting, and dependent on the individual experiencing them (D. L. Nelson & Burke, 2003). The causes relate not only to the individual but to the work group, the larger organization and its structure, and the societal context in which the work is embedded.

Job stress is expensive: It is estimated to cost U.S. industry $300 billion annually, as measured by absenteeism, lost productivity, turnover, direct medical costs, insurance fees, and legal fees (The American Institute of Stress, 2005).

Absenteeism

Job stress results in 416 million lost workdays per year, which translates into 9 days per employee per year. One employee in every 15 is absent at least once a week. These time losses translate into these direct dollar costs in the United States: $26.4 billion per year, $66 per day for each day lost to absenteeism, and $150 for each 1% of absenteeism per worker. For organizations, this means that a 1% increase in employee absence can cut profits by 4% (Brannon & Feist, 1997; Klarreich, 1998; Knaus, 1998). Workplace stress increases absenteeism, and Knaus (1998) lists several broad reasons why employees voluntarily miss work.

Hooky: People play hooky to have a day off to do other things (or just to do nothing), and to escape the responsibilities of adult life.

Substance use: A person may need to recover from a hangover or a night of partying, or may have serious problems with substance dependence (Bennett & Lehman, 2003).

Family obligation: An employee may need to take care of a sick child or go to the doctor with a family member.

Resentment: An individual may skip work as a form of "payback," a passive-aggressive maneuver because of anger or resentment about something that is happening at work.

Depressed pattern: Apathy, loss of energy, and poor concentration (often paired with a sense of hopelessness) are symptoms of depression that can cause workers to miss work. Depression is often felt as a "who cares" attitude.

Neurotic anxiety patterns: Some individuals have social phobias that cause them to feel discomfort or embarrassment when they are with people. Although some people prefer to keep to themselves, others deeply desire contact at work but avoid people or stress that may exist there.

Mental health day patterns: Some people have rationalized that they are entitled to a certain number of days of absence per year above and beyond their vacation as a part of their self-care.

Self-indulgence: An employee may just not "feel like" going to work. "I am out of vacation days, but I just feel like going to Kings Island and riding the roller coaster today."

Stress-related absences and costs related to stress have greatly increased in the last decade. Two-thirds of both men and women say that work has a significant impact on their stress level. One in four U.S. workers have called in sick or taken a "mental health day" as a result of work stress (American Psychological Association, 2005; Ritter, 2000).

Some jobs are more stressful than others. However, it is not necessarily top executives who are prone to stress and stress-related illness. The jobs most likely to lead to heart disease, hypertension, cardiovascular problems, anxiety, depression, and other illnesses are those that give workers very little control over their tasks or work conditions. This can include middle-level managers, who are expected to mobilize lower-level employees although upper management provides limited resources and time for this task.

Daily hassles also cause stress. In the long term, the stress induced by daily hassles actually has a stronger impact on health than the stress of traumatic events (Weinberger, Hiner, & Tierney, 1987). Survey data show the following commonly cited causes of work stress (Petry, Mujica, & Vickery, 1998):

Balancing work and family	52%
Poor internal communications	51%
Work hours/workload	51%
Poor leadership	51%
Effects of downsizing	33%

The study of conflict between work life and family life is a growing field that monitors societal trends. There are actually two types of conflict: work to family (where work interferes with family life) and family to work (where family life interferes with work). Researchers have emphasized work-to-family conflicts, as evidenced by there being three times more studies in this area than in the area of family-to-work conflicts (S. Lambert, 1990).

Organizational policies at some workplaces create additional stressors such as inadequate flexibility to manage work and family responsibilities, inadequate materials and equipment, and inadequate support from other people at work (including supervisors who lack respect for employees).

Research investigating positive and negative interaction patterns (Gottman, 1981, 1994, 2002; Losada, 1999; Losada & Heaphy, 2004) has determined that a 3-to-1 ratio of praise and encouragement to criticism is necessary to have a flourishing work team. Workplace team productivity will increase as the ratio moves up to 13 to 1, after which there is no change. This ratio is important to share with consultees, as it suggests that managers must be liberal with their praise of employee performance. It also suggests that some criticism or conflict is useful, even necessary, to stimulate growth and change.

Since a supportive, encouraging culture is vital not only to morale but for worker productivity, the most valuable support at work is not praise but ongoing regard. It is most powerful when we can express direct and specific appreciation or admiration to another person. Instead of simply saying "Good job," it would be more effective to say "Bette, I really appreciate the work you did on the work stress project. Without your research on the importance of work, the paper would have lacked an important focus." We feel better about ourselves when we think that what we do matters. It provides a kind of food that keeps us nourished at work. People frequently have a fleeting sense of appreciation for others, but fail to express these feelings. Expressing them is like bringing oxygen into an organizational system. It builds trust and motivates workers. One approach is to create a ritual during meetings when managers offer direct and specific admiration or appreciation, directly telling their people how their behavior makes a difference. This is a good way to release the energy of the team, instead of acting as if the leader is the only or even the primary source of most of the good things that are happening.

Employee stress affects many things:

- Well-being
- Physical health
- Mental health
- Job satisfaction
- Employee morale
- Motivation
- Organizational commitment
- Climate

Prolonged stress at work contributes to high blood pressure (hypertension), coronary artery disease, and depression. With prolonged exposure, the body may adapt to the toxic environment of many workplaces, leading to high blood pressure at work but not at the doctor's office.

The modern workplace contains a host of stressors. Unpredictability results from being available 24 hours a day, 7 days a week, by means of pagers, cell phones, and e-mails. Fear of change results from mergers, downsizing, and corporate restructuring. Workers are continuously given higher demands to do more with fewer resources in less time.

Compared with the 1970s, the typical length of the workweek has increased (work hours have been steadily rising in the United States and now average 48 hours per week; Dresang, 2005). Leisure time, which is very important for "decompressing" from a stressful work environment, has been decreasing. A comparison of the average U.S. vacation time is shown in Box 3.1.

Box 3.1

Average Annual Vacation Days Taken (2001)

U.S.	13 days per year
South Korea	25 days per year
Japan	25 days per year
Canada	26 days per year
Britain	32 days per year
Brazil	34 days per year
Germany	35 days per year
France	37 days per year
Italy	42 days per year

Source: From *Average Annual Vacation Days Taken,* by World Tourism Organization, 2001, available from http://www.world-tourism.org.

CASE EXAMPLE

Peter, a 55-year-old Caucasian executive for a large government contractor, presented in crisis after he walked off the job in Washington, DC, following a period of significant job stress. Peter was perfectionistic and felt that he needed complete control over his work environment to be effective. When his situation grew more complex, he tried the "work harder" approach, increasing his hours, which only served to create more work stress. Eventually, Peter collapsed and was no longer able to function. He had been on disability for 4 weeks before he was able to come in for help. He struggled over whether to leave the company or to ask for a transfer. He did not feel that he could continue in his current environment, so he chose to accept a transfer to another installation. The company did not want to lose him because of his high level of performance. His wife developed problems during the course of her husband's disability, partly because she had put her own needs and issues on hold to assist her husband. This ordeal brought the wife's career issues to the surface, and eventually, she made a change from being a hospice nurse to becoming a consultant.

This case illustrates how underlying personality dynamics can interact with job stress. In such cases, it can be difficult to determine if the consultee should change positions, or should persevere and learn better coping skills.

Burnout

Burnout is being increasingly recognized as a major issue—there have been over 5,000 studies on the topic. Burnout can be thought of as mild depression related to work. It occurs when job stressors exceed the worker's ability to cope. Job burnout is caused by accumulated stress associated with overwork. An early symptom of burnout is a sudden increase in work effort and hours without an increase in productivity. Subsequent symptoms include lowered productivity, loss of interest, loss of motivation, irritability, negativity, social withdrawal, and physical complaints (e.g., backaches and headaches). Workers experiencing job burnout tend to be inflexible about work rules and procedures and, as a result, are unable to identify alternative solutions to the problems they encounter. They often feel that their efforts are useless, ineffective, or unappreciated, and that their opportunities for advancement are limited. Highly motivated, goal-driven, overdedicated workers are most susceptible to job burnout (Freudenberger & Richelson, 1980).

Job dissatisfaction leads to higher absenteeism, which leads to yet lower job satisfaction. Burnout increases absenteeism. Burnout, especially emotional exhaustion, increases job dissatisfaction (see Box 3.2).

Burnout, depression, chronic fatigue syndrome, and posttraumatic stress disorder (PTSD) overlap. They all result from chronic stress and a gradual imbalance in the hypothalamic-pituitary adrenal axis as measured by the presence of cortisol. Depressive burnout is related to high levels of cortisol, whereas fatigue is related to lowered levels of cortisol (Freudenberger & Richelson, 1980; Sauter et al., 2002).

Box 3.2

Factors Related to Job Stress and Burnout

- *Control:* A sense of control is a core factor in job stress. The higher the degree of autonomy and the greater the decisional latitude, the lower the stress. The employer should enable employees to have greater choices, not complete independence. There is a positive relationship between job control and job stress, which affects work-related health outcomes. A combination of high job demand and low job decision latitude produces *job strain.*
- *Workload:* Employees must be able to handle their workload on a long-term basis without feeling exhausted.
- *Rewards:* Employees must be able to see a result for their efforts. This may range from high monetary pay to simple acts of recognition in the workplace.
- *Community:* Employees should feel a sense of community in the workplace. During restructuring and downsizing experiences, burnout becomes elevated (only one-half of such actions are successful).
- *Value congruence:* The individual's values must feel congruent with those of the organization. The greater the incongruence, the greater the feeling of tension in the employee.
- *Fairness and respect:* Democratic management techniques (ones in which employees feel that they have some say) are associated with low levels of stress, good general health, and less absence and illness. Justice is important in work.
- *Distributive justice:* This refers to whether resources are distributed fairly and represents the degree to which all people are treated the same under a policy, regardless of race, ethnicity, gender, age, or any other demographic characteristic.
- *Procedural justice:* The degree to which the rules and procedures specified by policies are properly followed in all cases under which they are applied (Schermerhorn et al., 2000). A teacher who randomly assigned grades would be violating both distributive and procedural justice.

CASE EXAMPLE: BURNOUT

A middle-level executive at a military base had worked on a difficult project for 18 months. During that time, he lost 60 pounds, started drinking heavily, and became increasingly depressed until his commanding officer transferred him to a less stressful assignment. He also experienced a divorce during the same time frame.

During consultation, it was discovered that this client suffered PTSD-like symptoms from the intensity of the work demands placed on him. He had also significantly withdrawn from outside activities, developing a mild agoraphobia. Over the course of therapy, he was able to reengage with a new work situation and found support through a relationship with a family where he became a boarder.

Measuring Burnout

There are many measures of burnout. The most dominant and commonly used instruments are the Maslach Burnout Inventory (MBI; Maslach, Jackson, & Letter, 1996; Maslach & Leiter, 1997) and the Burnout Measure (BM; Pines, Aronson, & Kafry, 1981).

Burnout typically follows a developmental progression. It begins with feelings of emotional exhaustion. Next, feelings of cynicism develop. Later, there is a loss of personal efficacy or feelings of accomplishment. This increases the risk for physical and psychological problems. Psychological problems usually precede physical problems (e.g., the person develops depression or anxiety, and later develops an ulcer or coronary artery disease). Once burnout starts, it tends to be self-perpetuating, unless active steps are taken to reduce it.

Therapist Burnout

Though they often counsel others in matters of stress management, therapists themselves are frequently susceptible to burnout; they may act tired and have difficulty listening to clients, who may seem to feel like "the enemy." Therapists may begin making fun of clients and can become cynical and pessimistic, believing that no one will ever really change. They may start to wonder if the therapy they provide will ever help anyone.

When intervening in a mental health setting experiencing burnout, the consultant ideally should work on improving institutional policies and training the supervisor(s) to recognize the signs of burnout and provide interventions before the burnout progresses too far. Though supervisors may feel that they are already too busy to do this, the consultant can point out that small, regular check-ins with proficient therapists (which should include recognition and appreciation of their work) is much more time-efficient than training new therapists after the current ones leave.

Reducing Work-Related Stress and Burnout

Empowerment in work is important for reducing workplace stress. It is crucial to create environments where the desire to perform comes from factors inside (intrinsic) instead of from rewards outside (extrinsic) the person. This process unleashes the untapped potential contribution that lies within each person. Build an empowered team through respect, information, control, decision making, responsibility, and development of skills (C. D. Scott & Jaffe, 1991). Empowerment counters the negative effects of workplace stress. The meaningful reduction of complexity is also important, as is the maintenance of a safe work environment.

Many cases of work dysfunction lead to workplace stress. Some are related to a mismatch of a person's abilities, interest, and personality with a job, others are secondary to psychological problems or spillover. Many result from the conditions of the work environment and organization. Demographics don't tend to predict burnout. You will see work-related problems frequently in organizations (Lowman, 1993).

People respond to workplace stress by searching for a new job or job transfer, quitting the job (sometimes quitting on the job to varying degrees), or by adopting stress management techniques.

Interventions can occur at the individual level, which might involve stress management, behavioral techniques, or changing positions to avoid boredom. Ideally, change should take place at the organizational level, which might involve changing policies to improve the work environment (Angerer, 2003; O'Driscoll & Cooper, 1996).

ORGANIZATIONAL INTERVENTIONS

Employers may need to be convinced of the value of promoting a psychologically healthful environment. Managers often feel a tension between productivity and health, believing that spending time, energy, and financial resources on health may lower resources that could be applied to productivity. Consultants should educate the employer on the potential effects of reducing stress in the workplace, such as reduced employee turnover, reduced absenteeism, increased productivity, improved morale, and lower health care costs. To create tangible bottom-line reasons to implement better institutional policies, ask the employer about the rate of turnover, and about how much it costs to hire a new employee (including search costs, administrative costs, training costs, and lost productivity while the new employee gets up to speed). In extreme cases, the consultant may need to prevent a psychologically unhealthy worker from becoming violent.

Healthy and happy workers tend to be more productive, treat customers better, and boost the company's image in the community. Health care costs for workers who report high stress are 50% higher than for other workers, and health care costs continue to accelerate (Aldana & Pronk, 2001). Employees who have less supportive workplaces feel overworked. Organizations should be responsive to employee expectations, and should be sensitive to the differing needs of a diverse workforce (see Box 3.3).

To reduce organizational stress, employers should promote employee involvement, provide consideration for family support, actively promote employee growth and development, and establish programs to monitor health and safety issues (Barling & Frone, 2004).

A healthy goal for an organization would be to receive the Psychologically Healthy Workplace award (American Psychological Association, 2005). This award is designed for any organization that maximizes the integration of worker goals for well-being and company objectives for profitability and productivity (Sauter et al., 2002). Pursuit of such an award helps workers meet their work goals, manage stress, and balance their work and family life for enhanced productivity. It also increases workers' job satisfaction and loyalty to their employer.

A psychologically healthy workplace should ideally have:

- Quality benefits plans
- Effective leadership and communication

Box 3.3

Tips for Employers to Prevent Burnout

- Provide workers with clear expectations and recognition for good work.
- Keep employees well informed and involve them in decision making as much as possible.
- Encourage employees to support each other.
- Measure work-family conflict.
- Consider creative strategies like job sharing or flexible scheduling to help workers balance work and family.
- Demonstrate concern for quality, service, and ethical behavior.
- Create an employee assistance program to help employees with stress management, and encourage employees to use it.
- Build empowered teams through respect, information, empowered control, decision making, responsibility, and skill building.
- Provide opportunities for employees to grow (continuing education).
- Create a culture that acknowledges family life.
- Avoid rewarding "workaholic mentality."
- Create task forces to address workplace stress.
- Conduct exit interviews and use the information to improve the workplace.

- Policies and procedures that support employee needs
- Training programs for employee growth and development
- Programs on how to cope with and reduce work stress
- Ongoing programs that monitor and evaluate job satisfaction
- Cultural diversity and workplace equity among employees
- Employee Assistance Programs (EAP)
- Input from employees
- A physically and emotionally safe work environment
- Methods for employees to demonstrate potential
- Systems that promote health and wellness
- Fair and honest treatment of employees

INDIVIDUAL INTERVENTIONS

Imparting the importance of managing workplace stress tends to be easier at the individual than at the organizational level, because employees are keenly motivated to reduce the discomfort of workplace stress. Stress affects physical and mental health, job satisfaction, morale, motivation, and self-esteem. Employees can implement the suggested interventions in the following list to prevent burnout and reduce stress:

- Reassess your values and determine what is essential and what is not.
- Evaluate use of time and align with values.

- Set limits and work time. Risk saying "no."
- Delegate, and consider the trade-offs between being in control and delegating.
- Maintain proper sleep, exercise, diet, and rest.
- Seek professional help if needed.
- Find work that fits your abilities, interests, personality, and values.
- Concentrate on the most important tasks first.
- Create greater balance in personal life. Invest more in family and other personal relationships, social activities, and hobbies (diverse interests and activities can help ensure that a job doesn't have an overpowering influence on self-esteem and self-confidence).
- Be a good team player.
- Open communications with coworkers and supervisors.
- Volunteer for things such as committees and projects.
- Don't deny stress and pressure.
- Avoid isolation.
- Change your circumstances.
- Reduce intensity in your life.
- Stop taking on everyone's problems.
- Learn to pace yourself.
- Take care of your physical self.
- Try to reduce unnecessary worrying.
- Keep a sense of humor.
- Maintain a positive attitude.

FAMILY-RESPONSIVE INTERVENTIONS

Work and family conflicts occur frequently and can have negative consequences on both work productivity and stress. Employers can adopt proactive interventions, either through integration (providing services directly) or through mutuality (allowing employees greater access and flexibility to needed services). Boxes 3.4 and 3.5 list possible interventions.

Significant obstacles may hinder the adoption of these practices. Relatively few employees may need any particular service. The business may also feel little need to provide such services, particularly if competitors are not providing them. There may also be negative effects, such as legal liability issues. Perceived cost will always be an issue for businesses, and business leaders may feel that providing such services (such as an on-site child care provider) represents an inappropriate corporate role. Lastly, the corporation may simply be antagonistic to change.

Even if some services are available, the employees may underutilize them, or not utilize them at all, because of poor quality control (leading employees to find better services elsewhere) and poor marketing (leaving employees unaware of the existence or benefits of services). Many employees may have an outmoded concept of work, and may not be willing to change the way they have always done things.

===== **Box 3.4** =====

Family-Responsive Interventions: Employee Focus

Integration	Mutuality
On-site or near-site day care center	Flexible work hours, flextime
Reserved spaces—local day care center	Supportive maternity, parental, adoptive, and family leave policies
After-school child care	Option to "buy" time off via salary or benefits trade-offs
Sick child care	Part-time and job share options
Respite care for the elderly	Condensed work week
Geriatric case management service	Pretax dependent care savings accounts
Elementary public school on-site	Child and elder care information and referral service
Warmline (telephone support service) for latchkey children	Child or elder care seminars
Company-sponsored summer camp	Child and elder care resource library
On-site holiday child care	Family care newsletter
Child care subsidy or voucher	Caregiver fair
Long-term care insurance	
Adoption benefits	
Convenience or concierge services	
Employee Assistance Program (EAP)—counseling	
Family, legal, or financial counseling	
Relocation counseling	
Parent or elder care support groups	
Children visiting the workplace	
Work at home/telecommuting	

To create family-friendly change in the workplace, employers need three things:

1. A sophisticated, research-based understanding of the relationships and interactions between work and family systems.
2. A complete vision of the organizational benefits of a healthy work-family interface.
3. An effective approach to marketing family-responsive policies and programs.

Consultants, particularly those with a mental health background, are in a good position to effectively educate employers on the value of creating a family-friendly environment.

========================= Box 3.5 =========================

Family-Responsive Interventions: Organizational Focus

Integration	Mutuality
Corporate funding for community child care and elder care programs	Regular consideration given to impact of company travel, work time, benefits, and personnel policies on family life
Corporate strategic plan that links work-family issues to corporate objectives	Supervisors trained in resolution of employee work-family conflicts
Family life workshops conducted with senior executives	Written policy on work-family benefits developed
Work-family coordinator appointed	Work-family needs assessments conducted

EMPLOYMENT STIGMA FOR INDIVIDUALS WITH MENTAL ILLNESS

Despite the progress that mental health professionals have made in educating the public about mental illness, stigma still pervades employment settings (Stefan, 2001, 2002). Many people with serious mental illness need work as an integral and beneficial aspect of everyday life. As discussed, work is important for overall health and promotes social inclusion. Among those diagnosed with serious mental illness, there is a high unemployment rate, despite a desire to work (Dorgan, 2002).

CAUSES OF UNDEREMPLOYMENT

Negative media images, combined with lack of public awareness, have perpetuated the stigma of mental illness. A person who is labeled as having a mental illness may face hostility and rejection in the workplace, leading to lowered expectations, isolation, exclusion, or a combination of these effects. Such discrimination makes it difficult to obtain and retain a job.

The stigma that society places on an individual with mental illness is related to the diagnosis, but the degree of rejection greatly exceeds the likely risk. One finding showed that 23% of people believed that a mildly depressed person is a danger to others. Employers are more likely to hire a person with diabetes than someone with mild depression. The majority of employers are uncomfortable with people who have a history of mental illness, so the individual must hide this fact from others, which adds more pressure to the stressors already present in the workplace (Corrigan & Kleinlein, 2005; Crisp, Gelder, Rix, Meltzer, & Rowlands, 2000; Herman & Smith, 1989; Major & O'Brien, 2005).

Such unfair treatment may lead to self-stigmatization. People may alter their behavior to be consistent with others' expectations. They may become apprehensive about being in the workplace, doubt their ability to do the job, and fear that symptoms may become unmanageable, creating a potentially embarrassing situation.

Interventions for these situations will likely involve educating the employer and debunking myths. Referrals for individual therapy may be needed if the stresses of work have created unmanageable symptoms in any employees. Employers may need to be warned about the consequences of engaging in discriminatory practices.

CASE EXAMPLE

A 50-year-old Caucasian mental health executive was fired after becoming somewhat disorganized on his job as the executive director of a community mental health center. He sought out consultation to understand himself better and prevent such an occurrence in the future.

This client was diagnosed as bipolar. The consultant worked with the executive to identify the stressors on the job and the course of his illness so that he could discern the early phases of a manic episode. He chose to move back to a less stressful position and away from management. His adjustment improved, and he was able to function without further incident.

FORMAL THEORIES OF JOB MOTIVATION

Motivation is an important concept in organizations; most managers feel that it is their role to motivate employees to be as productive as possible. Organizations may hire consultants, particularly with a mental health background, to help motivate their employees. Consultants should be familiar with the following formal theories of motivation because they are often still taught in graduate business schools, and consultees may ask specific questions about them. They will also serve as a solid foundation for consultants who want to motivate their consultees and client systems.

Motivation refers to the physical and mental energy that a person exerts to achieve a goal. Motivation can either be intrinsic (desire for achievement, accomplishment, or self-actualization) or extrinsic (bonuses, praise, and promotions).

$$Performance = f (Ability \times Motivation)$$

Performance is a function of ability and motivation. High motivation alone does not lead to high performance, but a high level of job performance requires both high ability and high motivation.

The Need-Hierarchy Theory of Motivation

Maslow (1970) viewed motivation as the result of five basic instinctual needs: physiological essentials, safety, belongingness, esteem, and self-actualization, arranged in a hierarchy such that each need acts as a motivator only when the previous needs have been satisfied. Once a need has been satisfied (except for self-actualization, which is never completely satisfied), it does not act as a motivator.

The implication for organizations is that employers should provide employees with opportunities to satisfy their unfulfilled needs. *Physiological* and *safety* needs are satisfied by job security, pay, benefits, and certain characteristics of the work

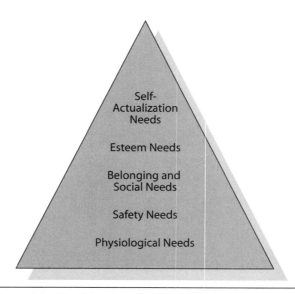

Figure 3.1   Traditional needs hierarchy (after Maslow, 1970).

environment. *Belongingness* needs and *esteem* needs are satisfied by quality relationships with supervisors and coworkers, and by recognition and opportunities for autonomy and self-control. *Self-actualization* needs are satisfied when employees perceive a job to be interesting and challenging. Lower needs (classically defined as physiological and safety needs—food, clothing, and shelter) are more directly fulfilled by monetary pay (see Figure 3.1).

Research shows little evidence that there are five distinct needs, that needs are always activated in the order described, that only one need can be activated at a time, or that a need becomes less important once it is satisfied. However, there is evidence that unfulfilled needs take precedence over filled needs and that the importance of needs seems to be related to job level (managers rate esteem and self-actualization needs as most important, whereas nonmanagers rate lower-level needs as more important).

Needs for Achievement, Power, and Affiliation

McClelland (1965, 1967, 1985) used the Thematic Apperception Test (TAT) to identify the needs that underlie motivation. He found that the need for achievement, the need for power, and the need for affiliation often act as motivators within organizational settings.

Need for Achievement

Employees with high levels of the need for achievement (nACH) prefer tasks of moderate difficulty and risk. They desire frequent, concrete feedback, and look to monetary rewards as a source of feedback and recognition. The need for achievement is highly related to entrepreneurial success (a tendency toward high nACH within a culture predisposes it to economic growth).

Need for Power

Employees high in the need for power (nPOW) desire control over others, visibility, recognition, status, and prestige. There are two kinds of power: personalized power (a self-aggrandizing need for power and dominance over others) and socialized power (which also involves dominance over others, but is expressed in socially acceptable ways). Managers who are high in the need for personalized power may have drinking problems, and they tend to brag about sexual and business exploits. Managers high in the need for socialized power make the most effective leaders, though they tend to have a high incidence of health problems.

Need for Affiliation

Employees high in the need for affiliation (nAFF) desire warm interpersonal relationships, are particularly sensitive to hostility and rejection, and avoid conflict and confrontation.

Two-Factor Theory

Herzberg's two-factor theory (Herzberg, Mausner, & Snyderman, 1959; House & Wigdor, 1967) is a theory of both satisfaction and motivation. Using a critical incidents technique (having engineers and accountants think of work experiences that had contributed to their satisfaction and dissatisfaction), he identified two basic needs: lower-level and higher-level. Lower-level needs have little effect on job satisfaction and motivation, but produce job dissatisfaction when they are unfulfilled. Factors that satisfy lower-level needs are *hygiene factors* and include pay, benefits, coworker relationships, supervision, job security, and physical work conditions. Higher-level needs increase job satisfaction and motivation when they are fulfilled but do not cause dissatisfaction when they are unfulfilled. Factors that satisfy higher-level needs are *motivators*. Motivators are related to the job itself, and include opportunities for challenge, responsibility, advancement, recognition, and achievement.

Providing employees with adequate hygiene factors will not increase their motivation but only keep them from becoming dissatisfied. Research suggests that although motivators appear to be more potent than hygiene factors in producing job motivation and satisfaction (especially for managers), the distinction between factors that produce satisfaction and dissatisfaction has not been confirmed. Instead, hygiene and motivator factors both seem to exert a strong effect on satisfaction and dissatisfaction. Herzberg's findings were method bound.

Herzberg developed the idea of *job enrichment* as a way to increase worker motivation. Job enrichment is a method of job redesign that involves combining several jobs into a larger job so that the employee performs a meaningful unit of work and has greater responsibility, freedom, autonomy, and control. Job enrichment tends to reduce turnover and absenteeism and improve job performance, especially work quality (Cascio, 1991). Its most positive effect is on job satisfaction, though effects vary. Younger and well-educated employees and employees high in nACH usually welcome enrichment. It is resisted, however, by employees who prefer security and stability to freedom and challenge, and by employees who have low self-esteem and low self-confidence. It may actually elicit anxiety and frustration in employees with low nACH.

Job enrichment involves increasing a job's *vertical loading* by giving the employee more high-level tasks. Job enlargement entails increasing the job's *horizontal loading* by increasing the number and variety of tasks. Although job enlargement can reduce monotony, job enrichment is more likely to have a positive impact on satisfaction and motivation.

The job characteristics model (Hackman & Oldham, 1980; Hackman, Oldham, Janson, & Purdy, 1975) places more emphasis on the worker's psychological state. A job is analyzed in terms of five core dimensions that help create three critical psychological states. Robbins (2001) defines the five core job dimensions as follows:

1. *Skill variety:* The degree to which the job requires a variety of different activities so the worker can use a number of different skills and talent.
2. *Task variety:* The degree to which the job requires completion of a whole and identifiable piece of work.
3. *Task significance:* The degree to which the job has a substantial impact on the lives or work of other people.
4. *Autonomy:* The degree to which the job provides substantial freedom, independence, and discretion to the individual in scheduling the work and in determining the procedures to be used in carrying it out.
5. *Feedback:* The degree to which carrying out the work activities required by the job results in the individual obtaining direct and clear information about the effectiveness of his or her performance. (p. 447)

The five core job dimensions influence three critical psychological states: experienced meaningfulness of the work, experienced responsibility for outcomes of the work, and knowledge of the actual results of the work activities. Three of the core dimensions contribute to the task's experienced meaningfulness: skill variety, task identity, and task significance. Autonomy produces feelings of personal responsibility and accountability. Performance feedback provides employees with knowledge about their performance. The three psychological states have an impact on internal work motivation, quality of work performance, satisfaction, and absenteeism and turnover rates.

The job characteristics model can be used to redesign jobs and determine whether jobs would benefit from enrichment. It applies well to people high in the need for growth. Research on this model suggests that all five core dimensions are important contributors to motivation, but that performance feedback is the single-most critical factor (Fried & Ferris, 1987; Rentsch & Steel, 1998).

Consultants can assist managers in enriching the jobs of their employees when it is appropriate to do so. Hackman (1977) made the following suggestions for designing an enriched job, based on the job characteristics model:

1. *Combine tasks:* Managers should seek to take existing and fractionalized tasks and put them back together to form a new and larger module of work. This increases skill variety and task identity.
2. *Create natural work units:* The creation of natural work units means that the tasks an employee does form an identifiable and meaningful whole. This increases employee "ownership" of the work and improves the likelihood that employees will view their work as meaningful and important rather than as irrelevant and boring.
3. *Establish client relationships:* The client is the user of the product or service that the employee works on (and may be an internal customer as well as someone outside the organization). Wherever possible, managers should try to establish direct relationships between workers and their clients. This increases skill variety, autonomy, and feedback for the employee.

4. *Expand jobs vertically:* Vertical expansion gives employees responsibilities and control that were formerly reserved to management. It seeks to partially close the gap between the "doing" and the "controlling" aspects of the job, and it increases employee autonomy.
5. *Open feedback channels:* By increasing feedback, employees not only learn how well they are performing their jobs, but also whether their performance is improving, deteriorating, or remaining at a constant level. Ideally, this feedback about performance should be received directly as the employee does the job, rather than from management on an occasional basis. (pp. 132–133)

Goal-Setting Theory

Locke (1968) believed that employees are motivated to achieve the goals that they have consciously decided to pursue. Participation in goal setting is necessary when employees are not likely to accept assigned goals. Assuming that employees have accepted the goals, moderately difficult goals (ones that have about a 50% chance of being successfully accomplished) and specific goals will produce higher levels of performance than easy, general goals. Providing employees with feedback about their performance is also critical for ensuring maximum productivity.

Locke incorporated the idea of self-efficacy (Bandura, 1986) into his theory. According to Locke, past success or failure in achieving goals affects self-efficacy beliefs that, in turn, determine future goals and the person's willingness to persevere in achieving them.

Research has supported goal-setting theory, but there are individual differences regarding its predictions. Workers high in nACH perform better when goals are specific and when they receive frequent feedback, whereas workers low in nACH perform best when they can participate in goal setting. Goal-setting techniques seem to be less effective with highly educated workers than with less-educated workers.

Goal-setting theory underlies Management by Objectives (MBO), a management strategy and method of performance appraisal that emphasizes the joint determination of goals by a subordinate and the subordinate's supervisor. MBO is based on the assumption that workers are more motivated to achieve goals when they have participated in their development.

In discussing the MBO concept, Lussier (2002) describes five criteria for setting the objectives: difficult but achievable; observable and measurable; specific, with a target date; participatively set when possible; and accepted:

Difficult but achievable: Employees perform better when they are given difficult objectives rather than easy ones or no goals, or simply are told "do your best" (Klein & Kim, 1988). Objectives must be challenging to motivate people to high levels of performance (Kotter, 1996a). If the objectives are set too high, however, people will not believe they are achievable and will not be motivated to work for their accomplishment.

Observable and measurable: People must be able to observe and measure their progress regularly to achieve their objectives (Forrester & Drexler, 1998). When progress is measured and evaluated, individuals perform better (Shalley & Oldham, 1985).

Specific, with a target date: Employees are more motivated to accomplish a task when they know exactly what they are expected to do and when it needs to be done

(Liccione, 1997). Though some tasks do not require or easily lend themselves to setting a precise target date, objectives should be specifically stated with a deadline whenever possible.

Participatively set when possible: Groups that participate in creating and setting their own objectives generally outperform groups that are assigned objectives (Erez, Earley, & Hulin, 1985). Employees with higher levels of capability and experience should be given a higher level of participation.

Accepted: Objectives must be acceptable to the individuals who are to perform them. People may not meet the objectives if they are not committed to striving for them (Dessler, 1999). Allowing employee participation in setting the objectives helps build acceptance (Erez et al., 1985).

Equity Theory

G. P. Adams (1963) theorized that employees compare the ratio of their inputs (skills, experience, education, etc.) to outcomes (financial and nonfinancial rewards) with the input/outcome ratios of others who are performing similar jobs. When employees perceive the ratios to be about equal, they will be comfortable with the situation and will attempt to maintain the status quo. If employees believe their input/outcome ratios differ from those of comparable others, they will experience a state of inequity and will try to make the situation more equitable by altering their inputs, outcomes, or both.

Studies have shown that for people on a piece-rate system (wherein employees are paid based on the number of pieces they produce rather than by the number of hours they work), underpayment results in increased quantity and decreased quality of output, whereas overpayment produces the opposite effect. In contrast, salaried workers respond to underpayment with reduced quality and quantity and to overpayment with increases in both quality and quantity. Underpayment has a greater impact on motivation than overpayment. Employees frequently regard situations as inequitable because of a tendency to overestimate their own performance and the outcomes of others.

Expectancy Theory

Expectancy theory states that employees will work hard if they believe (1) that high effort will lead to successful task performance (high expectancy), (2) that successful task accomplishment will lead to rewards (high instrumentality), and (3) that such rewards are desirable (positive valence). An employee's motivation is the result of a combination of these beliefs (Porter & Lawler, 1968; Vroom, 1964). Hence, this is also known as *VIE theory* (value or valence, instrumentality, and expectancy; Kesselman, Hagen, & Wherry, 1974).

Expectancy theory is useful for predicting job satisfaction, occupational choice, and job effort, at least in some situations. Predictions are limited because people do not always have sufficient information and often behave in irrational ways. There are some important methodological criticisms of expectancy theory (Heneman & Schwab, 1972; T. R. Mitchell, 1974; Reinharth & Wahba, 1975), as research has often included only highly educated professional or preprofessional subjects.

Reducing Obstacles to Motivation

Persico (1992) posits that rather than simply trying to motivate employees, employers need to focus on "de-motivators," or obstacles to motivation which cause employee frustration. He listed de-motivators that leaders should work to remove:

- *Thoughtless decisions:* Eliminate decisions made for personal reasons or made so that the department "looks good."
- *Lack of teamwork:* Teamwork is vital to the implementation of total quality management. The following are de-motivators to teamwork:
  —Autocratic decision making
  —Unkept promises
  —Too much reliance on one or two individuals
  —Poor staff utilization
- *Poor communication between managers and employees:* Employees who do not have all the information they need to do their jobs properly will become demoralized. They must know what is expected of them and how they are performing.
- *Invisible leadership:* Employees may feel out of touch with the organization if they do not know who is calling the shots, what top management actually does, and how they can approach top management.
- *Inaccessible leadership:* This creates an atmosphere of frustration and cynicism. Note that leadership includes not only top management but anyone who supervises or directs people.
- *Inconsistent instructions:* A lack of strategic direction and a lack of established priorities (e.g., not knowing your customers' needs) cause inconsistent orders and instructions. Also, a lack of a well defined decision-making process creates further confusion.
- *Lack of recognition:* Workers who are recognized and/or rewarded for their individual efforts are motivated to advance to an even higher level.
- *Lack of opportunity:* Employees will have no interest in the company's future, if they believe the company has no interest in their future. (pp. 80–81)

Persico (1992) also notes that there are other powerful de-motivators in the workplace, such as racism, sexism, differential treatment for hourly and salaried employees, and inflexible work rules.

JOB SATISFACTION

Job satisfaction refers to employees' attitudes toward their job or toward certain elements of the job. Surveys show that only 10% to 15% of respondents say they are dissatisfied with their jobs overall. However, when specific questions are asked, this figure increases. When workers are asked if they would choose the same job again, only about 43% of white-collar workers and 24% of blue-collar workers say that they would (Kahn, 1972). Some research suggests that job satisfaction reflects an enduring individual trait, finding it to be stable over 5 years across occupational changes (O'Reilly & Roberts, 1975).

Determinants of Job Satisfaction: Worker Characteristics

Age: Job satisfaction increases with age, especially among nonminority employees. Lower levels of satisfaction among younger employees may be due to a decline in the traditional work ethic or to higher initial expectations about the benefits of work. Younger workers are more likely to expect personal fulfillment from their jobs and opportunities for advancement, whereas older workers are more concerned with job security and opportunities for satisfying social relationships.

Occupational level: Satisfaction increases as occupational level increases. White-collar workers tend to be more satisfied than blue-collar workers and managers tend to be more satisfied than nonmanagers. Job content factors (motivators) are more important than job context (hygiene) factors for satisfaction among all employees regardless of occupational level. Among blue-collar workers, the primary cause of dissatisfaction is a lack of opportunity for promotion (Sheppard & Herrick, 1972).

Education and ability: Workers with higher levels of education are generally more satisfied than workers with lower educational levels. Employees who are too highly educated (or too skilled or too intelligent) for their jobs tend to be more dissatisfied.

Race: Members of minority groups tend to be twice as likely as members of the majority group to express dissatisfaction with their jobs. This discrepancy increases after age 45 when minorities exhibit their lowest levels of job satisfaction. This is likely due to continued institutional (and sometimes overt) racism that is often found in the workplace.

Gender: Some studies have found women to be more dissatisfied than men; others have found the opposite. There is some evidence that when women experience lower satisfaction, it is because they are more likely to feel exploited by their jobs, to be employed in lower-level jobs, and to be paid less, even when they are in jobs comparable to those of men. Men and women also seem to differ in the importance of specific job factors. Men are more likely to rate security and advancement as the most important factors when seeking a job, whereas women list type of work, company, and interpersonal relationships as most important (Jurgensen, 1978).

Job choice: People who feel that they chose their jobs freely and that their decision is irrevocable, tend to be more satisfied with and committed to their jobs (O'Reilly & Caldwell, 1980).

Determinants of Job Satisfaction: Job Factors

The nature of the job is an important determinant of job satisfaction. However, the use of one's skills and abilities is the most important contributor to both job satisfaction and mental health. Skill utilization is a better predictor of job satisfaction than other job factors for workers in a variety of occupations, including professional, administrative, clerical, and sales.

Pay: Research has given inconsistent results about pay. Some studies suggest that pay is a key determinant of job satisfaction; whereas in other studies, pay is less important than such factors as job security, opportunities for advancement, and type of work. Research suggests that pay contributes more to dissatisfaction than to satisfaction. There is some evidence that employees' perceptions that they are receiving the amount of compensation they deserve is most highly linked with satisfaction.

Effects of Job Satisfaction

Performance: The correlation of performance and job satisfaction is positive but weak (research studies average around .14; Iaffaldano & Muchinsky, 1985). There is evidence that performance leads to satisfaction but not vice versa, especially when employees perceive rewards to be contingent on successful job performance and believe that the organization distributes external rewards equitably (Robbins, 2001).

Turnover, absenteeism, and tardiness: Job dissatisfaction has been linked to high rates of turnover, absenteeism, and tardiness. The relationship between satisfaction and absenteeism has an average correlation of $-.40$ (Hackett & Guion, 1985; Locke, 1976; McShane, 1984; Robbins, 2001; K. D. Scott & Taylor, 1985). The negative correlation between satisfaction and turnover appears even stronger, though this is moderated by current employment rates (Mobley, Griffeth, Hand, & Meglino, 1979; Price, 1977; Robbins, 2001; Vroom, 1964).

Union activity: Job dissatisfaction is a major cause of unionization. Dissatisfaction with pay, job security, fringe benefits, treatment by supervisors, and opportunities for promotions are all significantly correlated with a vote for union representation. Other studies have found that dissatisfaction is associated with more strikes and high grievance rates (Berger, Olson, & Boudreau, 1983; Evans & Ondrack, 1990; Hammer, 1978; Robbins, 2001).

Physical and mental health: Job satisfaction is also related to both physical and mental health. In terms of physical health, job dissatisfaction has been linked to fatigue, headaches, sweating, and loss of appetite. It has also been linked to such illnesses as ulcers, arthritis, high blood pressure, alcohol and drug abuse, strokes, and heart attacks. Work satisfaction is a better predictor of longevity than either physical health or tobacco use. The mental health correlates of job dissatisfaction include anxiety, worry, tension, impaired social relationships, and irritability (F. W. Bond & Bunce, 2003; De Jonge et al., 2001; Dolbier, Soderstrom, & Steinhardt, 2001).

General life satisfaction: The research on the connection between job satisfaction and general life satisfaction is not clear. Some studies indicate that job satisfaction precedes life satisfaction; others suggest that life satisfaction is the cause of job satisfaction; and still other studies have found no relationship at all between the two variables (Klaus & Heinz, 2004; Kossek & Ozeki, 1998; J. D. Quick, Henley, & Quick, 2004; Rain, Lane, & Steiner, 1991; Tait, Baldwin, & Padgett, 1989).

WORK SCHEDULES

Traditionally, most employers have used the 40-hour workweek, consisting of five 8-hour days. However, work scheduling options have been increasing. The consultant should be familiar with various work schedules and should understand the advantages and disadvantages of each, including their effects on job motivation.

The Four-Day Workweek

The 4-day workweek compresses the usual 5-day schedule into just 4 days of 9 or 10 hours each. This schedule is associated with increased morale and satisfaction, especially among younger employees, lower-level employees, employees who have low job satisfaction or low organizational commitment, and employees who perceive the change in schedule as an upgrade of their jobs. It tends to lower absenteeism, but its effects on productivity are equivocal. Although productivity may improve initially, it usually returns to its original levels. The disadvantage of this work schedule is its potential for greater fatigue (due to longer work days), which can have a negative impact on productivity and safety.

Flextime

This schedule gives employees a choice of when to begin and end work, while providing a *core time* (e.g., 10 A.M. to 2 P.M.) when all employees must be present. This schedule appears to have no significant impact on productivity, but it is associated with increased morale and satisfaction and with lowered absenteeism and tardiness. The disadvantages of this approach are the problems it can cause in communication, scheduling, and work flow.

Shift Work

Companies that operate 24 hours a day usually have three work shifts: a day shift (e.g., 7:00 A.M. to 3:00 P.M.), a swing shift (3:00 P.M. to 11:00 P.M.), and a graveyard shift (11:00 P.M. to 7:00 A.M.). Some organizations permanently assign shifts to individual employees, whereas others rotate workers on shifts for set periods of time. Fixed shifts are generally preferred to rotating shifts since the latter tend to disrupt circadian rhythms increasing fatigue and sleepiness as well as causing concentration difficulties and more errors. The graveyard shift is associated with the most problems (e.g., higher accident rates and lower performance quality), apparently because of sleep deprivation. However, the swing shift has the most negative impact on social patterns.

Permanent Part-Time Employment

Some organizations have been experimenting with part-time employment options, such as job sharing and job pairing. In job sharing, two employees divide the hours and responsibilities of a full-time job by performing complementary tasks. In job pairing, each employee is responsible for all aspects of the job. These options have a positive impact on work quality, work quantity, and employee reliability. However, some studies have found that each job sharer actually ends up handling at least 80% of a full-time load (Frease & Zawacki, 1979). The primary disadvantage of permanent part-time work seems to be that it increases the costs of insurance and other benefits (Shellenbarger, 2001).

JOB PROBLEMS

Certain job problems can have a major impact on employee motivation. Consultants should be aware of these problems and be prepared to offer solutions when they are discovered in an organization.

Fatigue and Rest Breaks

Physical and mental fatigue can cause employee burnout, increased accident and turnover rates, and lowered job proficiency (especially on complex tasks and tasks requiring constant vigilance).

The effects of fatigue can be reduced by selecting workers who are least likely to be fatigued by the requirements of the job, by training workers in efficient job procedures, and by providing rest breaks. Rest breaks are most effective when their schedules are empirically determined. Generally, breaks should be provided during the fourth and eighth hours of work since these tend to be the times of greatest fatigue (McCormick & Ilgen, 1980). Frequent short breaks are more effective than longer, less frequent ones. Breaks produce an increase in overall productivity even though they involve time off the job (Bhatia & Murrell, 1969).

Arousal and Boredom

The highest levels of learning and performance are associated with moderate levels of arousal, especially when moderate arousal is coupled with moderate task difficulty. Excessive or inadequate arousal can lead to stress, fatigue, and greater variability in job performance.

Boredom (which is caused by a lack of arousal) can be alleviated in the following ways:

- Educating workers about the value of their jobs tends to increase interest and motivation.
- Job enrichment can make a monotonous job more challenging.
- Job rotation can provide employees with a greater variety of tasks.

ORGANIZATION STRUCTURE AND JOB EVALUATIONS

How organizations are structured and how jobs are evaluated also have a major impact on employee motivation. Consultants should research these issues for the particular organization for whom they are consulting, allowing them to assist in developing the optimal structure for the organization and in developing a method of job evaluation that both employees and managers perceive as being fair.

Organization structure defines how tasks are to be allocated, who reports to whom, and the formal coordinating mechanisms and interaction patterns that will be followed (Robbins, 1990). A formal organizational structure will manifest itself through a table of organization (which details the relationships of various offices and positions), specific job descriptions, and a formal appraisal or evaluation system.

Organizations have many reasons for assessing the performance of employees. It provides a basis for decisions about salaries, raises, bonuses, and promotions; it enables employees to receive feedback on their performance; it helps the organization determine its future training needs; and it helps the organization validate its employee selection processes (did the employee perform as the organization hoped?).

A variety of criteria can be used to assess job performance. A *job analysis* ascertains the skills, knowledge, and abilities the job requires. It explores what is done, how it is done, and why it is done. This information is obtained by actually performing the job; by interviewing employees, supervisors, or others who know the job well; by reviewing company records; by having employees keep a job diary that details the activities they carry out; or by using a combination of these approaches. Several formalized approaches to job analysis have been developed, such as the Position Analysis Questionnaire (PAQ; McCormick, Jeanneret, & Mecham, 1969), which has a strong research base and a wide breadth of application (Gatewood & Feild, 1998).

A *job evaluation* determines the relative worth of jobs in order to set salaries and wages. This can be done using either judgmental techniques (deciding what sounds right) or statistical techniques (e.g., using the average national salary for a specific position). These evaluations are based on the demands of the job in terms of skills and effort, the previous experience and education needed for the job and possessed by the employee, and the degree of autonomy and responsibility that the job entails (Milkovich & Newman, 2002).

Performance Criteria

Employees can be evaluated based on objective or subjective measures. Objective measures are quantifiable and direct. Examples include counting the number of units produced as a measure of production or using personal data such as absenteeism rates. However, objective approaches tend to be problem-biased (i.e., they often focus on what an employee is doing wrong or not doing right, rather than focusing on positive aspects such as the quality of the employee's work), and it is often difficult to quantifiably measure work behaviors (Borman, White, Pulakos, & Oppler, 1991; Hedge & Borman, 1995).

Subjective measures are the most frequently used form of employee evaluation. They are based on the judgments of raters, usually a person's immediate supervisor, though they sometimes include ratings by peers and the employee's own personal rating. Not surprisingly, self-ratings tend to be the most lenient, but they are less susceptible to the halo effect (described next). Supervisor ratings are generally the most reliable overall. Peer ratings seem to be particularly good for predicting training success and subsequent promotions. Peer ratings are most useful when there is a high degree of trust among employees, when the organization's reward structure is noncompetitive, and when information on the employee's performance is readily available to peers.

Problems with Subjective Ratings

Those who supply ratings are often poorly motivated to complete rating scales accurately and conscientiously, while those being rated often distrust performance ratings because they feel that they do not accurately measure their job performance. The reliability and validity of subjective ratings are threatened by phenomena that are well-known to social psychologists (Aronson, 1999; Baron & Byrne, 1991):

- *Halo effect:* The halo effect occurs when a rater's evaluation of an employee on one dimension of job performance affects the evaluation of that employee on other dimensions. For example, if an employer really likes a certain employee because she has never missed a day of work, the employer might rate her more highly on the quality of her work than would another evaluator.
- *Leniency/strictness bias:* This occurs when a rater tends to avoid the middle range of a rating scale and rates all employees as either "high" or "low" on all dimensions of job performance.
- *Central tendency bias:* This refers to a rater's tendency to use only the middle range of the rating scale.
- *Recency effect:* The recency effect occurs when a rater bases ratings on an employee's most recent job performance rather than on the employee's performance throughout the rating period.

- *Personal biases:* Personal biases are those attitudes and prejudices of the rater that affect performance ratings. Attractive employees, employees with longer tenure, and people who are perceived as more similar to the rater tend to receive higher ratings. Females performing "male" jobs are often rated less favorably due to unconscious (and sometimes conscious) biases.

Methods for Improving Subjective Ratings

Since subjective ratings are known to have great potential for bias, consultants can suggest specific steps to reduce the impact of bias. Consultants can share this information with supervisors and employers to create a sense of fair play that will likely reduce employee stress (Cardy & Dobbins, 1994; Hedge & Borman, 1995; Maddux, 2000; Murphy & Cleveland, 1995):

- Involving the rater in the entire rating process, including development of the rating scales, improves motivation.
- Accuracy of ratings can be increased with adequate training. Biases can be reduced through specific training aimed at identifying and distinguishing different levels of performance.
- Rating biases can be reduced by rating behaviors rather than traits ("John is 15 minutes late each morning" rather than "John is lazy"), and by rating specific behaviors rather than global behaviors ("John leaves important papers lying on the floor in the walkway" rather than "John is sloppy").
- Accuracy of ratings can be increased by using certain types of rating scales. The forced choice and paired comparison techniques (described next) reduce the central tendency and leniency/strictness biases.
- Making the results available to employees and encouraging employees to participate actively in the assessment enhances employee acceptance.
- Performance appraisal accuracy increases when top management supports the importance of doing appraisals.

Commonly Used Rating Scales

There are several commonly used types of rating scales. Each has its advantages and disadvantages, depending on situational needs (Cardy & Dobbins, 1994; Hedge & Borman, 1995; Murphy & Cleveland, 1995).

- *Paired comparison:* With this method, the rater compares each ratee with every other ratee in pairs on dimensions of job performance. The problem with this method is that it can be very cumbersome.
- *Forced distribution:* This method is based on the assumption that overall employee performance will follow a bell curve. Ratees are assigned to a limited number of categories based on a predetermined normal frequency. However, this method may yield erroneous data if performance is not actually normally distributed.
- *Critical incident technique:* With this method, a rater notes the specific job behaviors that lead to either successful or unsuccessful job performance. This provides direct, specific feedback to the employee. For example, an employee whose productivity has decreased may have been tardy more than three times per month. The disadvantages of this method are that it requires close supervision, accurate record keeping, and is time consuming.

- *Checklist:* The rater can use a checklist to mark those items that describe the ratee. Weighted checklists can weigh items in terms of importance to successful job performance.
- *Forced choice:* With the forced choice method, two to four alternatives that are considered to be about equal in terms of desirability are listed, and the rater selects the alternative that best or least describes the ratee. This method reduces bias, but the list is time-consuming to develop and raters often dislike it.
- *Graphic rating scale:* This is one of the most common rating scales. The rater indicates on a continuum the ratee's level of performance on one of several dimensions. This method is susceptible to rater biases, but can be improved by anchoring points on the continuum with critical incidents.
- *Behaviorally Anchored Rating Scale (BARS):* With this method, supervisors identify several independent dimensions of job behavior, identify several "behavioral anchors" for each dimension, and order and number the behavioral anchors within each dimension from least to most positive or desirable. The rater chooses the one behavior in each dimension that best describes the employee. This method provides employee feedback, increases reliability, and reduces rater biases; but accurately developing the scale is time-consuming.
- *Behavioral observation scales:* This method is similar to behaviorally anchored rating scales except that instead of marking a single critical incident in each job dimension that best describes an employee, the rater indicates for each critical incident how often the employee actually engages in the behavior.

LEGAL ISSUES IN EMPLOYMENT

Though human resources and employment law is a subspecialty all its own, consultants should have at least a basic familiarity with the laws that are relevant to the organization with which they are working. This will prevent consultants from inadvertently making suggestions that would violate the law. Such knowledge can also be used as leverage to promote better diversity practices in organizations that still contain subtle institutional discriminatory policies. Not all of the following laws apply to all organizations (e.g., some only apply to companies with more than 20 employees, or companies seeking government contracts). Brief descriptions of the most important employment laws are provided (Beatty & Samuelson, 2001; Mathis & Jackson, 2003).

- *The Equal Pay Act of 1963:* This act prohibits discrimination on the basis of sex in wages or benefits. Violations may occur if a different wage is paid to someone in the same job before or after an employee of the opposite sex has held that position.
- *Title VII of the Civil Rights Act of 1964:* This prohibits employment discrimination on the basis of race, color, religion, sex, ethnicity, or national origin, and covers all private employers and federal, state, and local government. Requiring employees to speak only English on the job may also be a violation unless the requirement is necessary to the business.
- *The Age Discrimination in Employment Act of 1967:* This act protects employees over the age of 40. It covers all private employers with 20 or more employees; federal, state, and local governments; employment agencies; and labor organizations.

An age limit may be required only where age has been proven to be a bona fide occupational qualification.

- *42 USC section 1981:* This prohibits race discrimination in all contracts, including employment.

- *The Immigration Reform and Control Act of 1986 (IRCA):* This act protects aliens "lawfully admitted for permanent residence" from employment discrimination. It requires employers to assure that they only hire employees who are legally authorized to work in the United States. All applicants and employees must provide verification. Employers who require citizenship or give preferences to U.S. citizens may violate IRCA.

- *Title I and Title V of the Americans with Disabilities Act of 1990:* This law prohibits discrimination against qualified individuals with disabilities in private employment and in state and local government. Qualified individuals are employees or applicants with disabilities who satisfy the requirements of the position. They must, with or without reasonable accommodation, be able to perform the job's essential functions. Employers must make reasonable accommodations, unless that would impose an undue hardship on the organization's operations.

- *Civil Rights Act of 1991:* This act prohibits subgroup norming, and provides monetary damages in cases of intentional discrimination.

- *The National Labor Relations Act:* This act, which is enforced by the National Labor Relations Board rather than by the courts, protects employees who have engaged in union activity from discrimination by their employers.

- *The Vietnam Era Veterans Readjustment Assistance Act of 1974:* This act prohibits discrimination and requires affirmative action in all personnel practices for all veterans who served on active duty in the U.S. military, ground, naval, or air service who are special disabled veterans, Vietnam era veterans, recently separated veterans, or veterans who served on active duty during a war or in a campaign or expedition for which a campaign badge has been authorized. It applies to all firms that have a nonexempt government contract or subcontract of $25,000 or more. An affirmative action program is required.

For more details on employment law, see Mathis and Jackson (2003) and Beatty and Samuelson (2001). Readers can also visit the web site of the U.S. Equal Employment Opportunity Commission at www.eeoc.gov or the Office of Special Counsel for Immigration-Related Unfair Employment Practices at www.usdoj.gov/crt/osc. For an overview of these government regulations, see the government publication, "Uniform Guidelines on Employee Selection Procedures and Regulations to implement the Equal Employment Provisions of the Americans with Disabilities Act."

After understanding the contexts in which organizations operate, and what motivates people, mental health professionals will be better equipped to work with organizational leadership, which is the topic of the next chapter.

Chapter 4

LEADERSHIP, MANAGEMENT, AND SUPERVISION

Mental health professionals are increasingly being called on to work with organizational leaders through coaching and consulting activities. Many clinicians will also find themselves actively serving in leadership roles. Management is a core competency of mental health professionals, but one for which most of us receive little formal training. Whether you will be working with leaders or simply want to improve your own management skills, this chapter provides useful theoretical knowledge and practical suggestions.

HISTORICAL BACKGROUND

When studying consulting, it is helpful to have some understanding of the history of organizational management psychology. One of the pioneers of the application of scientific principles to the workplace was Frederick Taylor (Wrege & Greenwood, 1991).

Scientific Management

Frederick Taylor, who wrote a book titled *The Principles of Scientific Management* (1911), is known as the "Father of Scientific Management." Taylor applied the scientific method to the study of job productivity, mainly through time and motion studies.
Scientific management is based on the following principles:

- Scientifically analyzing jobs into their component parts and then standardizing those parts
- Scientifically selecting, training, and placing workers in jobs for which they are mentally and physically suited
- Fostering cooperation between the supervisor and workers to minimize deviation from scientific methods
- Having managers and workers assume responsibility for their own share of the work

Taylor believed that employees are motivated by economic self-interest (pay is the best motivator). To increase worker productivity, he developed the idea of using piecework, which involved differential pay for those who produced more.

The often derided *efficiency expert*—someone who goes into a workplace to observe and improve on work processes—would be an example of this approach.

The scientific method was criticized by those who felt that the human side of the equation was missing. The Charlie Chaplin classic *Modern Times* is a satirical movie about scientific management, in which human needs are lost in the effort to be maximally efficient.

Classical Management Theory

That which came to be known as "classical management theory" emerged after the turn of the twentieth century. Like scientific management, it emphasized the importance of organizational structure.

Weber (1947) described the concept of *bureaucracy.* A bureaucracy is an ideal organizational structure consisting of hierarchical units that each perform a specialized function according to defined rules and regulations. This idea emphasizes the division of labor and the delegation of authority. Modern examples of bureaucracies include the Roman Catholic Church, the U.S. Army, and the federal government.

A bureaucracy has several major dimensions:

- A fixed division of labor
- A hierarchy of offices
- A set of rules governing performance
- Separation of personal from official property and rights
- Technical qualifications for selecting personnel (not families or friendship)
- Employment as a long-term career

Efficiency, freedom from nepotism, and freedom from favoritism are the ideal strengths of a bureaucracy. However, inflexibility and "lots of red tape" are well-known weaknesses.

Sometimes scientific management and classical management together are called the *structural perspective.*

Structural Perspective

Bolman and Deal (2003) describe six important ideas about the structural perspective:

1. Organizations exist primarily to accomplish established goals.
2. For any organization, a structural form can be designed and implemented to fit its particular set of circumstances such as goals, strategies, environment, technology, and people.
3. Organizations work most effectively when environmental turbulence and personal preferences are constrained by norms of rationality (structure ensures that people focus on getting the job done rather than on doing whatever they please).
4. Specialization permits higher levels of individual expertise and performance.
5. Coordination and control are essential to effectiveness. Depending on the task and environment, coordination may be achieved through authority, rules, policies, standard operating procedures, information systems, meetings, lateral relationships, or more informal techniques.

6. Organizational problems typically originate from inappropriate structures or inadequate systems and can be resolved through restructuring or developing new systems.

Organizational reorganizations are becoming more common as companies attempt to make structural changes to improve operations. It is often difficult to predict the potentially subtle and far-reaching impacts of organization-wide structural changes.

Furthermore, if an organization is too inflexible, it will be unable to adapt to the unpredictable changes in the external environment. Consultants can work with organizations to develop plans that deal with uncertainty.

Devices That Buffer an Organization and Reduce Uncertainty

A lot of uncertainty exists in the organizational world. While no one can directly control factors in the external environment such as the global economy, an organization can take steps to buffer itself from the shock waves of external changes:

Coding: Coding involves creating schemes for classifying inputs, allowing managers to have a better working knowledge of the work process. This allows managers to focus on the most essential aspects of operations.

Stockpiling: Companies can store raw materials and products so that the organization can control inputs and outputs. This is becoming less popular because maintaining inventory increases overhead costs.

Leveling: This involves motivating suppliers to provide inputs and creating a higher demand for outputs from customers.

Forecasting: Forecasting, which involves anticipating changes in supply and demand, allows a company to better flow with changes as they happen.

Growth: Small companies are more vulnerable to changes in the external environment. Growth requires striving for a scale of activity that will give the organization leverage over its environment.

Vertical Coordination

Vertical coordination relates to a company's table of organization. It provides a map of the organizational relationships and how higher levels control the work of subordinates (Bolman & Deal, 2003). This involves authority, rules and policies, and planning and control systems. Planning and control systems can be classified as either *performance control* or *action planning*. Performance control imposes outcome standards, without regard to how the outcomes are achieved. Subordinates are told what needs to be done, but are left to determine how best to do it. Action planning specifies the decisions and actions to be carried out in a particular way and/or at specific times. This method is useful when it is difficult to measure outcomes, and it is easier to assess how a job is done than to determine whether the objectives are achieved.

Lateral Coordination

Lateral coordination does not generally involve superior/subordinate relationships. Lateral forms of coordination are usually less formalized and more flexible than authority-based systems and rules. They can be simpler and quicker as well (Bolman & Deal, 2003). This method involves formal and informal meetings for developing plans, solving problems, and making decisions. It could also involve the creation of task forces that bring together representatives from different areas and specialties to work together through persuasion and information negotiation instead of through authority or rules. Another alternative is a matrix structure, in which employees have more than one boss. For example, a psychologist may work for the Psychology Department of a hospital, but be assigned to work on the Inpatient Unit.

Factors That Determine an Organization's Structure

The same structure will not work for the many different types of organizations. The following variables should be considered when trying to determine if a company is using an ineffective structure:

Size of the organization: Unless the organization's growth (or downsizing) is matched with corresponding iterations to the formal structures, problems will inevitably arise.

Core technology: Every organization has a central activity, which is referred to in the organizational literature as its "core technology." Organizations that forget what they are best at can end up being pulled in many directions by the myriad distractions that inevitably arise. For a college or university, teaching and research are the core technologies.

External environment: Suppliers provide raw materials to an organization and customers receive its outputs. Structures should be designed with suppliers and customers in mind.

Strategies and goals: Tactical day-to-day decision making and the strategic long-term health of the organization will greatly influence how an organization is structured.

Human Relations Movement

Elton Mayo, a psychologist at Harvard University, worked with Western Electric Company's Hawthorne Works in Cicero, Illinois, from 1927 to 1932 (Robbins, 1990). The purpose of these studies was to investigate the effects of physical conditions on job performance. Much to their surprise, the researchers found that productivity increased regardless of what changes they made. Follow-up interviews of the employees suggested the workers liked the novelty of the changes, liked the attention that they received, and were interested in the experiment. This finding was later replicated, and the change in performance that can result when people participate in a research study became known as the "Hawthorne effect."

This research sparked many subsequent studies, which found that informal group norms have a significant impact on performance. In any organization, there exists social pressure on people above and below the norm. When newcomers come along and "work too hard," senior workers will often tell them (covertly or overtly) to stop making the senior workers look bad. Likewise, employees who are slacking are often pressured into picking up their fair share of the workload. Consultants need to assess what type of work culture exists when designing individual, team, or organization-wide interventions. Failure to do so will make it difficult to effect any lasting changes.

The Hawthorne studies provided an alternative to scientific management, placing greater emphasis on worker needs, motives, and relationships. This became known as the Human Relations Movement.

Theory X and Theory Y

McGregor (1960) distinguished between the old views represented by Scientific Management, which he termed Theory X, and the newer views represent by the Human Relations Movement, which he called Theory Y. McGregor postulated that a manager's view of a task depends on the manager's assumptions about employee characteristics.

Managers operating under Theory X believe that employees dislike work and avoid it whenever possible, have little ambition, are passive and lazy, and must be directed and controlled. Managers who operate under Theory Y believe that employees view work as being "as natural as play," and assume employees are capable of self-control and self-direction. Theory Y posits that the essential task of management is to arrange organizational conditions so that people can achieve their own goals best by directing their efforts toward organizational rewards.

There is currently no evidence to confirm that Theory X or Theory Y is better at motivating employees. Which theory works best appears to be related to the particular situation in which it is applied (Robbins, 2001).

The International Perspective and Theory Z

Theory Z involves the incorporation of the Japanese business approach into American organizational philosophy (Ouchi & Jaeger, 1978). Basically, it suggests that involved workers are the key to increased productivity (Ouchi, 1981).

"Theory A" was used to describe the American way of conducting business. This typically involved short-term employment, individual decision making, individual responsibility, rapid evaluation and promotion, a specialized career path, and a segmented concern for the employee (only the employee's working life was of concern).

"Theory J" was used to describe the Japanese way of conducting business. This typically involved lifetime employment, consensual decision making, collective responsibility, slow evaluation and promotion, a nonspecialized career path, and a holistic concern for the employee.

Theory Z sought to combine the best of both worlds. It suggested long-term employment, consensual decision making, individual responsibility, slow evaluation and promotion, a moderately specialized career path, and holistic concern for the employee. Ouchi believed that the closer a company came to adopting a Theory Z strategy, the higher the levels of worker productivity and morale. The validity of this theory has not yet been proven.

LEADERSHIP

Leadership is the ability to influence a group toward the achievement of goals. People are said to have a leadership role when they have the power or ability to influence others (Northouse, 2001; Renesch, 1994; Zaccaro, 2001). Consultants are often called on to develop leaders or may discover that what ostensibly appears to be an organizational problem is in fact related to the leaders' lack of true leadership skills.

Leaders, Managers, and Supervisors

Although the terms are often used interchangeably, there are important distinctions between leaders, managers, and supervisors. A leader inspires others through a vision of the future, and works from a long-term strategic viewpoint. A manager allocates available resources to get things done from a short-term tactical viewpoint. A supervisor oversees the daily work functions of employees. Too often, the same person tries to perform two or even all three of these roles, which is extremely difficult (if not impossible) to do well. It is all too easy to get caught up in the daily tasks, which always seem urgent. An organization needs someone who can devote energy to planning for major issues, especially the determination of where the organization needs to be heading within the next few years.

In a traditional organization, the hierarchy is as follows, ranked from highest to lowest:

1. Board of Directors
2. Chief Executive Officer (CEO)
3. Chief Operating Officer (COO)
4. Vice Presidents
5. Directors
6. Managers
7. Supervisors
8. Line workers
9. Staff positions

Peltier (2001, p. 212) clearly differentiates the roles of workers (or professionals), managers, and leaders (see Table 4.1).

Consultants can work with organizations to make sure they differentiate these roles. Expecting one person to do all these functions will be ineffective at best and is likely to create a lot of strain on the person who is attempting to take on multiple roles. Consultants can work with leaders to make sure they are delegating daily maintenance tasks to others so they can focus on what is truly important to the long-term survival of the organization and its mission.

Delegating is an important skill for all leaders and managers, and consultants can coach executives in how to do this appropriately. Robbins (2001) makes five suggestions for delegating effectively:

1. *Clarify the assignment.* The place to begin is to determine what is to be delegated and to whom. You need to identify the person most capable of doing the task and then determine if he or she has the time and motivation to do the job. Assuming you have a willing and able individual, it is your responsibility to provide clear information on what is being delegated, the results you expect, and any time or performance expectations you hold.
2. *Specify the delegatee's range of discretion.* Every act of delegation comes with constraints. You're delegating authority to act on certain issues and, on those issues, within certain parameters. You need to specify what those parameters are so the individual knows, in no uncertain terms, the range of his or her discretion.
3. *Allow the delegatee to participate.* One of the best sources for determining how much authority will be necessary to accomplish the task is the person who will be held accountable for that task. If you allow employees to participate in determining what is delegated, how much authority is needed to get the job done, and the standards by which they'll be judged, you increase employee motivation, satisfaction, and accountability for performance.

Table 4.1   Differences between Workers, Managers, and Leaders

Worker/Professional	Manager	Leader
Performs basic tasks	Controls things	Creates things
Performs repetitive tasks	Keeps track of things	Changes things
Needs and uses resources	Budgets, makes ends meet	Finds resources
Develops specific task expertise	Plans	Gets the mission defined
Finds new business	Organizes	Creates an environment
Creates product/provides service	Solves problems	Shakes things up
In contact with customers	Copes with complexity	Sets the direction and tone
Enlists new clients, customers	Staffs jobs and tasks	Aligns people
	External locus of control	Internal locus of control
	Conservative and cautious	Creative risk taker
Follows rules	Rule oriented, system based	Imagination based
Needs managers (and leaders)	Needs leaders (and workers)	Needs managers (and workers)
Interacts with outsiders	Interacts internally	Interacts with outsiders
	Keeps people in line with systems	Inspires people
Responsible for own effort, production, and sales	Responsible for performance of organization	Responsible for overall outcome
Works independently	Deductive process	Inductive process
Lacks overarching viewpoint	Creates structures	Creates mandates
	Risk averse	Risk taker
Takes direction from others	Uses authority and rules	Uses influence
	Gives direction	Convinces
	Keeps everybody lined up	Shows the direction
Provides feedback to organization	Monitors organizational culture	Monitors outside culture

4. *Inform others that delegation has occurred.* Delegation should not take place in a vacuum. Not only do you and the delegatee need to know specifically what has been delegated and how much authority has been granted, but anyone else who may be affected by the delegation act also needs to be informed.

5. *Establish feedback controls.* The establishment of controls to monitor the employee's progress increases the likelihood that important problems will be identified early and that the task will be completed on time and to the desired specifications. For instance, agree on a specific time for completion of the task, and then set progress

dates when the employee will report back on how well he or she is doing and any major problems that have surfaced. (p. 421)

The Roles of Managers

Mintzberg (1973) believed that managers perform 10 different but highly related jobs that can be grouped into three areas: interpersonal, informational, and decisional (Robbins, 2001). Different roles will be more or less important in different settings and at different times.

Interpersonal

Interpersonal roles are very important for a manager. As a *figurehead,* the manager is a symbolic figure for the organization. As a *leader,* the manager must motivate and direct subordinates. As a *liaison,* the manager maintains a network of outside contacts who provide favors and information.

Informational

The manager must also handle information. As a *monitor,* the manager serves as a "nerve center" of internal and external information. In the role of *disseminator,* the manager transmits information to employees. As a *spokesperson,* the manager transmits information to outsiders about the organization.

Decisional

Managers must also be skilled at making decisions. As an *entrepreneur,* the manager searches for new opportunities and initiates projects. In the role of *disturbance handler,* the manager must take corrective action when the organization faces disturbances. As a *resource allocator,* the manager must make or approve resource decisions. As a *negotiator,* the manager represents the organization when dealing with other organizations.

It would be difficult to find someone with all these qualities. In fact, some of the abilities tend to be incompatible. Individuals must be selected based on the most important roles needed for a particular position.

The Skill Sets of Leaders

The *PDI Handbook* (D. L. Davis, Skube, Hellervik, Gebelein, & Sheard, 1996), which contains many great references for consultants and coaches, explores the skills and knowledge areas that are important for leaders (see Box 4.1). Consultants should develop at least a basic knowledge level in each of these areas, and have the resources to educate or refer a consultee for more information. Note that several of these areas are specialties of those of us trained as mental health professionals.

The degree of relative emphasis on each area will vary depending on the organization and the context in which the leader operates. Consultants should therefore clarify with the consultee which areas are strengths that can be expanded, and which areas need attention to improve organizational functioning.

The Four Managerial Functions

Consultants need to focus intervention efforts to improve the performance of tasks that managers do on a regular basis. Most managerial textbooks describe four basic activities for managers (DuBrin, 2000; Whetten & Cameron, 2002): planning, organizing, leading, and controlling.

=== **Box 4.1** ===

Skills and Knowledge Areas for Leaders

Administrative Skills

Establish plans
Structure and staff
Develop systems and processes
Manage execution
Work efficiently

Communication Skills

Speak effectively
Foster open communication
Listen to others
Deliver presentations
Prepare written communication

Interpersonal Skills

Build relationships
Display organizational savvy
Leverage networks
Value diversity
Manage disagreements

Leadership Skills

Provide direction
Lead courageously
Foster teamwork
Motivate others
Coach and develop others
Champion change

Motivation Skills

Drive for results
Show work commitment

Organizational Knowledge

Use financial and quantitative data
Use technical/functional expertise
Know the business

Organizational Strategy Skills

Manage profitability
Commit to quality
Focus on customer needs
Promote corporate citizenship
Recognize global implications

Self-Management Skills

Act with integrity
Demonstrate adaptability
Develop oneself

Thinking Skills

Think strategically
Analyze issues
Use sound judgment
Innovate

1. *Planning:* Planning involves setting future goals and figuring out how to achieve them. Planning pervades all aspects of being a leader and relies heavily on decision-making abilities.

2. *Organizing:* Organizing involves making certain that the necessary resources (human, financial, physical, and informational) are available at the right place and time to fulfill the goals of the organization.

3. *Leading:* Leading involves persuading other people to work toward the achievement of the goals of the organization. This includes inspiring and motivating others toward change, and showing them how to do so.

4. *Controlling:* Controlling involves ensuring that organizational plans are carried out properly by setting standards and monitoring performance against these standards. If standards are not being met, corrective actions must be taken.

The Major Activities of Leaders

Fred Luthans and his colleagues (Luthans, 1988; Luthans, Hodgetts, & Rosenkrantz, 1988) studied over 450 managers to find out what major activities they engaged in on a regular basis. The following activities were consistently found (Robbins, 2001):

- *Traditional management:* Decision making, planning, and controlling
- *Communication:* Exchanging routine information and processing paperwork
- *Human resource management:* Motivating, disciplining, managing conflict, staffing, and training
- *Networking:* Socializing, politicking, and interacting with outsiders

Luthans was also interested in knowing about the differences between "average" managers, "successful" managers (defined in terms of speed of promotion within their organization), and "effective" managers (defined in terms of the quantity and the quality of their performance and the satisfaction and contentment of their employees; Robbins, 2001). It was found that average managers did more traditional management; successful managers did more networking and less human resource management; and effective managers did more communication and less networking (Luthans, 1988; Luthans et al., 1988).

The Balanced Scorecard

Traditionally, the effectiveness of leaders has been measured by bottom-line financial results. However, the drive for monetary profits often leads to questionable treatment of intangible assets, like employee satisfaction. It also can lead to a tendency to create short-term profits at the expense of long-term growth. R. S. Kaplan and Norton (1996) developed the idea of the *balanced scorecard.* The organization can define the objectives it wants the leader to strive for, including both financial yardsticks (e.g., return on equity), and operational yardsticks (e.g., customer satisfaction and the ability to innovate). The organization can tie the leader's compensation to performance on all these measures (DuBrin, 2000).

R. S. Kaplan and Norton (1996) developed the balanced scorecard to monitor four processes that tie long-term strategic objectives with short-term actions:

1. *Translating the vision:* This process focuses on taking the long-term vision of the company and making it relevant to daily operations. This might take the form of fostering a sense of pride throughout the organization for having the highest quality product or service in the world.
2. *Communicating and linking:* The goal here is for the leader to make clear the long-term objectives of what employees are doing in their daily work. This might take the form of reminding even support staff of the valuable work the organization is doing to ultimately make the community a better place.
3. *Business planning:* This area includes typical financial indicators, but tends to focus on long-term measures to prevent the leader from engaging in "accounting tricks" to make short-term numbers look better.
4. *Feedback and learning:* This area focuses on getting feedback from customers and employees on how to make the organization run better.

The factors that an organization chooses to include on a balanced scorecard will depend on current organizational needs, past performance, and future goals. It is also important not to place too many measures on the scorecard, as it can be difficult to monitor and improve too many areas at once. Each item on the scorecard should also be measurable, though this may take the form of customer or employee ratings on a survey.

Outstanding Leaders

Outstanding leaders tend to have specific behavior patterns in common. They create a vision of where the organization is going and what they want to accomplish. They then align the organization to accomplish the vision, organizing resources to foster innovative learning (Senge, 1990). By reaching meaning through communication, they get people to buy into the vision and create motivation toward achieving it. Of great importance is the ability of the leader to build trust, which facilitates the development of a concrete strategy and plan to achieve the vision. The leader must then implement the plan. It is also crucial to monitor the outcomes of the plan and adjust implementation as needed.

LEADERSHIP THEORIES

Think about individuals who have been considered great leaders. What traits consistently appear among effective leaders? To what degree do these traits match research evidence on leader characteristics?

Many theories about leadership have been developed over the years. These can be grouped into the general categories of trait theories, style theories, behavior theories, contingency theories, situational theories, and those that attempt to integrate multiple ideas.

Trait Theories

Trait theories posit that there are differences in the traits possessed by leaders and nonleaders. Leaders are considered to have the following general traits:

- Ambition and energy
- The desire to lead
- Honesty
- Self-confidence
- Intelligence
- Job-relevant knowledge
- Stress tolerance
- Integrity
- Emotional maturity
- High self-monitoring

High self-monitoring refers to the capacity to be highly flexible in adjusting one's behavior in different situations. Individuals with this trait are more likely to emerge as leaders in groups than low self-monitors.

While the idea of leadership traits is intuitively appealing, research has shown that most correlations range between +.25 to +.35. Some researchers argue there is no stable pattern of traits (House & Aditya, 1997; Kirkpatrick & Locke, 1991; Yukl, 1998).

Judge, Bono, Illies, and Gerhardt (2002) conducted a meta-analysis of Leadership Correlation with the Big Five personality factors, and found the following correlations:

5 factor combination:	.48
Extraversion	.31
Conscientiousness	.28
Neuroticism	−.24
Openness	.24
Agreeableness	.08

In a meta-analysis of performance motivation, Neuroticism had a correlation of −.31, and Conscientiousness had a correlation of .24 (Judge et al., 2002).

Research has not supported trait theories very strongly, and the trait approach has at least four limitations (Robbins, 2001). First, traits only seem to predict leadership in selective situations, not in all situations (B. Schneider, 1983). Second, trait theories do not consider situational factors. They tend to predict behavior more in ambiguous situations than in situations in which the organization emphasizes and defines behavioral norms, incentives, and rewards and punishments (Barrick & Mount, 1993; Mischel, 1973). Third, there is little evidence to separate cause from effect in these studies. Does self-confidence lead to success as a leader, or does success as a leader lead to self-confidence? (Robbins, 2001). Fourth, traits seem to do better at predicting the appearance of leadership than predicting whether a leader is effective (Lord, DeVader, & Alliger, 1986; Lord & Maher, 1991; J. A. Smith & Foti, 1998).

Style Theories

Other theories of leadership focus on the styles of leaders, or the manner in which they interact with subordinates. Lewin, Lippitt, and White (1939) looked at autocratic, democratic, and laissez-faire leaders.

Autocratic leaders make decisions alone and then instruct subordinates what to do on the basis of those decisions. Democratic leaders involve subordinates in the decision-making process. Laissez-faire leaders leave it up to their subordinates to make decisions with little guidance or help.

Subordinates tend to be the most satisfied, motivated, and creative; are more likely to continue working in the absence of their leader; and have better relationships with their supervisor under democratic leadership. In terms of productivity, autocratic leaders are associated with greater quantity of output (at least while the leader is present; Robbins, 2001).

There has been an enormous increase in experiments in industrial democracy. Prior to the late 1950s, there were many experiments in benevolent paternalism, as well as state ownership of work organizations, but neither did much to increase employees' control over decisions.

Most of the empirical investigations of industrial democracy show more positive than negative consequences. Workers almost always prefer more power to less power.

Experiments with industrial democracy sometimes show an initial decline in productivity, but in the long run, most experiments either result in a gain in productivity or maintain a level of productivity roughly comparable to that under the previous system. The process is usually irreversible. When workers gain more power, they are rarely willing to give it up and often press for its expansion. Despite the mostly favorable evidence, many managers, scholars, and trade union leaders continue to oppose the idea (Hersey & Blanchard, 1982; Schermerhorn et al., 2000).

Behavioral Theories

Behavioral theories of leadership posit that specific behaviors differentiate leaders from nonleaders.

Ohio State Studies

Studies conducted at Ohio State University (Robbins, 2001; Schriesheim, Cogliser, & Neider, 1995; Stogdill & Coons, 1951) found that there are two primary dimensions of leadership behavior: *consideration* and *initiating structure.*

Consideration, which is person oriented, refers to the amount of warmth, concern, rapport, and support leaders display. Initiating structure, which is task or production oriented, refers to the extent to which leaders define, direct, and structure their own role and the roles of subordinates. Consideration is associated with greater subordinate satisfaction, although some studies suggest that initiating structure is important for productivity and satisfaction when tasks are ambiguous. Other studies suggest that effective leadership requires high levels of both consideration and initiating structure.

University of Michigan Studies

Similar to the Ohio State studies, the University of Michigan studies (Kahn & Katz, 1960) also found two dimensions of leadership behavior, which they termed *employee oriented* and *production oriented.* Leaders who were employee oriented took a personal interest in their employees and accepted individual differences among members. Production-oriented leaders focused on accomplishing the job at hand, viewing the employees basically as tools for accomplishment. The researchers concluded that leaders who were employee oriented fostered higher productivity and higher job satisfaction (Robbins, 2001).

The Managerial Grid

Blake and Mouton (1964) took the findings of the Ohio State and University of Michigan studies and created a matrix of 81 leadership styles, with "concern for people" on one axis and "concern for production" on the other axis. A 9,9 style (high concern for people, high concern for production) was considered best, rather than a 1,9 style (laissez-faire) or a 9,1 style (autocratic type).

As with trait theories, behavioral theories were also found to be weak because they did not address situational factors.

Contingency Theories

Fred Fiedler proposed a contingency model of leadership (Fiedler, 1967; Fiedler & Chemers, 1974, 1984; Fiedler, Chemers, & Mahar, 1976). He and his colleagues believed that effective group performance depends on the proper match between a leader's style of interacting and the degree to which the situation gives control and in-

fluence to the leader. He developed leadership dimensions of task and relationship behaviors. This theory later was developed into cognitive resource theory, which is a
leadership theory stating that stress unfavorably affects the situation, and intelligence
and experience can lessen the influence of stress on the leader (Robbins, 2001).

Fiedler developed the least preferred coworker (LPC) questionnaire (Fiedler &
Chemers, 1984) to measure an individual leader's style. More specifically, it is designed
to indicate a person's primary motivation or goal in a work setting. The LPC questionnaire asks test-takers to think of the person with whom they work least well. They then
proceed through a list of adjectives, arranged on either side of a Likert-type scale
with a rating from 1 to 8, and mark how they would rate that least-preferred colleague.
There are 16 items including "pleasant" to "unpleasant," "rejecting" to "accepting,"
"supportive" to "hostile," "boring" to "interesting," "efficient" to "inefficient," and
"gloomy" to "cheerful." The items are then added up (some are reverse scored), and a
score above 64 indicates a high LPC person, with a tendency to be relationship oriented.
A score below 57 indicates a low LPC person, with a tendency to be task oriented. Those
falling in between are told to determine for themselves if they tend to be more relationship or task oriented (Fiedler & Chemers, 1984).

According to Fiedler, the LPC score can help an individual find a situation match
and, therefore, become a more effective leader.

Situational control (or "favorableness") is the extent to which a leader determines
what the group of subordinates is going to do as well as the outcome of the group's actions and decisions (Schermerhorn et al., 2000). Situational control depends on the
amount of influence a leader has and is determined by the leader's relationships with
subordinates (when relationships are positive, the leader has greater influence), the nature of the task (the greater the task structure, the greater the leader's influence), and
"position power" (the greater the number of rewards available for subordinates, the
more influence the leader has).

The relationship between style and the favorableness of the situation is curvilinear,
with low LPC (task-oriented) leaders performing best in very unfavorable and very favorable situations, and high LPC (relationship-oriented) leaders performing best in
moderately favorable situations. Low LPC leaders are most effective when the situation provides them with either very little or a great deal of influence, while high LPC
leaders are most effective in situations that allow moderate levels of influence. Fiedler
recommended "job engineering" to alter the favorableness of the situation to ensure
leader effectiveness (Fiedler & Chemers, 1984; Fiedler et al., 1976).

Fiedler's theory was considered an improvement over trait and behavioral theories,
but it still contained gaps.

Situational Theory

Hersey and Blanchard (1982) emphasized that how a person leads depends on the situation. The abilities and motivational level of followers will determine the most efficacious leadership style. Four styles of leadership are distinguished, and are
differentiated by combinations of high and low task and relationship orientation
(DuBrin, 2000; Hersey & Blanchard, 1982; Schermerhorn et al., 2000).

1. *Telling: High task, low relationship orientation.* This leader is more concerned
   about "getting the job done" than about building relationships with employees.

The leader feels little concern for the needs or the level of satisfaction of the employees, who are seen as tools for the fulfillment of the leader's goals.

2. *Selling: High task, high relationship orientation.* This leader views task accomplishment and relationship development both as high priorities. Employees see this person as driven to accomplish tasks with high standards, yet considers the individual needs and concerns of subordinates.

3. *Participating: Low task, high relationship orientation.* This leader emphasizes relationships with subordinates over task accomplishment. This person tends to spend more time and energy on ensuring the satisfaction and growth of employee potential than on getting things done.

4. *Delegating: Low task, low relationship orientation.* This individual tends to not spend much time or effort on either task accomplishment or relationship building, leaving subordinates to work on tasks on their own.

Hersey and Blanchard also looked at *followers,* that is, those who were being led. They described four levels of readiness of followers (DuBrin, 2000; Hersey & Blanchard, 1982; Schermerhorn et al., 2000).

R1: People are *both unable and unwilling to take responsibility to do something.* They are neither competent nor confident.

R2: People are *unable but willing to do the necessary job tasks.* They are motivated but currently lack the appropriate skills.

R3: People are *able but unwilling to do what the leader wants.* They can but they do not want to.

R4: People are both *able and willing to do what is asked of them.* They can and they will.

By knowing the readiness level of the individuals with whom the leader is working, the consultant can help the leader operate most effectively in a given environment. Often a leader has been very effective in the past in other environments, but is not effective in a new setting due to a lack of sensitivity or awareness of the needs of subordinates. The selection of a leadership style should be based on the subordinates' level of job maturity (or readiness), which is determined by a combination of ability and willingness to accept responsibility for one's own behaviors.

- A telling leader is most effective for employees low in both ability and willingness.
- A selling leader is most effective for employees with low ability and high willingness.
- A participating leader is most effective for employees with high ability and low willingness.
- A delegating leader is most effective for employees high in both ability and willingness.

Situational theories of leadership, such as those of Fieldler (1967; Fiedler & Chemers, 1974, 1984; Fiedler, Chemers, & Mahar, 1976) and Hersey and Blanchard (1982), are limited in their conceptualization of leadership and lack strong empirical support. They usually fail to distinguish between leadership and management and typically assume that the domain of leadership is limited to the relationships between managers and their immediate subordinates.

Leader-Member Exchange Theory

Leaders develop relationships with each member of the group they lead. Leader-Member Exchange (LMX) theory explains how the relationships with various members can develop in very different ways (Dienesch & Liden, 1986; Education and Training Committee of the Society for Industrial and Organizational Psychology, 2005).

LMX theory is based on the idea that leaders treat different subordinates differently. Leaders develop relationships with each member of a work group. An "in-group" and an "out-group" form early in the leader's relationships with followers, and these groups remain stable based on compatibility with the leader and a higher level of competence. In-group members have higher performance ratings, less turnover, more responsibility, and greater satisfaction with their superior. Out-group members have a low-quality relationship with the leader, and tend to have less responsibility and lower job satisfaction (Graen & Cashman, 1975; Graen & Uhl-Bien, 1995; Robbins, 2001; Schermerhorn et al., 2000).

Relationships between leaders and followers develop from a series of exchanges or interactions. Phase 1 is known as the *role-taking* phase, when the member enters the organization and the leader assesses the member's abilities and talents. Phase 2 is known as the *role-making* phase, in which there occurs an informal, unstructured negotiation of what the roles of the member and the leader will be. Phase 3 is known as the *role-routinization* phase, in which a social exchange pattern emerges and becomes routine.

Precursors of LMX

The attributes of the member (or follower) will influence the relationship with the leader. Members who are extroverted, are high in ability (are good at what they do), and engage in ingratiating behaviors (e.g., offering to stay late to finish the leader's work) are more likely to be viewed favorably by the leader. By providing social support, the leader makes a relationship desirable for members. The affective responses of the leader or the members will have an impact on the relationship. Perceived similarity and attraction leads to increased interaction. Closer relationships also exist where there is trust.

Outcomes of LMX

When leaders and members have a good working relationship, it leads to job satisfaction and organizational commitment. This is moderated by other factors, such as the type of task (e.g., how challenging the tasks are) and by situational factors (e.g., the size of the group, the workload, and the financial resources of the organization).

Gender Fairness and LMX

Gender differences influence leader-member interactions. In mixed-gender relationships, supervisors rate performance lower, supervisors report liking subordinates less, and subordinates experience greater role ambiguity. The opposite is true for same-gender relationships (Fairhurst, 1993; Fairhurst & Sarr, 1996).

Several process phases develop in regard to gender issues:

- *Role taking:* In this phase, mutual respect is essential. Men and women may define respect differently, and social categorizing and stereotyping may occur.
- *Role making:* If respect is fostered, trust may begin to develop. However, a single violation of this trust may destroy any relationship that has developed. Such violations reinforce negative stereotypes.

- *Role routinization:* When trust is deepened, a sense of mutual obligation arises. At this point, gender fairness issues are usually resolved.

Perspective Taking

The ability to "read" the leader or members is important in LMX Theory. A consultant can encourage consultees to use role-taking skills to entertain the point of view of another. The ability to take on another perspective is positively associated with empathy, reasonableness, and sensitivity, and it is negatively associated with aggressiveness and sarcasm (Bardwick, 1991; M. H. David, Luce, & Kraus, 1994).

Path-Goal Theory

Path-goal theory is a contingency model of leadership. It states that a leader's behavior is acceptable to subordinates insofar as they view it as a source of either immediate or future satisfaction (House, 1971; Robbins, 2001). The theory proposes that the most effective leader is one who helps carve a path for subordinates that will allow them to achieve personal goals through the achievement of group and organizational goals. A leader's functions consist of (1) clarifying goals and the paths that will lead to their achievement and (2) providing rewards to subordinates through support and attention to their needs (House, 1971).

Robbins (2001) illustrates the predictions of path-goal theory:

- Directive leadership leads to greater satisfaction when tasks are ambiguous or stressful than when they are highly structured and well laid out.
- Supportive leadership results in high employee performance and satisfaction when employees are performing structured tasks.
- Directive leadership is likely to be perceived as redundant among employees with high perceived ability or with considerable experience.
- Employees with an internal locus of control will be more satisfied with a participative style.
- Achievement-oriented leadership will increase employees' expectancies that effort will lead to higher performance when tasks are ambiguously structured. (p. 325)

Meta-analysis of the research has generally supported the predictions of path-goal theory (Wofford & Liska, 1993). Employee performance and satisfaction are likely to increase when the leader compensates for what is lacking in the employee or in the workplace. However, a leader must also be aware that getting too involved for simple tasks or explaining things too much to someone who is already competent can be felt as redundant or even condescending (Robbins, 2001).

Charismatic Leadership

Charismatic leadership theory states that followers make attributions of heroic or extraordinary leadership abilities when they observe certain behaviors (Conger & Kanungo, 1988; Robbins, 2001). These characteristics include the following:

- Self-confidence
- Having a vision
- Ability to articulate the vision

- Having strong convictions about the vision
- Behavior that is out of the ordinary
- Being perceived as a change agent
- Environmental sensitivity

Transactional versus Transformational Leadership

Transactional leaders guide or motivate their followers in the direction of established goals by clarifying role and task requirements. Transformational leaders provide individual consideration and intellectual stimulation, and possess charisma (Bass & Avolio, 1990; Robbins, 2001). The research evidence supports the effectiveness of transformational leadership (Lowe, Kroeck, & Sivasubramaniam, 1996).

Bass (1992) succinctly describes the characteristics of transformational and transactional leaders:

Transformational Leader

- *Charisma:* Provides vision and sense of mission, instills pride, gains respect and trust.
- *Inspiration:* Communicates high expectations, uses symbols to focus efforts, expresses important purposes in simple ways.
- *Intellectual stimulation:* Promotes intelligence, rationality, and careful problem solving.
- *Individualized consideration:* Gives personal attention, treats each employee individually, coaches, advises.

Transactional Leader

- *Contingent reward:* Contracts exchange of rewards for effort, promises rewards for good performance, recognizes accomplishments.
- *Management by exception (active):* Watches and searches for deviations from rules and standards, takes corrective action.
- *Management by exception (passive):* Intervenes only if standards are not met.
- *Laissez-faire:* Abdicates responsibilities, avoids making decisions. (p. 210)

Leadership Versatility Index

Another recent approach to measuring and studying leadership is the Leadership Versatility Index developed by Robert E. Kaplan and Robert Kaiser (2003). The Index looks at the balance between *forceful, enabling, strategic,* and *operational* leadership. Forceful leaders assert themselves, take charge and make their presence felt, push others to perform, hold them accountable, and make the tough calls. Enabling leaders empower others, are receptive to their ideas, involve them in making decisions, and recognize their contributions. Strategic leaders see the big picture, monitor the external environment, think long term, position the organization for the future, and get people on board with the strategy. Operational leaders ground themselves in operational detail, have their fingers on the pulse of the organization, focus the organization on executing near-term objectives, are practical, street-smart, and realistic, and apply discipline and structure to move the organization forward.

The basic assumption is that every manager needs a mix of approaches, though most favor one over the others. Some leaders are lopsided, and overdo or underdo. Truly effective leaders are versatile and can adapt to the situation.

The Leadership Versatility Index (R. E. Kaplan & Kaiser, 2003) consists of a series of questions, answered on a scale from −4 (indicating much too little of that quality) to

+4 (indicating much too much of that quality), with 0 being just the right amount. Examples include: "takes charge—is in control of his or her unit"; "participative—involves people in decision-making"; "thinks broadly—pays attention to the big picture"; and "focused on meeting the immediate needs of customers."

Reframing Leadership

Bolman and Deal (2003) wrote extensively on four ways of framing organizations and leadership. They are known as structural, human resource, political, and symbolic. Structural Theorists emphasize organizational structure, boundaries, policies, and procedures. They fit the organizational structure to the mission. Human Resource Theorists emphasize the interdependence between people and organizations. They find the fit between people's needs, skills, and values and their formal roles and relationships. Political Theorists see power, conflict, and the distribution of scarce resources as the control issues. They utilize power, coalitions, bargaining, and conflict. Symbolic Theorists look at the problems of meaning. They rely on images, drama, magic, and sometimes the supernatural to bring order to organizations.

Table 4.2 shows how the organization and its processes can be viewed (Bolman & Deal, 2003).

A Structural Scenario

The fundamental responsibility of managers and leaders is to clarify organizational goals, attend to the relationship between structure and environment, and develop a clear structure that is appropriate to the goals, the task, and the environment. Without such a structure, people become unsure what they are supposed to be doing. The result is confusion, frustration, and conflict. In an effective organization, individuals understand their responsibilities and their contribution. Policies, linkages, and lines of authority are clear. When the structure is appropriate and people understand it, the organization can achieve its goals and employees can be effective in their roles.

Table 4.2   Ways of Framing Leadership

Effective Leadership	Structural	Human Resource	Political	Symbolic
Leader is:	Social architect	Catalyst, servant	Advocate	Prophet or poet
Leadership process:	Analysis, design	Support, empowerment building	Advocacy, coalition experience	Inspiration, framing

Ineffective Leadership	Structural	Human Resource	Political	Symbolic
Leader is:	Petty tyrant	Wimp, pushover	Con artist, hustler	Fanatic, fool (Jonestown)
Leadership process:	Management by detail and fiat	Management by abdication	Management by fraud, manipulation	Management by mirage, smoke, and mirrors

The job of a leader is to focus on tasks, facts, and logic, not personality and emotions. Most "people" problems stem from structural flaws rather than from flaws in individuals. Structural leaders are not necessarily authoritarian and do not necessarily solve every problem by issuing orders (though that will sometimes be appropriate). Instead, they try to design and implement a process or structure appropriate to the problem and the circumstances. Examples would include using downsizing or rightsizing, mergers, and acquisitions.

A Human Resource Scenario

People are the heart of any organization. When people feel the organization is responsive to their needs and supportive of their goals, leaders can count on their commitment and loyalty. Administrators who are authoritarian, uncaring, or insensitive, and who don't communicate effectively can never be effective leaders. The human resource leader works on behalf of both the organization and its people, seeking to serve the best interests of both.

The job of the leader is to provide support and empowerment. Giving support means letting people know that the leader is concerned about them, listening to find out about their aspirations and goals, and communicating personal warmth and openness. A leader empowers people through participation and openness and through making sure that they have the autonomy and the resources to do their jobs well. Human resource leaders emphasize honest, two-way communication to identify issues and resolve differences. They are willing to confront others when it is appropriate, but they try to do so in a spirit of openness and caring.

Political Scenario

Managers have to recognize political reality and know how to deal with it. Inside and outside any organization, there are always different interest groups, each with its own agenda. There are not enough resources to satisfy everyone, and there is always going to be conflict.

The job of leaders is to recognize the major constituencies, develop ties to their leadership, and manage conflict as productively as possible. Above all, they need to build power bases and use power carefully. They cannot give every group everything it wants, although they can try to create arenas for negotiating differences and coming up with reasonable compromises. They also have to work hard at articulating what everyone in their organization has in common. They must tell the people in their organization that it is a waste of time to fight each other when there are plenty of enemies outside that they can all fight together. Groups that fail to work well together internally tend to get trounced by outsiders who have their own agendas.

Symbolic Scenario

Symbolic managers believe that the most important part of a leader's job is inspiration—giving people something that they can believe in. People will give their loyalty to an organization that has a unique identity and makes them feel that what they do is really important. Effective symbolic leaders are passionate about making their organizations the best of their kind and communicate that passion to others. They use dramatic, visible symbols (e.g., the Golden Arches of McDonald's) that give people a sense of the organizational mission. They are visible and energetic. They create slogans, tell stories, hold rallies, give awards, appear where they are least expected, and manage by wandering around.

Symbolic leaders are sensitive to an organization's history and culture. They seek to use the best in an organization's traditions and values as a base for building a culture that provides cohesiveness and meaning. They articulate a vision that communicates the organization's unique capabilities and mission.

Finding the Appropriate Frame of Reference

Consultants can help managers determine what their fundamental focus should be by helping them determine the most appropriate frame of reference.

Consider the following scenarios. The most appropriate frames of reference are given in parentheses.

- Setting goals and policies under conditions of uncertainty (structural, symbolic)
- Achieving a delicate balance in allocating scarce resources across different businesses or functions (structural, political)
- Keeping on top of a large, complex set of activities (structural, human resource)
- Getting support from bosses (human resource, political)
- Getting support from corporate staff and other constituents (human resource, political)
- Motivating, coordinating, and controlling a large, diverse group of subordinates (structural, human resource)

Peters and Waterman (1982) listed characteristics of high-performing companies, which can be associated with the frames of Bolman and Deal (2003).

Characteristic	Related Frames
Bias for action	Structural, symbolic
Close to the customer	Human resource
Autonomy and entrepreneurship	Human resource, structural
Productivity through people	Human resource, symbolic
Hands-on, value-driven	Symbolic
Stick to the knitting	Structural, human resource, symbolic
Simple form, lean staff	Structural
Simultaneous loose/tight properties	Structural, symbolic

Consultants should consider the following questions when considering the different frames:

How Important Are Commitment and Motivation?

Structural Frame	*Unimportant*
Human Resource Frame	*Important*
Political Frame	*?*
Symbolic Frame	*Important*

How Important Is the Technical Quality of the Decision?

Structural Frame	*Important*
Human Resource Frame	*?*

| Political Frame | *Unimportant* |
| Symbolic Frame | *Unimportant* |

How Much Ambiguity and Uncertainty Is Present?

Structural Frame	*Low to moderate*
Human Resource Frame	*Moderate*
Political Frame	*Moderate to high*
Symbolic Frame	*High*

How Scarce Are Resources?

Structural Frame	*Moderately scarce*
Human Resource Frame	*Moderately abundant to abundant*
Political Frame	*Scarce (or getting scarcer)*
Symbolic Frame	*Scarce to abundant*

How Much Conflict and Diversity Is Present?

Structural Frame	*Low to moderate*
Human Resource Frame	*Moderate*
Political Frame	*Moderate to high*
Symbolic Frame	*Moderate to high*

Are We Working Top down or Bottom up?

Structural Frame	*Top down*
Human Resource Frame	*Top down*
Political Frame	*Bottom up*
Symbolic Frame	*Top down or bottom up*

Leadership Perceptions Approach

Leadership is hard to define, but people tend to know it when they see it. People must first be recognized as leaders before they can influence followers. Followers determine the ultimate success of leaders. Leader behavior determines follower perceptions, which are associated with positive or negative outcomes. Outcomes such as success can also shape follower perceptions.

All too often, identical behavior from men and women is interpreted differently. Perceivers attach different labels to the same behaviors enacted by men and women. One reason is gender stereotypes (expectations about members of certain groups). Gender-based stereotypes include beliefs about expected interpersonal behavior and about the types of roles or jobs best suited for men and women (Wellington, 1998).

The role of gender stereotypes in employment was at issue in *Price Waterhouse v. Hopkins* (Fiske, Beroff, Borgida, Deaux, & Heilman, 1991; *Price Waterhouse v. Hopkins,* 1989). Ann B. Hopkins was a high-performing, but "masculine acting," prospective partner at Price Waterhouse. Hopkins alleged she was denied partnership because of her gender. Price Waterhouse countered that Hopkins had interpersonal problems (e.g., she was "macho"). The court eventually ruled that gender-based stereotyping influenced perceptions of her behavior. Because Hopkins was a woman in a nontraditional role, her behavior was seen as more extreme than that of men who behaved similarly.

Controlling Our Stereotyping

Mental health consultants are especially well suited to working with organizations on issues of discrimination and stereotyping. Here are a few things to consider:

- Nearly everyone engages in stereotyping.
- Most recognize it is inappropriate to judge others based on a stereotype.
- One way to learn control is through awareness and conscious control.
- Identify organizational consequences of gender and race stereotyping.
- Train employees to gather individuating information about the stereotyped person (e.g., getting to know the person as an individual, understanding the benefits of diversity).
- Train employers to effectively manage diversity.
- Help to minimize the effects of stereotyping and unfair treatment of employees.

Women and Leadership

There is a lot of evidence of prejudice and discriminatory treatment of women in obtaining leadership roles and being evaluated as leaders (Butler & Geis, 1990; Eagly & Karau, 2002).

Women are more likely than men to be "transformational" leaders (Eagly, Johannesen-Schmidt & van Engen, 2003). Transformational leaders create the most productive and satisfying work environments. In Eagly's study (Eagly & Karau, 2002), which was a meta-analysis of 45 studies on leaders, women also scored higher than men on one measure of transactional leadership—rewarding employees for good performance. That is the only aspect of transactional leadership that has been associated with positive outcomes. The differences were small and the cause of the differences unclear. It could be that, because of the "glass ceiling" (Morrison, White, & Van Velsor, 1987; D. Smith, 2000), women have to be better leaders to make it into management positions. It could also be that women tend to use transformational styles because other, more forceful styles produce especially negative reactions when used by women (Eagly & Karau, 2002).

The following sections explore practical skills necessary for all leaders, which consultants should learn and pass along to their consultees.

SUPPORTIVE COMMUNICATION

As mental health professionals know from their work in psychotherapeutic settings, the ability to communicate accurately and honestly without jeopardizing interpersonal relationships is a crucial skill. Consultants can teach these skills to organizational leaders and their members.

Whetten and Cameron (2002) list the following attributes of supportive communication:

- *Problem oriented, not person oriented:* A focus on problems and issues that can be changed rather than on people and their characteristics. *Example: "How can we solve this problem?" Not "Because of you a problem exists."*
- *Congruent, not incongruent:* A focus on honest messages in which verbal statements match thoughts and feelings. *Example: "Your behavior really upset me." Not "Do I seem upset? No, everything's fine."*

- *Descriptive, not evaluative:* A focus on describing an objective occurrence, describing your reaction to it, and offering a suggested alternative. *Example: "Here's what happened; here is my reaction; here's a suggestion that would be more acceptable." Not "You are wrong for doing what you did."*
- *Validating, not invalidating:* A focus on statements that communicate respect, flexibility, collaboration, and areas of agreement. *Example: "I have some ideas, but do you have any suggestions?" Not "You wouldn't understand, so we'll do it my way."*
- *Specific, not global:* A focus on specific events or behaviors, avoiding general, extreme, or either-or statements. *Example: "You interrupted me three times during the meeting." Not "You're always trying to get attention."*
- *Conjunctive, not disjunctive:* A focus on statements that flow from what has been said previously and facilitating interaction. *Example: "Relating to what you just said, I'd like to raise another point." Not "I want to say something (regardless of what you just said)."*
- *Owned, not disowned:* A focus on taking responsibility for your own statements by using personal ("I") words. *Example: "I have decided to turn down your request because . . ." Not "You have a pretty good idea, but it wouldn't get approved."*
- *Supportive listening, not one-way listening:* A focus on using a variety of appropriate responses, with a bias toward reflective responses. *Example: "What do you think are the obstacles standing in the way of improvement?" Not "As I said before, you make too many mistakes. You're just not performing."* (p. 220)

DEALING WITH DIFFICULT EMPLOYEES

Another important skill that mental health consultants can teach managers is how to deal with difficult employees. Some managers have a difficult time confronting employees with problem behavior, even when that behavior is negatively impacting other employees or the organization as a whole. This may stem from the manager's natural human tendency to want to be liked, may stem from a fear of how the employee will react to confrontation, or may be due to the manager's internal struggle to confront an employee whose performance is excellent in many other areas. It can also be difficult for a manager to determine when coaching, counseling, or mentoring is needed to address an employee's lack of performance (Stone, 1999). The following strategy can be taught to managers who need to conduct a counseling session and is designed to keep the intervention focused on specific problem behaviors.

Preparation is the key to having a productive intervention conference with a difficult employee. Having an agenda set for yourself will help you conduct the meeting, and will keep you organized and in control. If you are not prepared, you will find it difficult to develop a corrective action plan with the employee.

As is true for any meeting, it is important to first clearly state the purpose of the meeting and what you want to accomplish. Since the employee is probably someone you work with on a daily basis, this is not an appropriate time to engage in small talk. It is best to keep a professional tone. You should identify and define the problem that needs to be addressed. Make the problem as specific as possible, preferably with something measurable. The problem should be defined with specific behaviors, and you should avoid vague terms referencing qualities of personality (e.g., "I've noticed you've been about 30 minutes late five times in the last two weeks" is better than "You're always late"). Also describe the impact of the problem on the organization as specifically as possible. This emphasizes that the issue is more than just a personal preference of the manager. The impact of the problem should also be described as specifically as possible, avoiding vague, generalized terms.

Next, explore the root causes of the problem. Begin by listening attentively to the employee's responses, reactions, and reasons for the behavior. A person who feels heard will be more open to feedback. The manager may also wish to submit any hypothesized reasons, discussing them with the employee. If the manager or some other aspect of the organization (such as a rule or policy) is also contributing to the problem, this should be openly discussed as well.

The next step is to define (or remind the employee of) the expected performance standard. Again, provide specific, measurable objectives ("Every line employee is expected to produce 80 widgets per day" is better than, "I want you to do better from now on"). Once the performance standard is set, and reasons have been explored for why those standards are not being reached, the manager and the employee should work collaboratively to develop a plan for reaching those standards considering the challenges that need to be faced. Multiple options should be considered and explored. Once a reasonable plan is established, it should be put in writing, with a copy for both the manager and the employee.

Before the meeting is ended, the manager should recap the key points and review the plan that was developed to meet the performance standards. A follow-up meeting should then be set, with clear expectations about what should be accomplished by that date. If the manager appreciates other aspects of the employee's work, stating this to the employee will end the meeting on a positive note.

One of the crucial points of this model is that it places the burden of change onto the employee to meet a defined performance standard, making it difficult for the em-

---

=== **Box 4.2** ===

Conference Agenda for Dealing with a Difficult Employee Behavior

I. Introduction.
   A. State the purpose of the meeting.
   B. State what you want to accomplish.
II. Report the Problem.
   A. Step 1: Identify and define the performance problem.
   B. Step 2: Explain the impact of the problem.
III. Explore the Causes of the Problem.
   A. Listen to employee's thoughts and reactions to what you have reported.
   B. Step 3: Analyze the reasons for the problem.
      1. Discuss reasons with employee; test your own ideas, as appropriate.
      2. Discuss your influence on the situation.
IV. Corrective Actions.
   A. Step 4: Define the expected performance standard(s).
   B. Step 5: Explore ideas for a solution.
   C. Step 6: Write the plan for improvement.
V. Close.
   A. Recap key points and review your plan to finalize it.
   B. Make sure to set a follow-up meeting.

ployee to view the manager as "the bad guy" who needs to "lighten up." Hence, if further managerial disciplinary action is needed in the future (up to and including termination), the employee will have a more difficult time blaming the manager for being discharged due to "personality issues."

Box 4.2 provides an outline summary of the agenda to follow when conducting a meeting concerning difficult employee behaviors (Brounstein, 1993; Shepard, 2005). Note that the overall agenda also incorporates the six steps of an intervention model.

CASE EXAMPLE: THE PAPERWORK-CHALLENGED THERAPIST

Simian is the managing partner of a group psychological practice. One of his therapists, Peter, is an excellent clinician who is loved by clients but is chronically late on paperwork (including therapy notes and treatment plans), which is driving the staff crazy. Simian decides to try to deal with the problem, and prepares an agenda for a meeting with Peter.

"Peter, the reason that I want to meet with you is to discuss your tendency to be late with your paperwork. I'm hoping we'll be able to find a way to get that paperwork filed in a timelier manner.

"The latest computer printout shows that you have five clients that you have seen for three or more sessions that do not have treatment plans yet. This makes it very difficult for support staff to work with the insurance company to approve future sessions for the client. They end up scrambling to get this taken care of without interrupting the client's treatment.

"The staff has also told me that you have a tendency to turn in your therapy notes one to two weeks late. As you know, one of the values of the therapy notes is to give you a quick reminder of what you covered in the previous session before you meet again with the client. Also, if one of your clients calls or walks in with a crisis situation, the on-call therapist won't know what has been happening with your client for the last week or two.

"What are your thoughts about all of this, Peter?"

Peter doesn't take much responsibility at first. "I just feel like I've got too much work to do, and the paperwork tends to fall by the wayside when I'm so busy taking care of clients. I'm really concerned about our waiting list, and I hate the thought of a client in need not getting therapy because I blocked off time to do paperwork. And with a new baby at home, I really don't want to stay late every day, or take work home with me."

Simian expresses understanding and admits that the organization contributes to the problem, but also reminds Peter of the expected performance standards. "We do have a bit of a waiting list right now, and I appreciate your concern about getting clients the help they need. But if we can't get the paperwork done on time, it affects the quality of the service we give to the clients we are seeing. The management team is working on some ideas for dealing with the wait list, so please don't feel pressure that it's your responsibility. I also do think it's important to keep good boundaries between your work life and your home life, so let's try to figure out a plan for how we can help you get that paperwork done.

"Let's start with the treatment plans. The policy is to have them on file by the third session. What can be changed to make that happen?"

Peter makes an honest effort to think about it. "I'm not sure. I don't have enough time between sessions, and I hate to take a whole lot of time out of somebody's therapy session to do it. It just seems like there's always some new problem that develops, which ends up taking the whole therapy session, and I just feel like it's not as important to take care of that administrative requirement."

"You should discuss this more with your clinical supervisor, but my thought is that your clients will always come up with problems to talk about. Unless a crisis situation has developed, it is up to you to structure the session, and to express the importance of coming up with a treatment plan so that both of you are clear on the goals you want to achieve, and so that you don't get as easily pulled off track by the inevitable minor problems that continually develop. Working on the plan with the clients in session helps them to focus on what they really want from therapy and serves as a foundation to work from when they feel pulled in many directions.

"Even though I know you hate to block off paperwork time, I think it would be helpful, especially as you are working to get caught up. Again, you should discuss this with your clinical supervisor, but rather than depriving a client of therapy time, perhaps you may have a current weekly client who is ready to be transitioned to being seen every other week. You could then use that time to catch up on paperwork, but let the client know the slot is available for therapy if a crisis develops."

Peter nods in agreement. "I can think of a couple clients that I believe would be ready for that."

"Good. Now what about treatment notes? Our policy is to have them in the system by the end of the day, or by the next workday at the latest."

"Well, as I said, I don't want to have to stay late every day, and my clients always seem to bring up important things at the end of session. Even when I end on time, I just don't have enough time to write down all the things I want to say about the session. Unfortunately, I admit, by the time I get around to writing the treatment notes, it is harder for me to remember everything that happened in the session."

"Again, you should talk to your clinical supervisor about this, but you need to take charge of the structure of the therapy session and make sure you wrap things up on time. You should process with clients why they choose to mention such important things at the end of the session, and model setting boundaries with them. In the ten to fifteen minutes between sessions, you should have enough time to write a brief note, review last week's note for the next session, and even take a quick bathroom break. Talk to your supervisor more about your note taking—you may be including far more information than you really need to."

"Okay, I'll give it a try."

Simian jots down some notes as he summarizes the meeting. "Okay, so you'll talk with your clinical supervisor about discussing treatment plans in session, shifting some clients to every other week to create time to work on paperwork, and ending sessions on time in order to get notes done. Anything else you'd like to add?"

"No, that sounds reasonable."

"Great. Let's meet again in one month to see how things are going. You know, you are one of our best clinicians. I agree that the paperwork is not much fun, but we have to get it in on time."

NETWORKING

Networks are composed of people, both internal and external to the organization, who provide one another with information, support, advice, and practical assistance to ac-

Box 4.3

Considerations for Managerial Networking

1. What do you need from a network?
2. Whom do you particularly want to help?
3. Recognize the reciprocal nature of networks. Help out in times of crisis. Stop by regularly just to talk.
4. Develop a systematic approach to networking. Develop a map of your potential network. Develop a plan to contact people to build rapport.
5. Networks are based on mutual interest and genuine concern.
6. Get to know higher-level executives.
7. Seek a mentor.
8. Attend social events to meet people informally. Invite people to lunch or call every month or two.
9. Establish networks outside your organization. Call key people in your field to ask for information, discuss an idea, or ask for advice.
10. Join professional organizations.
11. Join a peer support group who get together to exchange information.
12. Regularly touch base with network members to maintain your relationships.
13. State your needs to the individual whose help you need. Be prepared to negotiate if the other person cannot provide the assistance that you need.

complish individual or group goals. Leaders must learn how to effectively network. Building and nurturing a network is an ongoing process (see Box 4.3).

ORGANIZATIONAL POLITICS

Though "politicking" is considered a dirty word by many individuals, it is important for consultants to teach consultees how to function effectively within the political environment of an organization. The following suggestions are helpful for improving one's political effectiveness (Robbins, 2001; Robbins & Hunsaker, 1996):

- *Frame targets in terms of organizational goals:* Effective politicking requires camouflaging your self-interest. All the arguments you marshal in support of it must be framed in terms of the benefits that will accrue to the organization. People whose actions appear to blatantly further their own interests at the expense of the organization are almost universally denounced.
- *Develop the right image:* If you know your organization's culture, you understand what the organization wants and values from its employees—in terms of dress, associates to cultivate and those to avoid, whether to appear risk-taking or risk aversive, the preferred leadership style, the importance placed on getting along well with others, and so forth.
- *Gain control of organizational resources:* The control of organizational resources that are scarce and important is a source of power. Knowledge and expertise are particularly effective resources to control.

- *Make yourself appear indispensable:* Because we're dealing with appearances rather than objective facts, you can enhance your power by appearing to be indispensable. That is, you don't have to really be indispensable as long as key people in the organization believe that you are.
- *Be visible:* Because performance evaluation has a substantial subjective component, it's important that your boss and those in power in the organization be made aware of your contribution. Your job may require you to handle activities that are low in visibility, or your specific contribution may be indistinguishable because you're part of a team endeavor. In such cases—without appearing to be tooting your own horn or creating the image of a braggart—you'll want to call attention to yourself by highlighting your successes in routine reports, having satisfied customers relay their appreciation to senior executives in your organization, being seen at social functions, being active in your professional associations, developing powerful allies who speak positively about your accomplishments, and similar tactics.
- *Develop powerful allies:* It helps to have powerful people in your camp. Cultivate contacts with potentially influential people above you, at your own level, and in the lower ranks. They can provide you with important information that may not be available through normal channels. Additionally, there will be times when decisions will be made in favor of those with the greatest support.
- *Avoid "tainted" members:* In almost every organization, there are fringe members whose status is questionable. Their performance and/or loyalty is suspect. Your own effectiveness might be called into question if you're perceived as being too closely associated with tainted members.
- *Support your boss:* Your immediate future is in the hands of your current boss. Since he or she evaluates your performance, you will typically want to do whatever is necessary to have your boss on your side. You should make every effort to help your boss succeed, make her look good, support her if she is under siege, and spend the time to find out what criteria she will be using to assess your effectiveness. (Robbins, 2001, p. 368)

Bases of Power

Consultants can also help consultees understand the bases of power and can teach them how to recognize when it is being used inappropriately. Consultees will then be able to use power to serve the organization in the most effective way. French and Raven (1959) discussed five bases of social power: coercive, reward, legitimate, expert, and referent.

1. *Coercive power* is based on threats. This power rests on the ability to punish, constrain, or control rewards. This person takes and demands power. Needless to say, people resent this expression of power.
2. *Reward power* is based on an ability to distribute rewards that others see as valuable. People's compliance is based on the expectation that they will be rewarded.
3. *Legitimate power* is based on position. Power rests on the person's role. Here there is a need for balance of authority and responsibility.
4. *Expert power* is based on personal expertise. Power rests on the person's knowledge.
5. *Referent power* implies that a person is a model to be emulated. It involves personal relationships and characteristics. In this case, other people give the person power and credibility.

Yukl and Falbe (1991) developed five questions that can be used to determine which type of power is being used. Consultants can use these to assess what types of power an individual or organization tends to use:

1. Does the person make things difficult for people, and do you want to avoid getting him or her angry? If so, the person is exercising coercive power.
2. Is the person able to give special benefits or rewards to people, and do you find it advantageous to trade favors with him or her? If so, the person is exercising reward power.
3. Does the person have the right, considering his or her position and your job responsibilities, to expect you to comply with legitimate requests? If so, the person is exercising legitimate power.
4. Does the person have the experience and knowledge to earn your respect, and do you defer to his or her judgment in some matters? If so, the person is exercising expert power.
5. Do you like the person and enjoy doing things for him or her? If so, the person is exercising referent power.

One could probably also add information, attractiveness, alliances and networks, and track record to those bases of power.

Consultants should also keep in mind that women and minorities tend to suffer from a lack of power in all areas and all strata.

As a consultant, you should be consciously aware of the bases of power you are using. If you are working on a short time frame, it may be best to work in a directive, prescriptive, expert style (using coercive and expert power). If you are working with a longer time frame, it may be best to use a facilitative, nondirective approach (referent power), since you will have more time to develop relationships.

Kotter (1996b) developed four steps for dealing with the political dimensions in managerial work:

1. *Identify the relevant relationships.* Figure out who needs to be led.
2. *Assess who might resist cooperation, why, and how strongly.* Figure out where the leadership challenges will be.
3. *Develop, whenever possible, relationships with those people to facilitate the communication, education, or negotiation processes needed to deal with resistance.*
4. *When step three fails, carefully select and implement more subtle or more forceful methods.*

No strategy will work without a power base. To help consultees maneuver through political climates, advise them to see leaders alone on their territory, show them respect, be honest, and act as if each person were the most important one for any project's success. Once consultees have developed the relationship, they can move on to "horse trading," promising rewards in exchange for resources and support.

If someone resists a person's leadership, that leader should retaliate by aligning with others and keeping a distance from that person. It is better to develop a relationship with the resistant person, to facilitate the communication, education, or negotiation processes needed to deal with resistance. There is wisdom in the saying, "Keep your friends close, and your enemies even closer."

NEGOTIATION SKILLS

Consultants need to be skilled in the art of negotiation, for their own consulting practice, as well as to teach the art to consultees. Negotiation or "deal making" is an important skill for executives and is indeed something we all do throughout our lives in various ways (Fuller, 1991; Nierenberg, 1968). Many people think of negotiating in terms of "win-lose," wherein one person achieves desired goals at the expense of the other person. Such a situation, however, tends to be unstable, as the loser may create problems for the winner in the future. Another option is "lose-win," wherein one party chooses to give in to the other party's demands. Obviously, this is not the best strategy to use in all cases, but sometimes it may be necessary to save a long-term relationship. Sometimes a "lose-lose" strategy is employed. This is usually a passive-aggressive move in which a person sabotages things, thinking "If I can't have my way, no one will." This is the least desirable outcome.

A "win-win" outcome, in which both parties benefit, is being increasingly recognized as the best method for achieving a long-term positive outcome. There should be an attempt to make the best negotiation that is acceptable to both parties, particularly in an ongoing relationship. For example, if a company agrees to give a bonus to its employees based on an increase in profits, the employees will be motivated to perform better, and the company will likely have an even greater year-end profit.

THE ART OF NEGOTIATION

> Know the other and know yourself: One hundred challenges without danger;
> Know not the other and yet know yourself: One triumph for one defeat;
> Know not the other and know not yourself: Every challenge is certain peril.
>
> —Sun Tzu (Wing, 1988, p. 51)

You cannot always create win-win partnerships with everyone. When the time comes for negotiation, you must first know yourself. Know exactly what you want from the negotiation, including the optimum solution and the minimum solution you are prepared to accept. What factors are unimportant to you (things you are willing to concede)? What factors are important to you (things you are reluctant to concede)? What things do you consider nonnegotiable?

It is also important to know your opponent. Prepare your case by doing your best to determine ahead of time what your opponent wants and needs. It can be helpful to make an agenda, in which you list all the points you want to bring out during the negotiation. Prepare yourself by deciding the opening negotiation point, the fallback position, and the final offer. Don't make the initial offer if you're not sure of your opponent's interests and positions or if you need more time to probe for information. Never go beyond your final offer.

Negotiating caveats:

Never give something for nothing. "I can come down on the price, but I will have to eliminate some of the additional services I was offering."

Keep concessions small and infrequent. The other party will likely continue to push to see how much you will concede.

Make concessions progressively smaller. Again, this will discourage the other party from continually pressing for more concessions.

Sell your concessions. "I can move the due date up a week, but it will put a strain on the people currently allocated on the job." This also may help prevent the other party from pushing for more concessions.

CONFLICT IN ORGANIZATIONS

Conflict is inevitable in any organization. Mental health professionals can be helpful to organizations experiencing conflict by using the skills they have developed for handling conflicts.

Organizations can have either too much or too little conflict in an organization (Heffron, 1988). Some conflict is desirable, as it allows the organization to challenge old ideas and enables growth, but too much conflict results in reduced organizational effectiveness, wasted time, reduced quality of decision making, and the loss of group membership. The consultant can assist an organization by intervening when necessary to increase or decrease conflict, depending on the situational needs of the organization.

Conflict is particularly likely to occur at the boundaries, or interfaces, between groups and units within the organization, as they often have different goals. If the members of the clerical support staff in a mental health agency already are feeling overworked, they might resent the marketing department's efforts to bring in more clients. This situation, in which the conflict occurs in the interface between different departments or divisions in an organization, is known as *horizontal conflict.* If the support staff was angry at upper management for changes they made in policy, this would be a *vertical conflict,* defined as conflict between different levels in a hierarchy. Conflict that occurs between groups with different values, traditions, beliefs, and lifestyles is known as *cultural conflict* (Bolman & Deal, 2003).

Views of Conflict

There are several different ways to view organizational conflict. Each view is linked to a different set of assumptions about the purpose, process, and function of the organization.

The *functional view* considers conflict as a positive force that allows people to increase their knowledge, skills, and contributions to the organization for innovation and productivity. Keys to success lie not in structure and orderliness, but in valuing the creativity, responsiveness, adaptability, and feedback generated by conflict. The flexibility of this view allows the consultee to look at each conflict situation as an opportunity to improve and manage conflicts (not to completely eliminate them) in a way that enhances the organization as well as its members.

The *dysfunctional view* of conflict is embedded in the idea that the purpose of organizations is to achieve goals and create a structure that rigidly defines job responsibilities, authorities, and other job functions. Values of such organizations include orderliness, stability, and repression of conflict. The implication of conflict is that there is a fault in the design or structure of the organization. This belief fosters attempts to remedy the situation by implementing more elaborate job descriptions, responsibilities, and increased discipline.

The *escalation view* suggests that conflict tends to persist and eat away at the internal organization, performance, cooperation, and productivity of the organization. This may result in conflicts that exist between individuals in the organization for years, due to discouragement from giving up any attempts to resolve or address those conflicts. The workplace may become full of strife and private complaints, with little attempt to define, investigate, or fix the problem. Interest in working toward common goals tends to decrease as interest in self-protection increases.

Constructive versus Destructive Conflict

Conflict can be healthy and constructive, and can also be unhealthy and destructive. Consultants should work to help organizations shift from destructive to constructive patterns of conflict (Carpenter & Kennedy, 1988).

Conflict is destructive when it focuses mainly on people and "winning." Destructive conflict can have the following effects:

- Diverts energy from task or critical issues
- Produces barriers to cooperation or action
- Decreases productivity, quality, and improvement
- Deepens value differences, which polarizes groups, sets up "sides" and "us versus them" attitudes
- Destroys trust, morale, and self-esteem
- Produces irresponsible behaviors
- Prevents open discussions or confrontation of negative behaviors
- Builds doubt in people, teams, leadership, and organizations

Conflict is healthy when it leads to better decisions, creativity, and innovative solutions to either short- or long-standing problems. Within a conflict, there are seeds for the growth of ideas, positive relationships, and constructive change. Conflict can cause people to see the same issue in a new or different light, and sometimes in a better, more logical, effective, or more constructive way.

Conflict is beneficial or constructive when the focus is on finding the best solutions possible, or at least an equitable resolution for all parties. Conflict can have the following positive effects:

- Opens issues to constructive discussions and open communication
- Leads to positive solutions, decision making, and levels of understanding
- Opens people to spontaneous communication
- Increases productivity, prosperity, and growth
- Builds higher morale, self-esteem, and individual and company confidence
- Strengthens relationships for resolving conflicts
- Improves problem solving, allowing for more informed decision making
- Releases resentment, emotions, anxieties, and frustration

Five Myths of Conflict

There are many myths about conflict that tend to exacerbate problems when unchecked.

Personality

The personality myth suggests that conflict is due to personality styles, resulting in the belief that people are just "that way." Personality is given as a reason not to cooperate. The consequence is that by labeling a conflict as a "personality" issue, the conflict is redirected to a focus on changing the other person instead of resolving the issue.

Logic

The logic myth suggests that conflict is a simple breakdown in logic, resulting in the belief that there is a "right" and "wrong" way to do things. The consequence is that people will vehemently defend their positions by attacking alternative interpretations of the same events. Attempts to create a mutually agreeable definition of past events can obscure resolution of the issues.

Communication

The communication myth suggests that conflict is a matter of miscommunication, resulting in the belief that understanding another's perspective will eliminate conflict and result in increased openness. The consequence is that people may attempt to communicate longer and more forcefully in an attempt to resolve the conflict, which may cause the conflict to escalate. However, the quantity of communication is not as important as the quality, which involves mutual exploration and understanding rather than simply repeating oneself interminably until the other party "sees the light."

Justice

The justice myth suggests that the outcome of a conflict must be "just" or "fair." The consequence is that individuals take things personally if the result does not seem to be exactly what they want. To avoid the escalation of conflict, it is more realistic to search for acceptable rather than for perfect resolutions.

Win-Lose

The win-lose myth suggests that conflict results in only three possible outcomes: win-win, win-lose, and lose-lose. The consequence is that individuals attempt to get what they want at the expense of the other party. However, in win-lose outcomes, the losing party will immediately start to plan how to "win" the next conflict, so all win-lose situations eventually degrade to lose-lose situations. Win-win solutions should be sought whenever possible.

Managing Conflict

Viewing conflict as a natural phenomenon that exists for a reason allows the consultant to look for the underlying factors that are driving the conflict. A common source of conflict is simply resistance to change (Schaef & Fassel, 1988). Conflict may also come from the need to set boundaries, especially in terms of defining clear lines in relationships with authority and peers. Conflict sometimes arises from the need to establish priorities, especially when there is a need to cooperate with others to accomplish goals and objectives. Some individuals define their self-value through conflict with others, and use conflict to release their stress and anger.

The consultant can help individuals and organizations see that conflict can be an opportunity. Dealing directly with the sources of conflict can help to establish boundaries, reduce tension or stress, and establish clearer norms or standards. Openly working with conflict can prevent stagnation and improve decision making within an organization through the consideration of alternative points of view. Successfully managing conflict can increase group cohesion, leading to a greater commitment to working on problems and their solutions. Conflict reveals areas where communication and adaptation needs can be strengthened (Crum, 1987; Marcus, Dorn, Kritek, Miller, & Wyatt, 1995).

Conflict Styles

There are many ways to handle conflict. No one style is always appropriate in every situation, and people can learn to use a variety of styles depending on the situation (Katz & Lawyer, 1985; Whetten & Cameron, 2002):

Collaborator: A collaborator is concerned with the personal goals of both parties (self and other) and the interpersonal relationship; it is a win/win stance that uses appropriate conflict management techniques.

Compromiser: A compromiser assumes that each party must negotiate to achieve some goals with some compromise to the relationship; it is a mini-win/mini-lose stance that uses persuasion and manipulation.

Accommodator: An accommodator wants to maintain the interpersonal relationship and will sacrifice personal goals; it is a yield-lose/win stance that involves giving in, appeasing the other party, or avoiding the conflict.

Competitor/Controller: A competitor/controller focuses on meeting personal needs no matter how it affects the interpersonal relationship; it is a win/lose stance that uses whatever power is required to win.

Avoider: An avoider wants to avoid conflict. This style generally does not allow for meeting personal goals or maintaining the interpersonal relationship; it is a leave lose/win stance that involves postponing, diverting the issue, or withdrawing.

Ineffective Strategies in Conflict Management

Consultants should be alert for the ineffective strategies that organizations sometimes use for dealing with conflict. Consultants can help organizational leadership recognize these patterns and adopt more effective ways of coping with conflict:

Nonaction: Sometimes an organization is aware of conflict, but chooses not to do anything about it, perhaps because they do not want to get involved, or because they fear that interference will only escalate the situation. However, not doing anything about a problematic situation generally results in making things worse, as it sends the message that no one cares.

Administration orbiting: Organizations that engage in this type of strategy keep appeals for change "under consideration." Similar to the "nonaction" strategy, this strategy is often used in the hope that delaying will simply allow the problem to go way. The result is usually increased frustration.

Secrecy: Sometimes conflicts are simply not talked about. This is a common means of avoidance. The conflict may be delayed, but when it surfaces, many negative emotions will be attached.

Law and order: Managers may use this strategy if they believe that they can simply order subordinates not to be in conflict. This tactic only builds resentment toward the manager, and sends the conflict underground, where it is likely to continue to grow and fester.

NEGATIVITY IN ORGANIZATIONS

Goetsch and Davis (2000) defined negativity as any employee behavior that works against the organization's optimum performance. Below the level of actual conflict, negativity can permeate entire organizations, lowering morale and productivity. Goetsch and Davis (2000) list the most common categories of negative behaviors: control disputes; territorial disputes (boundaries); dependence/independence issues; need for attention/responsibility; authority; and loyalty issues.

In some organizations, negativity can become the norm, creating peer pressure that fosters similar negative attitudes in all employees that become part of the organization. Goetsch and Davis (2000) suggest symptoms of negativity that managers should monitor:

- *"I can't" attitudes:* Employees in an organization that is committed to continuous improvement have can-do attitudes. If "I can't" is being heard regularly, negativity has crept into the organization.
- *"They" mentality:* In high-performance organizations, employees say "we" when talking about their employer. If employees refer to the organization as "they," negativity has gained a foothold.
- *Critical conversation:* In high-performance organizations, coffee-break conversation is about positive work-related topics or topics of personal interest. When conversation is typically critical, negative, and judgmental, negativity has set in. Some managers subscribe to the philosophy that employees are not happy unless they are complaining. This is a dangerous attitude. Positive, improvement-oriented employees will complain to their supervisor about conditions that inhibit performance, but they don't sit around criticizing and whining during coffee breaks.
- *Blame fixing:* In a high-performance organization, employees fix problems, not blame. If blame-fixing and finger-pointing are common, negativity is at work. (pp. 427–428)

Once negativity has begun to appear in an organization, the consultant can help managers take specific steps to reduce it. Goetsch and Davis (2000) make the following suggestions:

- *Communicate:* Frequent, ongoing, effective communication is the best defense against negativity in organizations, and it is the best tool for overcoming negativity that has already set in. Organizational communication can be made more effective using the following strategies: acknowledge innovation, suggestions, and concerns; share information so that all employees are informed; encourage open, frank discussion during meetings; celebrate milestones; give employees ownership of their jobs; and promote teamwork.
- *Establish clear expectations:* Make sure all employees know what is expected of them as individuals and as members of the team. People need to know what is expected of them and how and to whom they are accountable for what is expected.
- *Provide for anxiety venting:* The workplace can be stressful in even the best organizations. Deadlines, performance standards, budget pressures, and competition can all produce anxiety in employees. Consequently, managers need to give their direct reports opportunities to vent in a nonthreatening, affirming environment. This means listening supportively. This means letting the employee know that you will not shoot

the messenger and then listening without interrupting, thinking ahead, focusing on preconceived ideas, or tuning out.
- *Build trust:* Negativity cannot flourish in an atmosphere of trust. Managers can build trust between themselves and employees and among employees by applying the following strategies: always delivering what is promised; remaining open-minded to suggestions; taking an interest in the development and welfare of employees; being tactfully honest with employees at all times; lending a hand when necessary; accepting blame, but sharing credit; maintaining a steady, pleasant temperament even when under stress; and making sure that criticism is constructive and delivered in an affirming way.
- *Involve employees:* It's hard to criticize the way things are done when you are a part of how they are done. Involving employees by asking their opinions, soliciting their feedback, and making them part of the solution are some of the most effective deterrents to and cures for negativity in organizations. (p. 428)

TERRITORIAL BEHAVIOR IN ORGANIZATIONS

Human beings and other primates appear to have evolved with a strong predisposition to protect their own territory. In the workplace, this usually takes the form of psychological territory rather than actual physical territory (Goetsch & Davis, 2000). Consultants can help managers recognize territorial behavior when it takes place within an organization. Simmons (1998) lists manifestations that suggest territoriality in the workplace:

- *Occupation:* These games include actually marking territory as *mine*; playing the *gatekeeper* game with information; and monopolizing resources, information, access, and relationships.
- *Information manipulation:* People who play territorial games with information subscribe to the philosophy that information is power. To exercise power they withhold information, bias information to suit their individual agendas (spin), cover up information, and actually give out false information.
- *Intimidation:* One of the most common manifestations of territoriality is intimidation—a tactic used to frighten others away from certain turf. Intimidation can take many different forms, from subtle threats to blatant aggression (physical or verbal).
- *Alliances:* Forming alliances with powerful individuals in an organization is a commonly practiced territorial game. The idea is to say without actually having to speak the words, "You had better keep off my turf, or I'll get my powerful friend to cause trouble."
- *Invisible wall:* Putting up an invisible wall involves creating hidden barriers to ensure that a decision, although already made, cannot be implemented. There are hundreds of strategies for building an invisible wall, including stalling, losing paperwork, forgetting to place an order, and many others.
- *Strategic noncompliance:* Agreeing to a decision up front with no intention of carrying out the decision is called *strategic noncompliance.* This tactic is often used to buy enough time to find a way to reverse the decision.
- *Discredit:* Discrediting an individual to cast doubt on his or her recommendation is a common turf protection tactic. Such an approach is called an *ad hominem* argument, which means if you cannot discredit the recommendation, try to discredit the person making it.
- *Shunning:* Shunning, or excluding an individual who threatens your turf, is a common territorial protection tactic. The point of shunning is to use peer pressure against the individual being shunned.

- *Camouflage:* Other terms that are sometimes used to describe this tactic are *throwing up a smokescreen* or *creating fog.* This tactic involves confusing the issue by raising other distracting controversies, especially those that will produce anxiety and such as encroaching on turf.
- *Filibuster:* Filibustering means talking a recommended action to death. The tactic involves talking at length about concerns—usually inconsequential—until the other side gives in just to stop any further discussion or until time to make the decision runs out. (p. 179)

Overcoming negativity involves fostering cooperation among employees (Goetsch & Davis, 2000). Simmons (1998) makes the following recommendations for overcoming territorial behavior:

- *Avoid jumping to conclusions:* Talk to employees about territoriality versus cooperation. Ask to hear their views, and listen to what they say.
- *Attribute territorial behavior to instinct rather than people:* Blaming people for following their natural instincts is like blaming them for eating. The better approach is to show them that their survival instinct is tied to cooperation, not to turf. This is done by rewarding cooperation and applying negative reinforcement to territorial behavior.
- *Ensure that no employee feels attacked:* Remember that the survival instinct is the driver behind territorial behavior. Attacking employees, or even letting them feel as if they are being attacked, will only serve to trigger their survival instinct. To change territorial behavior, it is necessary to put employees at ease.
- *Avoid generalizations:* When employees exhibit territorial behavior, deal with it in specifics as opposed to generalizations. It is a mistake to witness territorial behavior on the part of one employee and respond by calling a group of employees together and talking about the issues in general terms. Deal with the individual who exhibits the behavior and deal in specifics.
- *Understand "irrational" fears:* The survival instinct is a powerful motivator. It can lead employees to cling irrationally to their fears. Managers should consider this point when dealing with employees who find it difficult to let go of survival behaviors. Be firm but patient, and never deal with an employee's fears in a denigrating or condescending manner.
- *Respect each individual's perspective:* In a way, an individual's perspective or opinion is part of his or her psychological territory. Failure to respect the perspectives of people is the same as threatening their territory. When challenging territorial behavior, let employees explain their perspectives and show respect for them, even if you do not agree.
- *Consider the employee's point of view:* In addition to giving an appropriate level of respect to employees' perspectives, managers should also try to step into their shoes. How would you, as a manager, feel if you were the employee? Sensitivity to the employee's point of view and patience with that point of view are critical when trying to overcome territorial behavior. (p. 187)

After gaining an understanding of what it takes to be a good manager, supervisor, or leader, mental health professionals will not only be better prepared to help the current leadership within organizations, they will also be better prepared to assist in the selection and development of future leadership, which is the topic of the next chapter.

Chapter 5

EXECUTIVE ASSESSMENT, SELECTION, INTERVIEWING, AND DEVELOPMENT

This chapter provides guidance for mental health professionals who assist business clients in choosing executives for their businesses. Finding the right executive involves not only assessing the applicant for the job, but assuring a match between the individual and the organization. Once an organization has a winning team, the consultant can further the professional development of those executives, and increase their success.

This chapter focuses on executive selection for business clients because they are a fairly large market for such services. However, nonprofit settings such as mental health organizations also can use this information. The consultant simply varies the language appropriately for use with different clients. The suggestions here can even be useful for mental health professionals who never do formal consulting. If you participate in the hiring of an office manager, or if you need to decide which accountant to hire for your practice, this chapter may prove helpful.

This chapter also discusses how to do assessments for executives who are already employed, when organizations need to make decisions about training needs, coaching goals, or promotions. Mental health professionals, particularly those with strong assessment backgrounds, are well suited to these tasks. Finally, we discuss how to develop executives within an organization.

PREPARING FOR THE SELECTION TASK

How do you determine what type of selection information you need to obtain? What do you look for psychologically in a leader? Prior to the selection assessment, it is important to clarify with the hiring agent the type of position and the psychological requirements necessary for that position, and to determine the organizational context or culture in which the job is embedded. It is also helpful to identify the areas of assessment that are particularly important. Table 5.1 shows an assessment profile form that the hiring

Table 5.1   Assessment Profile

Candidate's Name:

Position:

Which of the following areas of psychological assessment are you particularly interested in regarding this candidate?

Descriptor	Yes	No	In Depth
Intellectual characteristics			
Articulation			
Presentational characteristics			
Emotional characteristics			
Motivational characteristics			
Insight into oneself and others			
Interpersonal characteristics			
Vocational characteristics			
Leadership characteristics			
Management style characteristics			
Capacity to delegate			
Decision-making capacity			
Projected fit with the job context			
Projected fit with company culture			

Do you want to fill out the "Position Analysis Questionnaire," which is a structured job analysis questionnaire that can be used for analyzing jobs?   Yes   No

If not, please fill out the attached Psychological Evaluation Job Description and Referral Sheet.

Thank you for clarifying the assessment task!

agent can fill out along with the Position Analysis Questionnaire (McCormick, Jeanneret, & Mecham, 1969).

INTRODUCTION TO THE APPLICANT

When first meeting applicants, consultants should clarify their role, just as mental health professionals do with therapy clients, and address issues such as confidentiality. You can use the sample script shown in Box 5.1 to introduce yourself to the job applicant.

Box 5.1

Sample Script

I've been retained by the _____ Company to assist them in the selection process for _____ . My primary job will be to learn to understand you as fully as possible so I can provide input into the selection process. It is in both the company's and your best interest that we find a good fit between your needs, interests, and personality and the psychological requirements of this position. In this case, I work for the _____ Company, so I will ask you to waive the right to confidentiality regarding what we discuss in our meeting. (Present release of information form with company name on it.) This will allow me to freely share what we discuss in an open fashion with your full knowledge and consent. Also, the testing results will be the property of the _____ Company, so you will not have access to the data unless you are hired. Do you have any questions?

RESUME REVIEW

The consultant should carefully review the applicant's resume or vitae. Are there any gaps in the employment history? If so, make a note to inquire about this during the interview. Also, look over the applicant's educational background (diplomas or certificates obtained, courses taken, and grades achieved), as well as the applicant's occupational background (past jobs and duties, history of career progression). Keep in mind that a large percentage of resumes contain exaggerated or inaccurate information (Bolles & Bolles, 2005). It is often helpful to assess what the applicant is trying to leave and what the applicant is going toward. It is also fruitful to explain why an applicant left previous positions and what they liked and disliked about the previous positions they held.

INTERVIEW DATA COLLECTION

Two major skill sets are important in psychological executive selection: (1) the ability to do a selection interview, and (2) the ability to do a psychological testing assessment.

There are many more aspects to selection from a human resources (HR) standpoint, such as contacting references and ensuring that applicants know the technical parts of their job, but these are typically done by individuals in the HR department and by others in the company. The consultant should simply make sure that someone is doing them and that the psychological evaluation is viewed as input into the hiring decision, not as the total basis for the decision.

SELECTION INTERVIEWING

When given a selection task, you should consider the following two questions:

1. What characteristics are you selecting for (what kind of person is required for this position at this time)?
2. What kinds of questions will best address these issues?

Preparation, as always, is important. Jotting down key questions beforehand will help guide the interview.

Typically, the interview has very low validity as a selection technique. *Behavioral interviewing* has been shown to be a much more effective technique than ordinary interviews in selecting people. The key principles of behavioral interviewing are based on the idea that past behavior is the best predictor of future behavior, so your questions should try to solicit as many examples as possible of the candidate's actual past behavior. To do that, you put candidates in actual situations asking them what they would do, or more often, put them in past situations to report what they actually did. Follow-up questions are important because many job candidates are rehearsed and able to give socially desirable answers to most questions.

Interviewer Responses

In addition to carefully choosing questions to ask interviewees, consultants should consciously decide how to respond to the interviewee's responses. The consultant can use two broad categories of responses to the candidate when conducting interviews—*probing responses* and *understanding responses* (which summarize and clarify the responses given).

Probing responses are given by the interviewer to gather more information, and consist of *general leads, binary questions, follow-up leads, cue-exploration leads, continuation leads, amplification leads,* and *testing questions.* General leads are nonspecific questions or requests (e.g., "Tell me about yourself"). Binary questions can be answered with a yes or a no (e.g., "Have you ever worked as a CFO before?"). Follow-up leads are specific questions based on prior responses (e.g., "You said you worked before at Acme Company. What was your job there?"). Cue-exploration leads are questions phrased in responses to cues given by the client (e.g., "I noticed that you cringed when you mentioned the name of your last supervisor—what was that about?"). Continuation leads are designed to keep the client talking about a particular topic (e.g., "Go on about what went wrong for you at your last job?"). Amplification leads are requests for further explanation (e.g., "You said you were unhappy—what was that like for you?"). Testing questions are those that test out theories that the consultant is forming (e.g., if the consultant is wondering if the person is introverted, she might ask "How do you recharge at the end of a hard day?").

Understanding responses express acknowledgment and empathy for the interview; they consist of *restatement, paraphrase, reflection,* and *summarization.* These four responses are well known to mental health professionals. Restatement involves repetition of the interviewee's words. Paraphrase is a restatement of the client's response in the consultant's words. Reflection involves mirroring back to the client the feelings that the consultant believes the client is experiencing. Summarization is a recapitulation of the data gathered thus far (Cormier & Cormier, 1998).

CASE EXAMPLE

A university asked for assistance in selecting candidates for the position of provost. Following are some of the questions that the consultant asked:

- Why are you considering leaving X, and what attracts you to this university? (When one person was asked this question, he revealed trouble with his boss and prejudicial attitudes.)
- Talk about the last time you had a dean or chair with a performance problem and how you dealt with it? (This question is behaviorally based, looking for what candidates have actually done, not what they idealistically believe they would do.)
- List some situations that illustrate your strengths, your weaknesses? (This question differs from the traditional "Tell me about your strengths and weaknesses" because it is also behaviorally based.)
- Talk about a time when you faced adversity on the job and how you coped with it?
- What are your most important guiding values/principles?
- What system do you use to allocate scarce resources among deans (chairs)?

Sample Interview Questions

Interview questions should flow from the information that needs to be gathered for the particular position that needs to be filled. To ensure fairness, all candidates should be asked the same general questions. The following provide some ideas for potential interview questions:

Tell me about yourself.

Describe some situations that illustrate your greatest strengths and weaknesses.

Cite what your boss, peers, and subordinates respectively would identify as your greatest strength and your greatest weakness.

How do you compensate for your weaknesses?

What is your reason for considering a career change?

What would you redesign about your last job, and why?

Describe a work situation that best illustrates your management style.

How would you describe the principles that guide your management style?

Describe a manager you have known who was successful. What qualities did this successful manager possess?

If you were hiring a person for this position, what qualities would you look for?

How do you assess the strengths and weaknesses of the company and its current executive team? Its personality?

Describe your career plan and how this job fits into it.

What do you really want to do in life?

What are your reasons for believing you can fill this position?

What are your job-related skills?

Tell me about your duties and responsibilities on your last job.

What are you looking for in this position?

What two or three things are most important to you in a job?

What are the most important rewards you want from your career?

What motivates you to put forth your greatest effort?

Describe a situation in which you were successful and felt satisfaction. . . . How do you determine or evaluate success?

What do you think determines whether someone is successful in a position like this one?

Describe the work environment you have been the most comfortable in. What did you like?

How have you tried to be a part of (or develop) the team in your last job? What was your role on the executive team?

Describe a pressured work situation and how you coped with it.

Give me an example of when you had difficulty getting along with a coworker and how you dealt with the situation.

Tell me about the last time you were faced with an angry consumer of your services.

Describe a situation with a difficult employee and how you handled it.

Describe a situation in which you initiated a change in your workplace on your own.

Describe an experience in which your values differed from those around you. What happened? How do you feel about diversity in the workplace?

Describe situations in which you have gone out of your way to show respect and concern for someone while at work. How did you feel about how people were treated at your last place of employment? Why?

Describe two mistakes you made and what you learned from them.

What values do you feel are most important?

What is your current understanding of the meaning of life?

What are some of the obstacles you have had to overcome to get where you are today? How did you overcome them?

What (subject, teacher, job, boss, life event) did you value (most, least)?

How would you describe your (mother, father, sibling, teacher, boss, friend, spouse, child, job, organization, management style, strengths, shortcomings, self, etc.)?

Where have you received the most (praise, criticism, success, failure, satisfaction, frustration)?

If you had three wishes . . .

If you could meet anyone in history . . .

What kind of animal would you like to be and why. . .

If you could relive your life . . .

What do you do for fun? (cultural interests, weekends/holidays, projects)

What kinds of activities depress you the most?

What is the last book you read? What do you typically read?

What are some areas that we may not have covered that you would like to emphasize?

Legal Considerations for Preemployment Interviews

In general, the consultant must remember that all questions should be job related, and any general question asked should be asked of all job candidates (Lussier, 2002). There are several things an employer (or the consultant as an agent of the employer) cannot ask about because of laws such as the Americans with Disabilities Act and Equal Employment Opportunity legislation. Such topics include questions related to marital status, health (e.g., such as whether someone is pregnant), religion, ethnicity, age, and so on. The exception to this is if the question is related to a *bona fide occupational qualification* (BFOQ), which allows employers to discriminate if necessary for the normal operation of a particular enterprise. For example, it would be legal for an employer to inquire about a candidate's weight if a fire department needed the firefighters to be more than a certain reasonable weight to be able to carry victims out of burning buildings.

Consultants involved in executive selection must be familiar with what they can and cannot ask the job candidates. Lussier (2002) presents a summary of these types of questions (see Box 5.2).

PSYCHOLOGICAL TESTING

Organizations that are interested in hiring individuals with the best fit realize that mental health professionals possess a valuable skill—they can administer and interpret psychological tests. As with clinical practice, it is important to clarify the requisites for the position to be filled and then to determine which tests will best measure those qualities (Lowman, 1989, 1991).

Example Psychological Testing Instruments

  I. Personality Assessment
    A. Objective Personality Inventory
       1. 16 PF (Russell & Karol, 1994)
       2. California Personality Inventory
       3. NEO-PI-R (Costa & McCrae, 1992)
       4. Guilford Zimmer Temperament Survey
       5. Hogan Personality Inventory
       6. Myers-Briggs Type Indicator
       7. Edwards Personal Preference Inventory
       8. Guilford-Zimmerman Temperament Inventory
    B. Projective
       1. Sentence Completion
       2. Thematic Apperception Test (TAT)
  II. Management Style Assessment
    A. Management Style Diagnostic Test (Reddin)
    B. Executive Profile Summary (National Computer Systems)
    C. Leadership Inventory (Kouzes & Posner)
    D. 16 PF Leadership Style Indicators
  III. Management Success
    A. Leadership Motive Pattern on Thematic Apperception Test
    B. Diagnosis Test for Management Development
    C. Leadership Opinion Questionnaire
  IV. Motivational Assessment
    A. Motivational Analysis Test (IPAT)
  V. Job Analysis/Description (filled out by employer)
    A. Executive Position Analysis Questionnaire (Consulting Psychologists Press, Inc.)

=== **Box 5.2** ===

Legal and Illegal Interview Questions

Name

Can ask: Current legal name and whether the candidate has ever worked under a different name.

Cannot ask: Maiden name or whether the person has changed his or her name.

Age

Can ask: If the candidate is between specific age groups, 21 to 70, to meet job specifications. If hired, can you furnish proof of age?

Cannot ask: How old are you?

Marital and Family Status

Can ask: If the candidate can meet the work schedule or job and whether the candidate has activities, responsibilities, or commitments that may hinder meeting attendance requirements. The same question(s) should be asked of both sexes.

Cannot ask: To select a marital status or any questions regarding children or other family issues.

National Origin, Citizenship, Race, or Color

Can ask: If the candidate is legally eligible to work in the United States, and if this can be proven if hired.

Cannot ask: To identify national origin, citizenship, race, or color (or that of parents and other relatives).

Language

Can ask: To list languages the candidate speaks and/or writes fluently. May be asked if they speak and/or write a specific language if it is a BFOQ.

Cannot ask: The language spoken off the job, or how the applicant learned the language.

Convictions

Can ask: If the candidate has been convicted of a felony and other information if the felony is job related.

Cannot ask: If the candidate has ever been arrested.

Height and Weight

Can ask: If the candidate meets or exceeds BFOQ height and/or weight requirements, and if it can be proven if hired.

Cannot ask: The candidate's height or weight if it is not a BFOQ.

Religion

Can ask: If the candidate is of a specific religion when it is a BFOQ. If the candidate can meet the work schedules or anticipated absences.

Cannot ask: Religious preference, affiliations, or denominations.

(Continued)

=== **Box 5.2 (continued)** ===

Credit Ratings or Garnishments

Can ask: If it is a BFOQ.

Cannot ask: If it is not a BFOQ.

Education and Work Experience

Can ask: For information that is job related.

Cannot ask: For information that is not job related.

References

Can ask: For the names of people willing to provide references. For the names of people who suggested the candidate apply for the job.

Cannot ask: For a reference from a religious leader.

Military

Can ask: For information on education and experience gained that relates to the job.

Cannot ask: Dates and conditions of discharge. National Guard or Reserve units of candidates. About experiences in foreign armed services.

Organizations

Can ask: To list membership in job-related organizations, like union or professional or trade associations.

Cannot ask: To identify membership in a non-job-related organization that would indicate race, religion, and so on.

Disabilities/AIDS

Can ask: If the candidate has any disabilities that would prevent him or her from performing the specific job.

Cannot ask: For information that is not job related. In states where people with AIDS are protected under disabled discrimination laws, you should not ask if the candidate has AIDS. (pp. 462–464)

Source: From *Human Relations in Organizations: Applications and Skill Building,* fifth edition, by R. N. Lussier, 2002, Boston: McGraw-Hill/Irwin.

VI. Team Involvement/Group Behavior
   A. Fundamental Interpersonal Relations Orientation-Behavior (FIRO-B; Schutz, 1977)
VII. Abilities Measures
   A. General Ability
      1. Wonderlic Personnel Test
      2. Wechsler Adult Intelligence Scale—Third Edition
      3. Wide Range Achievement Test
   B. Specific Abilities
      1. Miller Analogies Test
      2. Watson-Glaser Critical Thinking Appraisal (verbal reasoning ability)

3. Raven Progressive Matrices (nonverbal reasoning ability)
4. Bennett Mechanical Comprehension Test (mechanical reasoning)
5. Minnesota Paper Form Board (spatial ability)
6. Comprehensive Ability Battery (CAB), Flexibility of Closure (field dependence/independence; Hakstian & Cattell, 1982)
7. Meier Art Judgment (aesthetic judgment)
8. CAB-rd (artistic ability)
9. Musical Aptitudes and Abilities (artistic ability)
10. Interpersonal Problem-Solving Assessment Technique (social-related aptitudes and abilities)
11. Tests of Social Intelligence, Missing Cartoons (social-related aptitudes)
12. Minnesota Clerical Test (perceptual speed and accuracy)
13. Writing Sample (writing ability)
14. CAB-O (creative imagination)
15. CAB-Fi (ideational fluency)
16. CAB-Ma (memory)
17. Batteries of abilities
    a. Comprehensive Abilities Battery (IPAT)
    b. Differential Aptitude Test Battery
    c. Armed Services Vocational Aptitude Battery
18. Employee Aptitude Survey

VIII. Sales and Sales Management
   A. 16 PF Sales Success Indicators

IX. Interests/Career Issues
   A. Strong Vocational Preference Inventory
   B. Holland Self-Directed Search
   C. Vocational Aptitude Test
   D. Campbell Interests and Skill Inventory
   E. Kuder Vocational Preference Test

X. Values
   A. Rokeach Value Survey (Rokeach, 1973)

XI. Entrepreneurial Testing
   A. 16 PF Entrepreneurial Scale

XII. Emotional Intelligence
   A. Emotional Competence Inventory (Boyatzis, Goleman, & HayGroup, 2001)
   B. Mayer-Salovey-Caruso Emotional Intelligence Test (MSCEIT, Mayer, Salovey, & Caruso, 2002).
   C. Emotional Quotient Inventory (EQ-i; Reuven Bar-On, 2002)

XIII. Personality Disorder
   A. MCMI-III

XIV. Strengths
   A. Strength Deployment Inventory

XV. Symptoms (not for use in selection)
   A. Adjective Checklist

The consultant should be familiar with and qualified to administer and interpret an instrument before using it and should be aware of potential issues in applying it in different contexts. For example, the Minnesota Multiphasic Personality Inventory

(MMPI or MMPI-2) has not been included on this list. This instrument is used to assess psychopathology, but to make hiring decisions based on the presence of a mental illness would be considered discrimination under the Americans with Disabilities Act (ADA). The exceptions to this include selection for some forms of law enforcement and fire department personnel, which requires special training.

Brief descriptions of several popular instruments used in organizational consultation settings follow.

FIRO-B

The FIRO-B (Fundamental Interpersonal Relations Orientation-Behavior) (Schutz, 1977) is a measure of an individual's interpersonal orientation. It is based on Schutz's theory of group process (Schutz, 1958, 1992). Schutz hypothesized that the patterns of interactions among individuals can be explained largely in terms of three interpersonal needs: inclusion, control, and affection. From a group development perspective, as soon as a group is formed, the inclusion phase begins. People have concerns such as whether they want to remain a group member. After problems of inclusion are sorted out, control problems become the center of concern. At this point, the issue of decision making arises. Each person in the group is attempting to structure the situation to achieve just the right amount of responsibility in the group. Assuming that the control issues are resolved successfully, the group moves to the affection phase. At this point, when the group has been formed and the problems of responsibility and power distribution have been worked out, all that remains is the problem of emotional integration. Each member attempts to establish the most comfortable position possible for affectional interchange. The three phases are not discrete—all types of behavior occur in all phases. However, the phases represent periods in the group's history that emphasize particular problem areas.

The FIRO-B is a measure of an individual's level of need for inclusion, need for control, and need for affection. These three areas are measured in regard to how much they are expressed toward others and how much they are wanted from others. Hence, the FIRO-B results consist of six numbers.

An individual's interpersonal style can be important, especially in relationship to supervisors, peers, and subordinates. For example, if a supervisor has a strong need to express affection, and a subordinate scores low in wanted affection, difficulties may arise in their working relationship unless they can find a way to consciously work with this difference.

Values

Rokeach (1973) argued that people possess only a relatively small number of values, but differ in the importance that they ascribe to them. He divided them into two major categories: *instrumental values* and *terminal values*. Instrumental, or "means oriented" values prescribe desirable standards of conduct for attaining an end. Terminal, or "ends oriented" values prescribe desirable ends or goals for the individual (Rokeach, 1973; Whetton & Cameron, 2002). Table 5.2 lists the values "judged to represent the most important values in American society" (Rokeach, 1973, p. 29).

Consultants can administer the Rokeach Value Survey (RVS; Rokeach, 1973), or can simply ask applicants to list the values that they hold as most important and compare them with the values of the organization. A consultant who is working with two

Table 5.2   Important Values in American Society

Terminal Values	Instrumental Values
A comfortable life (a prosperous life)	Ambitious (hard working, aspiring)
An exciting life (a stimulating, active life)	Broadminded (open-minded)
A sense of accomplishment (lasting contribution)	Capable (competent, effective)
A world at peace (free of war and conflict)	Cheerful (lighthearted, joyful)
A world of beauty (beauty of nature and the arts)	Clean (neat, tidy)
Equality (brotherhood, equal opportunity for all)	Courageous (standing up for your beliefs)
Family security (taking care of loved ones)	Forgiving (willing to pardon others)
Freedom (independence, free choice)	Helpful (working for the welfare of others)
Happiness (contentedness)	Honest (sincere, truthful)
Inner harmony (freedom from inner conflict)	Imaginative (daring, creative)
Mature love (sexual and spiritual intimacy)	Independent (self-reliant, self-sufficient)
National security (protection from attack)	Intellectual (intelligent, reflective)
Pleasure (an enjoyable, leisurely life)	Logical (consistent, rational)
Salvation (saved, eternal life)	Loving (affectionate, tender)
Self-respect (self-esteem)	Obedient (dutiful, respectful)
Social recognition (respect, admiration)	Polite (courteous, well-mannered)
True friendship (close companionship)	Responsible (dependable, reliable)
Wisdom (a mature understanding of life)	Self-controlled (restrained, self-disciplined)

executives who are not getting along can ask each of them to rank their values, which might reveal that part of their conflict is due to a different prioritizing of values.

Emotional Intelligence

Emotional intelligence refers to an assortment of noncognitive skills, abilities, and competencies that affect an individual's ability to cope with environmental demands and pressures (Goleman, 1995; Robbins, 2001; Salovey & Mayer, 1990). It consists of five dimensions:

- *Self-awareness:* exhibited by self-confidence, realistic self-assessment, and a self-deprecating sense of humor.
- *Self-management:* exhibited by trustworthiness and integrity, comfort with ambiguity, and openness to change.
- *Self-motivation:* exhibited by a strong drive to achieve, optimism, and high organizational commitment.
- *Empathy:* exhibited by expertise in building and retaining talent, cross-cultural sensitivity, and service to clients and customers.
- *Social skills:* exhibited by the ability to lead change efforts, persuasiveness, and expertise in building and leading teams. (Robbins, 2001, pp. 332–333)

Organizations are increasingly recognizing the importance of how an individual handles emotions (Cherniss & Goleman, 2001). Mental health professionals are uniquely qualified to assist in assessing emotional intelligence and in intervening to

===== **Box 5.3** =====

EQ-i Scales

Total EQ
Intrapersonal EQ
    —Self-regard
    —Emotional self-awareness
    —Assertiveness
    —Independence
    —Self-actualization
Interpersonal EQ
    —Empathy
    —Social responsibility
    —Interpersonal relationship
Stress Management EQ
    —Stress tolerance
    —Impulse control
Stress Management EQ
    —Stress tolerance
    —Impulse control
Adaptability EQ
    —Reality testing
    —Flexibility
    —Problem solving
General Mood EQ
    —Optimism
    —Happiness

Standard Score	Interpretive Guideline
130+	Enhanced skills—atypically well-developed emotional and social capacity
102–129	Enhanced skills—extremely well-developed emotional and social capacity
110–119	Effective functioning—well-developed emotional and social capacity
90–109	Effective functioning—adequate emotional and social capacity
80–89	Effective functioning—slightly below average emotional and social capacity
70–79	Needs improvement—extremely underdeveloped emotional and social capacity, requiring improvement
Under 70	Needs improvement—atypically impaired emotional and social capacity, requiring improvement

Source: From *Bar-On Emotional Quotient Inventory,* by R. Bar-On, 2002, North Tonawanda, NY: Multi-Health Systems.

increase the emotional intelligence of members throughout an organization. The consultant must remember, however, to do this in the context of the workplace and be careful not to engage in psychotherapy. The emphasis should be on increasing an individual's skills and comfort with the preceding five areas, and in helping organizations structure their policies and procedures in a manner that is conducive to emotional health.

The Bar-On Emotional Quotient Inventory (EQ-i; Bar-On, 2002) is a popular instrument for assessing emotional intelligence. Similar to an IQ test, the EQ-i gives standard scores (mean = 100, standard deviation = 15) for a total Emotional Quotient (EQ), five composite scales, and 15 content subscales, as shown in Box 5.3.

Consultants can look at an individual's EQ scores to add incremental data to how an individual will perform in certain situations. For example, an applicant with a very low Stress Management EQ may not be the best choice for the position of general manager in a fast-paced organization.

ITEMS TO INCLUDE IN THE REPORT OUTLINE

Consultants can customize the final assessment report according to the consultee's needs, but most reports will include the following information:

- Identifying information
- Characteristics determined from assessment data
- Intellect
- Articulation and presentation
- Emotion
- Motivation
- Insight into oneself and others
- Interpersonal attitudes
- Vocational goals
- Leadership ability
- Management style
- Capacity to delegate
- Decision-making capacity
- Projected fit with organizational culture and job context
- Summary and recommendations

These areas parallel the example assessment profile (Table 5.1) that was given to the hiring agent. If the company is not interested in something, or it is not relevant to the task, omit it from the report.

As with other assessments performed by mental health professionals, the consultant must choose a testing battery that suits the needs of the referral question. Typically, consultants will have several core tests with which they feel comfortable, and will add other tests as needed. The career assessment battery discussed in Chapter 2 can help determine fit with a given job context: It includes one or two measures of interest and personality, tests for general intelligence (G), and necessary specific abilities. Of the instruments listed earlier, a typical battery might consist of the following:

- Wonderlic/portions of the Wechsler Adult Intelligence Scale
- Comprehensive Ability Battery (CAB) subtests (Hakstian & Cattell, 1982)
- NEO/CPI/16 PF
- Strong/Vocational Preference Inventory
- FIRO-B (Schutz, 1977)
- Leadership Inventory
- Values (Rokeach, 1973)

Although it is sometimes tempting to overload the client with a multitude of instruments, the assessment process should always follow from the assessment question. Also, just as clinicians can use assessment feedback as an intervention, consultants can sometimes use feedback with applicants to get additional information and insight (assuming the consultant has discussed this arrangement with the consultee).

When designing the assessment and selecting the instruments and methods to be used, the consultant should consider the specific preferences of the client or organization. The organization may have a standard battery that they prefer, based on past performance or perhaps based on the advice of their legal department. The consultant should also consider the administrative convenience of certain instruments or methods, such as the amount of time involved, and the ease of administration and scoring. Costs should also be considered, especially if the consultant will need to develop and use a customized instrument.

The consultant should also consider the acceptability of the assessment tools to all the stakeholders involved. Do the instruments unnecessarily invade a candidate's privacy? Does the instrument have face validity (does it appear to be measuring something that is relevant to its business purpose)?

As in clinical practice, mental health professionals conducting psychological testing in the workplace must also understand reliability and validity issues, which are the standards for evaluating criterion measures. Reliability refers to how well the instrument consistently measures the criterion. Validity refers to how well an instrument measures what it purports to measure. Consultants should take care to research the reliability and validity of all the instruments they use, and must remember not to base important decisions on only one assessment method.

CASE EXAMPLE

A school system in a major metropolitan area once approached a consultant asking for assistance in selecting an important leadership position. The consultant agreed, only to quickly find out that the school system did not really want much help from the consultant. The consultant was not permitted to interview the applicants or see any of their background information. The consultant was asked simply to administer the 16PF and interpret the results. Though this was not the preference of the consultant, he was able to make some tentative inferences based on the testing and offered some ideas about things to look for in particular applicants.

This case illustrates that in actual practice the consultant often is not able to work under ideal conditions.

OTHER TYPES OF EXECUTIVE ASSESSMENT

Besides using executive assessment when hiring new executives, you can use it to assess and improve the performance of current employees and to groom individuals for internal promotions.

When looking for sources of information to assess the functioning of current managers, the consultant should consider the following:

1. Get upward appraisals by asking the people who work for the manager to evaluate that person.

2. Ask the manager to complete an inventory of normal personality and one of the new inventories of personality disorders (thereby assessing the manager's bright and dark sides).

3. Get some sense of how the manager's unit is performing, relative to other, comparable units in that or other organizations.

4. Ask the subordinates to give you some critical incidents of notably good or poor performance by this manager.

The outline shown in Box 5.4 offers some guiding principles in conducting psychological assessments with executives (Miner, 1991). It is divided into the search for individual causes, group causes, and organizational/contextual causes of underlying difficulties.

Tobias (1990) offers a comprehensive list of questions to use in integrating data for a detailed psychological assessment report (see Appendix).

AN EXAMPLE PROPOSAL

Once the mental health professional has spoken with someone about being engaged with the organization as a consultant, the consultant's understanding of the agreement should be put in writing (see Box 5.5 on p. 132). The proposal should name the project specifically, describe its scope, give a time estimate, explicitly state the cost, discuss confidentiality, and give the background qualifications of the consultant.

JOB ANALYSIS

In addition to conducting a complete assessment of the executive, the consultant must analyze the job in which the executive is working or hopes to work, in order to consider compatibility factors. A *job analysis* involves systematically gathering and analyzing information about the content, context, and the human requirements of a given job (Mathis & Jackson, 2003).

The consultant should first review the human resource department's job description and job specification for that particular position. A job description is simply a written statement of what the jobholder does, along with how and why it is done. A job specification details the minimum qualification the employee must possess to successfully perform the job (Robbins, 2001).

When gathering data, consultants should focus on the knowledge, skills, and abilities (KSAs) needed for the position. The consultant is especially interested in collecting

Box 5.4

Scheme for Carrying Out Diagnoses in Psychological Assessment

Individual Causes

- Intelligence and Job Knowledge
  - —Insufficient Verbal Ability
  - —Insufficient Special Ability (Numerical, Mechanical, etc.)
  - —Insufficient Job Knowledge
  - —Defect of Judgment or Memory
- Individual Motivation
  - —Strong Motives Frustrated at Work
  - —Strong Motives Satisfied Through Means Not Job-Integrated
  - —Excessively Low Personal Work Standards
  - —Generalized Low Work Motivation
- Emotions and Emotional Illness
  - —Frequent Disruptive Emotions (Anxiety, Depression, Anger, etc.)
  - —Psychosis
  - —Personality Disorders
  - —Alcohol and Drug Problems
- Physical Characteristics and Disorders
  - —Physical Illness or Handicap
  - —Physical Disorders of Emotional Origin
  - —Inappropriate (to the Job) Physical Characteristics
  - —Insufficient Muscular or Sensory Ability or Skill

Group Causes

- The Groups at Work
  - —Negative Consequences Associated with Group Cohesion
  - —Ineffective Management
  - —Inappropriate (to the Job) Managerial Standards and Criteria
- Family Ties
  - —Family Crises (Divorce, Death, etc.)
  - —Separation from a Family
  - —Predominance of Family Considerations Over Work Demands

Organizational/Contextual Causes

- The Organization
  - —Insufficient Organizational Action
  - —Placement Error
  - —Inappropriate (to the Job) Organizational Style (Overpermissive, Excessive Training, etc.)
  - —Excessive Span of Control
  - —Inappropriate (to the Job) Organizational Standards and Criteria

---

Box 5.4 (continued)

- The Societal Context
  - —Application of Legal Sanctions
  - —Application of Societal Values
  - —Conflict between Job Demands and Societal Values (Morality, Fair Play, etc.)
- The Work Context
  - —Negative Consequences of Economic Forces (Competition, Recession, etc.)
  - —Negative Consequences of Geographic Location (Climate, Population, etc.)
  - —Detrimental Conditions in the Work Setting (Noise, Illumination, etc.)
  - —Excessive Danger (Real and Phobic)

Source: From "Psychological Assessment in a Developmental Context" (pp. 225–236), by J. B. Miner, in *A Handbook of Psychological Assessment in Business,* C. P. Hansen and K. A. Conrad (Eds.), 1991, New York: Quorum Books.

---

data on how the job is different from other jobs. Mathis and Jackson (2003) provide the following list to help make this distinction:

- Work activities and behaviors
- Interactions with others
- Performance standards
- Financial and budgeting impact
- Machines and equipment used
- Working conditions
- Supervision given and received
- Knowledge, skills, and abilities needed (p. 180)

Consultants can go about gathering this data in several ways. Robbins (2001) lists the following popular job analysis methods:

- *Observation:* An analyst watches employees directly or reviews films of workers on the job.
- *Interviews:* Selected job incumbents are extensively interviewed, and the results of a number of interviews are combined into a single job analysis.
- *Diaries:* Job incumbents record their daily activities, and the amount of time spent on each, in a diary or log.
- *Questionnaires:* Incumbents check or rate the items they perform in their jobs from a long list of possible task items. (p. 476)

The Position Analysis Questionnaire (PAQ; McCormick et al., 1969) is a standardized, structured job analysis questionnaire containing 195 questions (Gatewood & Feild, 1998). Primoff, Clark, and Caplan (1982) described the six basic sections of the PAQ:

1. *Information input:* Where and how a worker gets information needed to perform the job.
2. *Mental processes:* The reasoning, decision making, planning, and information-processing activities that are involved in performing the job.

=== **Box 5.5** ===

Selection of the General Manager Position

This proposal outlines an individualized "selection process" designed to im-proved the probability of selecting an outstanding general manager for X.

Scope of the Project

Consultant, with the consultation of X staff, will develop a position analysis for the General Manager position and design a selection test battery including a psychological interview for the candidate(s). One to three candidates will be evaluated with the selection process and results will be presented back to the company both orally and in written report format. As a part of a developmental process, the results of the psychological evaluation will later be shared with any candidate who is awarded the General Manager position. The meetings with staff will take place at X and the psychological assessment will take place at facilities provided by the University Psychological Services Association.

The purpose of the selection evaluation is to hire an outstanding general manager who:

• Fits the organizational culture,
• Has outstanding abilities,
• Holds interests consistent with the position,
• Has a personality that will be effective in the position,
• Has the motivation to be successful and productive,
• Evidences the requisite behavioral and interpersonal skills to work effec-tively in a leadership position.

Time Estimate

Work will begin on the position analysis immediately following approval of the proposal. The selection report will be submitted to the company 1 week after test materials are returned by the applicant (some time is required for the com-puter laboratory to score the materials). The developmental coaching session will be arranged at the convenience of the new General Manager.

Cost

$1,500 per executive evaluation.

Confidentiality

The applicants will be asked to waive their confidentiality and their right to see the final evaluation unless they are hired by X. The testing materials will re-main with the Division of Applied Psychology and the testing report will be the property of the Client Company.

Consultant

This proposal is presented by John R. Rudisill, PhD, Dean of the Wright State University School of Professional Psychology. Dr. Rudisill is an organizational and clinical psychologist specializing in corporate psychology issues. Support for the project will be provided by the Organizational Group of University Psy-chological Services Associates (UPSA).

Thank you for the opportunity to provide this proposal. For more informa-tion, please call (555) 555-5555.

3. *Work output:* the physical activities, tools, and devices used by the worker to perform the job.
4. *Relationships with other persons:* The relationships with other people that are required in performing the job.
5. *Job context:* The physical and social context where the work is performed.
6. *Other job characteristics:* The activities, conditions, and characteristics other than those already described that are relevant to the job (pp. 5–6).

Brumback, Romashko, Hahn, and Fleishman (1974) described the six types of rating scales used by the PAQ:

1. *Extent of use:* The degree to which an item is used by the worker.
2. *Amount of time:* The proportion of time spent doing something.
3. *Importance to this job:* The importance of an activity specified by the item in performing the job.
4. *Possibility of occurrence:* The degree to which there is a possibility of physical hazards on the job.
5. *Applicability:* Whether an item applies to the job or not.
6. *Special code:* Special rating scales that are used with a particular item on the PAQ (p. 19).

LEGAL CONSIDERATIONS FOR PSYCHOLOGICAL TESTING IN THE WORKPLACE

It is very important for the consultant to have some familiarity with the basic laws that apply to psychological testing in the workplace. Such information can be obtained from textbooks on human resources (Mathis & Jackson, 2003). For example, it is important to know that only work-related testing can be required prehire, but clinical testing can be administered post hire.

The consultant should be especially aware of laws that help to prevent discrimination in hiring practices, such as the following.

Adverse Impact

Title VII of the 1964 Civil Rights Act (as amended in 1972) prohibits discrimination in hiring, placement, training, promotion, and retention on the basis of race, color, religion, sex, or national origin; and more recent legislation similarly prohibits discrimination on the basis of age or disability. The provisions of Title VII and related laws are enforced by the U. S. Equal Employment Opportunity Commission (EEOC), which issues the "Uniform Guidelines on Employee Selection Procedures." These guidelines apply to any measure, combination of measures, or procedure used as a basis for employment decision and pertain to selection procedures ranging from traditional paper-and-pencil tests, performance tests, training programs, or probationary periods and physical education and work experience requirements through informal or casual interviews and unscored application forms (U.S. Equal Employment Opportunity Commission, 2005).

Eighty Percent Rule

According to the Uniform Guidelines, an employment procedure might be discriminating against a minority group when it is having an "adverse impact." Adverse impact occurs when use of a procedure results in a substantially different selection, placement, or promotion rate for members of a subgroup. The 80% (Four-Fifths) Rule is often used to determine if a procedure is having an adverse impact. Using this rule, the hiring rate for minority group members is divided by the hiring rate for non-minority group members; if the result is less than 80%, then adverse impact is occurring. For example, if use of a selection test results in a 50% hiring rate for African Americans and a 90% rate for Whites, the test would be having an adverse impact for African Americans since 50% divided by 90% is 55%, which is less than 80%. A shortcoming of the 80% Rule is that it can be used to determine discrimination only when the person is a member of a specific group. In other words, for a finding of adverse impact, the 80% Rule requires establishing a pattern of discrimination.

Differential Validity

Another cause of adverse impact is differential validity. This occurs when a measure is valid for one group but is not valid (or is significantly less valid) for another group. Recent validity generalization studies suggest that differential validity is quite rare.

Unfairness

Unfairness is another cause of adverse impact. It occurs when members of one group consistently obtain lower scores on a predictor than members of another group, but the differences in scores are not reflected in differences in actual job performance.

The employer can counter the adverse impact charge by pleading "business necessity." If this fails, the court usually recommends the employer either (1) use an alternative procedure that does not have an adverse impact; (2) revise the measure so that it is valid; (3) use the measure in a different way (e.g., use a lower cutoff score for minorities if the predictor consistently underestimates their job performance); or (4) provide training when adverse impact is the result of consistently lower criterion scores on the part of minority group members so that their criterion scores reach acceptable levels.

COMMON SELECTION PREDICTORS

Interviews

Typical selection interviews contain inadequacies. The content of interviews are rarely matched to the requirements of the job. The accuracy of an interview is highly affected by interviewer biases. Evaluations tend to be based on the interviewer's first impressions of interviewees. Interviews can be affected by a "contrast effect," which occurs when an interview's assessment of an applicant is influenced by impressions of previous applicants.

How do you improve the validity and reliability of interviews? Training interviewers in the interview process increases the accuracy of interviews. The job relatedness of interviews is improved by basing the content of interviews on the results of a job analysis and by using the interview to obtain only certain kinds of information, such as work motivation, interpersonal skills, and technical knowledge. Using a structured interview maximizes the reliability and validity of interviews. One can also include multiple interviewers in the selection process (e.g., board or panel interviews).

Application Forms/Biographical Data

The collection of biographical data ("biodata") is based on the assumption that the best predictor of future behavior is past behavior. Studies have found biodata more valid than many other predictors for predicting training program success, job proficiency, and turnover. Biodata should be systematically developed and job related.

Weighted application blanks are one type of empirically derived application form, in which items are weighted in terms of their correlation with a criterion measure, and an applicant's item scores are summed to yield a total score. It has been found useful for predicting job turnover, salary increases, and performance ratings.

Biographical Information Blanks (BIBs), which are also empirically derived application forms, contain multiple-choice questions that not only assess an applicant's job history but also such things as family background, economic history, health, attitudes, preferences, and values. BIBs have been found to be valid predictors of turnover and success for jobs ranging from unskilled to administrative and executive, and tend to be better predictors of job performance than intelligence and personality tests. However, their disadvantages are that they are susceptible to faking, and may be perceived by applicants as an invasion of privacy since they contain many items that are not obviously related to job performance. BIBs must be revalidated if they are to be used for different jobs or in different organizations. There is a slight tendency for applicants to respond in a self-serving, inflated manner, and such errors are usually constant across applicants. In terms of EEOC requirements, the questions must be job related. Questions related to race, religion, ethnicity, or age should be avoided, and the same questions should be asked of all applicants applying for the same job.

Tests

Ability and Aptitude Tests

Ability and aptitude tests are the most common assessments used in industry, and are generally more valid than personality or interest tests for predicting job performance. The various tests do not differ substantially in validity coefficients.

For measures of general intellectual ability, the Wonderlic Personnel Test, the Otis Self-Administering Tests of Mental Ability, and the Personnel Tests for Industry are the ones most often used. These tests, however, tend to be better predictors of training success than of job success. They have also been challenged on the basis of unfair discrimination against members of minority groups.

Aptitude tests measure more specific abilities than intelligence tests and are often used to assess an examinee's capacity to profit from training for a particular job. The validity of these instruments is in the low-to-moderate range, and they tend to work best in training programs. Examples include the Bennett Mechanical Comprehension Test, the Revised Minnesota Paper Form Board, and the General Clerical Test.

Multiaptitude batteries consist of several subtests, each of which measures a different aptitude. They are particularly good predictors of occupational choice or job success. Commonly used multiaptitude tests include the General Aptitude Test Battery, the Differential Aptitude Test, and the Flanagan Aptitude Classification Tests.

Psychomotor tests evaluate applicants for jobs requiring quick reaction time, finger dexterity, coordination, and other motor skills. Their validity is greater the more similar the tests are to the measure of job performance. However, they are susceptible to practice effects, which make their reliability and validity low. They are most useful for predicting training success. Examples include the Purdue Pegboard and the Crawford Small Parts Dexterity Test.

Personality Tests

Personality tests are more susceptible to faking and social desirability effects than ability and aptitude tests. They are generally poor predictors of job performance, but there has been a recent revival of their use for predicting the job success of sales personnel. The 16 Personality Factor Questionnaire has been found useful for selecting clerical personnel. Personality tests (such as McClelland's Thematic Apperception Test) can also be used to assess leadership ability and achievement motivation and to predict managerial and executive success. Other commonly used personality tests include the Edwards Personal Preference Schedule and the California Psychological Inventory. The EEOC is skeptical about the validity of personality and interest measures, and some of the questions on these instruments may be considered an invasion of privacy.

Interest Tests

Interest tests are based on the assumption that applicants whose interest profiles resemble those of successful employees will perform best on the job. Two of the most popular tests are the Strong Interest Inventory (SII) and the Kuder Occupational Interest survey (KOIS). However, they are very susceptible to faking, and tend to be more valid for predicting job choice, satisfaction, and persistence than job success.

Work Samples

Work samples require an applicant to perform tasks similar or identical to those actually performed on the job. They are commonly used to select applicants for jobs involving clerical, mechanical, or technical skills. They are generally better predictors than tests. They also tend to be fairer than written tests for minority-group applicants, and tend to be preferred to written tests by both minority and nonminority applicants.

Work samples are also used as methods of performance appraisal and as "job previews." Job previews are used to give applicants information on both the negative and positive aspects of a job, and have been linked to reduced turnover rates and increased job satisfaction.

Assessment Centers

Assessment centers primarily evaluate administrative and managerial-level personnel, and are most commonly used to determine whether current managers should be promoted. They make use of structured interviews, written tests, and situational tests (or work samples).

"In-Basket" is a situational test in which the executive is required to take action on letters, memoranda, reports, and statements typically encountered by managers. "Leaderless Group Discussion" occurs when participants are placed in a group without an assigned leader, and are asked to resolve a particular business problem. "Manufacturing Games" is a situational test in which participants are asked to organize a fictitious company and develop a plan for producing and marketing a product.

Participants are assessed by a team on such dimensions as leadership, human relations skills, oral and written communication, resistance to stress, decision making, and

```
========================= Box 5.6 =========================
```

Mean Validity Coefficients for Workplace Assessments

Work sample	.38 to .54
Ability composite (General mental ability + Psychomotor ability)	.53
Assessment center	.41 to .43
General mental ability	.25 to .45
Biodata	.24 to .28
References	.17 to .26
Interview	.14 to .23
Personality assessment	.15
Interest assessment	.10

Source: From *An Instructor's Guide for Introducing Industrial-Organizational Psychology,* by Education and Training Committee of the Society for Industrial and Organizational Psychology, 2005, available from http://www.siop.org/Instruct/inGuide.htm.

flexibility. Interrater reliability and correlations between assessment center predictors and measures of job performance are relatively high. They tend not to unfairly discriminate against women and minority group members. However, they are time-consuming, costly to develop, and costly to administer, and tend to be used only by large organizations.

Letters of Recommendation

Letters of recommendation are frequently used for higher level positions. However, they often do not have adequate information, and letter writers may not be honest. Letters are most reliable if they have a structured format, and if the questions included in the recommendation form ask about specific behaviors critical for successful job performance. Letters are most predictive of job success when they are from the applicant's previous supervisor.

Box 5.6 provides a list of validity coefficients for the various assessment tools used in organizational settings.

CASE EXAMPLE: PUTTING IT ALL TOGETHER

This case example of an executive assessment report combines much of the material discussed in this chapter. This assessment was prompted when Jeremy Drummer (the executive) was having significant interpersonal difficulties on the job, and the company wanted to clarify the factors involved in the situation. As with clinical assessments, this report, given to the consultee, describes and integrates the data gathered, conceptualizes the factors involved in the executive's difficulties, and makes suggestions for future action steps. For this particular case, rather than listing details about the testing instruments, the data gathered from the assessment are put into common language taking into consideration the organizational context and the referral question.

This report is intended to be an aid in this person's vocational and personal growth. Only this individual and those in a position to constructively influence the person's development should have access to the report—and only with the individual's consent. The report contents must be considered in light of other relevant data, and the author should be consulted on the report's proper interpretation and implementation. Safeguard the report by keeping it in a confidential file. Since it has been written for a specific time and place, the report can be understood only in that framework and should be destroyed when no longer timely.

Identifying Information

Jeremy is a 29-year-old white male who has been an employee of the Mason Company for approximately 7 years. He presented to the interviewer looking much more tense and defeated than when last seen by the same interviewer almost 3 years earlier. He was the middle of five children of German Lutheran parents. He always tried to please his parents by working hard and being a perfectionistic kid. He says he spent his whole life trying to be as good as his 16-month-older brother who was "better, more gifted." Jeremy recalls being beaten up by his brother most days growing up. Jeremy always felt he had to work harder than his brother and still did not get recognition. The incidents at his current work assignment in Elisabethtown have revived those childhood feelings. He recalls being taught, "If there's a job to be done, let's go do it!" He values his Lutheran religion and tries to be a good and honest person. He has had some personal losses (two friends and two grandparents) that have been difficult for him. He also feels badly that he may have disappointed his family whom he had always tried to impress.

Jeremy's health has been good except for frequent headaches. He has never smoked, drinks beer occasionally, and denies the use of drugs.

During his tenure at Mason Company, he has been assigned to several managerial level positions aimed at developing his skills and career potential. His most recent assignment was as Plant Superintendent of the Elisabethtown plant, where he helped in the start-up of the operation since June 2000. He has seen himself as an entrepreneur within the company. He has struggled with wanting to feel more appreciated and recognized for his abilities by the company. He recalls resenting others who were promoted ahead of him to high-level positions.

The present evaluation is prompted by Jeremy's interpersonal difficulty at the Elisabethtown assignment. Jeremy describes very much enjoying the early period of start-up at Elisabethtown, only to have great difficulty turning over some of his functions to the new managers who were added to the team. He recalls feeling very territorial and believes that this made it difficult for some of the people to get into their jobs. He felt that unless he pushed things through, others would "drop the ball," and he also noticed himself taking everything very personally. He aggressively complained about and couldn't understand others who didn't pour themselves into their jobs. His response was to try to control everything and do the job himself, saying he often averaged 16 to 19 hours a day on the job. He felt that his social relationship with the CEO, Mr. Smith, as well as his aggressiveness and his hard work, was threatening to his superiors. He received the feedback that he was overbearing and challenged too much. He felt an "Outward Bound" trip did not resolve the growing conflict among the management team. In March 2001, he was upset about the groundbreaking event, feeling that the plant manager got too much credit and his good start-up performance wasn't adequately recognized. He felt upset with the company, and was depleted and tired. Even though he couldn't give as much, he still felt dedicated to making the company's product, and continued to put in long hours of work. In May 2002, after Jeremy failed to stop a bad load of product that he had unrealistically promised he would prevent, Jeremy felt very much a failure, and requested another position from Human Resources. After receiving counseling from Mr. Jones regarding these issues and being instructed to talk to someone, he went to a mentor at the Universal Product Company, who suggested he was putting too much into the job, and encouraged him to figure out what was important to him. Jeremy responded by cutting back to a 12-hour day. In June 2002, he received an upsetting review after getting a positive one in January. He felt hurt and unrecognized. He particularly did not feel support from or trust the plant manager. In July 2002, he states that Human Resources told him he would no longer have a job at Mason Company by September 1, 2002. From July 2002 onward, he feels he did not function well; his supervisors did not understand his lowered productivity.

Jeremy, although devastated and angry at himself and by the chain of events, felt almost rescued from the situation. Jeremy has felt out of control for the past 4 to 5 months. He became obsessed with instilling the Mason ways and neglected his family for the job. He says that at one point he didn't take much time to sleep or eat because he was so driven. Friends and wife noticed a change in him. He got very talkative and did not listen as well. This behavior seems strange to him looking back. He had lost his sense of balance, and jeopardized his family relationships. He said that "this could be the best thing for me. I could have worked into a divorce or a heart attack." Jeremy has remorse about his mistakes, particularly the problems in the control system and his failure to stop a bad load of product. He further stated that he is angry at his motivations, his fear of failure, and his fear of being a human being. In retrospect, he believes a lot could have been avoided and that he needs to "learn to get back on the bike" and to "stop operating not to fail instead of to win."

The purpose of this evaluation is to provide input into action plans regarding Jeremy's future development within or without the company.

Intellectual Characteristics

Jeremy's basic intellectual capacity is average or slightly above. He is most comfortable with thinking about practical problems. He is not particularly well adapted for academic endeavors because he is action oriented. One of his major perceived failures is not completing his thesis requirement for his MBA degree. Jeremy's intellectual orientation is more concrete than abstract, and he tends to make decisions decisively and sometimes without thinking things through. He is pragmatically oriented and sometimes has difficulty understanding the subjective aspects of his evaluations and feedback. His drive and impulsiveness sometimes prevent him from completely carrying out logical thought processes. He is particularly interested in statistical processes and tends to be bottom-line oriented. Despite having a strong and likable interpersonal presence, he does not have strong empathy or understanding of others' motives and feelings. He sometimes interprets events differently than others, resulting in interpersonal conflicts. He has a tendency to "work hard but not smart," believing that his dedication, loyalty, and hard work will ensure success. Sometimes he has difficulty distinguishing between what is necessary and unnecessary. Although not particularly creative, inventive, or visionary, Jeremy is liberal and open about change, but tends to have fairly conventional attitudes. He seeks out new knowledge and experiences that will advance his ability. His work product is sometimes hasty and he tends to be careless about established protocols.

Emotional Characteristics

This is a difficult time in Jeremy's life. He appears to be going through a lot of uncertainly and self-doubt and is engaged in anxiety and worry about his future.

Jeremy is easily affected by his feelings. He is unusually sensitive to hurt and slight. When upset, Jeremy sometimes acts out his feelings in ways that are upsetting to those around him.

Jeremy is an extremely competitive, aggressive, and dominant person. He can be forceful and take the initiative to get things done. When faced with conflict or disagreement, he likes to directly challenge and clearly state his own views. He also strongly prefers a dominant leadership style in his superiors. He is socially bold, and can be persevering and even stubborn in his commitment to an idea. Even though he is not a particularly trusting person, he is straightforward in presenting his feelings and doesn't play politics well. His inner drive and commitment to task are so strong that he often has a kind of "get out of my way" quality. Despite his aggressiveness, Jeremy is sensitive to hurt and is careful of others' feelings as well. He often feels that he is being unfairly treated and is not properly recognized. He fears failure, and his self-concept is often variably high and low. When he is feeling good about himself he can be cocky and egotistical, and when he is feeling down, he can have serious doubts about himself. He needs a great deal of affirmation and social approval. One superior suggested that Jeremy distorts events at times to make himself look better. He sometimes has a difficult time bouncing back from defeat or mistakes. He tends to be anxious and worry a lot, and to have a high energy level, except when he is feeling defeated. He is generally active and enthusiastic. He likes excitement, stimulation, and adventure, and may impress some as being too daring. He has difficulty with personal and career integration, often crowding out his personal life with work involvement. Jeremy has not yet attained a high degree of emotional maturity and is still working out areas of insecurity in which he is trying to prove himself, "I want to see if I am really worth a shit out there." He has difficulty being his best without being the best.

Motivational Characteristics

Jeremy is motivated by a strong drive toward achievement, recognition, and winning. He often tends to approach life from the vantage point of sports. He admires "home run hitters" in baseball, people who change the game—who are important and make a difference. Jeremy often needs major projects to feel important. His deeper attachments appear to be in the form of heroes, mainly powerful and somewhat older men. He tends to form adoring relationships with these men and tries to carefully learn from them. He tends to have a sense of urgency about the goals before him. He tends to have a zest for change and becomes easily bored with routine. Jeremy wants to be someone to be emulated, a positive role model for children. He wants to "establish a message of my own and carry it out." Jeremy tends to feel guilty when he does not fulfill personal role relationships in his life.

Insight into One's Self and into Others

Jeremy has a good understanding of his own personality, and generally values his own traits. In past evaluations, however, he has been seen as not accurately assessing himself. More importantly, Jeremy sometimes has difficulty assessing the impact of his personality on others. He has less understanding of the needs and feelings of others, particularly when these conflict with his goals. He is not particularly psychologically minded, preferring to focus on pragmatic issues of what someone is doing rather than why. Jeremy is aware that he often ends up turning things into a struggle that he has to win. Jeremy often feels insufficiently recognized and advanced for his performance and contributions.

Interpersonal Characteristics

Jeremy is an extrovert (people-oriented) and has considerable interpersonal skills. He feels best when he is being helpful to others. He has a fair amount of charm and poise interpersonally, and initiates humor freely. He is also capable of relating to a broad range of types of people. Sometimes, however, he so strongly wants people to perform that he may try too hard and become pushy and demanding. Mostly, however, he is able to relate to people with ease and comfort. Jeremy is socially bold and is not afraid to state his feelings forcefully. He likes things to go his way, and prefers freedom from other people's influence. He may resent others interfering with his plans. At times, he can be oppositional and distrusting of the motives of others. Even in situations in which he feels distrusting, he tends to be forthright and exposes himself to others. He tends to be easily read by others. Jeremy is capable of a great deal of enthusiasm and is usually friendly to people he meets. He relates best to competitive people who are goal oriented. He has a need for the group to approve and be pleased with what he is doing, but is not very effective in winning their approval. Others often don't realize that approval is critical to Jeremy. He may be swayed by flattery from others.

Vocational Characteristics

Jeremy is highest in the (1) venturous-influential interest pattern and (2) nurturing-altruistic interest pattern. He likes activities in which he convinces, directs, or persuades others to attain organizational goals, and he also likes to show a genuine concern for other people. He is drawn to conventional and enterprising vocations, particularly in the world of business. Jeremy seems likely to enjoy and be interested in work in sales, marketing, and management, especially sales management. He tends to perform best in start-up and turnaround situations, and he tends to value power in himself and others, requiring a strong, dominant boss whom he respects. Jeremy also is curious about learning new skills and developing himself, although such development does not always come easily for him. When the workplace starts to develop a maintenance framework, and things begin to become institutionalized with clear boundaries, he tends to have difficulties. Jeremy likes to think of himself as self-directed and independent, but in actuality needs group support and approval for his decisions. His independence may be somewhat troublesome to some superiors, and Jeremy tends to have strong aspirations for the leadership position in the face of strong authoritative leadership. Jeremy can be a loyal and devoted follower. Despite his strong drive and action orientation, Jeremy sometimes has difficulty with staying organized and on top of things. He tends to keep a lot of things in his head instead of writing them down. He does not plan very far ahead. His accident-error proneness is also predicted to be above average.

In terms of management style, Jeremy is a goal-oriented manager who likes to connect strongly with the line worker and lead by example. Past superiors have suggested that when he gets frustrated, he becomes autocratic. He needs to guard against monopolizing situations and intimidating others by his competitive, aggressive style. Because of his decisiveness, he also needs to make sure that he has all his bases covered before jumping into a decision. He tends to like hands-on involvement in the projects he directs. He likes to deal with people on a direct, oral one-on-one basis rather than through written or memo formats (his least favorite subject is English). He likes visible, overt leadership with the attached high status. In past evaluations, he has been seen as having difficulty developing others and appropriately focusing on others. He sees his personal weaknesses as not being savvy to all opinions and being judgmental.

Jeremy needs to guard against several tendencies to be effective in his performance: (1) his tendency, at times, to act, with so much eagerness, energy, and optimism that he may overlook important details, fail to prepare himself for what he undertakes, or sufficiently anticipate consequences of his actions; (2) his tendencies to become overly impatient, demanding, and excitable if he is trying to get others to accept what he wants done, or if he is confronted with possible roadblocks to completing a task, when an organized approach to problems would allow him to work more constructively and with more meaningful purpose than he seems to be able to do at this time; (3) his pattern of giving up on, or letting go of, problems and situations too early, when he feels upset, angry, or unable to cope with things; (4) his likelihood of showing too much of his emotions or feelings in tense or stressful situations; (5) his feeling of being superior to or better than others or trying to force his ideas on them; (6) his tendency to be so natural and forthright in relations with others that he overlooks or dismisses the need to be critically insightful and/or politically and socially astute, and pressing so hard in work-related and other personal situations that he neglects opportunities to relax; (7) his willingness to take on activities or tasks that focus on theoretical issues and problems, since his strengths are much more in doing practical tasks; (8) his overestimation of his importance and abilities and belief of being entitled to positions of power and responsibility or of feeling cheated when he does not receive these accolades.

Climate Issues

Jeremy's characteristics meet some of the elements of the Mason culture over the years. He is task oriented and has a good work ethic. He tries to be open, honest, and have integrity in his dealings with others. Jeremy is committed to being a team member but his strong needs for recognition and status often create problems for him in this area. His impulsiveness and drivenness create quality problems for his performance, and his fears of failure sometimes inhibit innovation and risk taking. He is committed to people and loyal to the company but is sometimes too controlling and does not grant enough autonomy to subordinates. He also lacks trust in several people within the organization.

Conclusions and Prognosis

Jeremy is a sharply defined personality who will not be received as neutral by many. He has many strengths, particularly his energy level, dedication, loyalty, and willingness to work hard for the company. He also has the potential to create more problems with others than most managers. In such a person, the match between person and environment becomes extremely important. Jeremy tends to be a doer who at his best can be inspiring and charismatic, and at his worst can create system problems that baffle those around him. Continuing personal maturation, improving self-discipline, and developing ways to be flexible around his own shortcomings are imperative to his future success. He has strained some of his relationships within the company and will have to overcome negative impressions to achieve success. Despite his sense of urgency and his many experiences in the company, Jeremy is still only 29 years of age and capable of continuing development. Personal therapy might prove helpful with his extreme sensitivity and strong need for approval and recognition.

Suggestions for Corrective Actions

Miner (1991) suggested that after one makes a diagnosis of any problems found after performing an executive assessment, the following recommendations can be made as possible corrective actions:

- Job redesign and changed role prescriptions
- Promotion, transfer, or demotion
- Management development and training
- Changes in supervision (either the style of the existing supervision or the person holding the position)
- Changes in method or amount of compensation
- Personnel policy modifications (or exceptions to policy)
- Threats and disciplinary action
- Alcoholics Anonymous and other such group procedures
- Medical treatment
- Psychotherapy/Counseling (including assessment feedback)
- Employee assistance program (p. 233)

These intervention topics are discussed in the following section and in subsequent chapters.

CASE EXAMPLE: EXECUTIVE DEVELOPMENT REQUEST

Dr. John Johnson, a psychologist in private practice, recently had some successful consultation experiences with a large chemical company. The organization is so impressed with John's work in helping the organization select and hire new executives that they invite him to assist in developing the executives they already have on their team. John expresses that he would be interested in pursuing this further, and asks more about the specific needs of the executive team. The consultee replies that she did not have anything in particular in mind, just that it would be nice to have someone who can help their executives improve themselves, perhaps in a 1-hour weekly "development meeting." While John notes that this is a laudable goal, he tells the consultee that the time of so many executives is very precious (e.g., 20 executives making $40 per hour meeting one hour each week for 52 weeks is $41,600, not including overhead, consultant fees, and the opportunity costs of the executives not actively working on developing the organization). John goes on to provide some education as to typical executive development needs and goals, as well as typical methods for achieving those goals. The consultee says she will think about what their needs might be, and will ask the other members of the management team to do so as well. John agrees to meet with the consultee and the management team in 2 weeks, at which time they can discuss their goals and strategies and how John might help to achieve them, after which John will send the consultee a contract proposal.

Coaching, Counseling, and Training

In addition to helping an organization select new employees, a consultant can assist an organization in further developing the skills of current employees. The most common ways that mental health professionals can assist in the development of executives is through coaching, counseling, and training.

Development refers to the improvement of an employee's ability to handle tasks and assignments. It may also involve assisting the employee to grow and advance within the company. Although some agencies may be too small to facilitate consistent promotional opportunities, training and development may foster a more versatile employee, which will improve the quality of work performed. It will also help to alleviate boredom by allowing the employee to handle different types of assignments. It also helps to foster a higher sense of confidence and self-esteem.

A well-run organization knows that employees are its strength. Companies with this philosophy help employees build careers that make them more valuable to the organization. This effort starts by identifying an organization's current and future needs for particular types of employees and skills. Once these needs are identified, the next step is to assess current employees' abilities, performance, and potential. With this information, the company can establish career development plans that ensure employees receive the training needed. While training is essential to career development, a career development program involves more than training. Career development requires individualized counseling, from the initial needs assessment, through each training experience and job position, to the end of the employee's tenure with the company (Advisor on the Web, 2003).

Pipeline for Development

D. Peterson and Hicks (1996) outlined the following necessary and sufficient conditions for development, which they called the "pipeline for development." If these conditions are not met, any efforts at trying to develop executives will end in failure.

- *Insight:* Do people know what to develop?
- *Motivation:* Do people see a clear personal payoff for development?
- *Capabilities:* Do people have or know how to acquire the skills and knowledge they need?
- *Real-world practice:* Do people have opportunities to try their new skills at work?
- *Accountability:* Do people internalize their new capabilities to improve performance and results?

Forms of Executive Development

Executive development takes many forms within organizations. Consultants can recommend one or several of these methods, depending on the needs of the executive and the organization. Some of these methods can be used independently by the executive, some can be conducted by the consultant, and some can be referred out to other sources.

Mentoring

Mentoring is typically an informal process of development. As a formal method of development, however, mentoring involves pairing a junior employee with a senior employee. This allows the junior employee to seek advice without taking the time to contact the human resource department for every minor question that comes up. It also allows the senior employee to be sure that the junior employee is doing quality work. Junior employees can receive customized training from the expertise of the senior employees, without the additional expenditure required to bring in external consultants (Stone, 1999).

It is important to recognize that not all positions require the same type of mentoring, and there may be some positions for which there is no need for mentoring. For those positions that would benefit from mentoring, some general, progressive stages take place (see Table 5.3). A new hire does not need the same type of mentoring as a more experienced employee (Higgins & Fram, 2001; Mathis & Jackson, 2003, p. 330).

Observing or Shadowing Other People

Observing or "shadowing" another person for a day or other limited period can help an executive learn about the jobs of other members of the organization. A consultant can also shadow executives to better understand their daily functioning and give feedback about how they use their time, relate to others, and so on.

Table 5.3   Stages of Mentoring

Less-Experienced Employee	Stage	Length of Time	More-Experienced Employee
Admires the senior employee's competence: recognizes him/her as source of guidance	Initiation	6–12 months	Realizes younger employee is someone with potential and "is coachable"
Gains self-confidence, values, and styles of operation	Cultivation	2–5 years	Provides challenging work, coaching, visibility, protection, and sponsorship
Experiences independence but has feelings of anxiety, and loss at times	Separation	6–12 months	Knows when to begin to move away
Responds with gratitude for the early years; relationship becomes a friendship	Redefinition	Ongoing	Continues to be a supporter; takes pride in the younger manager's accomplishments

Coaching and Counseling

Coaching or counseling involves direct, one-on-one feedback given from a consultant to the executive. This topic is covered in detail in Chapter 6.

Appraisal

Appraisal is specific, performance-based feedback given to an executive by a consultant or by other members of the organization.

Internal Rotation, Attachment, and Placement

This method is frequently used for executives who are being groomed for important management positions. Executives are placed in various departments to more fully understand the operations of the organization at all levels. The rotations are strategically assigned based on the position for which the executive is being groomed. For example, a potential chief financial officer may spend time in accounts receivable and accounts payable, and work with employees knowledgeable about the general ledger system being used. These assignments must be somewhat challenging to the executive, to foster growth and development, but must not be so challenging that the executive feels overwhelmed. The purpose is to build the executive's sense of self confidence and mastery.

Knowledge Building

This development method increases the executive's breadth or depth of knowledge. This may involve reading assignments, attendance at workshops, or enrollment in local college courses.

Joining Special Projects

Executives who are accustomed to engaging in the same routines on a daily basis may benefit from taking on occasional special projects. These allow the executive to use different thinking processes, learn new things about the organization and its processes, and further build interpersonal connections.

Committee Membership

Joining a committee allows an executive firsthand experience in viewing the larger picture of the organization, and gives a sense of responsibility for the future course of the organization.

Discussion Groups

Formal or informal discussion groups allow executives to share notes on a variety of issues, allowing them to learn from each other's successes and mistakes.

Professional Meetings

Attending professional meetings and conferences allows executives to learn about the latest cutting edge technologies and provides opportunities to network with experts in their fields.

Learning from One's Own Job and Experience

Executives can practice self-monitoring and self-awareness exercises to learn from their jobs. They can also reflect back on their past experiences and note what contributed to past successes and failures. Consultants can help them set up experiments using different behaviors, encouraging them to try new things, such as how they interact with subordinates. The executive can learn to pay attention to the results and process which behaviors are effective and which are ineffective.

Special Activities

Executives may be asked to participate in certain activities to foster new knowledge and skills. An executive who needs to develop public speaking skills could join Toastmasters, join the local Rotary Club, take a Dale Carnegie course, or lead a United Way campaign.

Psychotherapy

Executives may wish to seek out individual psychotherapy. As mental health professionals know, this can provide a safe and confidential place to express feelings and process stressful events at work. It can also help executives deal with unresolved past issues that might interfere with their professional life.

Executive Development and Mental Health Professionals

Mental health professionals provide many forms of executive development today. Executive coaching, which is discussed in Chapter 6, is becoming increasingly popular.

During the 1960s, many mental health professionals ran sensitivity groups. However, they lost popularity because they did not produce lasting results. Today, places like the Center for Creative Leadership, which uses mental health professionals as staff, offer seminars and courses (such as giving feedback from 360 instruments and looking at the executive's management style and personality). Many mental health professionals offer management training seminars within training departments, as HR offerings, or on a freelance basis.

The Dynamic Nature of Development

The employment contract is changing from one of company paternalism; employees are now taking responsibility for their own careers and development. They need to prepare themselves for their own progression.

Development is a dynamic process. Strengths may become weaknesses, and flaws that went unnoticed before may suddenly become important. In the future, some strengths may not matter as much as they do now; and new, untested skills may be required. Executives who do not continue to learn and grow may become derailed.

CASE EXAMPLE: EXECUTIVE DEVELOPMENT PLANNING

After meeting with the management team, John feels that they were able to create workable executive development goals, and the consultee accepts his contract proposal. John begins by conducting a needs assessment on each executive of the management team, so that individualized development plans can be created. John also sets up group meetings for those goals that require the overall development of the entire team, such as the creation of a formal mentorship program, and a system that involves rotating executives through different departments to more fully understand the workings of the entire organization.

Things are proceeding smoothly, with the members of the management team giving John positive feedback, until the president of the company announces that the organization will soon be purchased by a large conglomerate corporation. The consultee calls John and says that she and the other members of the management team are experiencing a great deal of anxiety and uncertainty, since the new owners have been known to fire previous management teams. The consultee asks John to come in to meet with her and the management team, as they are all afraid that they will lose the jobs they have worked so hard to develop.

DERAILMENT

Since the help of consultants is most often requested in times when things are going badly, consulting mental health professionals often get involved with *derailed* executives. Derailment refers to the idea that executives who have been on the "track to success" become somehow dislodged and are no longer successful in the work environment. Whether they are working with individuals or larger organizations, consultants can learn to look for the warning signs of derailment, and can help an executive take action to get back on track.

Derailment can occur for many reasons:

Problems with interpersonal relationships: Executives can sometimes achieve a great deal of success due to their technical skills, but will not survive over a long period in most organizations without good people skills. For example, executives are held responsible for the performance of subordinates, and if an executive cannot effectively deal with problem subordinates, the organization will suffer.

Difficulty in molding a staff: An individual working alone can accomplish little within an organization. Executives rely on their subordinates and on the teams to which they belong. Ideally, executives can synergistically pull out the strengths of those who work for and with them. An executive who is unable to effectively develop a cohesive team will find it difficult to make noticeable positive impacts on the organization.

Difficulty in making strategic transitions: Sometimes an executive's skills, knowledge, and personal style fit in perfectly with a particular organization. Other times, executives work very hard to adapt to the needs and styles of the organization they have joined. In today's world, however, organizations must constantly change and adapt to environmental needs and circumstances. New company policies and strategies may make the old style of an executive less adaptive. Also, during organizational takeovers, new owners may decide to replace all of the existing management. If executives are not sufficiently flexible and adaptive to continuous strategic transitions, they will be replaced with those who are.

Lack of follow-through: Sometimes executives can progress in an organization because of their vision, creativity, ability to develop ideas, and their skill at inspiring others (Dilts, 1996; Dilts & Bonissone, 1993; Dilts, Epstein, & Dilts, 1991). To remain successful, executives must be able to follow through with what they communicate to others. Some executives get inspired and take on large projects for which they are unprepared, only to lose interest in the project. If executives cannot follow through on their responsibilities, they will not keep their positions long.

Overdependence on a mentor/advocate: As discussed, selection of and connection with a mentor can help executives as they climb the corporate ladder. Executives should also try to find advocates within their own and other departments and within the top levels of management. An advocate is someone with whom one has developed a close, trusting relationship who has the power to give the executive support (emotional as well as the provision of needed resources) and who has influence with top management. However, organizational politics constantly change. An executive's mentors and advocates may fall out of favor with upper management, get transferred, be terminated, or quit or retire. If an executive has relied too much on one or two mentors or advocates, the executive may quickly lose resources and power, becoming derailed.

Strategic differences with management: Displaying independent thinking skills and offering original ideas to an organization can help an executive move up in the ranks. However, if an executive's fundamental views on how the organization should do things conflict with the views of top management, an otherwise highly capable executive may become derailed.

Ways Individuals Derail Themselves

Just as mental health professionals often work with individuals who are unaware of their contributions to their presenting problems, consultants can help executives become more sensitive to the parts they play in derailment. Following are some common problems that could derail an executive.

Ignoring (or Being Blind to) a Notable Flaw

The executive may be completely unaware of the negative impact of certain presentation styles or behaviors. Such flaws can become the proverbial "elephant in the room" that everyone else in the organization is aware of but is afraid to discuss with the individual. Likewise, the executive may be aware of certain flaws but not believe that they have a significant impact. The executive may feel that certain behaviors are "just my style of doing things," and may expect others to "just deal with it." Successful executives must become aware of their strengths and weaknesses, and must be sensitive to their impact on others. Therapy experience often gives mental health professionals the skills they need to tactfully present difficult-to-hear information to defensive individuals.

Having Untested Areas

In today's world of dynamic organizational change, executives are likely to face many new challenges. It is inevitable that sometimes they will fail. The consultant can help executives become perpetual learners who prepare for new challenges and who deal with challenge and failure in a constructive and emotionally healthy way.

Overreliance on Strengths

Executives often achieve high-ranking positions due to their idiosyncratic strengths. While they should continue to build on their strengths, it is also important for them to acknowledge and work on their weaknesses. Too often, executives cling to old habits when the environmental requirements of the situation have changed (Bellah, Madsen, Sullivan, Swidler, & Tipton, 1996). As the old saying goes, when the only tool you have is a hammer, everything looks (and is treated) like a nail. Consultants can work with executives to identify and assess their areas of strength and weakness, and can create a developmental plan that addresses both areas.

Narrow Leadership Perspective

Frequently, executives are promoted due to the knowledge and expertise they have in their departments. Once they move up to higher levels, however, they must adopt a broader perspective of the entire organization as well as the external environment with which they interact. The specialized focus that served them so well in their departments may no longer be useful in their new role, and a narrow focus is likely to be harmful to the overall growth of the organization. Consultants can help executives develop the ability to look at the bigger picture by making them consciously aware of the processes and procedures of gathering the needed information and insights.

Failure to Learn from Experience

All too often, executives seem to make the same mistakes over and over again. They may feel that if they simply try a little harder next time, things will work out. As mental health professionals know, one cannot keep doing the same actions and expect a different result. Consultants can help teach executives how to be more scientific and empirical in their approach to things, monitoring their own and others' reactions and soliciting feedback.

Reasons for Success

Though sometimes executives are derailed for reasons beyond their control, several factors can help them successfully navigate the sometimes stormy waters of change. Consultants can help executives become aware of and cultivate these resiliency factors.

Track Record

A long history of successful performance will be helpful to executives when things do not go well temporarily. This is akin to the idea of the "emotional bank account," which allows a person to make an occasional withdrawal after a long series of investments. Even if executives lose their jobs, they may be able to rely on their past successful track records to secure new jobs. Consultants can work with executives to put things in perspective when things are not going well, reminding them of their many past successes. As therapists do in psychotherapy, consultants can also explore with executives how they dealt with challenging situations in the past, and what strengths they can bring forward into the future.

Interpersonal Style

How executives interact with other members of the organization on an interpersonal level has a strong bearing on how they handle difficult situations. Executives with terse or demeaning interpersonal styles are not likely to receive much support when their jobs become threatened. Executives who display warmth and foster interpersonal connections are more likely to be seen as valuable to most organizational members.

Though this does not mean that executives should try to be everyone's "best friend" at the expense of doing a good job, interpersonal relationships play a major role in career development. Consultants with mental health backgrounds can use their training to help executives develop more effective interpersonal skills.

Composure

The ability to retain composure under stress is an important skill in the fast-paced modern organizational world. Executives who snap at employees or who become angry at unpredictable times are viewed as unprofessional at best and are likely to build fear and resentment among employees. Executives who can remain cool during a crisis are inspiring and comforting to other members of the organization.

Handling Mistakes

Executives, like all human beings, make mistakes. The more innovative the executive, the more frequently mistakes will occur. Executives must acknowledge and rectify their mistakes in a responsible, mature way. Doing so displays a sense of integrity and fosters respect among colleagues. Resentment builds among other organizational members when executives will not admit their own mistakes. Blaming others, or making others responsible for correcting an executive's mistakes, also builds resentment. Consultants can work with executives to help them resolve the obstacles that may prevent them from openly admitting their mistakes, such as difficulties with low self-esteem or fears of appearing inadequate to others.

Solving Problems

Problem solving is another important skill among executives. Technical skill and knowledge are important for professional work, but managers are required to deal with situations that employees are unable to handle. An executive can get promoted for professional expertise, but must be good at problem solving to progress further. Consultants can work with executives on developing their problem-solving skills, such as through teaching them the problem-solving model that was presented in Chapter 1.

Many of the preceding factors are related to emotional intelligence (Goleman, 1997; Salovey & Mayer, 1990; Weisinger, 1998), and consultants can borrow tactics from the research on this topic for their intervention plans.

Lombardo and Eichinger (1989) found that a critical difference between successful and derailed managers of high potential was their ability to learn from experience. Consultants can give executives honest, open feedback and teach them skills for self-awareness and self-monitoring. Just as in therapy, mental health professionals can teach executives to be more aware of the impact they have on the world around them.

CASE EXAMPLE: MANAGING TRANSITIONS

John meets with the management team to talk with them about the upcoming takeover and how the management team will deal with it. He begins by applying some of the skills from his mental health background such as normalization, to help assuage their anxieties and fears, and prediction, to help them prepare for the future. He tells everyone that while it is a very real possibility that they will all lose their jobs, and that they should prepare for such an eventuality, they should also consider that finding, hiring, and training a management team with as much knowledge and expertise as this team will be very difficult for the new owners to do. He then allows everyone to talk about their concerns, and what they know about the new owners. This allows them to feel heard and reduces unreasonable ruminations. It also helps them to come up with a concrete plan for dealing with the situation. John asks each member of the executive team to reflect on the best-case scenarios, acceptable scenarios, and worst-case scenarios for their individual situations in this takeover. John then talks in general terms about derailment and how to prevent it.

General discussions reveal a wide variety of feelings and opinions about how best to go about managing this transition. Some think the takeover is a positive event that may allow them to have more resources and more opportunities to advance in a larger corporation. Others feel that such a large, out-of-state organization will not have much impact on the daily operations. Some believe it may be an opportunity to move into another field or industry; some feel a lot of distress and don't know what to do; some just want to quit or retire. Everyone agrees that it would be best for each team member to consider personal goals and options and to set up individual meetings with John on how to best achieve those goals and to have contingency plans based on how things turn out.

Chapter 6

EXECUTIVE COACHING AND PERFORMANCE ENHANCEMENT

Executive coaching is becoming popular among business executives and other individuals who are looking to improve themselves and their performance in life and on the job (C. Fitzgerald & Berger, 2002; Flaherty, 1999; Hargrove, 1995; Hargrove & Kaestner, 1998; Kilburg, 2000; J. Miller & Brown, 1993). Mental health professionals, with the proper training and with a background in interpersonal skills, are especially well suited for executive coaching. We are also skilled at assessing an individual's performance within the context of a larger system, and at giving constructive and sometimes delicate feedback.

After agreeing that executive coaching will be helpful for a particular client, the consultant should send a written proposal that outlines the understanding of what is to be accomplished. The proposal should define the scope of the project, the time estimate, all costs, expectations for the client, and should briefly describe the consultant's background and qualifications. Box 6.1 shows a sample proposal for grooming two managers who are potential successors to the company's CEO.

Box 6.1

Proposal
Executive Coaching

This proposal outlines an individualized "executive coaching" process designed to equip the two potential CEO successors with the tools, knowledge, and opportunities they need to develop themselves and become more effective.

Scope of the Project

Consultant will meet with each of the two managers to provide executive coaching according to the following process: Phase 1—Setting the foundation (clarifying understandings of the coaching process), Phase 2—Assessment phase (fact gathering), Phase 3—Planning and consolidation (developing a developmental plan), Phase 4—Implementation and development (implementing the plan). Meetings may be held at X Industries or at another agreed-on location dependent on the convenience of the participants.

The purpose of these sessions is to coach for development (learning focused on a person's future job) according to the developmental plan that will be based

(Continued)

Box 6.1 (continued)

on the data collection process. The sponsor and each participant will agree on the developmental plan. Typical goals involve increasing competencies/abilities/skills (e.g., interpersonal sensitivity, concern for personal impact, relationship building, leadership, use of influence strategies, directing versus developing others, group management, self-control, communicating vision, developing teams, managing conflict productively) relevant to enhanced leadership, improvements in managerial style, and interpersonal effectiveness (e.g., understanding communication styles, identifying and resolving specific issues that block effective leadership or teamwork, developing improvement strategies to work effectively in the future). An emphasis is placed on enhancing the strengths of each person.

Time Estimate

Monthly coaching meetings with each executive for one-to-two-hour sessions for 12 months to 2 years and a data presentation and planning meeting for ½ to 1 day. Quarterly meetings will be scheduled with the sponsor and as necessary with others in the organization. Observational meetings may also be held. An additional two-to-three-hour meeting will be held jointly with both executives.

Cost

$160 per consultant hour.

Requirements for Program Success

1. Data collection, feedback, and coaching processes will be ongoing activities.
2. Agreement must be reached with the sponsor and the executive regarding the specific coaching process.
3. Specific data belong to the executive and discussions of the data collection require the verbal release of the executive. To effectively employ the resources of others and to create the developmental plan, the executive will be encouraged to be open about the feedback and the issues on which they are working. The sponsor will be entitled to participate in the development and implementation of the developmental plan, but the executive has control over what specific data are shared with others.
4. The specific coaching process used will be agreed on with the executive and the consultant.
5. It is agreed that the consultant will have several opportunities to view the executive at work with his subordinates during the coaching process.

Consultant

This proposal is presented by Richard Sears, PsyD, MBA. Dr. Sears is a consultant and coach specializing in corporate work-related issues.

Thank you for the opportunity to submit this proposal.

Richard Sears, PsyD, MBA
richard@psych-insights.com
www.psych-insights.com

By having the coachee (or the organization representative if contracting through the coachee's company) sign and return the document, the agreement becomes a legally binding contract. For more information about contract law, see Beatty and Samuelson (2001).

WHAT IS COACHING?

Coaching is a one-on-one relationship, taking place as an ongoing process (involving multiple sessions), that focuses on improving an individual's insight into his or her own functioning and on improving his or her effectiveness in an organization (Kraiger, 2002; D. Peterson, 2002).

Coaching is considered by some as a form of consultation and is similar to consultee-centered mental health consultation. However, organizations such as the International Coaching Federation promote coaching as a separate field. Although mental health professionals can rely on many skills they have learned in doing therapy, there are some important differences between psychotherapy and coaching/consulting. Sperry (1996, p. 184) notes several major differences, as shown in Table 6.1.

Mental health professionals who are interested in coaching should also take some time to learn the language of the organizational world. In Table 6.2, Peltier (2001, p. 240) suggests changing the language that therapists customarily use.

Table 6.1   Comparison of Psychotherapy and Consulting

Psychotherapy	Executive Consultation
1. Client seeks out and chooses clinician; pays clinicians; one-to-one relationship.	1. Executive seeks out and engages consultant who is paid by the organization; one-to-one relationship.
2. Work on clinician's turf; rules of clinician prevail.	2. Work on client's turf; rules are usually negotiated.
3. More process oriented and client centered.	3. More likely to involve advising and to be expert oriented.
4. Agenda negotiated by client and clinician.	4. Agenda usually set by client.
5. Sessions usually involve 50-minute hour and scheduled weekly.	5. Sessions of variable length.
6. Confidentiality issues are relatively straightforward.	6. Confidentiality issues may be more complex; "double agentry" (working for two clients, such as the executive and the employer) is not uncommon.
7. Often involves working through characterological issues.	7. Usually involves working around defenses and characterological issues.

Table 6.2   Business Language for Consultants

Therapy Language to Avoid	Business Language to Learn
Issue ("What are your issues?")	Challenge, solution ("What challenges are you facing?" "What solutions are required?")
Why ("Why is this happening?")	How ("How does it happen?")
Sessions (with clients)	Meetings
Way I work, way of working	Method
Sense ("I get a sense that...")	Idea ("Here's my idea." "Here's what I think.")
Feeling ("What are you feeling?")	Reaction ("What is your reaction?")
Around ("I have feelings around this issue")	About ("I am concerned about this.")
Tasks ("What do we need to do?")	Results and deliverables ("What are the deliverables?")

Definitions of Coaching

Coaching is the process of equipping people with the tools, knowledge, and opportunities they need to develop themselves and become more effective (D. Peterson & Hicks, 1996).

Executive coaching is a consultative, relationship-based service provided by seasoned consultants who serve as advisors and objective sounding boards to senior executives. This type of coaching is intended for leaders who are wrestling with the implications of tough business decisions, who want to develop new strategic insights into how they can better manage the personal dynamics of their responsibilities, or who want to enhance their own development as they face greater obstacles in achieving organizational and personal goals (Milojkovic, 2001).

The role of the coach or counselor is to help the client learn and to teach the client how to learn. The focus may be on imparting specific skills, addressing performance issues on the job, or supporting broader changes in the executive's behavior. The consultant can coach for skills (learning that is sharply focused on a person's specific task), coach for performance (learning focused more broadly on a person's present job), coach for development (learning focused on a person's future job), and/or coach for the executive's specific agenda. Coaching interventions typically have two parts: the improvement of the executive's performance at the skills level, and the establishment of a relationship that allows for a coach to enhance the client's psychological development (Witherspoon & White, 1997).

Common Coaching Situations

Fix-it situations: In this scenario, the coach provides practical direction for "turning around" senior people who have performance problems. The typical case involves a technically competent person who is promoted to a position requiring management skills beyond his or her training and ability. According to the Peter Principle, "In a hierarchy, every employee tends to rise to his or her level of incompetence" (Peter & Hull, 1969, p. 7).

Onboarding: This situation involves getting someone into a new job, and socializing the person into the culture of that particular organization. This will likely involve joint sessions with the employee's supervisor.

Executive development: This encompasses developing an executive from where he or she *is* to where he or she *needs to be* in terms of knowledge and skill.

Succession: This involves grooming someone who has been designated for succession to a very high position in the company.

High potentials: This scenario may develop when a senior executive in the company recognizes the potential of a junior employee and wants to invest more resources into the person's growth for the future benefit of the organization.

International assignments: This involves helping prepare people for overseas assignments (expatriation) or helping people adjust after coming back from overseas assignments (repatriation). For this type of assignment, it is important to work with the executive's family whenever possible. This type of coaching can be very valuable; somewhere between 16% and 50% of international workers return early because of dissatisfaction with their assignments, often due to culture shock (DuBrin, 2000). Culture shock can involve physiological and psychological symptoms that develop when a person is abruptly placed into a foreign culture. Symptoms may include excessive hand washing, fear of contact with others, fear of being mugged, and strong feelings of homesickness (DuBrin, 2000; Triandis, 1994).

CASE EXAMPLE: SUCCESSION ISSUES

Related to executive development is the idea of developing a successor to an organization's current leader. Consultants often get involved with succession issues in family businesses (Gersick, Davis, McCollom, & Lansberg, 1997).

A large, family-owned manufacturing company once asked a consultant to help prepare the two "boys" in line for succession from their mother. Though the case was complicated, basically the previous consultants had suggested that the boys divide the company into two separate divisions, then compete for who would become CEO based on how each division performed. The family did not like this idea because it would damage family relationships. The new consultant worked out a less confrontational approach that allowed the mother to gradually withdraw her control of the company while each heir received increasing responsibilities. Although this was a slow and difficult process, the sons found it much easier to get along and share responsibility once they were no longer competing for mother's favor.

COACHING AND HUMAN RESOURCE SYSTEMS

Traditionally, an organization's human resources (HR) department is responsible for a wide variety of employee needs, including training and development. An executive coach will therefore frequently need to collaborate with the organization's HR department. Table 6.3 describes the different types of coaching necessary for organizational and HR needs.

Table 6.3   Coaching Needs

Organization Need	HR System	Type of Coaching
1. Ensure talent for current needs	Staffing	Transition coaching
2. Learn new skills	Training	Targeted coaching
3. Meet job requirements	Performance	Performance coaching
4. Ensure future talent	Succession planning	Developmental coaching
5. Retain talent	Career development	Career coaching
6. Build effective organization	Organization development	Executive coaching

WHY IS COACHING SO POPULAR?

Coaching has become popular because of the accelerating changes in today's business environment. There is a growing need for people to learn new things on a continuous basis. Coaching is uniquely suited to meet the demands of the ever-changing organizational environment. The coaching relationship is also increasingly being valued as meeting the human need for a safe place to talk to others about important issues (Kraiger, 2002; D. Peterson, 2002; Williams & David, 2002).

COACHING CUSTOMS

Aspiring coaches need to know the current customs in the coaching field, since clients come to expect these things of all coaches. CoachVille.com (2003) lists customs that they have found to be common to coaches:

Working weekly: Coaches tend to work with clients on a weekly basis, with an average of three to four sessions per month.

Pro bono work: Professional coaches tend to give away or charge a reduced fee for some of their time to those who need it, such as nonprofit agencies.

Client's needs are primary: Coaches do not take on a client if they are not qualified to handle the client's particular concern, and they help connect the client to other resources when necessary.

Networking with the community: Coaches stay in touch with a wide variety of people and resources in the community and share these connections and resources with clients when doing so is helpful.

Advance payments: Professional coaches are usually paid in advance for their services, on a monthly basis, rather than billing by the session.

A coach for the coach: Individual coaches often have a coach of their own, to help them with their own professional success.

Maintaining a full practice: Coaches strive to maintain a practice that provides revenue that is 50% greater than all expenses. By maintaining a reserve, coaches are empowered to provide service based on client need unbiased by personal monetary need.

Coaches stick to coaching: When it appears that clients are in need of other services, such as psychotherapy or financial planning, coaches make appropriate referrals to help the clients achieve their goals.

Confidentiality is maintained: Coaches take care not to discuss their clients with others and protect the confidentiality of any information they receive from clients.

Practicing without borders: Coaches often work with clients on the telephone, and can therefore work with clients from other states and other countries. Frequently, coaches provide their clients with a toll-free number.

Maintaining a coaching network: Coaches stay in contact with other coaches for support, referrals, and professional development.

Continuous development: Coaches continually work to grow themselves personally and professionally, and monitor trends and changes in the field.

Maintaining cash reserves: Coaches keep money in the bank so that they have a safety net when they need it. This helps the coach make decisions based on the client's best interests, not on the coach's need for cash.

Availability: Coaches understand the importance of the relationship with the client, and strive to be emotionally, physically, and mentally available to help the client.

Relationships are protected: Coaches do not interfere with the client's other relationships, and communicate openly and honestly with other professionals when requested to do so by the client.

THE COACHING PROCESS

As with other forms of intervention undertaken by mental health professionals, the coaching process takes place through a series of phases (Hargrove, 1995; Hargrove & Kaestner, 1998; Kilburg, 2000). In actual practice, these phases may overlap or occur in differing order. In general, Phase 1 consists of setting the foundation, Phase 2 involves data gathering, Phase 3 involves planning and consolidation, and Phase 4 involves implementation and development.

Phase 1: Setting the Foundation and Developing an Intervention Agreement

The coach should begin by meeting with the client to establish a focus and goals for the coaching effort. You should make a commitment of time to the process, identify and agree on the methods that will be used, set the confidentiality constraints and agreement, and establish the amounts and methods of payment (if appropriate).

Up-Front Understandings

As coaching is a long-term developmental process, the contract should be for an extended period, ideally 12 months or longer (though there are exceptions to this). You should let the client know that data collection, feedback, and coaching processes are ongoing activities. You should also come to an agreement regarding the specific coaching process with both the sponsor (the one who pays your bill) and the executive you will be working with.

It is also important early on to come to an agreement on who gets what; that is, what data will be privileged rather than public. Agree on what types of things the sponsor needs to know regarding the coaching process before going forward.

Contract with the executive to define the specific processes you will use during coaching. This should include the data to be collected as well as the structure of the tutorial process.

Ensure that all parties agree on the expectations and the format for developmental planning. Allow for regular (perhaps quarterly) review sessions with the executive and sponsor and for some three-way meetings during the process. You should also seek agreement that you will have several opportunities to view the executive at work with subordinates during the coaching process.

Be Prepared

Although at this point in time there are no legal licensure requirements for becoming an executive coach, some coaching certificates do exist. Probably the most accepted is from the Corporate Leadership Council, which offers a PCC (professional certified coach) and an MCC (Master Certified Coach). There is also Coaches U., an online training and certification course.

It is also important when coaching to have some understanding of the business the coachee is in, unless you are only doing personal coaching. Think about your coaching in the context of economics and a business. This will be important even if you are working with a nonprofit, though perhaps not to the same degree.

Here are some questions to ask especially if you need more education about the coachee's current situation (it is always important to ask when you don't understand something):

- What are the challenges for the organization now?
- What do they do?
- Whom do they serve (customers)?
- What is going on in the industry? The business itself?
- What are their goals and the goals of their boss for them, any P&L (profit and loss) responsibilities?
- Results are everything—what does the boss consider success?
- What are the coachee's most salient issues?
- What does the coachee do upon arriving at work at the beginning of the morning? (This is known as the "typical day" question)

Create a Profile of Success

Try to find out what it will take to be successful. What are the organizational imperatives (key challenges, growth mode, stage of development, emphasis)? What are the success factors for that particular role with the organization? What behavioral requirements are necessary to achieve these success factors (types of problem-solving requirements, types of constituencies, style of leadership required)? This profile of success should be created by talking to people who have a stake in the executive's success, such as the individual's boss, the board of directors, and the human resources department.

Build a Coaching Relationship

Mental health professionals are especially aware of the importance of establishing a working alliance with the client. The coach must identify and manage transferences, initiate and preserve a safe learning environment, and create and manage expectations of coaching success. As we know from meta-analyses of therapeutic outcome studies, the therapeutic alliance and the expectancy that things will get better account for approximately 45% of the variance in the change process (Hubble, Duncan, & Miller, 1999).

Client Confidentiality

Just as mental health professionals routinely do in psychotherapy, coaches must be clear about confidentiality when entering into a coaching relationship. This should be noted in the written proposal or the coaching agreement. CoachVille.com (2003) provides several examples of how to word such an agreement, such as the following:

> All of our interactions (conversations, e-mail, faxes, etc.) will remain strictly confidential, meaning that I will not share any information provided by you with anyone without your express consent. The exception to this will be that, from time to time, I may use a situation from your coaching experience as an analogy in another client's session, or in a public setting such as a newsletter or a seminar. In this case, I will not use your name and will refer to the situation in such a way that you will not be identifiable to others. (p. 49)

The coach may also add other exceptions to confidentiality, such as when the coach is made aware of illegal, unethical, or dangerous situations.

A further complication arises when the coachee is not the one who has directly hired the coach. Sometimes the organization is paying for the coaching services of one or more of its employees. In such cases, the coach should be clear to all parties involved about who owns the data being gathered, what information will or will not be shared with the organization, and what information will or will not be shared with the individual coachee.

Phase 2: Assessment Phase (Fact Gathering)

Data Collection for the Personal Development Plan

The coach can use GAPS Information (Goals, Abilities, Perceptions, and Standards) to comprehensively assess an executive's current level of functioning within the organization (Kilburg, 2000; D. Peterson & Hicks, 1996).

	Where the Person Is	**Where the Person Wants to Go**
Person's view	*Abilities:* What the person can do	*Goals:* What the person wants to do
Others' view	*Perceptions:* How others see the person	*Standards:* What others expect of the person

Goals can be clarified through personal reflection, a written personal mission statement, career counseling, values clarification exercises, and career interest instruments (Whitmore, 1992). Abilities can be assessed through performance evaluations, professional assessments, expert observation and feedback, or through personal observation over time. Perceptions can be gathered from people inside or outside the organization through face-to-face conversations or through 360-degree surveys, and through third-party interviews. Standards can be assessed through conversations with the organization's leaders, statements of corporate vision and strategy, competency models, job descriptions, performance evaluations, and statements of team goals. The coach should help prioritize the executive's development goals and develop a concrete plan for development and behavior change. All members of the coaching team, including the organizational sponsors, need to agree on the coaching plan.

Typical Goals of Executive Coaching

Though the goals of executive coaching vary widely based on client need, there are typical goals for those who engage a coach's services (Kilburg, 2000).

- Increase the range, flexibility, and effectiveness of what the client can do.
- Increase the client's capacity to manage an organization (using the skills discussed in Chapter 4).
- Improve the client's psychological and interpersonal competencies.
    —Increase psychological and social awareness and understanding, particularly in terms of how it might affect the client while at work.
    —Increase tolerance of ambiguity.
    —Increase tolerance and range of emotional responses.
    —Increase flexibility in and ability to develop and maintain effective interpersonal relationships within a diverse workforce.
    —Increase the client's awareness and knowledge of motivation, learning, group dynamics, organizational behavior, and other components of the psychosocial and organization domains of human behavior.
    —Decrease negative emotional and behavioral patterns.
    —Improve the client's desire and capacity to learn and grow.
    —Improve the client's stress management skills and ability to handle stress.
- Increase the client's ability to manage self and others in conditions of environmental and organizational turbulence, crisis, and conflict.
- Improve the client's ability to manage a career and to advance professionally.
- Improve the client's ability to manage the tensions between organizational, family, community, industry, and personal needs and demands.
- Improve the effectiveness of the organization or team.
- Improve self-efficacy (the person's belief in being able to do things well in a specific area) or sense of mastery/confidence.

Typical Assessments

The following subsections describe assessments that are commonly used in coaching.

Interview

The psychological study of executives should include an interview focusing on such things as work history and work life, experiences that have shaped managerial philosophy and style, views of challenges in the present role and the way the challenges are being met, personal and managerial style, family history, career aspirations, and current personal life. Explore the client's vision and values both as a person and an executive. How do the clients handle affection (the need to love and be loved), aggression (the attacking or mastery component of the personality), and dependency (the need to work interdependently with others)? What is their ego ideal (their imagined future best; Levinson, 2002b)? Ask for specific examples of behavior in the wide range of executive practices the coachees have experienced. What has provided special gratification, peak experiences, or highly gratifying achievement? Explore their disappointments, failures, and mode of recovery from them. When were the coachees not challenged in a role, and when were they in over their head? How have they dealt with authority figures, peers, and subordinates? How do the clients see themselves and their conscious rationale for the trajectory of their career? What do they recall of their growing-up period and relationships with parents and family? Ask them to discuss anything about themselves in any way they think would help you to understand them and the issues they want to deal with or the problems they must surmount. Have them explain their educational and career choices and their varied job experiences and relationships.

Whenever possible, gather collateral information by interviewing relevant others in the organization and in the executive's family who could offer information helpful to the client's development process. Reviewing past performance appraisals can also yield useful information.

Identify competencies required for the executives' position, identify competencies possessed by the executives (including managerial style and their impact on the organizational climate), and identify the executives' motivation (including the social motives of achievement, affiliation, and power).

360 Feedback

A 360 feedback involves getting input from the executive's peers, subordinates, and superiors, and comparing the information to look for consistencies and inconsistencies. Several 360 feedback instruments are available. The Hay/McBer Executive 360 is a comprehensive planning process that assesses critical competencies and guides the development of the executive. PROFILOR is another 360-degree feedback survey. Nordli is a 360-degree feedback instrument with a checklist and open-ended questions. Skillscope is available from the Center for Creative Leadership (R. E. Kaplan, 1997). Some coaches prefer doing interviews for the 360 instead of using survey instruments.

Benton (1999) suggests that even if the coach does not use a formal 360 feedback instrument, a great deal of information can be gathered through having the coachee informally reflect on questions such as the following:

- How well do I look for ways to meet or exceed customer needs?
- How well do I look for ways to meet or exceed management's needs?
- How well do I take a positive approach to business?
- How well do I work effectively with people in a wide variety of circumstances?
- How well do I analyze complex situations accurately and in a timely manner?
- How well do I minimize activities that do not add value to the organization?
- How well do I value others' thinking; champion others' thoughts?
- How well do I understand how to get things done in the organization?
- How well do I have in-depth industry knowledge?
- How well do I overcome obstacles?
- How well do I quickly act when I see an opportunity?
- How well do I demonstrate intellectual curiosity?
- How well do I make sure I can be counted on?
- How well do I remain in control when stressed or pressed?
- How well do I gain trust?
- How well do I admit responsibility for failures or mistakes?
- How well do I help others?
- How well do I follow through to get results?

- How well do I set a good example?
- How well do I see and understand the broad view of business? (pp. 104–105)

Psychological Testing

Mental health professionals are accustomed to looking for psychopathology when performing assessments. However, when performing assessments during the coaching process, you should use a battery that helps you get a comprehensive picture of the normal personality.

CASE EXAMPLE: HELPING A COACH

A professional coach I had met a few years before (a former executive) called and wanted help with the psychological assessment of someone he was coaching. What do you think of first? Why? How will an assessment be of benefit? Is he unclear about the person, or is he looking for an objective way to deliver bad or hard news? What does he need?

The Situation

A community college in another city had a change in administration and more recently a new vice president (VP) of finance/administration. The new VP is changing and modernizing the expectations for the directors of that area. The former VP did all the leadership and management tasks; the directors did what they were told and did project-management-level work. When the new VP raised expectations, one director did not seem to get it—in the facilities area. Professionally, the director is an architect who had worked as a contractor and is now running facilities management. The director is having a hard time understanding what the new VP wants. The VP is committed to giving the director a chance, but she doubts he can turn it around. If he fails, he will move into a lower job or move on. They have already done a review, goal setting, examination of staffing, and benchmarking. The coach's question is "Where is this person?"

What Kind of Coaching Situation Is This?

This is a "fix-it" situation with doubts about success.

What Should You Ask the Coach?

What are the expectations and how is the director failing? What is judged to be the cause of the failure? What is the coachee's explanation? Is the VP really committed to giving the director a chance? What has been tried so far?

What Is Working against the Coachee?

The coachee is associated with the old regime by a new VP and president. The VP wants the director to be proactive, and the director is doing project management and responding to crises. The VP is hard-driving and works harder than the director. She has no children and is in her early 40s; he has a family, is in his late 40s, and works fewer hours. She feels that he does not provide enough follow-through, or that he provides her with the wrong things. She resents having to tell him what to do. Does he have the capacity, interest, desire, and personality to do the job? The coachee sees everything as his job and feels he has too much to do, at a time when he needs to delegate more since he is filling a vacant position. Coaching goals will include helping him to become more organized and efficient, but what should the other coaching goals be? Perhaps assessment will help him clarify his own interests and goals. Does he want to function at this level, or does he prefer to function at a project level (construction of individual buildings or other more proactive work)?

Assessment Instruments Given

- 16PF
- NEO
- Strong
- FIRO-B
- Campbell Abilities and Interests
- Watson Glaser Critical Thinking
- Wonderlic
- Comprehensive Ability Battery (CAB)
- Elliot Jaques questions (These are questions that look at how conceptually sophisticated someone is about dealing with complicated issues; e.g., "Tell me how you would handle an employee who develops a drug problem.")

How Do We Set Things Up?

Working with other consultants can be tricky—you must make sure that they stay in charge and that you don't undermine them. Give feedback to the coachee with the coach present.

Assessment Results

During the interviews, it was discovered that the coachee was waiting for his manager's planning and direction, while she was waiting for him in terms of planning and direction. He has been dealing with depression, anxiety, and work/family issues since he became seriously depressed 3 years ago. His resolution was to lessen perfectionism, take things less seriously, and to favor more family priority and less work priority.

On the Wonderlic Personnel Test, the coachee scored a 33 (missing only two items). In the normative group, upper level management score 28 and over, with a standard deviation of 6. Hence, the coachee's score suggests that he is able to gather and synthesize information easily, and he can infer information and conclusions from on-the-job situations.

The coachee scored lower on the 16PF reasoning subtest, which indicates that he was more in the concrete direction than expected.

The coachee's Watson-Glaser Critical Thinking Appraisal raw score was 71. This is a high score, and is important where careful, analytical reasoning is an important part of the job.

Overall, his span of thinking tends to be operational in scope.

In terms of personality, the coachee tends to be nonassertive, acquiescent, and passive. He is tradition-bound, conventional, and dogmatic. He tends to be detail-oriented, somewhat perfectionistic, and likes routine and organization. He is high on agreeableness. He is not very assertive or dominant for a leader or manager, and he is less drawn to leadership or control. He has a high level of compliance, and is high in tender-mindedness. He is very straightforward. He is below expected levels of proactivity, exhibiting considerable reactivity.

According to the Strong Interest Inventory, this architect is Realistic, scoring high on Artistic, and scoring average in the Investigative area. The Campbell showed him to be analyzing, producing, and creating. His level of influencing others was low.

In looking at his abilities, he was found to be low in his ability to influence. He avoids leadership and public speaking situations.

Interpersonally, he prefers to keep a low profile.

In looking at his leadership skills, he was highest at enabling (fostering collaboration and strengthening people) and modeling (setting the example and achieving small wins). He was lowest at challenging (searching out opportunities, experimenting, and taking risks) and inspiring (envisioning an uplifting future and enlisting others in a common vision).

Since this was only a diagnostic consultation, the case was turned back over to the original coach. As with many consulting situations, how things eventually turned out was left unknown.

Phase 3: Planning and Consolidation

After completing the assessment, you should plan to meet for a long "insight session" during which you present all the collected information to create a comprehensive portrait (strengths and shortfalls, perceptions of motivation, use of power and influence, decision making, expectations, handling of conflict, integrity, emotional competence, discipline, planning/organization, coping with stress at work or home, selling ideas, etc.). You can present the findings yourself or prepare participants to present findings. It will be important to provide clarification for the feedback and to set up change possibilities. Consolidate the assessment information and target the most important areas for development, including the leveraging of identified strengths. Produce a plan that details specific and measurable goals and action steps. Identify prospective situations to apply what is being learned. Use ongoing data collection and a continuous feedback process.

Phase 4: Implementation and Development

With the executive's approval, data from the information-gathering process are shared in a meeting involving the executive, the organizational sponsor, and the consultant. A plan is then agreed on, which may involve additional meetings with others in the organization. Plans may involve the following:

- Providing an experience of behavioral mastery or cognitive control over the problems and issues
- Assessing, confronting, and solving problems and issues
- Identifying and working with emotions
- Identifying and managing resistance, defenses, and operating problems

- Identifying and managing conflicts in the organization, in the working relationships, and in the unconscious life of the client
- Using techniques and methods flexibly and effectively

As in psychotherapy, it is important to get the issues on the table. Use feedback, disclosure, and other communication techniques to maximum effect. Emphasize the reality principle—what will work most effectively with the best long-term outcomes. Be prepared to confront acting out, moral issues, or ethical lapses in a tactful way. Try to use and engage in yourself and in your client the highest level of defensive operations—sublimation, learning and problem solving, communication, curiosity, humor, and creativity.

Typically, you will meet monthly with the client for a 2-hour session for the first 12 months to 2 years. Additional feedback instruments can be used when needed. A coaching contract, similar to a treatment plan, calls for formal development plans with specific goals and targets, reviewed and signed off on by the reporting official. Goals and expectations are made explicit in terms of needed competencies (e.g., interpersonal sensitivity, concern for personal impact, relationship building, leadership, use of influence strategies, directing versus developing others, group management, self-control, communicating vision, developing teams, managing conflict productively, developing specific strengths, improving management style). The executive may be asked to keep a personal journal of important interactions. Meet with the reporting official quarterly. After the first 12 months to 2 years, you may wish to cut the sessions back to bimonthly for another 12 months. You should regularly perform an evaluation and attribution of coaching success or failure by assessing your coaching sessions together periodically, looking back over what has been accomplished.

There is also a growing trend to conduct coaching sessions by telephone. This allows the consultant to coach individuals from across the country and around the world. Phone sessions typically last either 25 to 30 minutes or 45 to 55 minutes, and are usually billed in advance on a monthly basis. Recruiting clients from such diverse areas requires creative marketing strategies, such as effective use of the Internet (CoachVille.com, 2003).

THEORETICAL APPROACHES TO COACHING

Mental health professionals who are well trained in a particular theoretical orientation, such as psychodynamic, cognitive-behavioral, or humanistic-existential, can bring these skills with them into the coaching setting. The consultant must take care, however, to modify the techniques as appropriate to the setting and the needs of the individual and the organization, and must not cross the line into psychotherapy. Use of techniques can sometimes feel rather artificial, so consultants must consider the context of the situation when using them. These methods are often simply ways to help the coach conceptualize a case, and are not necessarily overtly described to the coachee.

Psychodynamic Approaches

The basic premise of the psychodynamic approach is that past experiences have a significant impact on current patterns of behavior. People learn various ways to deal with their anxiety (defense mechanisms), and frequently they continue to use defense mechanisms that no longer work very well in particular settings. Individuals who grew up in abusive environments may have learned that they could not rely on authority figures: Those who were supposed to take care of the child's needs were the people who were most dangerous. A certain degree of distrust and suspicion was adaptive in such a situation, but will no longer work well when the individual is an adult in a work setting.

Kilburg (2000) and Peltier (2001) have discussed defense mechanisms in a coaching context. Peltier divides them into adaptive defense mechanisms (positive ways of handling anxiety), defense mechanisms that deny, defense mechanisms that twist reality, and defense mechanisms that cause people to behave strangely.

Adaptive Defense Mechanisms

Though any defense mechanism can be seen as adaptive or maladaptive depending on the context, several defense mechanisms are generally seen by society as more adaptive and functional when an individual is experiencing a high degree of stress. Coaches should take note when they see clients using them, and help clients to become aware of when and how they are using them. Sometimes clients may use these defenses without even knowing that they are methods for coping with distressing situations, or they may use them in extreme ways that are maladaptive. Coaches can work with clients to deal with the root causes of the anxiety when appropriate, and can help them optimize their use of these coping devices to be most productive:

Altruism: Altruism is the desire to rise above selfish personal needs for the greater good of the community. Those who have experienced the rewards of community service know that helping others tends to help one put one's own problems in perspective.

Coaching example: The director of an agency that is experiencing significant budget cuts may be more worried about her employees and helping them find new jobs than about her own possible job loss.

Sublimation: Sublimation involves channeling anxiety and energy into areas that are creative and acceptable to society. Rather than seeing strong emotions as negative forces that must be eliminated, the energy involved with emotions is harnessed for the client's work.

Coaching example: A man who had a very unstable and emotionally tumultuous childhood later decided to become a child psychologist. He felt that his past experiences gave him a gift—he was able to quickly connect and empathize with the experiences of small children who had been mistreated. He devoted his life to helping children with these experiences, and worked to make changes in the community systems to prevent and reduce future harm to other children.

Humor: Humor can also be a healthy way to discharge anxiety. To see a situation as humorous requires the person to take a step back and put things in perspective, which can be difficult to do. Of course, someone who constantly makes light of serious situations is likely avoiding taking responsibility for action, and this may irritate peers. The coach can use humor on some occasions to help a client shift perspectives, but this can be very risky if the coach has not established a strong alliance with the client.

Coaching example: A coach was speaking with an executive who went on for a long time describing all of her (not directly business related) concerns about her executive peers. The coach listened attentively, then responded, "It must be hard work carrying all those people around in your head all day long." The executive paused for a moment, then laughed at herself. A productive discussion followed about the difficulties in controlling others for whom one is not accountable, and on the action steps she could take to protect herself and do her job effectively.

Substitution: Substitution occurs when someone replaces an anxiety-producing activity with a more comfortable one. While keeping occupied with productive activities is better than wasting time worrying about something, the minor activity may be doing nothing more than delaying something unpleasant that must be faced.

Coaching example: An executive who was a bit of a perfectionist continually had trouble completing proposals on time, due to her desire to do them perfectly. Rather than struggling to work on them, she continually found things to file, cleaned off her desk, made phone calls, and responded to unimportant e-mails. Coaching helped her to assign priorities to her tasks, and to allot a specified period of the day for checking e-mails, and so on.

Compensation: Sometimes an individual may have serious deficits in an area, but will compensate by using some other strength. While creatively using strengths can be adaptive, weaknesses can go unrecognized and undeveloped. The coach should be sensitive to an individual's desire to not appear weak, and can reassure the client of the confidentiality of the coaching relationship.

Coaching example: An executive with a "math phobia" had somehow managed to avoid dealing with financial statements for over a year before his direct supervisor began to hold him more accountable. The executive was able to use his well-developed interpersonal skills to compensate for his phobia—he was able to persuade others who were more expert in the area of finances to give him brief explanations of the reports. However, as the organization began losing profits, the executive needed a more detailed understanding of what was going on in the company's financial statements. The coach worked with the executive to reduce his anxiety and assisted him in getting through an online course in basic finance and accounting.

Rituals: In a world that is constantly changing and presenting myriad complex variables, rituals give an individual a sense of structure and stability. An executive may always listen to Mozart when reading financial statements, a basketball player may always bounce the ball four times before taking a free throw, or a counselor may always check the previous week's therapy note before a session. Organizational rituals, such as always having a pitch-in lunch on the last Friday of the month, give employees a sense of structure and predictability. Coaches can help clients find a good balance so that rituals do not become unwieldy and unproductive.

Coaching example: A consultant was once called in to help with "employee morale." During her assessment, she discovered that the new manager forbade them to spend the first 15 minutes of the day drinking coffee in the break room, as they had customarily done. The manager felt that this was a frivolous waste of time, not recognizing the ritualistic value of everyone coming together and connecting socially before starting the day.

Identification: This defense mechanism involves identifying oneself with a person or an organization. Role models can inspire self-development, and identifying with one's organization fosters a sense of team spirit. Consultants can help individuals and organizations consciously choose good role models.

Coaching example: A manager once called in a consultant to do some team building. As the consultant met with the manager to discuss the situation, she noticed an entire shelf of books by a certain "iron-handed" managerial writer. When she casually commented on this, the manager proudly announced that he greatly admired this writer, and his ability to whip his employees into shape. The consultant tactfully worked to explore with the manager the possibility that such a managerial approach might not be appropriate for his particular organization.

Affiliation: This defense mechanism involves seeking the comfort of others when one is experiencing negative feelings, reinforcing the old saying that "misery loves company." This can be adaptive as long as employees and supervisors maintain appropriate boundaries.

Coaching example: A coach working with the client in a particularly difficult situation felt that he was not contributing much. He approached the client and told her his thoughts, asking if she would like to terminate the coaching relationship. She replied that she still very much wanted to continue with his services, valuing his emotional support and skills at being a good sounding board.

Defense Mechanisms That Deny

Some defense mechanisms are designed to push the problem completely out of the individual's conscious awareness. The individual is likely to know about the problem at some level but is unlikely to openly admit it. Coaches must take note when they see such defenses and try to determine if it is worthwhile to subtly bring the problem to conscious awareness:

Denial: Denial occurs when a person strongly wishes that something is not so. The individual ignores or refuses to seek out any information that would confirm that the undesirable situation really exists.

Coaching example: The CEO of a company in dire financial trouble refused to acknowledge how bad the situation was. When her subordinates tried to bring the financial statements to her attention, she would simply say, "I don't put much faith in numbers." The coach worked with her to help her understand that the numbers did not reflect any negative qualities in her leadership abilities, but were guideposts to help her focus on the areas of the business that most needed her attention.

Repression: A form of denial, repression involves completely pushing a thought out of one's consciousness. In an organization, this can be seen when certain topics are completely taboo. When topics cannot be discussed, they cannot be dealt with effectively.

Coaching example: A coach was called in to work with a newly promoted supervisor. His immediate subordinates were treating him very disrespectfully. At first, it was suspected that jealousy was the reason; then the coach discovered that no one really wanted that job anyway. Eventually, it came out that the new supervisor's brother had once held the position, and had treated everyone poorly. When these memories openly surfaced and were talked about, resentment for the new supervisor lessened.

Isolation: This defense mechanism involves separating emotions from behaviors. This is sometimes necessary, as when a manager must fire an employee, but also can be detrimental to the organization when it is regularly used as a defense against anxiety.

Coaching example: A certain manager was once asked to fire someone on behalf of his boss. Though she really did not want to do this, she felt that it would be a way of gaining favor with the boss. She worked hard and spent a lot of energy to steel herself so that she would not appear emotional when she reported back to the boss. The boss was so impressed (and relieved that he did not have to do it) that he made her the "axe person" of the organization. She further developed her ability to cut off her emotions, but in so doing, also damaged all of her other work relationships.

Defense Mechanisms That Twist Reality

When reality is hard to accept, and we just can't ignore it, the human brain is capable of coming up with some clever ways to distort reality to something that is more acceptable:

Rationalization: This defense involves creatively coming up with "good reasons" for past actions or results. Someone who has treated another person badly can think of several reasons the person might have "deserved it." Similar to the "sour grapes" fable, a person who doesn't get a desired thing may decide it probably wasn't any good anyway.

Coaching example: A manager with poor interpersonal skills once hired a coach to help him be more influential over others. After shadowing the manager for a day, she noticed that the manager did not treat his employees very respectfully. When she brought this to his attention, he replied with several rationalizations, such as, "Why should I treat them with respect when they don't treat me with respect?" Instead of trying to argue with the manager's rationalizations, the coach shifted to a discussion of the results of the manager's behaviors, noting that regardless of the manager's intentions, the results of his current behaviors were reducing employee productivity.

Intellectualization: This defense involves cutting off emotions and arguing about complex situations in a purely intellectual way. When dealing with human beings, emotions play an important role in the decision-making process.

Coaching example: A senior manager once called in a coach to help him learn how to make better decisions. When he was a lower ranking supervisor, he felt that he was very much in touch with the needs of his employees and made important decisions on a regular basis. However, as he moved up the managerial ladder, he found it increasingly difficult to make even small decisions. Explorations with the coach revealed that the manager was extremely anxious about affecting so many other people's lives, and so he attempted to be very intellectual in his decision-making process. The coach worked with the manager to take better control of his emotions, and to use them as effective decision-making tools.

Projection: An individual who very much dislikes a certain aspect of self may project this quality onto someone else or onto the organization itself. This can create confusion for the coach who is called in to determine where the real problem lies.

Coaching example: A manager once called in a coach to help his employees with anger management. However, during her assessment, the coach discovered that the employees were only reacting to the behavior of the manager. The coach worked tactfully and collaboratively with the manager to bring this to his attention.

Defense Mechanisms That Cause Strange Behavior

The preceding defense mechanisms, while they can sometimes take extreme forms, are generally understandable to most people, since there is usually an obvious connection between the defensive behaviors and the problem itself. However, some defense mechanisms can seem confusing or even frightening to those who observe them, creating a lot of tension within the organization:

Reaction formation: This defense mechanism involves treating someone in a manner that is the exact opposite of the way we feel. When expressing our true feelings seems inappropriate, it creates anxiety, and behaving in the opposite manner is a misguided attempt to reduce that anxiety. An individual who despises a coworker may go out of his way to do special favors for him.

Coaching example: An executive invited a coach to help him get along better with his boss. The boss was frequently treating him in a rude manner, and the executive wondered if he was somehow contributing to this situation. The boss agreed to also work with the coach, and it was soon discovered that the boss was actually very fond of the executive. The executive did great work, and he also reminded the boss of his son. The boss was afraid that allowing his feelings to show would give the appearance of favoritism, creating resentment among the other executives.

Help-rejecting complaining: Individuals who use this defense mechanism are perpetual complainers. However, they almost always reject helpful offers or suggestions for one reason or another. Such individuals are likely covering up feelings of inadequacy or anger, and they may have a distorted sense of fulfilling their need for attention by constantly complaining to others.

Coaching example: The coach who was asked to work with a perpetual complainer decided to first "join with" the employee, acknowledging how difficult the employee's situation was. Eventually, the coach had built enough rapport to be more direct with the employee, and talked about alternatives to complaining and different ways the employee could seek social support.

Displacement: When it is inappropriate to display strong emotions in a particular situation or to a particular person, these emotions may be displaced onto someone else. If a manager feels a lot of anger toward her boss, she may take it out on her administrative assistant.

Coaching example: An executive who was complaining about his subordinates was helped by a coach to see that his feelings were actually stemming from the actions of the company president. Meetings were later set up with the executive and the president to bring the issues out into the open.

Regression: This defense mechanism involves reverting to older, less effective ways of handling situations. The anxiety involved is so overwhelming that the person can no longer act responsibly. The classic example is that of a mature adult throwing a temper tantrum.

Coaching example: A newly elected president was under an enormous degree of stress to fix the problems left by the previous president. He found himself frequently pacing the shop floor, which had worked well to reduce stress when he was a line supervisor, but now was causing him to miss important phone calls and meetings. The coach worked with him to develop better ways of handling his anxiety.

Conversion: When some individuals are unable to deal directly with their anxiety, it expresses itself physically through somatic symptoms. Employees who get sick before important presentations, become hoarse and unable to make phone calls, or who break out around the neck if they are required to wear a tie may be experiencing conversion.

Coaching example: A manager asked a coach for advice on how to deal with an employee who continuously broke out into a coughing fit when she was asked to make presentations at staff meetings. The coach suggested that after getting a medical examination, the employee should consider seeking counseling through the organization's Employee Assistance Program.

Passive aggression: Strong aggressive feelings, which are inappropriate to display in the workplace, sometimes manifest themselves passively. An administrative assistant who is angry at her boss may "forget" to create the handouts for the boss's presentation to the company's CEO. Anger is expressed indirectly, and the individual can claim that they really "didn't do anything."

Coaching example: A psychologist was resentful that he was required to attend a multidisciplinary staff meeting every day. He chose not to attend, always finding something else to do or some reason that he was unable to make it. When confronted, he would politely apologize and promise to try to make it the next time. A coach worked with the psychologist and his supervisor to bring the resentments out into the open.

Provocative behavior: Commonly seen in adolescence, this behavior is sometimes seen in adults as well. These individuals provoke others around them and then use those reactions to justify their own behavior. They may sometimes even sabotage their own work.

Coaching example: A coach was once called in to work with an executive who continuously pushed others to the point of making them angry, whereupon he would respond with anger, feeling justified to do so. The coach worked with the executive and his supervisor. The supervisor made it clear that the executive's angry outbursts were unacceptable, and outlined the disciplinary consequences of such continued behavior. The coach also made suggestions to the executive to help him repair the relationships with his peers.

Cognitive-Behavioral Approaches

The essence of the cognitive-behavioral approach is to explore the connections between one's thinking and one's behavior, and to understand how they influence each other. Coaches can use this framework to help individuals work through ineffective patterns of thinking and believing, and can work to build more optimal ways of conceptualizing situations that facilitate more productive action.

Irrational Ideas

Albert Ellis developed a list of what he called "irrational ideas" (Ellis & Harper, 1961) that he believed must be recognized, evaluated, challenged, and changed. It is our attachment to these ideas that causes problems, not life itself (Peltier, 2001):

Irrational idea 1: It is a dire necessity for an adult to be loved or approved by almost everyone for virtually everything he or she does.

Irrational idea 2: One should be thoroughly competent, adequate, and achieving in all possible respects.

Irrational idea 3: Certain people are bad, wicked, or villainous and they should be severely blamed and punished for their sins.

Irrational idea 4: It is terrible, horrible, and catastrophic when things are not going the way one would like them to go.

Irrational idea 5: Human happiness is externally caused and people have little or no ability to control their sorrows or rid themselves of their negative feelings.

Irrational idea 6: If something is or may be dangerous or fearsome, one should be terribly occupied with it and upset about it.

Irrational idea 7: It is easier to avoid facing many life difficulties and self-responsibilities than to undertake more rewarding forms of self-discipline.

Irrational idea 8: The past is all-important and because something once strongly affected one's life, it should indefinitely do so.

Irrational idea 9: People and things should be different from the way that they are, and it is catastrophic if perfect solutions to the grim realities of life are not immediately found.

Irrational idea 10: Maximum human happiness can be achieved by inertia and inaction or by passively "enjoying oneself." (Peltier, 2001, p. 88)

Cognitive Distortions

One of the values of the cognitive-behavioral approach is its techniques of recognizing and correcting cognitive distortions. Cognitive distortions are misguided beliefs about reality, which are usually internalized by the client, who does not recognize their irrationality. These distortions can be either positive or negative. For example, the client can believe that everyone loves all of his jokes (positive overgeneralization distortion), thereby helping him to feel comfortable with his coworkers (even though he may actually be offending them with his jokes), or he could feel that nobody would ever find him funny (negative overgeneralization distortion), causing others to see him as cold and aloof. A coach can help the client see situations more rationally and objectively. Freeman and Fusco (2000, pp. 38–39) present some cognitive distortions, with example statements of what a mental health professional might hear in therapy. In each case, an example has then been added to show how this might manifest itself in an organizational coaching setting:

All-or-nothing thinking: "I'm either a success or a failure." "The world is either black or white." The therapeutic response needs to move the patient from the extremes to a more moderate belief. The modification here is minimal. Accept the patient's position and try to offer the smallest possible modification.

Coaching example: "I don't like what's happening here. I'm going to have to quit my job." The coach can explore with the client if there are any options between the extremes of expecting the perfect workplace and quitting.

Mind reading: "They probably think that I'm incompetent." "I just know that he or she disapproves." The therapist needs to offer a challenge by asking the patient to identify the evidence of their mind reading ability.

Coaching example: "My boss must really hate me. She gave the assignment to Jim." The coach can ask the client about other situations and interactions with the boss. If the client has gotten consistently good reviews from the boss, has received other special assignments, and has always done good work, the client's thought is likely to be a distortion.

Emotional reasoning: "Because I feel inadequate, I am inadequate." "I believe that I must be funny to be liked, so it is fact." Challenging the client to produce evidence that supports this distortion can effectively break down this irrational belief style.

Coaching example: "I feel so nervous about this presentation. I'm going to do terribly, and people will laugh." The coach can discuss the naturalness of feeling anxiety before important presentation, and how simply having that feeling does not mean the presentation will go poorly. If the person has given major presentations before, and felt very nervous before them with the end result that they went pretty well, discussing this with the client may help correct this distortion.

Personalization: "That comment wasn't just random, it must have been directed toward me." "Problems always emerge when I'm in a hurry."

Coaching example: "The boss is really out to get me. I felt so humiliated in front of everybody when she said that our sales figures were down this quarter during the meeting." Here again, the coach can explore what evidence there is for this assertion. If the client is simply one of a number of salespeople, none of whom did well last quarter, the coach can help the client see that it is irrational for him to accept all of the blame personally.

Overgeneralization: "Everything I do turns out wrong." "It doesn't matter what my choices are, they always fall flat."

Coaching example: "Frank didn't like my idea. He must think I'm stupid." The coach can ask the client to produce evidence that Frank thinks the client is stupid just because he did not like one idea.

Catastrophizing: "If I go to the party, there will be terrible consequences." "I'd better not try because I might fail, and that would be awful." The therapist may suggest the patient produce a "disaster" continuum and realistically identify the exact consequences of each perceived catastrophe.

Coaching example: "I missed the deadline on that report. Now the boss is going to fire me, I won't be able to find another job, and my wife is going to leave me." The coach can help the client see that his wife leaving him is a pretty big stretch from missing a report deadline (assuming the client is not experiencing any actual marital difficulties). The coach can help put things into perspective by asking him such things as how important the report truly was, and what the true chances are of him getting fired just for missing one deadline.

Should statements: "I should visit my family every time they want me to." "They should be nicer to me." Challenging the patient to "leave all shoulds outside" can assist the patient in identifying what their own needs are versus what has been expected or dictated by others' rules.

Coaching example: "I should work harder. The boss keeps giving me more assignments, and I should be able to get them all done." The coach can help the client see the impact of these "should" statements. The client may need to explore setting boundaries, since there are limitations as to how much work human beings can be expected to do, and if the client is working too much and too hard, it will affect the quality of her work as well as the quality of her home life.

Control fallacies: "If I'm not in complete control all the time, I will go out of control." "I must be able to control all of the contingencies in my life." Encouraging the patient to view a less-controlled atmosphere creates additional options and may assist the patient to feel less constricted and hopeless in their situation.

Coaching example: "I'm working my butt off trying to make sure my employees do everything right, and I'm falling behind in my own duties." Coaches can help supervisors see that they don't need to be involved in every aspect of what their employees are doing for the operation to run successfully. It can be difficult for supervisors to let go of that sense of needing to control everything when they feel overly responsible for their employees' performance. Coaches can help these clients reframe their role as facilitators rather than as taskmasters.

Comparing: "I'm not as competent as my coworkers or supervisors." "Compared to others there is clearly something flawed about me." The therapist may encourage self-appraisal versus other-appraisal as a mechanism to challenge the patient to progress on an internal rather than external basis.

Coaching example: "Everyone else seems so calm and together when they make their presentations during our meetings. My presentations are so poor I feel foolish." As with all cognitive distortions, the coach can approach this in many ways. First, the coach can discuss how the important thing is to get information across to other members, not to compete with them on how best to do it. Second, the coach may ask the client to videotape herself giving a presentation. Chances are that even though she feels nervous on the inside, she will appear more confident from the outside.

Heaven's reward fallacy: "If I do everything perfectly here, I will be rewarded later." "I have to muddle through this life, maybe things will be better later." The patient needs to be redirected to experience life's events in the "here-and-now" versus putting all his or her eggs in the future basket.

Coaching example: "I really can't stand my job. But if I stick with it for a few years, my boss may give me a good promotion." Some people feel that if they are not suffering, something is wrong, and it is hard for them to conceptualize that things don't have to be that way. Some people may unconsciously think that their suffering will get them more attention. A coach can help challenge some of these assumptions, and help the client look at them objectively. The client in this case may simply not be suited for the job she is in and may serve the company better doing a job that she is more excited about.

Disqualifying the positive: "This success experience was only a fluke." "The compliment was unwarranted." "I'm really a fraud and everyone will find out." The therapist can challenge the patient to list the positives or achievements that have actually occurred.

Coaching example: "I'm really lucky that this project went as well as it did, considering that I was involved with it." If a client has a habitual pattern of not taking credit for accomplishments, the coach can bring this to the client's awareness. The client may have been taught that it is important never to take credit for one's work. While it is important to always recognize other people's contributions to one's own success, continually putting oneself down can become annoying to others. The coach can help the client practice saying things like "Thank you, I worked very hard on that project" when given a compliment. (As in all consultation work, the coach needs to make sure that this intervention is appropriate given the client's cultural background and the context of the situation.)

Perfectionism: "I must do everything perfectly or I will be criticized and a failure." "An adequate job is akin to a failure."

Coaching example: "I know you want that article for the company newsletter tomorrow, but I'm going to need at least two weeks to write it." Individuals engaging in perfectionism tend to have a difficult time in a work setting, as their need to be perfect causes them to take a great deal of time with everything they do. Such individuals may also put off doing work for fear that they may not be able to do it perfectly. A coach may help the client to choose his or her battles, and help the client to let go of things that are less important to free up more time for the important things.

Selective abstraction: "The rest of the information doesn't matter. This is the salient point." "I must focus on the negative details while I ignore and filter out all the positive aspects of a situation."

Coaching example: "I've got far more education than my employees. Why don't they just shut up and do things the way I think they should be done?" While we all tend to look for information that supports our position and ignore information that doesn't, this can be dangerous in the business environment. The coach can help the client to see that if one knows one is right, there is no harm in hearing about the opinions of others. This allows other people to feel heard. Sometimes even very inexperienced people can have brilliant, fresh perspectives on a situation.

Externalization of self-worth: "My worth depends on what others think of me." "They think, therefore I am."

Coaching example: "I feel terrible. Bob was unhappy with my proposal this morning. Sally seemed upset that I didn't go to lunch with her. The customer I spoke with this morning seemed angry that I couldn't help far more." The coach might respond by saying, "It must be hard work carrying all those people around in your head all day." While it is natural for people to want others to like them, if one's entire sense of self-worth is based on others, one is likely to live on an emotional roller coaster. The coach can help the client explore other, more internal sources of self-worth.

Fallacy of change: "You should change your behavior because I want you to." "They should act differently because I expect it."

Coaching example: "It irks me to no end that my boss continues to insist that I give presentations at every meeting, when I keep telling him that I don't want to." While a desire to change things in our favor is a desirable coping skill, we truly do not have the power to make other people change. If the client seems to be continually pushing against an immovable brick wall, the coach can suggest that it might be better to try another tactic. In this case, the coach could explore with the client other options that may be available, such as getting the boss fired (not likely if his performance is otherwise good), learning to like presentations (or at least to tolerate them), getting transferred to another department, or looking for another job.

Fallacy of ignoring: "If I ignore it maybe it will go away." "If I don't pay attention I will not be held responsible."

Coaching example: "I know the employees are complaining about the new policies, but they'll eventually get used to them." The coach can explore with the client how well ignoring tactics have worked in the past. Generally, they tend to reduce anxiety in the short run, but increase problems in the long run. By opening up to employee feedback now, the employees will at least feel heard and will be less likely to build up their resentment. They may even have some viable suggestions for improvement. A small amount of effort now can save a lot of hassles down the road.

Fallacy of fairness: "Life should be fair." "People should all be fair."

Coaching example: "I've been here for three years, and George has only been here for six months. It's not fair that he got promoted and I did not." While we all feel unfairly treated from time to time, one of the signs of maturity is being able to recognize that life is simply not fair. If an individual continuously complains about the fairness of things, the coach can point out that this is common and redirect the client's energies toward strategies for helping him get what he wants and needs in the future.

Being right: "I must prove that I am right because being wrong is unthinkable." "To be wrong is to be a bad person."

Coaching example: "The predictions I gave were inaccurate because the team gave me bad numbers." Some people feel a need to always be right, perhaps due to the need to feel important in the eyes of others. However, no one likes people who cannot admit they are wrong, and this damages working relationships. The coach may be able to help clients take the reverse point of view—how would they feel if they knew someone else who was wrong, but would not admit it? The coach can help clients nurture a new belief that admitting when one is wrong actually strengthens relationships. Clients can begin to practice doing this, noting how people are reacting to that approach.

Fallacy of attachment: "I can't live without a man." "If I was in a relationship, all of my problems would be solved."

Coaching example: "I know I've been fired four times in the last year, but I just haven't found the right boss to work for." Similar to a romantic relationship, some individuals may feel that they need the perfect relationship with their supervisor. The coach can help clients explore more of their own contributions to being happy and productive in the workplace.

As mental health professionals know from their work in psychotherapy, one should look for pervasive patterns of cognitive distortions before labeling them as such. Sometimes clients simply need to emote, and the coach does not necessarily need to intervene. It is also important to consider that these cognitive distortions may have roots in traumatic past events. The coach should attempt as much as possible to base interventions on the impact that such distortions have on clients' performance in the workplace and should refer clients for psychotherapy if they desire to do more work on dealing with traumatic past events.

CASE EXAMPLE: INITIATING STAGES OF CHANGE

Jarrod, a senior manager of Cosmos & Chaos, approaches Cheyenne, a counselor who has become an executive coach, and asks for help in how to deal with the members of his staff. They all seem to be dismissive, talking behind his back, and somewhat disrespectful. Jarrod wants Cheyenne to teach him some "simple techniques for how to deal with such problem employees." He says that his employees are very good at what they do, and he does not want to fire them, but he wants them to treat him with more respect. After further discussion, Cheyenne begins to sense that Jarrod's personality and lack of interpersonal skill are the real problems. She knows that teaching him "techniques to use on the employees" will only make matters worse. Cheyenne contemplates how she will help Jarrod to change his current interpersonal style to improve the performance of his employee team.

The Stages of Change Model

The Stages of Change model stresses the importance of meeting clients where they are before moving them to a new level of functioning and recognizes the importance of understanding that clients may be at differing levels of readiness for change with different presenting issues (Prochaska, 1999; Prochaska & DiClemente, 1992; Prochaska, DiClemente, & Norcross, 1992).

It is important for a consultant to consider where the organization currently is in relation to readiness for change. Trying to force change when the members of the organization are not yet ready can produce frustration and resentment. Prochaska's research identified six stages of change: precontemplation, contemplation, preparation, action, maintenance, and termination. Prochaska (1999) also describes techniques to move the individual to the next stage of change.

Precontemplation

Precontemplation is the stage in which people are not even considering changing. They may be unaware of the need for change, may be in denial, or may not be aware of the impact and consequences of not changing. Hence, exhortations from others that change is needed will not be heeded, and coaches or consultants will only feel frustration in their attempts to force change to happen. The coach must first help the client reach the next stage of change. Prochaska (1999) has found that to progress to the next stage (contemplation), the pros of changing must increase. Clients must begin to see that there will be advantages and benefits to changing.

To help the consultee or client system progress to the next stage of change, the consultant can use *consciousness raising, dramatic relief,* and *environmental reevaluation.* Consciousness raising involves providing information to the clients about the current situation, carefully bringing up issues that they may have been ignoring in their attempts to avoid change. The coach can do this by observing the clients' current situation and providing feedback and interpretation regarding their present pattern of behavior. Direct confrontation can be used if the coach has built a solid relationship with a client.

Dramatic relief involves engaging the clients' emotions to encourage them to begin contemplating that change might be necessary. Fear, inspiration, guilt, and hope may provide an impetus, and the consultant can do this through telling stories, using analogies, and through discussion of the human impact of the current pattern of behavior.

Environmental reevaluation involves helping clients understand emotionally and cognitively how their behavior affects their social environment. This environment can be improved by working with clients on building empathy, clarifying the clients' values, and exploring the systems affected by the current pattern of behavior.

Using Precontemplation

Before their next meeting, Cheyenne joins Jarrod during a routine staff meeting to observe the dynamics of the interactions. Cheyenne sees that though the employees are rather antagonistic, Jarrod's haughty personality and biting comments tend to exacerbate the situation.

Later, Cheyenne meets with Jarrod alone in his office. "Do you see what I mean? It's a wonder I ever get anything done! Please let me know what thoughts you have after observing this."

Cheyenne carefully chooses her words. "I can understand your frustration. The environment really felt adversarial in there."

"It's been that way for months."

"Then it is probably no wonder that you react the way that you do."

"What do you mean?"

"I just notice a big contrast between the way you are in a one-on-one situation, as you are with me right now, and how you were during the meeting. I understand your level of frustration, but the way you spoke sometimes appeared to exacerbate things. For example, when Diane said she did not like the last proposal, you told her that she does not know enough about such matters to comment. This would naturally build resentment in her and the other members. Do you remember a superior ever making you feel that way in front of your peers?"

"I guess I went a bit over the line on that one. They just really frustrate me."

"They would frustrate me too. But maybe if we can find a different way for you to respond to them, we can begin to change how these meetings go."

Contemplation

In this stage, clients actively consider the prospects of change. Though the advantages of changing may lead them to consider change, they will also begin to consider all the things they must give up to change. Since change always involves loss, the ambivalence of this stage may be difficult to overcome. Prochaska (1999) has found that to progress to the next stage, the cons of changing must decrease.

To help the consultee or client system progress to the next stage of change, the consultant can use *self-reevaluation.* Self-reevaluation involves making a cognitive and emotional assessment of how things will be and how a person will feel once the change has occurred. This can be done through imagery, use of role models, and clarification of the client's values. Prochaska (1999) has found that people first tend to look back into the past to reevaluate the impact of their past behaviors, and develop a sense of regret. As they progress toward the preparation stage, they begin to take on more of a future focus.

Contemplating Change

At their next meeting, Cheyenne notes that Jarrod has moved into the contemplation stage. "I've been thinking a lot about our last session. I took a long walk that evening, and began to remember what it was like for me to be embarrassed in front of my boss. I thought about all the different verbal blows I was given over the years. I then thought about the things I had been saying the last few months. At first, I felt like they deserved it. After all, I was the boss, and they should be the ones to change and show me respect. But the more I thought about it, the more I realized that as the leader, I should be the role model. I was abusing some of my power."

Cheyenne listened attentively and provided empathy. She also suggested that he next think about the bosses he has had in the past that empowered him and made him feel good about himself, and how they might respond in his current situation.

Preparation

In this stage, people are ready to begin the change process in the near future. They have begun to make plans and may do considerable research about how exactly to undertake change, but have not yet taken concrete action. Prochaska (1999) has found that to progress to the next stage (action), the pros must outweigh the cons of doing so. If clients still hold on to what they will lose by changing, or see too many negatives in the future change condition, they will not be motivated to take action.

To help the consultee or client system progress to the next stage of change, the consultant can use *self-liberation*. Prochaska (1999) describes self-liberation as the belief that one can change and the commitment to act on the belief. Publicly making a commitment to change appears to enhance motivation more than privately making such a commitment. Research also shows that people are more motivated to change if they have two or three choices of action from which to choose (W. R. Miller, 1985). Prochaska (1999) used the example that for a smoking cessation program, this might involve the client considering either quitting "cold turkey," using nicotine replacement (e.g., patches), or using nicotine fading.

Preparing for Change

At their next meeting, Jarrod expresses his desire to change his own behaviors when interacting with his employees. Cheyenne sits down with him and creates a list of concrete behaviors that he can focus on and begin to use during the staff meetings. They also plan how they will assess improvement. Cheyenne advises Jarrod to publicly announce his desire to change the way he is treating everyone, and to pass out surveys asking for honest feedback on his current and past behaviors, so that he can monitor his progress.

Action

In the action stage, clients have made specific, observable modifications in their behavior related to the goals for which change is sought. The consultant must be conscious of the criteria for desirable action, since gauging how much change has taken place depends on how it is measured. To help the consultee or client system make change happen, and to help them progress to the next stage once the desired change has occurred (maintenance), the consultant can use *contingency management, helping relationships, counterconditioning,* and *stimulus control.* Contingency management involves the systematic use of reinforcements and punishments for taking action toward the desired behavior change. Positive reinforcement tends to work better than punishment, and this can take the form of small rewards (given by the organization, the supervisor, or by the clients to themselves), verbal praise, or group recognition. Self-reinforcements are better to use for long-term maintenance of the change, since others cannot always provide reinforcement (Prochaska, Norcross, & DiClemente, 1994).

Helping relationships involve having supportive people around during the change process. The consultant can provide this directly, by building rapport and being present and available throughout the change process, or indirectly, by helping consultees build supportive relationships both within and outside the organization. A consultant who provides significant support must be certain to replace that support lest the client deteriorate at the termination of the coaching relationship.

Counterconditioning involves replacing problem behaviors with better alternatives. Rather than simply trying to get rid of bad habits, clients must cultivate new habits. This can include the use of techniques such as desensitization, assertion, and cognitive counters to irrational, distress-provoking self-statements (Prochaska, 1999).

Stimulus control involves changing one's external environment to reduce cues that might trigger old behaviors and increase the cues that might trigger the desired thoughts, feelings, and behaviors. This could also include avoiding negative situations and surrounding oneself with positive role models.

Taking Action

At their next meeting, Jarrod tells Cheyenne about some of the things he has been working on. One thing he has done is to avoid hanging around the watercooler, a place where he used to overhear a lot of gossip that irritated him. Also, before each staff meeting, he sits alone in his office for a few minutes and reflects on what he wants to accomplish. He thinks about each member of the team and the valuable contributions they have made in the past. During the meeting, he makes a conscious effort to include everyone and does not ridicule anyone's input. He also consciously works not to retaliate if he feels he has been personally attacked, choosing instead to either reframe the statement or ignore it and get back to the issue at hand. Jarrod reports that the meetings are now going more smoothly than they were before, but says that several members are still speaking in sarcastic tones much of the time. Cheyenne tells Jarrod he is on the right track, letting him know that it will take time to undo the patterns that have been developing over the past several months.

Maintenance

In the maintenance phase, clients work to hold on to the gains they have made. For some, it is tempting to think that complete change has been accomplished, which may result in "relapsing" to old patterns of behavior. Consultants can work with clients to help them practice the new skills, thoughts, and beliefs they have learned until they are thoroughly ingrained. Consultants can also stay in touch with clients to help them fine-tune the changes and progress they make.

Maintaining the New Skills

Jarrod tells Cheyenne that he has noticed a marked difference over the past month. His staff meetings have been much more productive, and his employees have been volunteering more and better ideas for improving the organization. He can literally sense that the atmosphere around the office is much calmer, and he himself feels much less stress. However, he feels that there are still two or three individuals who continue to be disrespectful.

Cheyenne congratulates him on all the progress he has made. She offers to come in once per month over the next few months to sit in on meetings and to observe how things are going, to help him fine-tune his new skills. She also offers to discuss with him ideas for dealing with the employees who are still causing him problems.

Termination

In the termination phase, the client has completely internalized the new pattern of behavior, almost as if the old pattern had never existed. For many individuals, this is difficult to truly achieve, and they may need to adopt a lifetime maintenance pattern.

Several months later, after observing him during a routine staff meeting, Cheyenne tells Jarrod that he is doing wonderfully, and she no longer has anything to offer him. She spends the rest of the session reviewing with Jarrod all the progress he has made, summarizing what he has learned, and they agree that Jarrod no longer requires Cheyenne's guidance on this issue. Cheyenne leaves with an open invitation for Jarrod to contact her at any time in the future if the need ever arises again.

The stages of change approach can also be useful for consultants to incorporate into other models and techniques, at both the individual and the organizational level. Assessing a client's or an organization's readiness for change, especially in consideration of the multiple levels involved with most issues, is an important skill for all consultants to have.

The Existential Approach

The existential approach involves facing the big issues of life. There are four main issues that this approach boldly explores: death, freedom, isolation, and meaninglessness (Batchelor, 1983; Bugental, 1965, 1987; Frankl, 1963, 1969; May, 1953, 1975; Yalom, 1980). Looking at death is to confront our own mortality and the inevitability of death, loss, and change. Looking at freedom is to accept that we must take responsibility for the choices we have and have not made in our lives. Looking at isolation is to face our need for social interaction while acknowledging that we can never truly merge with another person, and hence are ultimately always alone. Looking at meaninglessness is to question why we are here and what to do with the life we have.

Wrestling with these questions is not always pleasant, but these issues are always present, and facing them directly helps to lessen our fears about them. Knowing that life is short gives us a sense of urgency and motivation to change. Awareness of our isolation motivates us to treasure our interactions with others. Awareness of our freedom to choose, and of our ability to create our own meaning inspires us with visions that we can create more fulfilling lives.

The existential approach respects the autonomy of the individual and considers that the therapist's job is to assist in removing obstacles and restoring the client's will to make decisions to change (Yalom, 1980). Research underlying the Common Factors approach (Hubble et al., 1999; M. J. Lambert, 1992) shows that regardless of theoretical orientation, extratherapeutic factors (factors that occur outside of the therapy session) account for 40% of therapeutic change, relationship factors account for 30%, expectancy factors account for 15%, and technique accounts for only 15%. The existential approach also emphasizes the importance of the therapeutic relationship. Indeed, a book written by Bugental (1987) on psychotherapy consists almost entirely of how to deepen the relationship. Also like the Common Factors approach, the existential approach regards the building of hope as important to motivate someone to change and sees specific techniques as playing a comparatively small role in outcome. Consultants can adapt these theoretical ideas to coaching and consultation settings.

Death

The existential approach views death as an inevitable, unavoidable aspect of life. Here we mean death both literally, as the end of life, and as a metaphor for change, which involves the loss of something and the birth of something new. Normally, we are able to suppress thoughts of death, and ignore the signs of death and decay that are all around us. However, when we unexpectedly lose a loved one, or are otherwise made aware of the pervasiveness of death, we tend to experience great anxiety.

In organizations, death may represent the shutting down of the company, the loss of one's job, the anxiety of losing coworkers to layoffs, or simply the unpredictable changes that continuously occur in the business world. Coaches can help clients bring these anxieties and fears out into the open, where they can be talked about and dealt with directly.

CASE EXAMPLE: EXISTENTIAL INTERVENTION

Frederick, who was recently promoted to the position of chief executive officer of Mega Pharmaceuticals, calls in Cheyenne to do some executive coaching with him. As they begin to talk, Frederick describes his current thoughts and feelings about becoming chief executive officer. Though he has dreamed of a position like this all his life, he somehow feels disappointed and empty. He wonders what he can really do for his company and for his stakeholders, what he can give to the customer, and how he should deal with current and future issues facing the company. As Cheyenne listens, she realizes that Frederick has all the technical skills he needs to run the company, but is dealing with existential issues.

After talking with Frederick for a while, Cheyenne asks him a direct question. "Are you afraid that you might make the wrong decisions and send the company into bankruptcy?"

At first, Frederick seems surprised by the question, and then he turns to gaze out the window. "Yes," he admits, "though I never thought about that directly before. All these years, I've had input into the decision-making processes of this organization, but someone else was always responsible for the final decision."

Cheyenne responds with empathy. "We've both read of other pharmaceutical companies who could not keep up with the times, and ended up out of business. It's a very natural concern for you to have."

"I just get so overwhelmed by the number of variables in terms of where to take the company in order to survive, I suddenly find myself feeling like I shouldn't make any changes."

"Which of course is not a satisfying solution, since the world will go on changing regardless of whether you or your company does."

Isolation

Relationships are an important part of being human. Many times, clients enter therapy because of relationship difficulties, or because they feel that their social support is inadequate (perhaps due to the uniqueness or the severity of their presenting problem). The relationship with the therapist, whereby clients can feel that they are worthy of being listened to and cared for, works to undo previous or present occasions wherein the clients' social or family relationships have been unsupportive. This sense of support enhances self-esteem, and the client comes to see that things can be different, after all. This sense of hope, this contrast with "how things could be" versus "how things have been up to now" works to pull, inspire, and motivate clients to engage in new behaviors and new ways of thinking. Coaches can also apply these principles in organizational settings.

The Client's Relationship with Employees

In their next coaching session, the topic revolves around Frederick's relationships with his employees. "I've known some of these employees for twenty years, and I feel a strong obligation to take care of the employees, in addition to making sure the company survives."

"It's a heavy but noble burden to bear," says Cheyenne, "but you know the world won't come to an end for any of them if you fail."

"Yes, but I do feel I should try to do my best." Frederick looks up from his reports and smiles at Cheyenne, "I do appreciate being able to talk with you about this. I feel a great sense of support from my employees, but I also feel I cannot burden them with everything I must be concerned about."

"You might consider joining one of the local CEO groups, which I believe are still being offered by the Chamber of Commerce. You'll likely find others that are struggling with the same business and personal concerns that you have."

Freedom

If we believe we are free to make choices in our lives, we are burdened with the responsibility to determine and create those changes. Many individuals long for freedom, but may be overwhelmed by it. When we make our own free choices, we have no one else to blame for our failures. Coaches can work to empower clients, building up their self-esteem so that they will be more proactive in making positive life choices.

The Client Learns to Make Decisions

Another session focused on Frederick's difficulty in making major decisions. Over the years, he had much experience in making big decisions, but now he was having a lot of difficulty doing so.

"It was always easier to make decisions when someone else was in charge," Cheyenne noted. "You could make valuable contributions to the decision-making process of the organization, but you never had any responsibility for the final outcome."

"I'd never thought about it that way before."

Cheyenne continued, "When someone else was in charge, he gave you only a few possibilities to work with in coming up with what the company should do. Now you have the freedom to choose any of a wide number of possibilities, and it can be pretty overwhelming. Though it's nice to have the freedom to make choices, once you make a decision, you automatically shut off other possibilities. Once you decide to make Drug A, for example, you have to divert company resources away from research into Drug B, and you may never know if drug A would have been better than Drug B."

Frederick asked thoughtfully, "So, all I can really do is try to make the best decision I can based on the current data I have, and based on input from my employees, and press on?"

Cheyenne reminded him, "Sometimes it's better to make a decision, tweaking or changing it later on, than to hesitate too long and miss all opportunities. No decision will ever be perfect."

Meaninglessness

Many people spend their whole lives trying to find some kind of meaning or purpose in the external world, only to find that they never feel fulfilled. The existential viewpoint posits that the meaninglessness inherent in the external world is not a cause for despair, but an opportunity for us to create our own meaning. Individuals who are "simply doing their jobs" are more likely to be unhappy. Workers who are able to see, believe in, and feel passionate about the larger purpose of what they are doing are more likely to be motivated to do well, and are more likely to feel contentment about what they are doing.

The Client Finds Meaning

Cheyenne has felt that the last few sessions focused on more of the problems Frederick has been working through since becoming CEO. "In this session, I'd like to focus more on the bigger picture, on why you believe the company is in existence and where you think it should be going."

"One of the reasons I stayed with this company, beyond the advancement opportunities, is that I really believe in what we're doing. We've already created three brand-new drugs that the world had never seen, and our research staff tells me we've saved more than 10,000 lives over the years, and made countless lives more comfortable."

"When you speak about this organization's purpose, you do it with real passion. I wonder how well this is reflected in the company's vision and mission statements?"

Frederick pulled out a copy of the vision and mission statements. "In looking over them again, they sound rather corporate and uninspiring. I think it would be worthwhile to improve on these."

"And how well is your passion communicated to everyone in the organization? Are they keenly aware of all the lives they are saving?"

"My guess is that the employees lose sight of that bigger picture as they work on a daily basis. Can you help me figure out a plan to better communicate these things with everyone?"

Family and Systems Therapy

Mental health professionals who have worked with families know that sometimes the dynamics of the system can push certain individuals into playing particular roles within that system. Even when the individuals involved know that a role has become dysfunctional, it can be difficult to move away from it because doing so will affect the entire system. These roles often are remnants from the individual's family of origin (Blevins, 1993).

Peltier (2001) lists a number of roles that adults seem to take on in the workplace (see Box 6.2).

Coaches can help clients understand the dynamics of the role they have been forced into, in order to adopt a healthier role within the organization. The coach can also think about how systems theory plays itself out among executives in the organization (Gladding, 2002).

Box 6.2

Adult Roles in the Workplace

Star: This person is accorded star status in the organization. He or she is treated as special, and he or she generally performs at a very high level. Inadequacies are minimized and mistakes are ignored. The star's future is assumed to be quite bright.

Blamer: This person always seeks to blame someone for everything that goes poorly. When things don't come out the way the organization wants, someone must be to blame. This person reliably points this out.

Hero: This person's job is to "save the day." Whenever the organization is in a tight spot, he or she gets involved and makes things work out. The hero makes the big sale or gets the team through an accreditation or inspection.

Rebel: These people don't quite fit in. They are highly autonomous, and they usually don't follow the rules. They dress differently, think differently, and behave differently, and they get away with it, for the most part. Top management finds them annoying, but they are often good at what they do.

Martyr: This person endures constant suffering on behalf of the organization or its members, typically to get and keep a certain kind of attention.

Scapegoat: This person bears and accepts the blame for the team when things go poorly.

Box 6.2 (continued)

Distracter: This person does things that take attention away from the team's problems or difficulties. He or she finds other things to which the team should attend.

Cheerleader: This person stays on the sidelines most of the time and encourages others to take action. He or she does not take risks or get directly involved in anything difficult.

Jester: This person creates humor compulsively. Jokes and laughs distract the team from difficulties and problems. This can be delightful and it can be annoying.

Invalid: This person is often sick or damaged or impaired in some way, so that he or she cannot always take on or complete difficult assignments. Additional stress is too much for the invalid.

Placater: This person can be counted on to appease people when things get difficult. He never confronts things.

Oldest/favored son: This person is given special treatment and has extra responsibility. He or she often serves as a trusted go-between for leadership and other layers of an organization. He or she gets subtle benefits and opportunities that others don't get, but is expected to take some responsibility for the behavior of the "younger siblings."

Mascot: This person is kept around for good luck. Mascots are treated as if they were cute and somehow good for the team, but they are not actually expected to contribute much of substance.

Saint: These people never think, say, or do anything wrong. They are above it all, and behave virtuously, even when such behavior is not completely appropriate or realistic. They behave as if they are better than others. People treat them this way.

Skeptic: This person can be relied upon to cast doubt, especially when optimists or creative people come up with new ideas for the team.

Source: From *The Psychology of Executive Coaching: Theory and Application* (pp. 107–109), by B. Peltier, 2001, New York: Brunner-Routledge.

AN ABBREVIATED LIST OF COACHING METHODS AND TECHNIQUES

Aside from any theoretical orientation, Kilburg (2000) lists methods and techniques commonly used by coaches:

Assessment and feedback: This involves the assessment of such things as intelligence, leadership style, personality dimensions, interpersonal style and preferences, conflict management and crisis management approaches, knowledge, ability, and skills. As mental health professionals know, giving someone direct feedback can also be an intervention in and of itself.

Education: Sometimes the coachee simply needs to gain knowledge about a certain area, and the coach can provide a psychoeducational intervention.

Training: A coachee lacking specific skills may need experiential training.

Skills development: A coach can develop a coachee's skills through description, modeling, demonstration, rehearsal, practice, and evaluation of life experiences.

Simulations: Simulations allow a coachee to practice skills or new behaviors with the coach.

Coaching example: A high-level executive in a major corporation presented with a speech phobia in which he would sweat profusely during presentations. This was a source of considerable anxiety and embarrassment and finally avoidance. Behavioral techniques were used with him, including speaking simulations (in vivo desensitization). He also received pharmacological support and was able to improve considerably in his anxiety regarding speaking.

Role playing: Rehearsal of a coachee's developing skills can help build self-confidence for real-world applications.

Coaching example: A university faculty member came to a consultant feeling conflicted about serving on her chair's search committee. She was aware of problems in the Chair's performance, and felt a sense of responsibility to the Department, but did not want to reveal her feelings to the Chair, feeling that to do so would risk retribution in terms of merit pay or other rewards. After the consultant helped her clarify her feelings and values, she chose to serve on the committee.

Organizational assessment and diagnosis: A clearer understanding of an organization's contextual situation can help coachees operate more effectively within the environment, or may empower them to change and improve their environment.

Brainstorming: A coach can serve as a "sounding board" for coachees to consider strategies, methods, approaches, diagnostics, problem solving, intervention plans, evaluation approaches, hypothesis testing, and worst case analyses.

Conflict and crisis management: Sometimes executives are going through emotionally draining times, and appreciate the support of an objective outsider.

Communications: Coaches can use communication as an intervention in and of itself. This could involve active-empathic listening, judicious use of silence, free association, open and closed questions, memory, translation, interpretation, analysis, synthesis, and evaluation questions.

Clarifications: Restatements of the client's communications can help them feel understood, and may help them clarify their own thinking. Coaches also need to be able to clarify their own ideas.

Confrontations: As in psychotherapy, once rapport is established, coaches can use frank verbal interventions to direct the client's attention to issues, behaviors, problems, thoughts, or emotions that are evident to both the client and the coach, but that are not often openly talked about.

Interpretations: Coaches can also carefully use verbal interventions to direct the client's attention in a meaningful way to issues, behaviors, problems, thoughts, or emotions that are evident to the coach but are out of the client's conscious awareness.

Reconstructions: The coach can make attempts based on what is present in and missing from the client's communications, memories, and so on, to fill in an apparently important gap in recollection of some life event along with its actual emotional and reality repercussions. For example, if a coach notices that a coachee gets very nervous whenever she speaks to the boss on the telephone, the coach can inquire about where and when this first started happening.

Empathy and encouragement: In the competitive modern organizational environment, executives often appreciate someone who will offer unconditional acceptance and support.

Tact: Coaches need to be able to talk about difficult situations and sensitive emotional topics in a delicate way.

Helping to set limits and maintain boundaries: Sometimes the executive possesses the necessary skills and resources, but is simply overwhelmed. Setting limits and boundaries with one's superiors and subordinates can be difficult.

Depreciating and devaluing maladaptive behaviors: Sometimes an executive engages in maladaptive behaviors, defenses, attitudes, values, emotions, and fantasies, simply because they are effective in short-term situations. Coaches may need to call executives on the long-term negative consequences of such behaviors, and help the executives extinguish these behaviors.

Behavioral analysis: Coaches frequently gather and assess information about how the executive performs on the job, which may involve "shadowing" the executive during the workday.

Group process interventions: This involves direct coaching in how to effectively work well in groups.

Coaching example: A young chief executive officer (CEO), only 26 years of age, suddenly inherited the family business. This CEO needed more didactic instruction on the characteristics of highly functioning groups and how to facilitate groups (including task and maintenance leadership functions). Coaching work also focused on how to set group goals and action steps and how to monitor these in a way that would encourage participation and group productivity.

Working relationship interventions: This involves helping the coachee get along better with others in the workplace (usually with key subordinates or superiors).

Project- and/or process-focused work: This involves a collaborative effort to work on specific structure, process, and content issues in the organization, or on input, throughput, or output problems or issues.

Journaling, reading assignments, conferences, and workshops: These activities can be done outside of coaching sessions, and allow the coach to leverage his or her time and effectiveness.

Improve self-efficacy: Self-efficacy is a person's belief in the ability to do things well in a certain specific area. The coach can help the coachee develop self-efficacy or sense of mastery through performance accomplishment, vicarious learning, emotional arousal, or through verbal persuasion. Verbal persuasion appears to be the least effective method. To build self-efficacy: Identify and define clear parameters of success; build and structure situations which have potential for success; identify factors which lead to success; and identify inner sources of success. Listening, explaining, demonstrating, and imitating are required. Simple and concrete tasks require a "follow me" approach, and more abstract or complicated tasks require joint experimentation and reflection.

Other interventions using organization development or training technologies: The coach can also apply other consultation methods, such as those of organization development, on an individual-level coaching basis (Hanson & Lubin, 1995).

One of the most important things a coach should do is build a relationship and forge a partnership with trust and understanding so that the coachee will feel safe. The coach should inspire commitment (by building insight and motivation to focus energy on the goals that matter), grow skills, promote persistence, and shape the environment. The coach should help the coachees see the impact of their managerial style on both individual effectiveness and team effectiveness. Coaches can help executives make rapid progress and effectively adapt to change. Coaches should highlight the key strengths in coachees, and educate them on key dimensions of superior performance to enhance their organizational performance (Hicks & Peterson, 1999).

Coaching is a rapidly changing field, and coaches need to be continuous learners. They should not try to impress the client with psychobabble, but should explain things in terms that are easily understood. The coach should try to go where the energy is, and should translate insight into action whenever possible. The effective coach teaches people to develop themselves and to listen for and ask for feedback.

Coaches build a learning community by providing and creating a safe zone that encourages and supports reflection, creative exploration, and self-examination—be self-responsible and self-challenging; listen, listen, listen, and respond; lean into discomfort; experiment with new behaviors to expand your range of response, take risks, make some mistakes—then let go; accept working through conflict to its resolution as a catalyst for learning; be crisp and say what is core; be open-minded.

Coaches make the unsaid said and the unconscious conscious. Keep in mind that organizations and their people often know or perceive precisely what the problems are with individuals or systems, but they often collude to keep silent or to employ nonproductive, and at times symptomatic compromise formations, instead of describing what is happening and engaging in constructive problem solving.

CASE EXAMPLE

In a large accounting firm, the managing partner was having an affair with another partner. The relationship was going sour, and other colleagues were overhearing arguments. It was the elephant in the living room. It is usually helpful to identify the elephant and allow people to perform the adaptive work surrounding the problem to solve the issue. The consultant in this case was able to do this, and it allowed the firm to reinvent itself. It has become a regional firm and it is now the second largest accounting firm in the area. The female member of the affair left the firm shortly after the intervention.

Coaches often emphasize one side of the partnership between the client and the organization: person-centered (insight-oriented, motivational, human potential), or oranization-centered (feedback-oriented, behavioral focus, well-developed methodologies, a well-stocked "tool kit"). It is important for coaches to balance both. If you are too organization oriented, you compromise your effectiveness with the client. In such cases, clients feel less free to explore their issues, and they sometimes don't trust that you are there for them and devoted to their development. If you are too client oriented, the company wonders if you are on the side of the company and will produce benefits for the company; they may see your consultation as less relevant to their outcomes, and not invite you back into the organization.

DIVERSITY ISSUES IN COACHING

As in all consulting situations, consultants should be keenly aware of diversity issues involving their coachees and the organizational environment. Hodgson and Crainer (1993) discussed important considerations when coaching women:

- Stereotypes and role preconceptions
- Challenges in finding understanding mentors
- Difficulty accessing senior networks
- Difficulty getting honest feedback (males may fear being accused of sexual harassment)
- Lack of visible line jobs
- Having to be twice as good (having different standards from men)
- Differential interpretations of behavior (the same behavior may be viewed as "assertiveness" in men and "bitchiness" in women)
- Less tolerance for child-care issues in the executive ranks

Hodgson and Crainer (1993) also noted special issues that the coach should consider when coaching people of color:

- Difficulty getting honest feedback
- Never sure if feedback is real or racially motivated
- Difficulty knowing who to trust
- Absence of corporate role models
- Having to constantly prove and repeatedly demonstrate competence (working against stereotypes)
- Wondering if position/promotion is a token gesture to meet affirmative action requirements (Robinson, 1995)
- The burden to make others feel comfortable (Kochman, 1981)
- The fear that an individual's mistakes may negatively impact opportunities for other members of one's ethnic group
- Still some closed doors despite modern laws
- Difficulty obtaining access to opportunity at the right level with the right people

Diversity Tips for Coaches

Mental health professionals likely have a good deal of training in diversity issues, but should always be open to learning more. The following is a list of diversity tips that coaches should bear in mind when working with executives in an organizational setting:

- Be open to learning about the other person's culture and worldview.
- Resist the temptation to know more about them than they do.
- Understand that their experiences really are different.
- Take time to establish and build trust.
- Take the time to get to know someone different from you. Having the social time is a foundation and is crucial to build trust. Take the time to make a connection before developing a task orientation.

- Focus on empirical data and observable behavior to help validate feedback.
- Help coachees to get information that may be unavailable to them.
- Use your differences to offer alternative viewpoints and perspectives.
- Expand and develop your own perspectives through the relationship.
- Learn what happens in different cultures—people have to feel that the coach cares about them. One person is not an expert on a whole culture and shouldn't be made to feel the burden of teaching the whole culture.
- Take risks to give tough feedback to the organization.
- Treat diversity as a business issue.

Advancement for African Americans

Several writers (D. A. Thomas & Gabarro, 1999; R. R. Thomas & Woodruff, 1999) have discussed important issues regarding the advancement of African American executives in the workplace. Because African Americans must prove themselves, advancement through the early stages of their careers is slower than for whites. However, African Americans tend to do well once they make it into middle and upper level management. Some get promoted on performance and others on potential. Clarity and consistency are important—organizations should clearly identify what it takes to be successful. Consultants should try to move the organization away from its subjectivity bias by challenging them to bring in objective data. For example, some organizations do well on recruitment but not retention, so objective data can be helpful (e.g., "Your HR records show that African Americans stay only about half the time that white employees do—do you think the environment here is uncomfortable with diversity?"). Determine what development supports are needed within organizations.

Ask people what is racial for them. Don't stereotype them or the forces they deal with. Keep individualizing and talk about the experiences and perspectives of the person with whom you are working.

Coaches are an example of a role model. Help people sort out what is "me" and what is racism. This is difficult—after a lifetime of exposure to racism, it is difficult to differentiate what is "me" and what is the environment, what the individual is in control of and not in control of. Acknowledge what is going on as a result of differences, and remember that people are often searching for a reason to be racist (D. A. Thomas & Babarro, 1999; R. R. Thomas & Woodruff, 1999).

Executive Coaching with African American Senior Executives

Pennington (2002) discussed that in some ways, race is important to consider in the workplace, and in other ways, race should not matter.

Race Matters

Most often, the "race card" is present, even if it is face down (Pennington, 2002). Coaches are more likely to understand its impact if they can find ways to raise it. It is too costly for the executives to play it. Find a way to open discussion about race. Most executives will not volunteer to do so. Understand that behaviors are interpreted differently when demonstrated by blacks compared with nonblacks (West, 2001).

Rumors of intellectual inferiority flourish. Innate intellectual ability is still the predominant belief in companies and in people: "Some folks are born smart and some folks are not." The focus has moved from questions about IQ to questions about "strategic thinking." The coach should force others to define "strategic thinking" to be certain it is not being used as a euphemism for the questioning of innate intellectual ability (Hammond & Howard, 1988).

The coach should insist on defining behavioral characteristics and performance rather than indicators (e.g., "able to synthesize a wide range of information and identify overall themes" versus "a Harvard graduate").

Though a title and socioeconomic status give a person more options, it does not change core identity. One cannot look at African Americans and not see the color of their skin. They cannot deny their color, and their self-identity will always include race.

Translate the "black tax" into a "flat rate tax." Use more "how to" than "hugs"— help clients figure out how to deal with situations instead of having them try to always smooth things over. Give coachees an overall goal of increasing their impact on the organization. There is more value in a coach who provides directions to navigate the environment than there is in a coach who is exploring for insight. Navigation includes mapping the environment, charting the paths of least resistance and most impact, and running interference to minimize obstacles.

The coach should explore the person's interests outside of work activities, comparing, contrasting, and leveraging those skills and interests. The coach can help to identify the written and unwritten rules of success within the organization, asking and helping to answer the question, "Where and how will race be perceived as an obstacle for this coachee?"

Race Does Not Matter

Ultimately, minority executives understand that they must contribute to the bottom line of the organization (Pennington, 2002). Ideally, the evidence of their contribution and success will be measurable and objective. Nevertheless, the coach must accept the paradox that it is critical to consider race to get to the point where race does not matter (R. Lewis & Walker, 1997; Livers & Carver, 2002).

The coach must actively listen to the person's perspective about race, and try to help distinguish between those areas where race matters and where it does not (G. David & Watson, 1982; Pennington, 2002).

STUMBLING BLOCKS FOR COACHES

It is crucial to be aware of potential stumbling blocks when engaging in executive coaching. Next, we look at both client factors and coach factors that can lead to failure.

Hypothesized Factors in Clients Contributing to Negative Coaching Outcomes

Regardless of the skill of the coach, the coaching process may fail due to problems inherent in the client. Kilburg (2002) lists five major reasons that coaching may fail because of the clients:

1. *Severe psychopathology:* The client may be experiencing psychotic symptoms, major character problems, obsessive-compulsive disorder, and so on, and may refuse to seek treatment.

2. *Severe interpersonal problems:* The client may be unwilling or unable to develop or maintain working relationships, or may have significant or protracted negative transference onto the coach.

3. *Lack of motivation:* The client may experience little pressure to change from self or others.

4. *Unrealistic expectations of the coach or the coaching process:* The client may expect the coach or the process itself to substitute for or actually do the work of the executive. The client may also make major or repeated violations of the coaching agreement.

5. *Lack of follow-through on homework or intervention suggestions:* As in therapy, no matter how brilliant the insights or how well thought out the plan, lasting change will not take place unless there is a change in behavior.

Factors in Coaches Leading to Negative Coaching Outcomes

Regardless of the readiness of the client, the coaching process may fail due to problems inherent in the coach. Following are six major reasons coaching may fail because of the coach (Kilburg, 2002):

1. *Insufficient empathy for the client:* The client will sense when the coach does not truly care about the client's well-being or future.

2. *Lack of interest or expertise in the client's problems or issues:* Again, if the client senses that the coach does not care, or is not competent, the client is not likely to risk trying something new.

3. *Underestimating the severity of the client's problems or overestimating the coach's ability to influence the client:* Sometimes as mental health professionals, we can be lulled into overconfidence in our abilities to handle things. It is always important to do further assessments or seek consultation from peers when in doubt.

4. *Significant or protracted negative countertransference:* Sometimes the coach may overreact to the client emotionally, stemming from echoes of past significant, problematic relationships, which the coach does not manage appropriately.

5. *Poor technique:* The coach may use inaccurate assessment, may lack clarity on the coaching contract, and may make a poor choice or poor implementation of methods.

6. *Major or prolonged disagreements with the client about the coaching process:* The coach may believe that the client's views of the agreement, problems, methods, implementation, or evaluation of the coaching efforts are flawed in major ways, and may be unable to reach an understanding with the client.

Characteristics of Successful Coaches

Though mental health professionals must possess many positive traits to be good at what they do, some qualities may be differentially valued in coaching situations. The successful coach tends to demonstrate the following characteristics:

- Shows devotion to profession
- Is dedicated to achievement
- Has nonpunitive attitude

- Gives direct and down-to-earth feedback
- Takes into account the needs of the trainee and coach's needs
- Gives specific rather than general feedback
- Is descriptive and not judgmental
- Aims feedback at behaviors that can change
- Checks to make sure remarks are understood in the way they were meant
- Conveys the message that it is always possible to improve performance
- Emphasizes long-term goals, stressing the ultimate aim
- Always emphasizes successes and treats failures as opportunities for improvements that will lead to success
- Focuses on strengths
- Appreciates and acknowledges environmental factors
- Affirms feelings

Characteristics of the Successful Coaching Relationship

Meta-analyses of psychotherapeutic factors that help clients change has shown that building a good relationship is one of the biggest factors leading to a successful outcome (Hubble et al., 1999; M. J. Lambert, 1992). Communicating basic respect for clients and their efforts to improve themselves and their organizations, and encouraging exploration, toleration of frustration, and the anxiety that comes with risk-taking are all appropriate and part of the basic relationship. Courting favor with unnecessary compliments, encouragements, and flattery will usually lead to trouble in the coaching relationship. Consultants must gauge the extent to which a client is ready to receive such information or engage in a real dialogue. Use a "good news/bad news" format in the feedback session, or ask the client if it is a good time to move into some difficult material. The consultant should be prepared to reduce the tension if the situation seems to call for it. In addition, humor, metaphor, and personal examples in these situations can be extremely useful.

Kilburg (2000) has listed important characteristics necessary for a successful coaching relationship:

- The relationship is predictable and reliable for the client.
- The issues of time, fees, places of meetings, confidentiality, requirements for self-report, participation, practice, follow-through and homework, cancellation policies, information exchange, and goals are made clear in a formal agreement.
- The consultant consistently displays the following behaviors toward the client:
  —Respects the client as a person, a learning manager, and a striving performer in the organization.
  —Displays consideration and understanding for the complexities of the client's life at work, at home, and in his or her inner world.
  —Maintains courtesy in managing the various technical and interpersonal issues that arise.
  —Possesses accurate empathy for the client and his or her struggles.
  —Provides an experience of nonpossessive regard, of friendly, and, when possible and desirable, tender feelings that can approximate the early learning acquired with nurturing parents or teaching others in the client's life.
  —Consistently and, at times, playfully challenges the client to change, grow, explore, reflect, be curious, and ultimately be responsible for participating fully in the coaching process.

—Engages in tactful exchanges with the client.
—Provides assistance for the regulation and direction of attention.
—Interacts with the client in a nonphony, nondefensive, authentic, and genuine fashion.
—Provides knowledge, skill, and technical assistance on the client's organizational systems, behavioral interfaces, working relationships, and psychological components of institutional, managerial, and, at times, personal lives.
—Uses coaching interventions in an appropriate, timely, and effective fashion.
- Emotions such as shame, anxiety, sadness, anger, and sexual arousal are monitored, identified appropriately, and regulated in such a way that the client can use them productively in the work of personal and professional growth.
- The client and consultant constantly and consistently reflect on and explore issues and methods that either impede or improve the executive's or the organization's performance, especially the manifestations of defensive operations, resistance, and conflict. (p. 72)

CASE EXAMPLE: THE CASE OF THE NONLISTENING HR PROFESSIONAL

A hard-working, extremely valuable HR professional in a large social service agency was viewed as needing people skills. A brief (6 sessions) focused coaching process was conducted following an assessment. Since the company had been using the same consultant for a number of coaching situations, the vice president wanted the consultee to get to know the consultant and how the coaching process worked firsthand.

Assessment Results

- Strong Interest Inventory
  —Conventional (very high interest)
  —Enterprising (average)
  —Artistic (average)
  —Social (average)
  —Investigative (average)
  —Realistic (average)
- Basic Interest Scales
  —Office services (very high interest)
  —Data management (very high interest)
  —Computer activities (very high interest)
  —Athletics (very high interest)
  —Mathematics (very high interest)

What can we predict about her from the preceding information? Note that her Strong type is very similar to that listed for a Human Resources Director, Enterprising, Artistic, and Social (EAS), though her highest score was in the Conventional category.

16PF (Selected Subtests)

C (emotionally changeable)	3
E (dominant, assertive)	8
I (unsentimental)	4
L (accepting, trusting)	4

M (practical, grounded)   4
N (private, discreet)   8
Q1 (open to change)   7
Q2 (self-reliant, individual)   7
Q4 (tense, driven)   8
Producing (high)/Venturing/Helping Interests

Based upon the above data, she appears to have a good knowledge of her own personality.

Myers-Briggs

ISTJ (administrative)

What do the personality tests tell us about her style as an HR professional?

FIRO-B

	Inclusion	Control	Affection	Total
Expressed	5	8	2	15
Wanted	0	0	2	2
Total	5	8	4	17

The FIRO-B suggests that she prefers to keep a low profile (wanted inclusion), frequently takes on the task of providing structure and direction for others (expressed control), and seeks out wide degrees of autonomy to do her work (wanted control). It also suggests that she is cautious about how much support and closeness she shows others (expressed affection) and that she keeps a distance from situations where people want to be close and supportive (wanted affection). She is not comfortable relying on others for what she needs (her Total Wanted Behaviors is only 2, which is a very low score).

Skillscope (98 Items)

Highest Strengths

- Makes her point effectively to resistant audience (she and boss agree)
- Troubleshooter; enjoys solving problems (she and boss see her as in the middle)
- Has good relationships with superiors (she and boss agree)
- Sizes up people well; has a nose for talent (she and boss agree)
- Doesn't let power or status go to her head (she and boss agree)
- At home with graphs, charts, statistics, budgets (she and boss agree)

Worst Areas Needing Improvement

- Isn't abrasive; doesn't usually antagonize people (she agrees, boss disagrees)
- Listens well (she disagrees, boss agrees)
- Avoids spreading self too thin (she and boss agree)
- Participative manager; shares responsibility and influence with direct reports (she and boss agree)
- Readily available to others (she agrees, boss doesn't)

After going through the testing with her alone, the Strong 360 was then done with her boss present. Based on the testing results, the goals that were established in the first coaching session were:

1. Change the perception that "I don't listen well." (When she is stressed, she listens even less well, shuts down more, distances herself, internalizes and thinks things out and comes back.)
2. Change my abrasiveness, shortness, insensitivity, lack of tactfulness. (She becomes frustrated with things not getting done, she tends to carry her feelings on her sleeve, and she reacts quickly.)
3. Increase availability. (She multitasks and tends to cut people off quickly.)

The coaching became focused on the first goal of changing the perception that she doesn't listen well because it was important to her, and the coach decided to go where the energy was. As it turned out, most of her problems in the workplace were related to this first goal.

Based on the data gathered from the assessment, an intervention plan can be formulated. She thinks she listens well but is not perceived to listen well, so the coach chose to have her learn the skill of affirmation (through the use of role playing) and active listening. It was suggested that when she is too busy or stressed to listen, she could "call a time out." She should work to drop everything and pay attention when people come to see her, and she should limit her availability to times she is willing to listen.

PERFORMANCE ENHANCEMENT

Mental health professionals who have skills in sports psychology can use these skills to enhance the performance of executives on the job (Cox, Qi, & Liu, 1993; Raalte & Brewer, 2002; Suinn, 1997; Weinberg & Gould, 1999). Clinicians can also make use of knowledge and skills in motivational interviewing (W. R. Miller & Rollnick, 1991), self-monitoring (systematic recording of observations about his or his own behavior), self-management techniques, and stages of change (Prochaska & DiClemente, 1992). Performance enhancement is often a part of the skill set for coaching—either personal or executive coaching (Garfield, 1989; Hays & Brown, 2004). It involves the following considerations:

- Who is involved? (individual, team, authority figure, intrusive third party)
- What kind of problem is it? (academic, behavioral, emotional, medical, mental, lack of skill or resources, poor communication, conflicting values, insufficient support system, confusion over goals, disagreement on policy or procedures— fundamentally the consultant needs to decide whether the situation involves a training problem, a motivational problem, or a characterological problem)
- What is the goal? (stretch, realistic, attainable, clear)

CORPORATE "COUPLES" COUNSELING

The following case study nicely integrates many of the issues and methods discussed in the preceding chapters. It involves a consultation request in which two executives were having trouble with their working relationship.

CASE EXAMPLE: GREEN CHEMICAL

Green Chemical is a small (approximately $50,000,000 in annual sales), privately held manufacturing company located in a rural, mid-Western area.

Jeff Green is the entrepreneurial founder and chief executive officer of Green Chemical. He founded the company 25 years ago after leaving a large chemical company where he was employed as a chemical engineer.

Green Chemical has been successful both in terms of profitability and in the provision of stable jobs for its dedicated employees. During his leadership, Jeff has emphasized innovation and focused on the aspects of the business related to marketing, chemical processes, financial systems, and computer technology. Approximately 15 years ago, Jeff hired Mark Harvey as a salesperson. Mark tripled sales during the past 15 years and was promoted by Jeff to chief operations officer (COO) and president of the company. Four years ago, Jeff brought on Bob Apples as a consultant. Bob is also a chemical engineer who has advised the company on management issues, and has served on the company's board of directors. Recently, Jeff started "open-book management" (Stack, 1994) to create increased involvement and participation among employees. Jeff has been increasingly trying to "back away" from the company to begin to explore other interests and leisure activities.

The Consultation Request

The referral came from a sales executive recently downsized by Green Chemical with whom I had worked during his stay in outplacement. During my initial meeting with the owner, Jeff Green, he complained that he was experiencing conflict with Mark Harvey, his president, COO, and potential successor. Jeff described Mark as "dead serious and not spontaneous." He was concerned about Mark's tendency to direct employees without communicating information to them. He was afraid employees weren't having fun anymore. Although Jeff is not present in the office daily, many employees still come to him with problems concerning Mark's leadership. Eight years ago, Mark started a customer service department with June Davis in charge. Jeff viewed June as a very competent employee, but saw her as dictatorial and "rubbing people the wrong way." Jeff saw Mark and June as extremely close, and viewed Mark as supporting June even when her behavior was inappropriate. Jeff also remarked that Mark is closed and resistant to change, and has objected to such things as the open-book management approach. Jeff described Mark as a manager but not a leader. Despite Mark's ability to build sales volume and customer relationships, Jeff felt Mark has failed to effectively select employees or develop them once on board. Jeff was concerned about Mark's inability to keep June from violating the culture by micro-managing and preventing input from others. Jeff was also upset by Mark's inability to hold celebrations, to give credit to others for achievements, and for his failure to join in on the goal-setting meetings. He worried that Mark expected everyone to be like himself (to work and not complain). Jeff wanted Mark to share power rather than to centralize the decision-making power of the organization.

Mark, on the other hand, saw Jeff as undermining his leadership, fraternizing and showing favoritism with employees by going out drinking with some of them. He also viewed some of Jeff's preoccupations with technology and innovation as esoteric, costly, and nonbusiness related. Mark had difficulty talking to Jeff and felt criticized, unsupported, and generally unappreciated for his efforts and contributions. He wondered if Jeff was having a hard time turning over the business, and if he still wanted to control the business without providing the day-to-day leadership for the company.

Despite these long-standing concerns, Jeff and Mark had little open conflict. Each described himself as being conflict avoidant. By sharing their concerns regarding each other with selected employees, however, their conflict had affected the larger organization. Jeff was particularly concerned about protecting certain people in the organization, especially those in MIS (management information systems) and finance, while Mark was concerned with the fate of other people in the organization, especially those in customer service. The organization seemed to perceive Jeff and Mark as dividing the organization and showing favoritism toward each one's own people and less support toward the other people. Lately, Jeff had become more confrontational with Mark as the conflict had escalated.

Many individual differences troubled Jeff about Mark. Jeff is sloppy and Mark is neat. Jeff loves trade organizations and being the up-front leader, whereas Mark prefers to stay in the background, avoiding nonwork-related social situations.

They believed they compensated for each other's weaknesses. With Jeff wanting to pull back from the business, however, he was concerned about how his contribution would be replaced and his people treated. Jeff had previously attended the Center for Creative Leadership in an attempt to resolve the issue, but did not have any success in doing so.

For Jeff, his relationship with Mark is the most important issue facing the company. He felt that he must resolve the issue or sell the company. He wants to keep the company for 10 years with the same culture and not lose Mark. If he could not resolve the issue this time, he planned to return Mark to sales manager and hire a new president. For Jeff, this would be a difficult action since Mark works so hard and does so many things well.

At 64, Jeff is also dealing with retirement issues. Jeff now lacks passion with Green Chemical, except possibly marketing (making Green known) and innovation. Lately, he has been able to get away from work for several brief periods because good systems are in place. He has bought a fruit farm in Florida where he hopes to get into growing. To be able to retire in peace, he wants to feel secure in the leadership of the company.

The goal of this consultation was to improve satisfaction and harmonious functioning between the two executives, and with those changes, increase teamwork within the larger company. I decided to attempt to intervene by applying a modification of the Executive Fit Rehearsal methodology described in a previous issue of *Consulting Psychologist* (Rudisill, Hempy, Eddy, Zimmerman, & Rudisill, 1998).

Meeting with the Consultant

Bob (the company's current consultant) shared his perspective on Green Chemical. He saw Jeff's strengths as his relationships with employees and his emphasis on innovation. His drinking with employees and failure to give feedback were seen by Bob as shortcomings. He saw Mark's strengths as focus and drive and his weaknesses as being nonentrepreneurial and being fearful of risk. He saw June's strength as getting things done and her weaknesses as ruffling feathers and calling attention to herself.

His goal for the consultation was to help Jeff and Mark become more accepting of each other. He had been trying to resolve the conflict between Jeff and Mark for several years. We discussed the issue of triangulation, in which he had become the message carrier between Jeff and Mark, attempting to smooth the conflict by explaining each to the other. In the process, Jeff and Mark failed to dialogue with each other or resolve their issues on their own.

I attempted to involve the consultant at each stage of the conflict resolution process, not only to use his expertise, but also to reduce any potential resistance to the intervention and to simulate the actual interactions that existed on a day-to-day basis. Everyone hearing the same message was anticipated to stabilize the changes to be made.

Intervention

The intervention consisted of three half-day meetings with Jeff, Mark, Bob, and myself, spaced 1 month apart. They would then be followed by another half-day meeting 6 months later. Prior to the sessions, Jeff and Mark completed several psychological tests (some of the tests had been taken previously at the Center for Creative Leadership) and a 360 degree feedback exercise.

At the outset, I stated the following: "We will be working together in several sessions over the next few months. Today's agenda will be to identify, understand, and begin to discuss the implications of the individual differences between the two of you. The middle session will focus on the changes you would like each other to make and negotiating those changes. The final session will be devoted to contracting with each other to create a new relationship that will be much more satisfying than the previous one. Is everyone comfortable with this agenda?"

Session 1: Problem Identification Session

Goal: To improve your working relationship, reduce your discomfort with each other, and agree on a coherent management approach to move Green Chemical into the future. Is that your understanding?

Working assumption: Both of you value each other's contribution and would like to work things out so that Green Chemical can continue to receive the benefit of your expertise. Is that your understanding as well?

Today's agenda: We will begin to discuss the implications of the individual differences between the two of you. Is everyone comfortable with this agenda?

Rationale: Differences can be very valuable in a work setting. They ensure that different viewpoints and approaches are covered and that things don't fall between the cracks. Ideally, they are valued and treasured. In the context of a relationship, however, differences are a liability. Each difference typically becomes a point of contention, an issue of negotiation, and may result in a sense that the other person is not doing it the "right way." By definition, many of the differences we will be discussing are not likely to change but must be managed by accommodations in your behavior and largely by understanding and accepting them in each other.

Ground rules: Be as open as possible. Respect the feelings and perceptions of the other person. Be accountable rather than blaming. Look to see what changes you can make to improve the relationship instead of focusing on changes needed in the other person. Any additional ground rules from your perspective?

Exercise: The consultant briefly presented the key findings of the psychological assessment. Some of the scores, particularly personality scores were plotted on tables to help the participants focus on potential differences in style, outlook, and approach. When both individuals scored in an extreme but similar range, this finding was explored as suggestive of possible mutually reinforced blind spots. It is important to present such data and discuss it in a nonjudgmental fashion, fostering an atmosphere that is speculative and exploratory rather than dogmatic. If the consultant allows the data to be perceived as "good" or "bad," the session can degenerate into competition or dominance struggles. The consultant strongly encouraged the participants to discuss and amplify the data.

Testing Results: 16PF (A Measure of Normal Personality with Workplace Implications)

Table 6.4 graphically illustrates how Jeff and Mark scored on the 16PF. This table can prove useful in assessing how the two individuals are getting along. Note that to Mark (MH), Jeff (JG) will seem very suspicious, even though he actually scores in the average range for the normative group. Use of these normalized measures helps each partner put the other's behaviors in perspective, and to view them as differences in style and personality rather than as deliberate attempts by the colleagues to be annoying.

Two major differences appeared on the 16PF:

1. Interpersonal style (Jeff was more bold, direct, and thing oriented; Mark was more shy, indirect, but focused on people.)
2. Control (Jeff was imaginative, creative, less disciplined, and expedient, whereas Mark was more practical, rule governed, structured, and grounded.)

We discussed the human tendency to value what we are, to assume that others should act the way we act, and not to fully appreciate the value of another perspective. We processed a number of previous misunderstandings and disappointments in terms of these differences.

Strong Vocational Inventory (Interests)

Mark had considerably more interest in the world of work than Jeff at this point in their respective careers. Mark's very high interests involved enterprising and social themes with conventional and artistic themes of high interest; Jeff's highest interests (at the average level) were conventional, investigative, enterprising, and artistic in that order. Much of Jeff's dissatisfaction with Mark's lack of interest in management information systems (MIS) and new projects was reflected by their differences in interests. Whereas Mark most enjoys selling, Jeff likes financial analysis and working with computers. Both enjoy the management of people. Again, we were able to reattribute much of their conflict to legitimate differences in focus and interest instead of the more malignant motives they had previously ascribed to each other.

Values Clarification Exercise (Values)

In processing this exercise, we discussed the following questions: "What kinds of behaviors or concerns would be generated from this value? What kinds of conflicts of priorities would be generated by these competing values?"

Jeff and Mark showed a remarkable similarity in values. Both executives rated independence—to have freedom of thought and action (rated number 1 by both), improvement (to optimize personal development), friendship (to share companionship), wealth (to earn a good deal of money), and pleasure (to enjoy life, to be happy and content) among their top 5 values. Jeff rated achievement (to obtain significant accomplishments), recognition (to be commended for results), and leadership (to advance and

Table 6.4 Scores on the 16PF

Left Meaning	Average										Right Meaning
	1	2	3	4	5	6	7	8	9	10	
Cool				JG					MH		Warm
Concrete thinking									JG/MH		Abstract thinking
Affected by feelings		JG			MH						Emotionally stable
Submissive					JG		MH				Dominant
Sober					MH		JG				Enthusiastic
Expedient							JG/MH				Conscientious
Shy			MH				JG				Bold
Tough minded						MH	JG				Tender minded
Trusting	MH					JG					Suspicious
Practical						MH	JG				Imaginative
Forthright			JG			MH					Shrewd
Self-assured				JG	MH						Apprehensive
Conservative								JG/MH			Experimenting
Group oriented						MH			JG		Self-sufficient
Undisciplined				JG	MH						Following self-image
Relaxed					MH	JG					Tense

become influential) more highly than Mark, whereas both Jeff and Mark rated power (to have control of others), prestige (to become well known), and expertness (to become an authority), among their lowest ratings (see Table 6.5).

Jeff's disappointment in Mark's involvement in the trade association as well as his lack of interest in up-front leadership appeared related to differing values. For the

Table 6.5   Values Clarification

Jeff Green's Values	Mark Harvey's Values
Independence (to have freedom of thought and action)	
1	1
Improvement (to optimize personal development)	
2	2
Achievement (to obtain significant accomplishments)	
3	9
Friendship (to share companionship)	
4	3
Wealth (to earn a good deal of money)	
5	5
Pleasure (to enjoy life—to be happy and content)	
5	4
Recognition (to be commended for results)	
6	12
Leadership (to advance and become influential)	
7	13
Security (to have a secure and stable position)	
8	10
Service (to contribute to the satisfaction of others)	
8	6
Parenthood (to raise a family—to have heirs)	
9	7
Expertness (to become an authority)	
10	11
Duty (to dedicate oneself to something)	
11	8
Prestige (to become well known)	
12	15
Power (to have control of others)	
15	14

most part, however, Jeff and Mark were told that they held similar values. Each held dear many of the same things. Their differences appeared to be mainly a matter of personality, preferences, and style. The fact that they agreed on what is important (just not on how to get there) served as a uniting factor.

Skillscope for Managers

The Skillscope for Managers (R. E. Kaplan, 1997) was introduced by telling the participants that the 360 degree exercise measures perceived ability, or how one is viewed by others in the organization. It represents a portrait of managerial abilities and not a photograph of reality. At times, feedback can be used to play out politics or to send messages, but it is always useful and interesting. It is important to be open to feedback, or at least to consider how perceptions arise. The importance of how employees tend to act on their perceptions of reality as opposed to reality was also highlighted.

The 360 degree feedback exercise painted the following picture of the participants: Jeff and Mark were perceived as having strengths in all the broad areas of management: information skills, decisional skills, interpersonal skills, personal resources, and effective use of self. Jeff was unanimously acclaimed as having strength in "Brings out the best in people." Development was needed (a majority view of the respondents) in the following areas: "Structures subordinates' work appropriately," "Sets priorities well; distinguished clearly between important and unimportant tasks." Mark was perceived as having no unanimous strengths. Development was needed (majority view) in the following areas: "A good public speaker," "A team builder; brings people together successfully around tasks," "Can easily handle situations where there is no pat answer, no prescribed method for proceeding," "Effective at managing conflict," "Builds warm, cooperative relationships," "Has good relationships with superiors," "Competent at dealing with people's feelings," "Tolerant of the foibles, idiosyncrasies of others," "Brings out the best in people," "Inspirational; helps people to see the importance of what they are doing," "Astute sense of 'politics,'" "Able to inspire, motivate people; sparks others to take action," "Accepts criticism well; easy to give feedback on his performance," "Avoids spreading self too thin," "Strikes a reasonable balance between his work life and private life."

The 360 degree exercise revealed that they held a much more negative view and experience of each other than others in the organization held of either of them. The failure to give each other the benefit of the doubt, and acknowledge each other's strengths, probably represented a negative bias toward each other based on their relationship difficulties, especially in light of the relatively positive evaluations of their subordinates. The testing, particularly the 360 degree feedback, became important data for coaching and collaborating on a developmental plan.

Participant Reactions

Initially, the participants were combative and blaming. After supportive confrontation and norm setting about focusing on one's own contribution to the problems, the session became constructive. Jeff and Mark were impressed with their differences. They seemed to begin to understand some of their difficulties in terms of differences in style and personality. The idea that they could appreciate their differences while working on and compensating for their weaknesses became important.

At the end of the session, both participants agreed to allow the other to see their testing packets to further increase their understanding of each other.

Session 2: Problem Exploration Session

The middle session focused on the changes Jeff and Mark wanted each other to make and on negotiating those changes.

Goal: To improve the prospects for productive collaboration by identifying obstacles to mutual respect and the working relationship.

Working assumption: By identifying and negotiating desired behavioral changes in the relationship, the productivity of the working relationship will improve.

Today's agenda: Today we will focus on exploring some of the changes both of you would like in the relationship, and preferences you have for how to relate.

Rationale: By improving the relationship between the two of you, we will improve the leadership and clarity of direction for the entire company.

Exercise (Dyer, 1987): We started with an exercise that was designed to help us focus on desired possible behavioral adjustments or changes that Jeff and Mark could both make that would strengthen their relationship in the best interests of Green Chemical.

They first made some notes to themselves regarding three areas:

1. Behaviors you would like the other person to do more of
2. Behaviors you would like the other person to do less of, and
3. Behaviors you would like the other person to do at the same level as now.

After allowing time to make notes, I asked them to share their wish list one item at a time in the following sequence:

Mark what would you like Jeff to do more of? (The leader encouraged behavioral responses, and concrete examples.)
Jeff what would you like Mark to do more of?
Mark what would you like Jeff to do less of?
Jeff what would you like Mark to do less of?
Mark what would you like Jeff to do about the same?
Jeff what would you like Mark to do about the same?
Bob what would you like from Mark and Jeff?

We then focused on some specific areas for discussion and further identification of their wish list as time allowed (Rudisill et al., 1998):

- Culture (What is the company culture? How would each of you like to change the culture?)
- Mission and goals (What is the mission of the company? What are the personal goals of the participants? How do they fit with the overall mission of the company?)
- Mutual expectations (What do we need from each other to be successful?)
- Hot buttons (What behaviors are experienced as provocative and disruptive in the pursuit of success?)
- Role clarification (What are our respective roles and boundaries? For what are we responsible respectively? What are the criteria for our success? What are the limits of our respective authority?)

- Working relationship (How will we organize our work together and maintain our communication? How can we best address conflicts and problem situations as they arise?)
- Failure and disappointment (How will we deal with disappointments and a sense of not being successful? What will we do if the relationship is unsuccessful?)
- Success (How will we reward success?)

The consultant's role during these presentations and discussions was to (1) listen closely for clarity and resolve ambiguity by asking questions; (2) look for uncertainty in the listener and help the participants formulate their questions; (3) look for hidden messages and agendas and surface them for discussion; (4) look for and discuss potential interaction problems between the participants; (5) manage conflicts that arise and help participants view conflict as positive in terms of the potential for prevention of future problems; and (6) help participants create working cultural norms that will encourage ongoing resolution of problems (e.g., "we will both welcome openness with each other about our concerns even if it will hurt the other person"). Many of the clinical skills developed from couples counseling are helpful in conducting this dialogue.

The discussion yielded the desired changes listed in Box 6.3.

Participant reactions: The participants started to make explicit their feelings for each other and work on improving the relationship by asking for specific behavioral changes. They began to talk more openly and freely with each other and discussed the possibility of a more open and engaged relationship.

Session 3: Problem Resolution

The final session was devoted to Mark and Jeff contracting with each other to create a new relationship that would be more satisfying than the previous one. Prior to the beginning of the session, the participants were asked, "Are there any reflections or comments that came to mind as you thought about our last session?" "I would be particularly interested in any other things you would like to change about the other, particularly anything you would like less of in the other?" "Any other reflections?"

Goal: To create an action plan to resolve the interpersonal problems in the relationship.

Working assumption: By committing the participants to a behavioral action plan with an increased understanding of the origin of their difficulties, the relationship will move forward in a positive direction.

Today's agenda: Today, we will focus on negotiating behavioral changes in the relationship.

Exercise (Christensen, Jacobson, & Babcock, 1995): "We have discussed findings based on each other's personality, interests, feedback from others, values, and preferences that would be helpful to each of you. To make each of you happier, all we need to do is to increase the frequency of those actions happening that you desire. Some of them have minimal cost, like not asking Mark to do speeches, or showing appreciation to each other. I would like you to try to figure out what you could do or give to the other that would improve the relationship. Take a few moments and write down your thoughts."

Jeff and Mark were asked to share their lists while Bob and I helped them operationalize (the facilitator made sure the items were clear, doable, and, behavioral) and

=== Box 6.3 ===

Desired Changes

Behaviors You Would like Jeff to Keep the Same

- From Mark's perspective:
  - —Continue as the Green Chemical spokesperson with trade associations and the public.
  - —Continue your involvement on the IT side of the operation.
- From Bob's (consultant) perspective:
  - —Continue to grow and learn and to make things interesting for me.

Behaviors You Would like Jeff to Do More Of

- From Mark's perspective:
  - —More communication relevant to the business (vision, goals, expectations, action items, personal direction).
  - —Bring in customer service.
  - —Allow me to maintain my involvement with sales.
  - —See how the current alignment works before making more changes (we sometimes make corrections before seeing if the changes we have made will work).
  - —Let's get on the same page and support each other and show solidarity with the other employees.
- From Bob's perspective:
  - —Increase the number of compliments and increase your support of Mark.
  - —Provide Mark with a clear level of security by providing a contract for him.

Behaviors You Would like Mark to Keep the Same

- From Jeff's perspective:
  - —Remain the Chief Sales Officer (CSO), but delegate the grunt work.
  - —Continue to grow in your new areas of responsibility: finance and appreciation of the use of information technology and systems.
- From Bob's perspective:
  - —Continue to stay focused. Continue to be a person who, when he sets a goal, achieves that goal.

Behaviors You Would like Mark to Do More Of

- From Jeff's perspective:
  - —Increase your enthusiasm, encouragement, and validation of the process in meetings. Join in more and seem more involved.
  - —Confront people when needed and deliver the difficult messages when needed.
  - —Grow more in the nonsales aspects of the business such as finance and information technology.
- From Bob's perspective:
  - —Ask for more help and guidance from Jeff.
  - —Create a structure to help you coach, confront, and set goals with your people.

========================= **Box 6.3 (continued)** =========================

Possible Action Items

- Hold regular meetings between Jeff and Mark. Make discussing issues part of the daily fabric of working, as a matter of fact.
- Discuss negative feedback that arises from others about each other. Give each other the benefit of the doubt and find out the other person's perspective on the issue before jumping to negative conclusions.
- Offer Mark a contract.

---

add to the lists. During the sharing of the lists, the other person was asked to remain silent and merely listen at that point in the process. Later the recipient of the gifts provided input into the process by validating or modifying items on the list.

Following the process of solidifying the lists, it was pointed out that it is also important to recognize and acknowledge the behaviors that the other has done for you. This will encourage the other person to keep up the intended changes.

The participants were also asked if there were any other action items for which they would like to hold themselves accountable. These items were added to the list of action items.

The exercise yielded an examination of both Mark and Jeff's weaknesses and areas of potential development and improvement as well as contracts for each person to follow to improve the relationship (see Box 6.4).

The participants were informed that another follow-up meeting would be held in about 6 months to help hold themselves accountable. At that time, we would go over how they had done with their assignments and with improving their relationship.

Finally, participants were asked, "Has this been valuable for you? Any feedback for me to help me improve what I do?" They were also told, "Thank you for the opportunity to work with you. Let me know if I can help in any other ways, otherwise I'll see you in 6 months."

> *Participant reactions:* Jeff and Mark seemed pleased with their work. They felt that they had come a long way in confronting and resolving their differences. Both had taken responsibility for the necessary changes that were involved in continuing to develop and improve the relationship.

Contracting and Coaching

As an initial follow-up to the problem resolution meetings, we focused on the items of perceived weakness and developed goals for a coaching plan to work on the areas over the next 6 months. For Jeff, the coaching plan addressed the target areas of time management/procrastination/self-indulgence (his words) through developmental suggestions and homework with reading and seminars. For Mark, the coaching plan addressed the target area of managing conflict more effectively, and included developmental suggestions, readings, and tapes on conflict management, negotiation, and assertiveness along with suggested seminars. He also targeted the area of becoming a more effective team builder with developmental suggestions and readings on teams, management, and leadership along with seminars. The coaching plan included many choices and ideas on how to work on the respective problems. The participants were encouraged to pick and choose what appealed to them. They were encouraged to seek

=== **Box 6.4** ===

Areas for Improvement (Using Language from Skillscope)

Jeff's Perceived Deficits

- Decisive; doesn't procrastinate on decisions
- Structures subordinates' work appropriately
- Confronts others skillfully
- Sets priorities well; distinguishes clearly between important and unimportant tasks
- Makes the most of the time available; extremely productive

Mark's Perceived Deficits

- Good public speaker; skilled at performing, being on stage
- A team builder: brings people together successfully around tasks
- Can easily handle situations where there is no pat answer, no prescribed method for proceeding
- Effective at managing conflict
- Builds warm, cooperative relationships
- Has good relationships with superiors
- Competent at dealing with people's feelings
- Tolerant of the foibles, idiosyncrasies of others
- Brings out the best in people
- Inspirational; helps people to see the importance of what they are doing
- Astute sense of "politics"
- Able to inspire, motivate people; sparks others to take action
- Accepts criticism well; easy to give feedback on his or her performance
- Avoids spreading self too thin
- Strikes a reasonable balance between his or her work life and private life

Source: From *Skillscope for Managers,* by R. E. Kaplan, 1997, Greensboro, NC: Center for Creative Leadership.

---

further help or to discuss their progress at any point. We agreed to discuss their progress when we met in 6 months.

Following the formal workshop sessions, Jeff and Mark signed the contracts outlining the changes to which they had committed (see Boxes 6.5 and 6.6).

Coaching Plans

Individualized coaching plans were developed for Jeff and Mark that included assigned readings, tips, and suggestions for improving their work performance (see Boxes 6.7 and 6.8).

Six-Month Follow-Up

The 6-month follow-up session reviewed the outcome of problems identified in the initial meeting, and solicited and addressed current problems reported by the dyad. The

===== Box 6.5 =====

Mark Harvey, President and COO
Personal Contract with Jeff Green

On the basis of my understanding of Jeff's personality, interests, abilities, values, and preferences, I will attempt to make Jeff happier by trying to do more of the following behaviors:

- Overcome my fear of Jeff, don't shut down around Jeff, open up with him, both ask for and give feedback to Jeff.
- When Jeff is present, stay involved and committed to the discussion, but not redundant.
- Confront people when needed and deliver the difficult messages.
- Spend more time conversing with managers and departments.
- Continue to learn more about other facets of the business, for example, finance and information technology. Learn better how to tie the business together.
- Take responsibility for initiating meetings with Jeff.
- Request Jeff's help with the most important problems; allow Jeff to mentor me.
- Share regularly my ideas with Jeff about the direction of the 5 top concerns so that Jeff is aware of my thinking.
- Listen to Jeff's brainstorms.
- Bring negative feedback received from others to Jeff; don't triangulate.
- Give Jeff the benefit of the doubt, especially in front of others.
- Do more celebrating of successes.
- Support Jeff's conviviality within the limits of my schedule.
- Recognize and acknowledge the behaviors that Jeff does for me, encouraging him to continue his positive changes toward me.

Sincerely,

Mark Harvey, President and COO, Green Chemical

---

follow-up found the relationship much improved, and the contracts being followed. They continued regular (at least weekly) breakfast meetings that were described as open and productive. They agreed that things were going very well in terms of climate. An attitude of mutual respect and appreciation was apparent between the two executives. These attitudes were appreciably different from the climate they had previously created. Both executives appeared to be working on their sides of the conflict. I was asked to do coaching and team building with Mark's executive team. During the session, the focus was on how Jeff and Mark had attempted to fulfill the behavior exchange/contract and recognize the attempts of the other. They were asked a series of questions: (1) How did you attempt to do the behavioral exchange? Be specific; (2) Did you notice these attempts? (3) Was there was anything in the contract that was hard to do? Why? (4) Was there anything in the contract that didn't make sense when you tried to do it? Why? (5) List the two best interchanges you have had and tell me why they

========= Box 6.6 =========

Jeff Green, Chief Executive Officer
Personal Contract with Mark Harvey

On the basis of my understanding of Mark's personality, interests, abilities, values, and preferences, I will attempt to make Mark happier by trying to do more of the following behaviors:

- Congratulate the positive successes (e-mail, notes, etc.).
- Initiate regular meetings with Mark that include more communication relevant to the business and that focus on positive agenda items. As a part of this, I will make requests rather than criticize.
- Avoid triangulation with 3rd parties and bring feedback to Mark without accusation.
- Be more regular about initiating phone meetings when I'm out of town.
- Attend to Mark's material needs (e.g., contract, bonus), trying to anticipate his needs so he is not forced to ask.
- Be the spokesperson for Green Chemical, the external representative; avoid putting Mark on stage.
- Take the lead in information technology.
- Deal with conflict whenever possible (e.g., talking to Bob), especially when the problems lie with people perceived to be in my camp, also try to support people whenever possible who are perceived to be in Mark's camp.
- Listen, draw out Mark's perspective and perceptions on issues.
- Allow Mark to pursue the Chief Sales Officer (CSO) role and continue his involvement in sales.
- Give Mark autonomy and independence by fostering a COO role with which Mark is comfortable. Help Mark by correcting the misperceptions of his role by others.
- Give Mark the benefit of the doubt, especially in the presence of others.
- Recognize and acknowledge the behaviors that Mark does for me, encouraging him to continue his positive changes toward me.

Sincerely,

Jeff Green, Chief Executive Officer, Green Chemical

were good for you; (6) List the two worst interchanges you have had and tell me why they were bad for you; (7) What additional things would you like for each other? Say it in terms of what you want more of, the same, or less of.

Following the discussion of the behavioral exchange contract, the focus shifted to the progress of their personal coaching plan. The following questions were processed: How have you progressed with your personal coaching plan? What additions to the plan would be helpful? They were thanked for their involvement and complimented on the improvement in the relationship. The changes were attributed to their creative implementation of behavioral change.

Box 6.7

Coaching Plan
Jeff Green

Target area: Time management/procrastination/self-indulgence
Developmental suggestions:

Readings on Time Management

First Things First by Stephen Covey, New York, Simon & Schuster, 1994.

Managing Management Time by William Oncken Jr., Englewood Cliffs, NJ, Prentice-Hall, 1989.

How to Get Control of Your Time and Your Life by Allen Lakein, New York, Signet, 1973.

Right on Time! The Complete Guide for Time-Pressured Managers by Lester R. Bittel, New York, McGraw-Hill, 1991.

The Time Trap by Alec R. Mackenzie, New York: AMACOM, 1990.

Audio Tapes for Time Management

Working Smarter: How to Get More Done in Less Time by Michael Le Boeuf, Chicago, Nightingale-Conant Audio.

The Organized Executive by Stephanie Winston, New York, Simon & Schuster.

Reading for Procrastination

Overcoming Procrastination by Albert Ellis, New York, NAL/Dutton, 1978.

Seminars

Time Management. American Management Association, P.O. Box 319, Saranac Lake, NY 12983, Telephone: (800) 262-9699.

Managing Management Time. William Oncken Corporation, 18601 LBJ Freeway, Suite 315, Mesquite, TX 75150, Telephone: (214) 613-2084.

Tips/Suggestions

- Finish what you start, avoid jumping around between several unfinished projects.
- Designate a spot for the paperwork, books, and so on that you use most frequently and keep them there.
- Keep your desk clear of noncurrent projects and paperwork.
- Make a list of your goals and objectives at the beginning of each day (a "to do" list).
- Break large jobs into smaller pieces. Be sure to get started on parts of the job that you dislike early. Reward yourself periodically by doing a part of the job you really enjoy.
- Attempt your highest priority items at your best time of the day.
- Set firm deadlines for having a job done.

(Continued)

=========== **Box 6.7 (continued)** ===========

- Make the decision to get started on a project and go public by announcing it to others.
- Reward yourself for persistent effort with short breaks.
- Set short-term goals that lead to project completion.
- Be willing to make decisions based on partial information.
- Record due dates for assignments on your calendar.
- Sort your in-basket according to priority, and work on high-priority items first. Skim or throw away low-priority items.
- Before leaving work each evening, list the things that need to be done the next day.
- Monitor how you spend your time for a week. Use the insights to adjust your schedule so it is in line with your priorities.
- Delegate as much as possible.
- Return phone calls early in the day or near the end of the day to increase your chances of getting through.
- Use a daily planning tool.
- Look at time as a financial investment and monitor how you spend it.
- Assign a "process observer" for meetings to help keep the group functioning effectively.
- If you procrastinate on follow-up tasks, block out time on your weekly schedule and dedicate it to following up.
- If you put off projects that seem too difficult or overwhelming, make a list of the small, easy tasks involved in the project and do these tasks first. Their momentum may carry over into the more difficult tasks.
- If you find a particular project unpleasant, consider delegating it, or do the most interesting tasks involved in the project first. Let the momentum of these tasks carry over into the less interesting tasks.
- Tell yourself you'll work on a project for a half hour to see how it goes (knowing that you can handle it for a short period of time). By the end of the half hour, you may have found that the task isn't so difficult or distasteful after all.
- Establish ways to reward yourself along the way—for example, a coffee break after writing the introduction to a report or a change of pace after completing a major project.
- Think differently about undesirable tasks. Instead of focusing on your dislike for the task, focus on the sense of accomplishment you'll feel after you've finished the task.
- Simply do the undesirable tasks first to get them out of the way.
- Ask your staff to give you feedback about how your procrastination affects them. If that input concerns you, write it down on a note card and keep it in sight on your desk as a reminder.
- At the beginning of each day, plan—in detail—the work you expect to complete that day. List the tasks according to priority, and determine the amount of time you expect to spend on each. At the end of the day, review your list to determine how much of the work you accomplished and how long it took to accomplish it. If your analysis reveals a considerable discrepancy, look for reasons for the discrepancy between what you planned to accomplish and what you actually accomplished.

=== **Box 6.8** ===

Coaching Plan
Mark Harvey

Target area: Managing conflict more effectively

Reading on Managing Conflicts

Learning to Manage Conflict by Tjosvold, Dean, New York: Free Press, 1993.

Readings on Negotiating

Getting to Yes: Negotiating Agreement Without Giving In by Roger Fisher and William Ury, New York: Penguin Books, 1991.

Getting Past No: Negotiating Your Way from Confrontation to Cooperation by William Ury, New York, Bantam Books, 1993.

Audiotape on Negotiating

The Secrets of Power Negotiating by Roger Dawson, Chicago, Nightingale-Conant Audio.

Readings on Assertiveness

Managing Assertively: How to Improve Your People Skills by Madelyn Burley Allen, New York, Wiley, 1983.

Developing Positive Assertiveness by Sam R. Lloyd, Los Altos, CA, Crisp Publications, 1988.

Seminars

Team Building and Conflict Management, Arthur Andersen & Company, 1345 Avenue of the Americas, New York, NY 10105, Telephone: (212) 708-8080.

Managing Differences and Agreement: Making Conflict Work for You, Designed Learning, Inc., 1009 Park Avenue, Plainfield, NY 07060, Telephone: (908) 754-5102.

People Skills, Ridge Associates, Inc., 5 Ledyard Avenue, Cazenovia, NY 13035, Telephone: (315) 655-3393.

Attend an assertiveness training course at your local community center, community college, university, or other source of adult education.

Tips/Suggestions

- Observe your style in relation to conflict. Do you withdraw/avoid, agree to end the conflict, become disagreeable/win-lose, or do you constructively work toward collaboration?
- Use active listening as a conflict management technique (avoid interruptions). Listen carefully to what is being said without judgment, showing interest nonverbally. Ask for clarification of the position (e.g., tell me about, explain, how do you feel about, describe, what). Periodically rephrase the speaker to ensure understanding.

(Continued)

Box 6.8 (continued)

- Try to discuss the real reasons underlying the problem rather than focusing on the symptoms.
- To deal with a conflict collaboratively, ask the other person to meet in a non-threatening place such as his office or a conference room. Begin the session by defining the purpose of the meeting. When you have pinpointed the problem, together investigate alternative solutions, remain nonjudgmental, evaluate the possibilities picking the best alternative and committing to the best solution; follow-up the meeting.
- Look for win-win solutions. Try to find a common goal on which you both agree and keep focusing on that goal.
- List two or three people or departments who tend to "lock horns" on the job. For each source of conflict, determine its cause; decide if you need to meet. If so, announce the purpose, allow both sides to state their problems and move into a problem-solving mode.
- When possible, allow employees to resolve conflicts with each other (coach them on how). If it is necessary for you to get involved, help the individuals define the problem in specific, observable terms. Ensure that each person listens to the other. Help them identify areas of agreement. Have them brainstorm alternative approaches and determine viable solutions, creating a problem-resolution plan. Set up future meetings during which they can discuss how things are going and whether the chosen approach is working.
- Never avoid conflict, but approach it early so that it will be more manageable.
- Approach conflict situations as opportunities to strengthen interpersonal relationships.
- At the beginning of a conflict discussion, express your desire for a resolution that is acceptable to both or all of you.
- Ask the person, "What is the minimum you will accept? What would you prefer?"
- Restate the positions held by those on both sides of a conflict to ensure that the conflict is not just a misunderstanding and to show that you understand the others' perspectives.
- Encourage people to depersonalize the conflict; look at it as a conflict of ideas or approaches, rather than of people.
- Bring conflict into the open without feeling that you are doing something wrong. When people disagree with you, analyze the reasons for their positions.
- Continue to seek feedback from peers in both formal and informal situations about your effectiveness in handling interpersonal conflict.
- Ask a neutral third party to help you and the conflicting party talk through the problem.
- Allow others to vent their anger. Venting frustrations allows people to set them aside while you work through the conflict.
- Clearly tell the other person the things you both agree on before dealing with the points of disagreement. This approach provides a positive starting point by building bridges between people.

Box 6.8 (continued)

- If the other person feels like he or she is losing something or that you are being unfair, listen to what the person is saying. Don't try to convince the person that he or she is wrong.
- Attack problems, not people.
- If a conflict escalates, call for a time-out. Reconvene when both people have reduced tension to a productive level and have regained their perspective.
- Be willing to give and take in dealing with tough conflicts.
- Instead of showing your frustration with the conflict, talk about it.
- Be willing to confront others when you feel they have made an error.

Target area: Become a more effective team builder

Readings on Teams

Tips for Teams by Kimball Fisher, Steven Rayner, and William Belgard, New York: McGraw-Hill, 1995.

The Wisdom of Teams by J. R. Katzenback and D. K. Smith, Boston: Harvard Business School Press, 1993.

The Team Handbook by Peter R. Scholtes, Madison, WI: Joiner Associates, Inc., 1993.

The Skilled Facilitator by Roger M. Schwarz, San Francisco: Jossey-Bass, 1994.

Readings on Management and Leadership of People

Bringing Out the Best in People by Alan McGinnis, Minneapolis, Augsburgh Fortress, 1985.

The One Minute Manger by Kenneth Blanchard and Paul Hersey, New York, William Morrow, 1982.

Seminars

Team Building and Conflict Management, Arthur Andersen & Company, 1345 Avenue of the Americas, New York, NY 10105, Telephone: (212) 708-8080.

Leadership and Teamwork, Center for Creative Leadership, One Leadership Place, P.O. Box 26300, Greensboro, NC 27438-6300, Telephone: (910) 545-2810.

Team Builder, Personnel Decisions International, 2000 Plaza VII Tower, 45 South Seventh Street, Minneapolis, MN 55402-1608.

Leadership and Teamwork, The Leadership Development Center, 4541 Prospect Road, Suite 102, Peoria, IL 61614-6529, Telephone: (309) 685-1900.

Tips/Suggestions

- Convince yourself that you do not need to "do it all." It is okay to rely on others.
- Make a conscious effort to involve others in the decision-making process. Subordinates and peers (or others less capable or less knowledgeable than

(Continued)

Box 6.8 (continued)

you) may not make decisions as good as yours the first time they try. How-ever, they will improve with the practice they will get if you involve them. Furthermore, as they grow in their capabilities, you can spend more of your time on more important issues, more complex problems, and so on. Think of this as a short-term investment for long-term gain. Look for opportunities to use a more participative approach.

- Schedule an annual retreat to build team spirit and commitment to goals.
- Make a list of the key strengths and limitations of each person on your team. Find ways to utilize the strengths.
- Find ways to involve quiet team members without embarrassing them. Try using open-ended questions and reflective listening to draw out quieter members of your team.
- Use active-listening skills to acknowledge, summarize, and reinforce the contributions of your team members.
- Avoid premature judgment of others' ideas and suggestions.
- Reward team accomplishment.
- Value and show appreciation to your administrative and support staff, not just your "line" or professional people.
- Celebrate as a team.
- Pull your people together as a group to solve problems.
- Foster an environment of trust by ensuring that all criticism is constructive and is focused on individuals' behaviors, not personalities.
- Use your team to develop the group's vision, mission, and goals.
- Share success with team members.
- Show your trust by sharing information beyond what is necessary.
- Have fun while working.
- Provide structure conducive to teamwork—avoid too much hierarchy.
- Include an appraisal of team performance, in addition to individual performance, as a part of your performance management system.
- Reward successful team contributions, as well as individual contributions.
- Ask yourself the following questions designed to build a healthier team environment. If you answer "no," this is an area of opportunity for improvement for your present team environment:
  —Do the members of my team trust me and each other?
  —Are my actions consistent with my words?
  —Are my team members and I honest with one another? Is information readily shared?
  —Do I keep my commitments to team members? Do they keep commitments to each other?
  —Do my team and I listen effectively to one another?
  —Do we address disagreements and other conflicts proactively and responsively?
  —Do we value differences (e.g., do we value introverted members to the same degree as extroverted members)?

========= **Box 6.8 (continued)** =========

—Is my work environment inclusive, engaging, and empowering (versus exclusive, controlling, and patronizing)?

—Do I foster cooperation and information sharing with other departments?

—Does my team have fun at work? Do we celebrate together as a team?

—Ask your team members the same questions, and then discuss their responses.

- Value the work everyone does.
- Provide verbal recognition for everyone's contributions.
- Include team members at all levels in as much planning, decision making, and problem solving as possible.
- When you want input from the team, ask for comments and suggestions from everyone.
- Establish the norm of group interaction at meetings. Redirect comments that are inappropriately directed to you. Ask different team members to lead discussions of particular topics or points.
- When involving others, identify everyone who is affected. Check with others to be sure that you haven't missed anyone. Meet with these people and give them the big picture of what is happening. Ask for the help you want from them—inform them about the plan, how they will be affected, get help in identifying the problem or opportunity, have them determine a course of action. With the team members' mutual investment in the objective, you will be better able to get others to buy into your goal.
- As the group leader, facilitate, rather than direct, the group discussion. Group interaction allows the resources of all members to be used most fully.
- Protect minority opinion. The most obvious or popular suggestions are not always the best.
- Make sure the team does not jump to solutions before adequately considering the problem.

One-and-a-Half-Year Follow-Up

The relationship had continued to go very well (several employees had remarked that the tension had eased and a sense of "oneness" was developing within management). Problems arose again, however, when an employee named Lisa, whom Jeff had admired, decided to leave the company and blamed Mark for allowing June to be problematic and disruptive of her functioning. The fact that the company had experienced a brief downturn in profitability added to Jeff's concern.

We met again and discussed the situation as a learning opportunity, looking at the event as feedback to the system. The issue had polarized Jeff against Mark again, triggering some of his initial concerns. Jeff again viewed June as a very competent employee but dictatorial and "rubbing people the wrong way." Jeff repeated his concerns that Mark and June were so close that Mark could not view June objectively, even when her behavior was inappropriate. Mark countered with the problems Lisa evidenced, as well as the improvements June had made in her interpersonal relationships.

Jeff was able to openly express his concerns, and Mark, although feeling somewhat defensive and unappreciated, was able to suggest some organizational changes that might avert problems in the future. The potentially volatile conflict was handled without excessive incident.

Coaching is a vast field, and this chapter only briefly touches upon some of the potential contributions of mental health professionals. There are a number of other ways to conceptualize and conduct the coaching process that we were unable to discuss in this chapter, such as the approach based on Martin Seligman's book Authentic Happiness (2002). Those interested in pursuing coaching should seek more detailed resources such as the International Coaching Federation or Coachville.com.

PART TWO

CONSULTING TO SMALL SYSTEMS

Chapter 7

WORKING WITH TEAMS AND GROUPS

This chapter describes how mental health professionals can work with teams and groups. We explore the nature of teams and groups (using systems theory, role theory, and group theory) and explain how to effectively conduct a meeting and facilitate a group (including feedback, basic skills, methods and tools, and effective design).

ANALOGIES TO CLINICAL SKILLS

As mentioned, mental health professionals can modify the skills they have developed in individual, couples, family, and group therapy situations for use in consulting and organizational settings.

Couples Therapy Skills and Consulting in Dyadic or Small Group Work

The principles of couples therapy are helpful in dealing with any two people trying to get along in an organization. The common issues for couples (communication, power, equity, control, negotiation, etc.) are important in dyadic and small group work and are basically similar. However, the focus is different. Instead of working on achieving intimacy or emotional closeness, the focus is on working together on task effectiveness. There are also no contracts for therapy. The organizational roles structure the work—especially the power aspects of the relationship (as in a subordinate-supervisor relationship).

Family Therapy Skills and Consulting with Small Groups or Teams

The analogy in organizations and family therapy is that male leaders may be viewed as the father (the authority figure) and female managers as the mother (the role of sexism should also be explored with this). Subordinates can be viewed as children (brothers and sisters) in the family, with issues of sibling rivalry and the development of a relationship with the parents while working out competition/cooperation issues with each other. Just as in ordinary families, weak or inconsistent parents create feelings of insecurity and striving to become a parent or parentified children. The psychoanalytic view of organizations relies heavily on the notion that people replay their struggles with their families of origin in organizational settings. People look in their organizational families for what they did not get in their childhood families (Gladding, 2002; McGoldrick, 1998).

Just as in families, pathology or dysfunctional patterns of behavior exist in teams and organizations.

Group Therapy Skills and Consulting with Small Groups or Teams

The group therapy analogy is important in terms of looking at the interaction between the role the leader plays and the behavior of the members of the group. The norms of the group are important, and what is subtly communicated about rewards is often more important than what is said. Groups always operate at two different levels: an overt, conscious level where they focus on the task, and a subtle, implicit level of process that focuses on group maintenance and interpersonal dynamics (Corey, 2000; Yalom, 1995).

Central Issues to Note in Group Process

- Informal roles
- Informal norms
- Interpersonal conflict
- Leadership and decision making

Dealing with Groups as a Leader

- Create structure by agreeing on the basics (task and process)
- Create the appropriate norms by talking and walking the talk
- Depending on the group, create empowerment and participation
- Value and embrace group differences

SYSTEMS THEORY AND CONCEPTS

A system is a set of interacting and interrelated parts. A consultant cannot intervene in one small part of a consultee system without affecting the larger context within which the intervention takes place. The following items are important for the consultant to consider when operating at a systems level (Bolman & Deal, 2003; Haines, 1998; Von Bertalanffy, 1976).

CHARACTERISTICS OF A SYSTEM

All systems are considered within the context of their larger system and its interactions with the environment. Human organizations are appropriately viewed as "open" systems. Their boundaries are permeable, and they are continually engaged in importing, transforming, and exporting matter, energy, information, and people.

Entropy is the universal law under which all organisms tend to run down and die. Social systems may arrest the entropic process by importing excess energy from the environment and storing it to build a reserve. Human systems also have entropy, but human organizations are capable of negative entropy; they can survive and grow, rather than decay and die, if they are able to work out a mutually beneficial relationship with their environment. The organization, for example, provides goods or services in return for the resources it needs to survive and prosper.

Systems are arranged hierarchically, so that every system is a supersystem for systems constrained within it and a subsystem for systems containing it. (A classroom is a supersystem for teacher and students but a subsystem for the school, and so on up and down the hierarchy.)

A system is more than the sum of its parts: its properties emerge from the relationship among its parts and from the system's relationship to its environment.

Organizations move in the direction of growth and expansion while maintaining steady states of dynamic equilibrium in which diverse forces are approximately balanced. Such steady states have the property of ultrastability: The more that a system is threatened with disequilibrium, the more resources it will marshal to maintain or restore its balance. Systems attempt to maintain homeostasis, preserve their welfare and needs, and resist change.

To maintain a steady state, open systems need adaptive processes, including feedback loops that enable the systems to sense relevant changes in the internal or external environment, and they need to be able to adjust their properties accordingly. Open systems also tend to move toward increased differentiation and elaboration (e.g., agencies tend to grow more specialized).

Boundaries are characteristics of systems, and must be considered at the personal level, the subsystem level (team/group), and the system level (division/company). *Enmeshed boundaries* refers to a relationship in which the boundaries are not well defined. There is little autonomy, and there are many personal boundary intrusions. *Disengaged boundaries* refers to a situation in which there is distance between the subsystems and therefore little support or engagement.

An open-systems analysis includes a review of salient environmental systems and internal subsystems. A *technological subsystem* is devoted to the organization's central technology or process. A *supportive subsystem* supports the organization's central processes. A *maintenance subsystem* maintains the organization's systems in good working order. An *adaptive subsystem* monitors the environment and assesses the effects of impending changes on the organization.

In a university setting, a technological subsystem would include the faculty and the teaching activities; a supportive subsystem would be the admissions department; the maintenance subsystems would include the formal policies and procedures; and the adaptive subsystems would include lobbying campaigns to win government funding.

THE PSYCHODYNAMIC APPROACH TO TEAM DEVELOPMENT

To help clients understand how past experiences influence current behaviors, mental health professionals use the psychodynamic approach, even if it is not adopted as a formal therapeutic orientation. This approach can also be useful when consulting with teams, as the group's past experiences, as well as those of each member, will influence their current functioning. Such a perspective can assist the consultant in understanding why team members may have overly strong reactions to what appear to be trivial issues.

In writing about the psychodynamic approach to team development, Koortzen and Cilliers (2002) list assumptions about this approach:

- Experiential learning is one of the best ways to facilitate adult learning (Neumann, Kellner, & Dawson-Shepherd, 1997). The interventions in this approach therefore take the form of experiential group relations workshops. Adult learning about interpersonal relationships occurs by making use of available opportunities in this dynamic environment. Team members take responsibility for their own learning by using these opportunities. Consideration of the here-and-now behavior enhances learning. It also provides the consultant with valuable information on the processes and dynamics in the team.
- We also believe that the individual's and team's behavior (such as needs and anxieties) are both conscious and unconscious, and that consultants should work on both levels.
- Human and personality development start with individual intrapersonal awareness, and the consultant also provides opportunities to individuals to study their own dynamics within the team.
- Intrapersonal awareness forms the basis for interpersonal awareness and relationship building.
- A group of workers—or work team—has a unique life of its own with the individuals (the microsystem) forming the basic component.
- Group behavior follows predictable processes as well as specific, collectively developed conventions, thus creating the team's dynamics.
- Group dynamics refers to the study of how individuals and teams relate to each other, and the implied assumptions and myths. Consciously determined policies are sometimes supported and often subverted by less-conscious factors.
- The group process and dynamic consultant interprets this behavior in order to help move the group along its path to maturity and interdependence. (pp. 264–265)

Koortzen and Cilliers (2002) go on to describe the specific behaviors that consultants should address to improve the functioning of work teams:

- The way individuals and teams manage their anxiety by making use of various defense mechanisms
- The way individuals and teams exercise their authority in the different systems of the team and organization
- The nature of the interpersonal relationships within the team and the organization
- The relationships and relatedness with authority, peers, and subordinates
- Leadership practices and the management of boundaries
- Intergroup relationships between subsystems or departments
- Identity, roles, tasks, space, time, and structures as boundaries, and the management thereof in coping with anxiety (p. 276)

BASIC SCIENCE RELATED TO GROUPS

As mental health professionals know from their studies of social psychology, individuals in a group act differently than they do when they are alone. Since work groups, such as committees and task forces, are a vital part of every organization, the consultant should review the small group phenomenon relevant to consultation to teams (Aronson, 1999; Baron & Byrne, 1991).

Types of Groups

Groups can be classified into several types, depending on their structure and function:

- *Formal group:* A designated work group defined by the organization's structure.
- *Informal group:* A group that is neither formally structured nor organizationally determined; appears in response to the need for social contact.
- *Command group:* A manager and immediate subordinates.
- *Task group:* Those working together to complete a job task.
- *Interest group:* Those working together to attain a specific objective with which each is concerned.
- *Friendship group:* Those brought together because they share one or more characteristics.

Why Do People Join Groups?

A person often has multiple reasons for joining any particular group. Being aware of these reasons can help a consultant assess why the members are in the group, allowing the consultant to more effectively work with the groups. Robbins (2001) describes six of the most important reasons people join groups:

1. *Security:* By joining a group, individuals can reduce the insecurity of "standing alone." People feel stronger, have fewer self-doubts, and are more resistant to threats when they are part of a group.
2. *Status:* Inclusion in a group that is viewed as important by others provides recognition and status for its members.
3. *Self-esteem:* Groups can provide people with feelings of self-worth. That is, in addition to conveying status to those outside the group, membership can also give increased feelings of worth to the group members themselves.
4. *Affiliation:* Groups can fulfill social needs. People enjoy the regular interaction that comes with group membership. For many people, these on-the-job interactions are their primary source for fulfilling their needs for affiliation.
5. *Power:* What cannot be achieved individually often becomes possible through group action. There is power in numbers.
6. *Goal achievement:* There are times when it takes more than one person to accomplish a particular task—there is a need to pool talents, knowledge, or power in order to complete a job. In such instances, management will rely on the use of a formal group. (p. 218)

GROUP PROCESSES IN ORGANIZATIONS

Just as in psychotherapy groups, groups that form in organizations also move through varying stages of cohesion. A working knowledge of these stages allows a consultant to move organizational work groups along to more productive stages.

Predictable Stages of Group Development

For mental health professionals who have studied social psychology and group dynamics, the following information on Tuckman and Jensen's (1997) stages of group development will serve as a quick review:

Forming stage: In this stage, members become acquainted with each other and attempt to establish ground rules with respect to both the job and the interpersonal relationships within the group.

Storming stage: This stage is characterized by a high degree of conflict as members resist the control of the group leader and act hostile toward one another. If this stage is successfully resolved, the third stage begins.

Norming stage: At this point, the group becomes more cohesive, and individuals identify themselves as members of the group. Feelings of camaraderie, friendship, and shared responsibility develop.

Performing stage: When the group reaches this stage, it is devoted to achieving the group's specified tasks and goals.

Adjourning stage: The group disbands when the group's goals have been met, or when many of the group members have left.

Punctuated-Equilibrium Model

The punctuated-equilibrium model suggests that there is no standard pattern of group development and that groups do not develop in a universal sequence of stages. However, it predicts that the timing of when groups form and change the way they work is highly consistent. The first meeting sets the group's direction. The first phase of group activity is one of inertia, and a transition takes place at the end of the first phase that occurs exactly when the group has used up half its allotted time. The transition initiates major changes, and a second phase of inertia follows the transition. The group's last meeting is characterized by accelerated activity.

ROLE THEORY

Janet is a humanistically oriented therapist who is asked to fill out insurance forms on her clients for insurance reimbursement. How would you explain her distress in giving a *DSM-IV* diagnosis and GAF (Global Assessment of Functioning) score in role theory terms? Janet is experiencing role conflict: a situation in which an individual is confronted by divergent role expectations.

Role theory can be very helpful for mental health professionals when consulting with small groups. A role can be defined as a set of expected behavior patterns attributed to someone occupying a given position in a social unit (Aronson, 1999). The roles that individuals take on, and the concomitant aspects of that role, greatly affect how an individual performs within an organization. Consultants should have a working knowledge of role theory. The following is a brief overview of the many aspects of roles:

Role identity: Certain attitudes and behaviors consistent with a role.

Role perception/conception: An individual's view of how he or she is supposed to act in a given situation.

Role expectations: How others believe a person should act in a given situation.

Role acceptance: What the individual is willing to do and the extent of his or her acceptance of others' expectations of the role.

Role behavior: What the individual actually does.

Role efficacy: An individual's effectiveness in occupying a particular role in an organization.

Role conflict: A situation in which an individual is confronted by divergent role expectations. A single mother may be expected to put in long hours at work, but also may be expected to be actively involved with her child's school activities.

Role overload: When the demands of a role are too great for the adaptive resources of the person. Graduate clinical students, who are often expected to be good students, clinicians, leaders, and parents, can be overwhelmed by the expectations that are placed on them.

Psychological contract: An unwritten agreement that sets out what management expects from the employee, and vice versa. A major change in our society is the erosion of the employment contract.

IMPORTANT GROUP PHENOMENA

Mental health professionals know that important phenomena are at play in group settings. Following is a review of the most important aspects of groups that commonly come up in consultation settings.

Group Norms

Norms are the standard rules of conduct that groups use to maintain uniformity of behavior among group members. When people obey norms, they engage in *conformity.* When they disobey norms, they are often labeled *deviant.* Consultants should be aware of the factors that lead to conformity and deviance, so that they can assist teams and workgroups when they become dysfunctional. Following is a list of contributors to conformity in groups and teams (Aronson, 1999; Baron & Byrne, 1991; Corey, 2000; Yalom, 1995):

Task demands: Conformity is greater in ambiguous situations, highly complex situations, and situations involving a problem that has no solution; also when group members must work together to achieve a common goal.

Group characteristics: Conformity increases as the unanimity (consensus) of group members increases. The presence of even a single dissenter can significantly lower conformity. Conformity also increases when the group uses surveillance or close supervision to enforce its norms and when group members are perceived as being highly credible and trustworthy.

Individual characteristics: Conformity is associated with authoritarianism, rigidity, and low self-esteem, whereas low levels of conformity are associated with high intelligence, tolerance, and ego strength.

Active participation: Members conform more to the group's norms when they have helped define those norms. They understand the norms better, feel more "ego-involved" with them, and are more likely to perceive the norms as equitable.

Fear of being ostracized: Ordinarily, a person who violates group norms faces disapproval or rejection. However, a person who has gained prestige, status, and respect by functioning competently in the group, by serving as the group leader, or by previously conforming to group norms may be allowed to occasionally violate them because the person has accumulated "idiosyncrasy credits" (Hollander, 1960).

Status

Status is a prestige grading, position, or rank within a group. Status can be a significant motivator, and is a common feature of groups. It can be organizationally imposed or may be granted by a particular group. It could come from a number of characteristics, such as:

- Education
- Age
- Sex
- Skill (such as vocabulary or speech)
- Experience
- Organizational affiliation
- Profession
- Titles, relationships, pay and fringe benefits, work schedule, office amenities

As an example of how status can be denoted in many different ways, we can look at how guests are treated on the *Tonight Show,* with Jay Leno, or the *Dave Letterman Show.* These shows denote status in the following ways, ranked from lowest status to highest status:

- Someone appearing late in the show
- Someone who does a comedy routine
- Sitting down and bantering with the host
- Whether the guest stays or departs after the interview (high-status guests get up and leave)
- Filling in as guest host
- Being guest host for a week rather than a night

It is important for consultants to quickly learn and appreciate the status symbols that consultees have acquired or aspired to in the organizational culture.

Group Cohesion

Groups develop cohesion based on perceived common interests, and after the members gain a sense of familiarity with each other. Groups tend to elevate themselves and denigrate outside groups, splitting things into "we-they."

Cohesion refers to a group's "solidarity." To do team building, you need to know the factors that affect group cohesion (Aronson, 1999; Baron & Byrne, 1991; Yalom, 1995):

Group size: Groups are most effective when they include 5 to 10 members, though this depends on the nature of the task. Smaller groups tend to be more cohesive than larger groups, and they ordinarily have fewer communication problems, less member dissatisfaction and alienation, less need for supervision and surveillance, and more per capita communication and productivity. As groups get larger, subgroups (cliques) tend to form, communication becomes more formalized, and leadership becomes more autocratic.

Homogeneity: Groups whose members are similar in terms of socioeconomic status, interests, values, attitudes, abilities, and personality characteristics are more likely to be cohesive. Group homogeneity is associated with greater member satisfaction in socially oriented groups and greater productivity in task-oriented groups when the task is simple. When the task requires originality and creativity, however, greater productivity is associated with heterogeneity (diversity).

Goals: Cohesiveness is maximized when members participate in goal norm-setting, and when members must depend on one another to achieve their common goals. Cohesiveness is also increased when members believe that participation in the group will help them achieve their own personal goals, and when the group has a previous history of successful goal achievement.

Difficulty of entry into the group: Difficult application procedures and severe initiations are associated with greater cohesiveness. For example, the tougher the pledge program, the more the members value the fraternity or sorority. This is also true for elitist branches of the military, such as the Marines and the Navy SEALS.

External threats: Competition or other external threats tend to increase group interdependence and cohesiveness.

Communication: High cohesiveness is linked to more frequent communication among group members, greater participation in group activities, reduced conflict, and higher levels of morale, interpersonal attraction, and conformity.

Group norms: Since high cohesion leads to greater group norm conformity, members of cohesive groups are more likely to adhere to informal work group norms. Whether this results in higher or lower performance depends on those norms.

Gender: On the whole, women report greater cohesion than men.

Effects of Groups on Individuals

Groups have numerous effects on the individuals who compose the membership of the group (Aronson, 1999; Baron & Byrne, 1991; Yalom, 1995). These effects can be both positive and negative, and a consultant can serve as an outside, objective observer of the group process to provide feedback on how to improve the group's functioning.

Among the positive aspects of group influence, groups can provide members with task-related or interpersonal skills through direct instruction, feedback, and modeling. Groups can also satisfy members' affiliative needs, especially when members share interests and values. Groups can also reduce members' anxiety, since no member will feel alone in tackling the tasks at hand.

"Social loafing" is a potential negative outcome of group participation (Latane, Williams, & Harkins, 1979). It occurs when group members exert less effort within the group than they would have exerted if working alone. Social loafing is most likely to occur when members know their effort (or lack of effort) will not be recognized and, consequently, feel no relationship between effort and outcome. For example, some employees never put forth the effort to engage in conversations about how things are going because they know somebody else will always speak up.

Social facilitation and social inhibition occur in groups. Social facilitation occurs when the mere presence of others increases task performance, and is most likely to occur when the task is simple or well learned. Social inhibition occurs when the presence of others decreases performance and is more likely when the task is complex or new (unlearned). The causes of social facilitation and social inhibition are not clear. Zajonc (1965) believes that the mere presence of other people heightens arousal, which, in turn, increases the likelihood that a dominant response will be made. If the dominant response is the correct one, then social facilitation occurs, but if the dominant response is incorrect, social inhibition is likely. Others argue that it is not the mere presence, but the fear of being judged by others that causes arousal (C. F. Bond, 1982; Bray & Sugarman, 1980; C. S. Carver & Scheier, 1981).

Group Process and Productivity

Group performance depends on three classes of variables: task demands, resources, and process. Actual group productivity is equal to potential productivity minus losses due to faulty process (Steiner, 1972).

Groups versus Individuals

Considering the preceding phenomena, there are both advantages and disadvantages in using groups. Advantages include:

- More complete information and knowledge
- An increased diversity of views
- Increased acceptance of a solution
- Increased legitimacy

Disadvantages involved in the use of groups include:

- More time consuming
- Greater pressure to conform
- Possible dominance by a few individuals
- Ambiguity about responsibility

PARTICIPATION

Participation and participatory management are becoming popular in businesses today. This refers to the idea that when the staff of an organization is involved in developing a change program, the members see it as belonging to them, and not to some outsider, and there is no "monopoly on wisdom." Rank-and-file staff can have important insights about how a program will work, or will not work, that may escape everyone else.

Participation leads to significant improvements in both morale and productivity; this is one of the very few ways to increase both morale and productivity at the same time. Even when it works, however, participation can have unfortunate side effects because it may create the need for changes that are resisted by other parts of the organization. Many efforts at fostering participation have failed not because participation did not work, but because it was poorly implemented.

Of course, there are times when even the best-intentioned employees will make bad suggestions (Goetsch & Davis, 2000). Milite (1991) recommends rejecting bad suggestions in a way that keeps the communication process open (see Box 7.1).

=== **Box 7.1** ===

How to Reject Suggestions Tactfully

Listen carefully: Give employees an opportunity to explain their suggestions in greater detail. Aspects of the suggestion that have merit or could be developed to make the suggestion more viable may not have been completely explained on the suggestion form.

Express appreciation: Be sure to let employees know that their suggestions are appreciated. Encourage future suggestions. The message to leave them with is this: "This suggestion didn't work out, but your effort is appreciated and your ideas are valued. I'm looking forward to your next suggestion."

Carefully explain your position: Don't make excuses or blame the company, higher management, or anyone else. Explain the reasons the suggestion is not feasible, and do so in a way that will help employees make more viable suggestions in the future.

Encourage feedback: Encourage feedback from employees. You may have overlooked an aspect to the suggestion, or the suggester may not fully understand the reasons for the rejection. Solicit sufficient feedback to ensure that you understand the employees and they understand you.

Look for compromise: It may be possible to use all or a portion of a suggestion if it is modified. Never adopt a bad idea, but if a suggestion can be modified to make even part of it worthwhile, a compromise solution may be possible.

Source: From "When an Employee's Idea Is Just Plain Awful," by G. Milite, October 1991, *Supervisory Management,* p. 3.

EMPOWERMENT

Empowerment is one of the organizational ways to increase performance. Empowerment is a core value in the quality movement. The root of the English word empowerment is *power*—the ability to do, to accomplish, to perform, or enable. The prefix *em* comes from the Latin and Greek, meaning "in" or "within." Empowerment, therefore, refers to the power within people. That power is related to intrinsic motivation, which increases one's feelings of self-efficacy and energy. Put another way, empowerment is the humanistic process of adopting the values and practices of enlightened self-interest so that personal and departmental goals may be aligned in a way that promotes growth, learning, and fulfillment. Empowering leaders strive to create environments where the desire to perform comes from factors inside (intrinsic) rather than rewards outside (extrinsic) the person. This process unleashes the untapped potential contribution within each employee.

In practice, empowering leaders often delegate responsibility to others with insufficient understanding, resources, or supportive guidance to be effective. People who think they are empowered too often resist the limitations and guidance that must accompany any responsibility. True empowerment is not a blank check or freedom "to do your own thing" without limits or accountability (Covey, 1996).

COMMUNICATION IN GROUPS: COMMUNICATION NETWORKS

A communication network is a pattern of communication between group members or between positions or departments in an organization. In *centralized networks,* all communication must pass through a central person or position. In *decentralized networks,* information can more freely flow between members without going through a central person. Centralized networks are more efficient for simple tasks, and decentralized networks are better for complex tasks because they provide greater flexibility and exchange of ideas. Overall satisfaction tends to be higher when the communication network is decentralized.

Communication is also affected by the organizational structure, which can also be centralized or decentralized. In centralized organizations, vertical communication is stressed, with patterns of communication being determined by established lines of authority and power (e.g., superior/subordinate). In decentralized organizations, the work units are distributed horizontally, rather than vertically, and there is greater interdependence and integration between units and less emphasis on power and control. Communication networks may or may not coincide with the structure of the organization.

WORK TEAMS

A work team is an interdependent, intact social system, with one or more tasks to perform, that operates within an organizational context. This concept is now pervasive in industry, and examples include quality control circles, task forces, safety committees, sales teams, and research and development (R&D) groups.

Types of Work Teams

Natural Work Teams form around natural work processes. An example would be a radiology department in a hospital:
   Cross-Functional Teams form with an ongoing purpose that crosses multiple organizational boundaries such as a safety team to address the reduction of lost-time accidents.
   Small Project Teams form to work on a particular task until it is completed, and then disband. An example would be a team brought together within a department to redesign the department's workspace.
   Special Purpose Teams are temporary teams that disband on task completion. In contrast to a small project team, special purpose teams work on a task having a larger scope with implications that cross multiple natural work groups. An example would be engaging in customer problem-solving activities.

The Rise of Work Teams

Surveys of Fortune 1000 companies indicate they will be placing more emphasis on teams and teamwork in the future. In today's hypercompetitive environment, old organizational structures can be too slow, too unresponsive, and too expensive to be competitive. Work teams can yield quality, productivity, and cost improvements, and workers can benefit from increased autonomy and empowerment. When properly implemented, a team-based approach can produce superior results on virtually every measure—from productivity to morale; from quality to shareholder return (Rayner, 1997). The challenge is to properly implement teams.

The move to teams is also driven by the continuing advances in information technology, the increasing importance of the knowledge economy, and the growing movement toward "worker empowerment" in general.

Work teams are not always the best way to do things. To help an organization determine whether to use work teams, the consultant should ask the following questions:

- Do people need to work together to get the task done effectively?
- Is expertise limited to a few people?
- Is there a sense of shared purpose and a commitment to that purpose?
- Is there strong formal leadership support for the teams?
- Can information and expertise be readily shared? If not (perhaps due to security constraints), this operation is probably not a good candidate for the team approach.

Qualities of a Successful Work Team

There are three important aspects of a successful work team: quality/quantity/timeliness of the work performed; the ability of members to work together; and the personal growth and well-being of the members. The relative weights that should be assigned to these three dimensions vary across situational circumstances.

Why Work Teams Fail

Anecdotal evidence indicates that teams are successful only about half the time (Johnson, Beyerlein, Huff, Halfhill, & Ballentine, 2002). This is likely due to the inappropriate use of teams, a lack of support from organizational leaders, a lack of good information, or a lack of team member skills. A work team's success can be affected as much by what is happening outside the team (e.g., managerial support, relations with other teams) as it is by what is happening inside the team (team development, process, conflict management, etc.).

How Do Consultants Help Organizations Use Work Teams?

Mental health professionals can use their knowledge and skills to consult with organizations on the use of work teams in several ways:

- *Personnel selection:* Consultants can use their knowledge of group dynamics and team functioning to help the organization select a well-balanced team, which depends on the type of team and its purpose. This can take the form of informal suggestions, such as using a "devil's advocate" role that rotates among members of the team, or can be done more formally, such as through psychological testing, if a diverse mix of personality types is needed.
- *Training:* Consultants can also provide training to team members. This could involve training in job-specific skills, such as how to effectively handle customer complaints, or could involve training in how to make the team run as optimally as possible. Many individuals are accustomed to working alone, So consultants can help in the transition to a team-based approach, which involves an entirely different set of dynamics to make full use of the synergistic properties of teams. A team

made up of individuals who wish to continue working as individuals actually tends to reduce productivity. Consultants can provide psychoeducation on group dynamics or can observe the group process and make intervention suggestions specific to that particular team and its individual members.

- *Performance appraisal:* Individual performance can be difficult to assess in team settings. Sometimes specific individuals carry the workload of the team, and sometimes there is a great deal of social loafing. In many cases when teams are running well, individuals contribute to the team process in myriad subtle ways. Hence, organizations must be careful not to covertly discourage altruistic behavior or to overly reward individual heroic behavior that undermines the functioning of the team. Consultants can help organizations develop fair and equitable appraisal systems.

- *Compensation:* Systems of compensation are very important to employees and to managers. If the incentive system is entirely based on individual performance, there will be little motivation to put forth the effort required to make an efficient team. If the incentive system is entirely based on team performance, individuals may feel that their efforts have no major impact on their compensation and that it would be unfair for them to work harder than other members of the team. There is also a great deal of uncertainty in this type of compensation system, as an individual can work extremely hard in a team that is still performing poorly overall,

---

Box 7.2

In their research on teams, Katzenbach and Smith (1999) discovered some interesting commonsense and "uncommonsense" findings:

Commonsense Findings

- A demanding performance challenge tends to create a team.
- The disciplined application of "team basics" is often overlooked.
- Team performance opportunities exist in all parts of the organization.
- Teams at the top are the most difficult.
- Most organizations intrinsically prefer individual over group (team) accountability.

Uncommonsense Findings

- Companies with strong performance standards seem to spawn more "real teams" than companies that promote teams per se.
- High-performance teams are extremely rare.
- Hierarchy and teams go together almost as well as teams and performance.
- Teams naturally integrate performance and learning.
- Teams are the primary unit of performance for increasing numbers of organizations.

Source: From *The Wisdom of Teams: Creating the High-Performance Organization* (pp. 2–5) by J. R. Katzenbach and D. K. Smith, 1999, New York: HarperCollins.

causing stress in an individual's mind about how to predictably provide for his or her family. A consultant can provide help to the organization in determining the proper mix between individual and team-based incentives.

- *Organizational development:* Whether developing one team for a specific purpose, or transitioning to a team-based approach for all employees, teams will have an impact on the entire organization. Consultants can help the organization prepare for the implementation and maintenance of a team-based approach, which will likely include assisting organizational leadership in redesigning various policies, procedures, and functions within the organization (see Box 7.2).

Handling Diversity in Teams

Consultants can help those who lead or coach teams to attend more closely to the matters of diversity that are likely to arise in teams with diverse membership. Goetsch and Davis (2000) give the suggestions listed in Box 7.3.

=== Box 7.3 ===

Suggestions for Handling Diversity

Conduct a cultural audit. Identify the demographics, personal characteristics, cultural values, and individual differences among team members.

Identify the specific needs of different groups. Ask women, ethnic minorities, and older workers to describe the unique inhibitors they face. Make sure all team members understand these barriers, then work together as a team to eliminate, overcome, or accommodate them.

Confront cultural clashes. Wise coaches meet conflict among team members head-on and immediately. This approach is particularly important when the conflict is based on issues of diversity. Conflicts that grow out of religious, cultural, ethnic, age, and/or gender-related issues are more potentially volatile than everyday disagreements over work-related issues. Consequently, conflict that is based on or aggravated by human differences should be confronted promptly. Few things will polarize a team faster than diversity-related disagreements that are allowed to fester and grow.

Eliminate institutionalized bias. A company whose workforce has historically been predominantly male now has a workforce in which women are the majority. However, the physical facility still has 10 men's restrooms and only two for women. This imbalance is an example of institutionalized bias. Teams may find themselves unintentionally slighting members, simply out of habit or tradition. This is the concept of *discrimination by inertia.* It happens when the demographics of the team changes but its habits, traditions, procedures, and work environment do not.

Source: From *Quality Management: Introduction to Total Quality Management for Production, Processing, and Services* (p. 295), by D. L. Goetsch and S. B. Davis, 2000, Upper Saddle River, NJ: Prentice-Hall.

The Future of Teams

The current trend appears to be that teams will become less physical and more virtual. In a wired, knowledge-based economy, we will likely see fewer "neighborhood teams" (teams composed of individuals in the same or a nearby physical location) and more "virtual teams" (teams that may be physically distant but are connected through technological means such as the Internet). However, virtual teams face challenges: They are more difficult to form and sustain than a neighborhood team; there is an increased possibility of incomplete communication (e.g., nonverbal cues that convey meaning are lost); and there are limited relationship-building opportunities. A face-to-face initial meeting can be crucial to building trust among team members.

One form of virtual team involves telecommuting; employees on the team work from home to avoid the hassle of commuting, but stay connected to fellow employees and supervisors virtually.

Virtual teams are so popular because they have several distinct advantages: More information can be examined in a shorter amount of time using e-mail compared with voice communication; having team members in many different time zones can literally keep a project running around the clock; the cost of electronic communication is far cheaper than that of transportation; and virtual teams allow for far greater organizational flexibility (Rayner, 1997).

Connell (2002) developed a list of sample questions that managers tend to ask consultants concerning issues that arise on virtual teams:

- Can people successfully work remotely in this organization?
- How do I know who will be successful at telecommuting?
- How do I create a fair system for letting some people telecommute?
- How do I know my remote employees are working and not off shopping at the mall?
- How do I keep remote employees visible in the organization?
- How do I know there is a problem with a remote employee?
- How often do I need to see the employees face-to-face?
- I want to have regular staff meetings, but it is impossible to coordinate everyone's schedules. How do I balance flextime with availability?
- Some of my team members don't like working remotely. Some complain that they don't feel as much a part of the team as the on-site employees. What should I do?
- How do I remain accessible remotely?
- How do I keep from being interrupted by remote employees calling in, and overwhelmed by the number of e-mails?
- One of my employees never responds to my e-mails. What should I do?
- One employee e-mails at the last minute to cancel meetings, and I don't get the messages in time. What should I do?
- How can multiple employees access documents all at once?
- How do I ensure that remote employees internalize the corporate culture?
- How do I know remote employees have a safe work space? (p. 291)

Connell (2002) suggests that these questions are worked through by dealing with issues of organizational policy and culture, employee selection and performance, trust, tools, and communication.

The Elements of Effective Feedback

A crucial aspect of effective team functioning is the ability of the member to give and receive effective feedback on how individuals are performing and contributing to the team effort. Consultants can use their knowledge of interpersonal communication skills to help employees and teams function more efficiently. The following considerations are important for giving feedback effectively, especially in team settings (London, 1997).

Effective Feedback

- *Describes the behavior that led to the feedback:* "You are finishing my sentences for me . . ."
- *Comes as soon as appropriate after the behavior:* Feedback should be given immediately if possible, though it can be given later if events make that necessary (something more important is going on, you need time to "cool down," the person has other feedback to deal with, etc.).
- *Is direct, from sender to receiver:* Messages from third parties can easily be miscommunicated, and receivers will feel resentful if you send someone else to give tough feedback.
- *Is "owned" by the sender:* The person giving feedback should use "I messages" and take responsibility for the stated thoughts, feelings, and reactions.
- *Includes the sender's real feelings about the behavior:* Most people will be sensitive to incongruence between stated and felt emotions, so the speaker should be authentic about feelings insofar as they are relevant to the feedback: "I get frustrated when I'm trying to make a point and you keep finishing my sentences."
- *Is checked for clarity:* The sender should ensure that the receiver fully understands what is being conveyed. "Do you understand what I mean when I say you seem to be sending me a double message?"
- *Has a problem-solving quality:* The sender should ask relevant questions that seek information, with the receiver knowing why the information is being sought and having a clear sense that the sender does not know the answer. Feedback should not be used to demonstrate the sender's knowledge or to "punish" the receiver.
- *Specifies consequences of the behavior for the present and/or the future:* "When you finish my sentences I get frustrated and want to stop talking with you." "If you keep finishing my sentences, I won't want to spend much time talking with you in the future."
- *Is solicited or at least to some extent desired by the receiver:* As in therapy, the receiver must be ready and open to receiving feedback for it to be effective.
- *Refers to behaviors about which the receiver can do something (if the person wants to):* "I wish you'd stop interrupting me."
- *Takes into account the needs of both sender and receiver:* Feedback is a "process," an interaction in which, at any moment, the sender can become the receiver. Sender: "I'm getting frustrated by the fact that often you're not ready to leave when I am." Receiver: "I know that's a problem, but I'm concerned about what seems to be your need to have me always do what you want when you want."
- *Affirms the receiver's existence and worth:* The sender should acknowledge the receiver's right to his or her reactions, whatever they may be, and should be willing to work through issues in a game-free way.
- *Acknowledges and, where necessary, makes use of the fact that a process is going on, that it needs to be monitored and sometimes explored and improved:* "I'm getting

the impression that we're not listening to each other. I'd like to talk about that and try to do this more effectively."

Hence, a suggested model for an effective feedback statement might be: "When you . . . (specific behavior), I felt . . . The consequences are that . . . Does that make sense to you? What are your reactions?"

Elements of Ineffective Feedback

Ineffective feedback can kill a team's functioning. Consultants frequently overhear consultees giving ineffective feedback. Consultants should be alert for such statements to assist consultees in being more effective in their communication, and in preventing negative reactions in the person receiving the feedback.

Ineffective Feedback

- *Uses evaluative or judgmental statements:* Feedback that is perceived as a personal attack is never well received. "You're being rude." You should also avoid generalized judgmental statements: "You're trying to control the conversation."

- *Is delayed, saved up, and "dumped":* This is also known as *gunny-sacking* or ambushing. The false belief is that as more time passes, it becomes safer to give the feedback. This induces guilt and anger in the receiver, because after time has passed, there is usually not much the person can do about it.

- *Is indirect or ricocheted:* This involves giving feedback as if it came from someone else, or presenting it in a subtle manner so as not to be perceived as feedback. Individuals giving feedback should be direct and take personal responsibility for what they say. "Tom, how do you feel when Jim cracks his knuckles?" This is also known colloquially as "let's you and him fight."

- *Transfers ownership:* Rather than taking personal responsibility for what one is saying, ownership is vaguely transferred to "people," "the book," "upper management," "everybody," "we," and so on.

- *Conceals, denies, misrepresents, or distorts feelings:* One way to do this is to transfer ownership. Another way is to smuggle the feelings into the interaction by being sarcastic, sulking, competing to see who's "right," and so on. Other indicators include speculations on the receiver's intentions, motivations, or psychological problems: "You're trying to drive me nuts"; "You're just trying to see how much you can get away with"; "You have a need to get even with the world."

- *Is not checked for accuracy:* The sender either assumes clarity or is not interested in whether the receiver understands fully: "Stop interrupting me with 'Yes, buts!'"

- *Asks questions that are really statements:* "Do you think I'm going to let you get away with that?" The questions may also sound like traps: "How many times have you been late this week?" Experts at the "question game" can easily combine the two: "How do you think that makes me feel?" or "Do you behave that way at home, too?"

- *Provides vague consequences:* "That kind of behavior is going to get you into trouble." The sender may also fail to specify any consequences, substituting instead other kinds of leverage, such as "shoulds": "You shouldn't do that."

- *Is imposed on the receiver:* This often occurs with the feeling that the feedback is for the receiver's "own good."
- *Refers to behaviors over which the receiver has little or no control:* This may be especially true if the receiver is to remain authentic: "I wish you'd laugh at my jokes."
- *Is distorted by the sender's needs:* These needs are usually unconscious or unconsidered, and likely stem from (1) a fear of rejection or a need to feel safe: "Now, I don't want you to get angry, but . . ."; (2) a desire to punish: "Can't you ever do anything right?"; (3) a need to win: "Ah-ha, then you admit that you do interrupt me?"; A desire to be virtuous, which can be very subtle: "I'm going to level with you, be open with you . . ."; and so on. Most ineffective feedback behaviors come either from lack of skills or from the sender not seeing the process as an interaction in which both parties have needs that must be taken into account.
- *Denies or discounts the receiver by using statistics, abstractions, or averages:* Here, the sender is using tactics to avoid accepting the receiver's feelings: "Oh, you're just being paranoid." "Come on! You're overreacting." "You're not really as angry as you say you are."
- *Either does not value the concept of process or does not want to take time to discuss anything other than content:* Consequently, the sender does not pay any attention to the process, which can result in confusion, wasted time and energy, and lots of ineffective feedback.

IMPORTANCE OF MEETINGS

A great deal of our professional lives is spent in meetings, so knowledge of how to optimally conduct and participate in meetings is an important professional skill. As many as 4 days a week are spent in meetings by high-level executives, so it is important for consultants to develop competence for intervening in this context. Consultants and managers will often be evaluated according to their ability to employ these skills.

How to Conduct a Meeting

There is a great deal of variability in meeting purpose and format, but there are generally seven steps in conducting a meeting:

Step 1: Determine if a meeting is necessary. Since meetings are expensive, do everything possible outside the meeting and before the meeting begins. Do you need to have your meeting? Consider opportunity costs: if 12 clinicians are to meet, and each charges $120 per hour to see clients who cannot now be scheduled, is the meeting worth $1,440? Also consider the time and other resources expended in preparing for the meeting.

Step 2: Determine the purpose of the meeting. In most cases, the more specific the stated purpose of the meeting, the better. This saves time and ensures that members are clear about what needs to happen and will work together toward the same end. This will also help members prepare so they can make more salient and substantial contributions.

Step 3: Determine who should attend the meeting. Determine the type of leadership the meeting requires and the type of involvement expected of the membership, including the method that will be used to make decisions.

Step 4: Determine the method for achieving the purpose of the meeting. Work to develop a meeting plan. This may include distribution of specific reports, assignment of presentations by specified employees, and completion of opinion surveys.

Step 5: Prepare materials for the meeting. Be sure all necessary items will be available (presentation aids, refreshments, etc.) so that the participants can focus their energy on the topics of the meeting. Nothing is more distracting than members searching for the coffee creamer during an important presentation.

Step 6: Script the meeting. Send out an agenda and ask for comments and additions before holding the meeting. By doing this, members can contribute valuable suggestions, and everyone will be better prepared to make the best use of the time available.

Step 7: Evaluate the effectiveness of the meeting. Gather feedback on how well the meeting fulfilled its purpose and use the data to adjust how future meetings are conducted. This could take the form of a short written survey, or informally by just asking, "How did you think this meeting went today?"

In the classic business meeting, the CEO talks (announcements, etc.) and then goes around the room calling on each person in turn. Mental health professionals with training in group dynamics will know that there are both strengths and weaknesses with this business format.

Leader Behaviors in Meetings

A leader's actions have a major impact on the members of a group. Consultants can assist team leaders to be more effective by working with them on the following behaviors:

Attend early to the norms that you want to develop in the team. Set the standard early on by paying attention to such things as ideas about time (e.g., starting and ending on time), decision making, communication, and treatment of fellow members (competition versus cooperation). State the purpose, objectives, and estimated time for the meeting. Make boundaries clear about each member's role.

Be responsible for the outcome. Be active, directive, and prepared for the meeting, but make members feel responsible for the outcome.

Leaders should structure the meeting. The leader should keep things moving, and should actively encourage member input and discussion. Remember the main value of a meeting is the generation of synergy, involvement, and commitment, as groups make more complete decisions than individuals.

Avoid using a meeting to provide information. There are better, more efficient methods for the delivery of information than a meeting (such as a memo or a telephone conference). The exception to this is if confidential information needs to be discussed.

Be open to member input and ideas. The most powerful teams are characterized by shifting leadership and shared responsibility.

Listen for consensus and check things out with the group so the group can move on. Don't allow the group to recycle arguments or comments over and over.

Don't play "guess my agenda." Be clear with all members about what is going on.

Each group has a task and a maintenance/process function. Attend to both the task that needs to be done, and the group process that is going on. If you are not good at attending to both, allow supplemental leadership to develop from within the team.

Be generous with support and praise. Publicly give credit to contributions and affirm the feelings members are experiencing.

Evaluate everything you do so you can get better at what you do. Remember to ask yourself and others, "If I could do it again, how could it be improved?"

Establish a meeting environment consistent with your goal. Make sure the members are comfortable and are not distracted.

Summarize periodically in the context of the purpose. This helps members stay focused.

Show courtesy and respect. Listen attentively and demonstrate your attention to others. Make people feel important.

Don't allow the meeting to go on when its work has been completed. Don't allow the energy of the meeting to drain away nonproductively.

Select the membership carefully. Include those individuals or representatives who will be affected by the outcome of the meeting, but try to include only the members necessary to effectively achieve the goal so people will not feel that their time is being wasted.

TYPES OF DECISION MAKING

To help groups and teams function effectively, one must understand the decision-making process. There are several types of decision making, and each has its advantages and disadvantages in any given context. As a leader, you should be clear about the type of decision making you will be using. If you have already made your decision, then asking for participation will only create resentment among your subordinates:

Command: This decision-making style is authoritarian and does not take other viewpoints into consideration. This style works best in emergency situations.

Consultative: This style takes into consideration how a decision affects the people involved (known as *stakeholders*). The message conveyed is "I want your input to help me make the best decision possible."

Consensus: The consensus decision-making style is empowering to employees. It conveys the message that "it is important that this be our decision." It can be difficult to achieve consensus in a reasonable amount of time.

Voting: In voting, the majority rules on what decision is made. The opinion of the majority may not take into consideration all of the facts in any given matter.

DECISION MAKING IN ORGANIZATIONS

Mental health professionals can use their knowledge of psychology and group dynamics to help individuals within an organization understand the processes involved in making sound decisions. Decision making is a critical task in organizations, and it occurs at both individual and group levels.

Individual Decision Making

The Rational-Economic Model: This model assumes that the decision maker attempts to maximize benefits by systematically searching for the best possible solution or alternative. The decision maker must have complete information about all possible alternatives and be able to process information in an accurate, unbiased way. This is often not feasible since the decision maker does not have all of the necessary information or the time to consider all alternatives.

The Administrative Model: This model posits that decision makers often exhibit "bounded rationality" rather than perfect rationality; that is, they make decisions under conditions of external and psychological constraints. As a consequence, decision makers tend to "satisfice" rather than "maximize." They consider solutions as they become available and then select the first solution that meets the minimum criteria of acceptability (Simon, 1955).

Group Decision Making

Although group decision making tends to be slower than individual decision making, it is generally superior. Having several people involved in the decision-making process increases the information available. Group decision making tends to produce a greater number of alternative solutions and approaches. Participation in group decision making also increases individual morale. It also increases understanding and acceptance of and commitment to the decisions that are made.

Group decision making tends to be most effective when groups consist of heterogeneous members who have complementary skills, and when the problem has multiple components that allow for a division of labor among group members.

Disadvantages of Group Decision Making

Groupthink (Janis, 1982) is the suspension of critical thinking that can occur in highly cohesive groups. It leads to illusions of invulnerability and superior morality, suppression of doubt and disagreement, strong pressure toward uniformity, rationalization of negative and discrepant information, and insulation from outside input. The leader can reduce groupthink by playing devil's advocate, encouraging skepticism and dissent among group members, and bringing in outside opinions.

Group polarization: Group judgments and decisions tend to be more extreme in the direction of the views initially held by group members than decisions that would have been generated by individual members alone. This is attributed to a bandwagon effect—to increased confidence among group members as a result of their participation in the group, to mutual reinforcement among group members, or to a diffusion of responsibility. This is also called the "risky shift phenomenon."

Overresponding: Groups sometimes overrespond to social pressure or individual domination, and personal goals can smother collective purposes. The members of a group must feel safe enough to call each other on things when they see individuals attempting to carry out personal agendas that will be detrimental to the group as a whole.

Methods for Improving Group Decision Making

Brainstorming.   Brainstorming involves encouraging group members to verbalize all ideas that come into their minds, regardless of how absurd these ideas may seem. To be effective, brainstorming requires members to refrain from evaluating each other's ideas until after the brainstorming session is over. Individuals brainstorming alone produce more and better ideas in the same amount of time than the same number of individuals brainstorming as a group, perhaps due to social inhibitions. Group brainstorming is more effective when group members are heterogeneous in terms of skills, when members know and feel comfortable with each other, and when members have been adequately trained in brainstorming (Osborn, 1957).

To keep the free flow of creative thoughts coming during a brainstorming session, the consultant should advise members to avoid the statements shown in Box 7.4 (Lussier, 2002, p. 353).

The Nominal Group and Delphi techniques are brainstorming methods that de-emphasize direct face-to-face contact by group members.

Nominal Group Technique.   With this technique, group members first brainstorm alone and then discuss and evaluate the ideas presented by all members. This is followed by a secret ballot (though it can also be an open ballot) in which each member ranks the proposed solutions. The idea that receives the highest ranking is taken as the group's decision.

Box 7.4

Responses That Kill Creativity

- It isn't in the budget.
- Don't be ridiculous.
- We've never done it before.
- Has anyone else ever tried it?
- It won't work in our company/industry.
- That's not our problem.
- We tried that before.
- It can't be done.
- It costs too much.
- That's beyond our responsibility.
- It's too radical a change.
- We did all right without it.
- We're doing the best we can.
- We don't have the time.
- That will make other equipment obsolete.
- We're too small/big for it.
- Let's get back to reality.
- Why change it? It's still working okay.
- We're not ready for that.
- You're years ahead of your time.
- Can't teach an old dog new tricks.
- Let's form a committee.

Source: From R. N. Lussier, 2002, *Human Relations in Organizations: Applications and Skill Building,* fifth edition (p. 353), Boston: McGraw-Hill/Irwin.

Delphi Technique.   This technique involves pooling the judgments of experts who respond independently and anonymously to questionnaires. The results are then summarized and returned to participants for further comments. Eventually, all participants vote independently on the various solutions or decisions.

Although the Nominal Group and Delphi techniques seem to improve decision making, the drawback is that neither technique involves true interaction between group members, which may reduce acceptance of and commitment to the group decision.

TASK AND PROCESS

Consultants always operate on two levels when working with groups and organizations, and these skills can be taught to client team and group members and leaders to improve their functioning. The *task* or *substance* level involves problem solving, rationality, and investigation of the explicit, real problems. The *process* or *maintenance* level refers to the relationship level, and considers feelings and implicit processes. It involves putting into words what you are feeling about the relationship that is going on in ways that decrease the defensiveness of the client.

The distinction between task and process is so important that consultants and leaders have been classified according to how task- or process-oriented they are. Ideally, a consultant or leader should be balanced, or have the ability to adapt as necessary, but if a person strongly favors one over the other, it will be necessary to find the work environment for which that preference is most suited.

IMPROVING GROUP FACILITATION SKILLS

Group facilitation skills are important for consultants to develop, and can be taught to consultees as well. Effective group facilitation skills brings out the synergy of groups (Hunter, Bailey, & Taylor, 1995). Mental health professionals can rely on their clinical group facilitation skills and should also consider the following:

- *As the group leader, facilitate, rather than direct, the group discussion.* Group interaction allows the resources of all members to be used most fully.
- *Use active listening skills to draw out the ideas and creativity of others.* Be careful to reserve your judgment and provide ample opportunity for others to develop their ideas (Stacey, 1996; Sternberg, 2004).
- *Promote minority opinion.* The most obvious or popular suggestions are not always the best. To ensure that innovative suggestions are given full consideration, provide those who propose minority solutions with an environment in which they feel comfortable voicing their ideas.
- *Encourage sessions that are problem oriented rather than solution oriented.* Too often, participants in problem-solving sessions jump immediately into the generation of solutions before fully defining the problem. This process leads to solutions that may solve only part of the problem—or the wrong problem. To ensure adequate emphasis on problem definition, use a sequential structure (e.g., "We will spend 15 minutes on problem definition, then 20 minutes on the generation of solution alternatives").

- *Use brainstorming techniques to generate alternate solutions.* When brainstorming, group members strive for quantity rather than quality, piggyback on the ideas of others, and avoid judging alternatives. This approach results in increased quality of the ultimate decisions and greater creativity in problem solving.
- *Seek an additional solution.* Look for a second solution after arriving at a first solution to encourage additional creative approaches.

The group facilitator should always ascertain the purpose of the group and how best to keep the group moving along productively. Both members and facilitators can use open-ended questions and should practice active listening skills. When appropriate, the facilitator should use other members' own words. This shows them that the facilitator is paying attention and values their contributions. Likewise, be quick to publicly give credit to and appreciation for other members' work.

As in group therapy, silence can also be a powerful tool. Sometimes enduring that first long pause can stir members to speak up when they would have otherwise hesitated too long to do so.

SMALL GROUP INTERVENTION

The following is a list of important points for consultants to remember when intervening in small group settings.

- Employees become more involved in organizational decision making and problem solving if they are placed in groups and teams.
- Interest in small groups has evolved through the advent of employee empowerment to include autonomous work groups, quality circles, and self-directed teams (Orsburn, Moran, Musselwhite, Zenger, & Perrin, 1990).
- A small group comprises 12 or fewer members and focuses on a common goal.
- When the membership of a group exceeds 12 people, the dynamics change from small group to large group.
- Basic skills include observing, listening, presenting, and challenging.
- Advanced skills include timing, delivery, tone, emphasis, and selection of interventions.
- Design skills involve creating an intervention for optimal effect, easy sequence flow, and continuity from one segment to another. A consultant must relate an intervention's design to its objectives, time constraints, and participant expectations.
- Self-knowledge skills require consultants to know and be able to manage themselves. They must know what makes them angry, happy, or afraid, as well as what motivates them to select a particular intervention. They must know what they do well and what they need to improve on as facilitators (Rees, 1998; Schwarz, 1994).
- Facilitative roles include being a model; being a force that is played to, off, or against.
- Themes (Dyer, 1987) around which interventions center are confronting, engaging, and encountering; silence; being open, being authentic, disclosing oneself; struggling to develop trust; helping the group become sensitive to the "here-and-now," and displaying care and affection.

- Questions consultants should ask themselves: How am I feeling at the moment? What physical sensations accompany this feeling? What images and metaphors come to mind? What aspects of myself or my behaviors do I criticize? What aspects and behaviors of group members do I criticize? What assumptions do I make about the group or its members? What expectations do I have about the group or particular members? Do I resist members' suggestions or feedback? How do I react to criticism? What arouses my anxiety? Do I encourage or discourage self-disclosure about myself or group members? Where and what do I rationalize? What do I dream about after a group session?

- A small-group intervention is intended (consultant consciously makes a statement or suggests an activity) to help the group reach its goals and purpose (consultant has a theoretical framework and a deliberate plan to work from).

- Small Group Intervention (Reddy, 1994):
  —Explicit goal
  —Clarify who the client is
  —Clarify the contract
  —Assess the group
  —Collaborate with the client
  —Set obtainable goals
  —Model appropriate behavior
  —Provide follow-up

- The consultant must be able to make relationships, bond, and yet maintain a separate perspective.

- The effectiveness of a given intervention is primarily related to the degree to which it facilitates forward movement in the team. The worst thing a consultant can do is to intervene in a manner that disrupts, delays, or otherwise interferes with the client's agenda and sense of direction. The consultant must figure out where the client is trying to get and help move the group there.

- Do active, interested listening. Listen for process: who talks, who talks to whom, what communication style is being used, who interrupts whom, how people react to interruption, what kind of group problem-solving process and decision mechanisms are being used, and so on. Listening leads to interventions such as clarification, summarizing, and consensus testing. These all aid task process.

- Forcing historical reconstruction is used when a group is puzzled about unexpected and undesired outcomes. "Well, let's look back over the meeting and see if we can reconstruct what we did the last couple of hours. How did we set our goals, how did we decide how to work on the issue, what can you remember happening early in the meeting?" Self-discovery can be used to determine how a bad result was produced.

- Force concretization. Instead of speaking in vague generalities, you should seek specific, concrete examples of a behavior. Rather than saying, "I am sick of your dishonesty and hostility!" which makes a person defensive, a more constructive way to communicate this would be, "Your expense report did not match the numbers on the corporate credit card, and the way you raised your voice to the clerk in the accounting department made him uncomfortable. This behavior is unacceptable."

- Sometimes structured exercises can "break the ice" or help move a group along (Pfeiffer & Jones, 1978).

- Giving and encouraging others to give open and honest feedback allows the group to grow and develop (Yalom, 1995).

Chapter 8

TRAINING AND TEAM BUILDING

Training consultation provides a great opportunity for professional psychologists to influence and help people. There is no other form of consultation that will reach more people than training can. In the year 2000, U.S.-based organizations alone spent $54 billion on educating and training their employees (Education and Training Committee of the Society for Industrial and Organizational Psychology, 2005).

TRAINING IN ORGANIZATIONS

The key idea of training is to change the way people behave on the job in some fashion. Training is not just learning—it also involves behavior change. After the training is done, trainees should actually do something differently than they did before. Consultants can assess the pretraining environment, conduct needs assessments, design training modules, evaluate training programs, and administer the entire training program if so desired by the contracting organization. Alternatively, the organization can have one of their own employees deliver or manage the training after the consultant has designed it (Education and Training Committee of the Society for Industrial and Organizational Psychology, 2005).

Ongoing training is often required to keep employees performing optimally and to maintain high-quality service. Consultants may do this by conducting training, by assisting in the development of in-house training for senior and appropriately qualified employees, or by referring the employees for training at outside facilities. Topics should not only directly relate to the job (e.g., recertification credits to maintain licensure), but may also include training to improve the quality of service and increase employee retention. Popular training topics include time management, stress reduction, burnout prevention, and interpersonal communication skills. Follow-up evaluations, both in terms of employee satisfaction with training and improved performance or retention rates, are important to assess the impact of training. Though this is often difficult, since results may be hard to quantify or may take years to manifest, it is important for consultants to help consultees make certain that training dollars are well spent.

Example of Management Training Topics

Mental health professionals can draw from their diverse backgrounds and knowledge base in psychology and interpersonal relationships to create training programs of interest to organizational leaders. Following is a list of common presentation topics:

- Self-development
- Employee development
- Effective leadership
- Decision making
- Team building
- Communication
- Diversity training
- Interviewing skills
- Stress management
- Conflict management
- Supervisory training
- Workplace violence
- Career transitions

More recently, Critical Incident Stress Management (CISM), which involves Critical Stress Incident Debriefing (CISD), has been offered to organizations (J. T. Mitchell & Everly, 2000). Usually, however, this is presented as a response to an acute crisis, such as after an organization has experienced a death or a robbery.

Consultants may work to customize their training presentations for the intended audience, rather than simply imparting factual information. For example, mental health professionals who have been trained in assessment may often give a test (such as the Myers-Briggs) to help people and teams understand individual differences and their implications for working together.

Some enlightened companies also offer workshops to enrich their employees' lives. This may include training presentations on parenting, taking care of aging relatives, HIV, and balancing home and professional life.

The offering of training programs can also be an effective marketing tool for consultants. It is a way to make connections with organizations. After hearing a consultant speak, potential consultees may feel more comfortable considering consultants for other types of organizational work.

Making Seminars Successful

Success is greatest when seminars are part of an integrated whole, consistent with explicit company goals, when a critical mass of seminar graduates return "home," when the organizational culture encourages learning and growing, and when there is follow-up that constantly reinforces the mentality and performance the seminar attempts to create.

Typically, seminars consist of some combination of lecture and discussion, along with exercises that involve participants. Some training programs focus more on education (passing along facts or information), and others focus more on growth (giving participants an opportunity for a transformational experience; Kelly, 1994).

TRAINING: THE FACILITATION PROBLEM

The facilitation problem refers to the challenge the consultant faces when choosing the particular method for conducting a seminar to meet the needs and objectives of the sponsoring organization.

The Design of Training Programs

When designing a training program, a systems approach is likely to be most effective. The systems approach involves specifying the instructional objectives, determining the specific learning experiences needed to achieve those objectives, and determining the evaluation criteria for each objective. This requires ongoing feedback as the basis for decisions about training program modifications. The consultant must also be careful to recognize the impact of interactions between components of the training program and between the training program and characteristics of the organization on the program's effectiveness.

The consultant should begin with a needs assessment, or an analysis of what will be most beneficial to the organization. The needs assessment involves (1) determining if it is actually training that is required to solve the organization's problems; (2) doing a task/job analysis to identify the skills, knowledge, and abilities required for successful job performance; and (3) doing a person analysis to determine if employees have deficits in the areas identified by the task analysis.

Principles of Effective Training

As mental health professionals know from their course work and experiences in human learning, many factors can facilitate participant learning:

Maximize motivation: Whenever possible, the consultant should strive to maximize the intrinsic motivation of the employees. However, extrinsic motivation (e.g., monetary rewards, recognition, praise, Continuing Education credits) can also be useful.

Motivation is maximized when the material to be learned is made meaningful to the learner. Meaningfulness is increased when learners are provided with an overview of the material at the beginning of training, and when the material is presented in a logical, well-organized manner.

Provide feedback: Feedback should be immediate and ongoing to be most effective. Feedback enhances motivation and reduces future mistakes.

Foster overlearning: Too often, an individual will stop practicing a new skill immediately after learning to do it correctly. The new skill will be soon forgotten if it is not practiced regularly (this is common for university students, who quickly forget the material they have just learned once an exam is over). Overlearning occurs when an individual practices a new skill or studies material beyond the point of mastery, which is useful for tasks that will be performed infrequently or will only be used under stressful conditions.

Provide frequent opportunities for active practice: Active learning (having the participants practice the new skills they are hoping to acquire) is more effective than passive learning (allowing the participants simply to watch or listen to the facilitator).

Whenever possible, the consultant should also have the participants practice the new skill at various times throughout the seminar. "Distributed" or "spaced" practice is more likely to be effective in the long run than "massed" practice (trying to master the new skill in only one sitting). This is especially true for tasks involving motor skills and certain cognitive skills (e.g., memorization).

Emphasize the appropriate type of learning: "Whole" learning (learning a task as a complete entity) appears to be most effective for tasks consisting of highly interrelated parts (e.g., driving a car). "Part" learning (learning parts of a task separately) is more effective for tasks that are highly complex or that consist of relatively independent components. When dividing into parts, each part should cover a cohesive and meaningful segment of the task.

For example, if a consultant were teaching interviewing skills, part learning might involve training in microskills such as reflection, summarizing, and paraphrasing. Whole learning might involve having a participant conduct an entire interview, with feedback given afterward.

Promote transfer of learning: The entire purpose of conducting a training seminar is to influence how the participants will later perform in the "real world." Positive transfer results in improvements in on-the-job performance. It occurs when training and job situations are similar, when training includes exposure to relevant stimuli (e.g., several types of problems that are likely to occur on the job), when training emphasizes general principles that can be applied to the job, and when the skills acquired in training are subsequently reinforced on the job.

Methods of Training

Organizational training methods can be roughly classified into two categories: on-the-job techniques and off-the-job techniques. The consultant can use both techniques, depending on the consultee's needs and desires.

On-the-Job Techniques

On-the-job techniques are the most widely used form of job training. It permits active participation and ongoing feedback, has obvious job relevance, and provides maximum opportunities for transfer of training. Problems arise with this technique if trainers are inexperienced job incumbents, if the training is unsystematic, or if mistakes made on the job are very costly to the organization. On-the-job training techniques include internships, apprenticeships, coaching (matching a trainee with a mentor), and job rotation (having the trainee learn several jobs, which is usually used to train managers).

Off-the-Job Techniques

Training employees before they engage in the job provides more opportunity to use professional trainers, to tolerate learning errors, to focus on specific job elements, and to receive supplemental information. Problems arise with this technique if the motivation of the trainees is lower, there is a restricted transfer of training due to the nature of the job, or if it is costly for the employee to take time away from the actual job. Off-the-job training techniques include lectures, programmed and computer-assisted instruction, role-playing, games, behavior modeling, and "vestibule training" (the use of a simulated job environment).

Keys to Training Presentations

Some individuals are natural presenters. For the rest of us, there are three keys to delivering good presentations: preparation and planning, delivery, and follow-up.

Preparation and Planning

In preparing for a presentation, the consultant should answer the following questions: "What is the goal of this training? What is the desired change in the learner? Have I used an approach appropriate to my audience?" The method of instruction should be determined by the desired learning outcome and the background and experience of the learners. The opening discussion questions should be planned in advance. A lesson plan should contain not only the content of the material to be covered, but the manner in which it will be taught so that the desired learning can most easily occur.

Delivery

As mental health professionals know from their experiences in psychotherapy, sometimes how something is said is almost as important as what is being said. Utilize the principles of adult learning. Establish why something should be learned, and be student centered in your approach. Remember that the goal is learning, not impressing the audience with a presentation. The student does the learning, not the presenter. Try to be engaging, "bigger than life," and animated to keep the attention of the audience. Most listeners can only concentrate for about 10 minutes of lecture before they need a break provided by active involvement of some kind. People learn best by doing, although the question is the trainer's most valuable learning technique. Make sure that visual aids are introduced as well, that they fit the learning objectives, and that they are processed with the audience appropriately.

Follow-Up

The consultant should design some way to reinforce the learning to facilitate long-term adoption of what is being taught. This may range from a simple e-mail or questionnaire to assess how things have been going since the seminar, to a full follow-up seminar to reinforce the learning objectives and to address any problems that people may have encountered since the previous presentation. Box 8.1 provides an example of a feedback questionnaire that the consultant can use to improve future training sessions. It can be modified to suit particular needs.

CASE EXAMPLE

A petroleum company was experiencing large cutbacks and decided to move away from the local area. A concerned member of management wanted to sponsor a training program through the safety department to help individuals deal with their anger (apparently this was the last in a series of transitions employees had already experienced).

What questions would you ask before accepting this consulting job? How would you proceed?

The consultants decided to do a transition management program. In the meantime, however, the company brought in a specialist to do a 3-hour workshop on transition management. Now what would you do?

The consultants got the specialist's presentation material to see what she had already done, and then provided a workshop that built on what had already been done.

TRAINING RESOURCES

For consultants who are interested in getting more involved in training, a good way to learn more and develop professional networks is through the American Society of

=== **Box 8.1** ===

Training Feedback and Rating Form

Rater _____

Presenter _____

Topic _____

Circle your agreement with the following statements:

1. The objectives were easily understood.

   Strongly Disagree   Disagree   Agree   Strongly Agree

2. The training was well organized.

   Strongly Disagree   Disagree   Agree   Strongly Agree

3. The training was important to my development.

   Strongly Disagree   Disagree   Agree   Strongly Agree

4. In general, the training was well presented.

   Strongly Disagree   Disagree   Agree   Strongly Agree

5. The training was engaging and held my attention.

   Strongly Disagree   Disagree   Agree   Strongly Agree

6. Almost all of the material presented was useful.

   Strongly Disagree   Disagree   Agree   Strongly Agree

Please give specific feedback on the presentation.

Training & Development (ASTD). Box 8.2 lists principles for delivering a training presentation. The following are further resources.

Publications

The Encyclopedia of Games for Trainers
Human Resource Development Press
22 Amherst Road
Amherst, MA 01002
Phone: (800) 822-2801
Fax: (413) 253-3490
Internet: http://www.hrdpress.com
E-mail: info@hrdpress.com

======================================= Box 8.2 =======================================

Important Principles for
Delivering a Training Presentation

- Establish why something should be learned.
- Be student centered.
- Remember the goal is learning, not presenting.
- Try to be engaging and animated.
- Most listeners need a break provided by involvement every 10 minutes.
- People learn best by doing.
- The question is the trainer's most valuable learning technique.

Guide to Simulations/Games for Education and Training
Sage Publications
2455 Teller Road
Newbury Park, CA 91320
Phone: (805) 499-9774
Fax: (805) 499-0871
Internet: http://www.sagepub.com
E-mail: webmastersagepub.com

General Training Materials References

The ASTD Models of Learning Technology
American Society for Training and Development
1640 King Street
P.O. Box 1443
Alexandria, VA 22313-2043
Phone: (703) 683-8100
Fax: (703) 683-8103
Internet: http://www.astd.org

The Training and Development Sourcebook
Human Resource Development Press
22 Amherst Road
Amherst, MA 01002
Phone: (800) 822-2801
Fax: (413) 253-3490
Internet: http://www.hrdpress.com
E-mail: info@hrdpress.com

Training Resources Buyer's Guide
American Society for Training and Development (ASTD)
1640 King Street
P.O. Box 1443
Alexandria, VA 22313-2043
Phone: (703) 683-8129
Fax: (703) 683-8103
Internet: http://www.astd.org

Film, Video, Audiovisual References

ASTD Video Directory
1640 King Street
P.O. Box 1443
Alexandria, VA 22313
Phone: (703) 683-8129
Fax: (703) 683-8103
Internet: http://www.astd.org

Management Media Directory
Gale Group
27500 Drake Road
Farmington Hills, MI 48331-3535
Phone: (800) 877-GALE
Internet: http://www.gale.com

Groups That Produce Training Materials

American Management Association
135 West 50th Street
New York, NY 10020
Phone: (212) 586-8100
Internet: http://www.amanet.org

American Media Incorporated
4900 University
West Des Moines, IA 5026
Phone: (800) 262-2557
Internet: http://www.ammedia.com

Bureau of Business Practices
24 Rope-Ferry Road
Waterford, CT 06385
Phone: (800) 243-0876 or (860) 442-4365
Fax: (800) 772-7421
Internet: http://www.bbpnews.com

Phoenix Coronet
2349 Chaffee
St. Louis, MO 63146
Phone: (800) 621-2131
E-mail: phoenixfilms@worldnet.att.net

CRM Films
2215 Faraday Avenue
Carlsbad, CA 92008-9829
Phone: (800) 421-0833
Fax: (760) 931-5792
Internet: http://www.crmfilms.com

Lakewood Publications Inc.
Lakewood Building
50 South 9th Street
Minneapolis, MN 55402
Phone: (612) 333-0471
Internet: http://www.lakewoodpub.com

Video Arts Inc.
8614 West Catalpa Avenue
Chicago, IL 60656
Phone: (800) 553-0091
Internet: http://www.videoarts.com

Mentoring Program Guide

Mentoring: A Guide to Corporate Programs and Practices
Catalyst 120 Wall Street, 5th Floor
New York, NY 10005
Phone: (212) 514-7600
Internet: http://www.catalystwomen.org

Visual Aid References

How to Prepare and Use Effective Visual Aids
American Society for Training and Development
1640 King Street
P.O. Box 1443
Alexandria, VA 22313
Phone: (703) 683-8129
Fax: (703) 683-8103
Internet: http://www.astd.org

Corporate Universities

Corporate University Review
(a magazine about organizational learning and performance published by Securities
Data Publishing, a division of Thomson Financial Services)
40 West 57th Street, 11th Floor
New York, NY 10019
Phone: (212) 765-5311
Internet: http://www.traininguniversity.com

WRITING THE TRAINING PROPOSAL

Because so many other individuals and companies are offering training to organizations, the consultant should consider sending training proposals to prospective consultees to differentiate the consultant's training programs from the competition. The training proposal is a planning document that presents the consultant's credentials and training plans. Most proposals include five items: (1) consultant's credentials and experiences, (2) purpose of the training program, (3) design of the training program, (4) training schedules and time frames, and (5) logistical arrangements (Holtz, 1993). Wallace and Hall (1996) describe what these five areas entail:

1. *Consultant credentials:* Of necessity, consultees are interested in the consultant-trainer's professional qualifications, formal training background, and consultation experiences. Such data provide a documented and visible record that facilitates a correct match between the consultee's training needs and the consultant's professional characteristics. Psychological consultants must adhere strictly to ethical principles when documenting descriptions of professional competencies and characteristics.
2. *Rationale:* Training proposals include a statement of purpose or rationale that elucidates the need for training. The written proposal reflects the consultant's understanding of consultation problems and any assessment data that have been synthesized or categorized. From the rationale statement, the consultee evaluates the trainer's assessment and understanding of training needs.
3. *Training design:* The training design is a brief account of how the training intervention is to occur; that is, it identifies the training program's methods and desired results. The training design is a planning draft that ensures that the training intervention is specially tailored to the consultee's setting and problem. Even polished, sophisticated trainers risk unsuccessful training when they fail to design properly matched training content and methodologies.
4. *Schedule:* Training programs occur in myriad time frames—hours, days, or weeks. A principal consideration is the expediency with which training programs are delivered; to be cost effective, training must be delivered efficiently enough that the benefits outweigh the losses associated with the trainees' time away from routine work activities. Further, training programs must be scheduled in convenient time frames that avoid unnecessary intrusions or disruptions.
5. *Logistical arrangements:* Training interventions often entail a range of logistical issues and arrangements. Clarification of such matters prior to training prevents confusion or inappropriate arrangements. Consultants should include logistical information that appears essential to training planning and implementation (e.g., information about fees, required media equipment or materials, copying, and training space). (pp. 242–244)

Training proposals will vary greatly depending on the consultant, the consultee's needs, and the training program. A sample proposal is provided in Box 8.3.

TEAM BUILDING

An extremely popular modality, team building uses all the group dynamic material covered in the previous chapters as well as all the facilitation skills previously discussed.

Since the early 1950s, in the heyday of the human relations movement, team building has been a foundation of consulting. Gradually, the focus changed from concern for

===== **Box 8.3** =====

Training Proposal for Ashemy, Inc.

- *Trainer credentials and experience:* Richard Sears received his doctorate in Clinical Psychology from the School of Professional Psychology and his Master of Business Administration from the Raj Soin College of Business at Wright State University in Dayton, Ohio. Richard has performed consultation services for individuals, businesses, and nonprofit agencies on a wide variety of topics, including executive coaching and development, strategic and tactical business planning, training and development workshops, mental health issues in the workplace, stress reduction, change management, and self-defense and security issues. References are available on request.

- *Purpose of the training:* Ashemy, Inc. has expressed interest in providing a training seminar for the 25 members of its human resource department regarding mental health issues in the workplace. Ashemy, Inc.'s human resource department has been dedicated to continuously working to establish a fair and healthy working environment for all its employees. The proposed training program is designed to build awareness of mental health issues in the workplace, to promote making appropriate referrals to employee assistance programs, and to provide a basic overview of the legalities involved in mental health issues in the workplace.

- *Design of the training program:* The proposed training program consists of a 1-day training session involving lecture and discussion of issues that are most relevant to Ashemy, Inc. Participants will each receive a training packet containing written materials that summarize the content of the lectures. Participants will also view videos describing case scenarios, and participants will discuss the cases and will have the opportunity to discuss issues faced by their own department.

- *Schedules and time frames:* The program is eight hours long, and it is suggested that the training be scheduled from 8 A.M. to 5 P.M., with one hour for lunch. Currently, May 10, May 24, and June 9 are available.

- *Logistical arrangements:* A meeting room that can comfortably seat the 25 participants is needed, with bare space on the wall for the computer projector. The trainer will provide the projector, all computer equipment, and all handout materials. The fee of $2,000, payable 30 days before the training event, will cover all costs, including materials, travel, meals, and other expenses.

Thank you for your consideration. Attached is a course outline for more details about the training content. Please contact me to arrange a date, or if you have any further questions or concerns.

Richard Sears, PsyD, MBA
richard@psych-insights.com
www.psych-insights.com

social interaction (process-oriented, e.g., "T-groups") to the achievement of specific results (task-oriented). Modern team building focuses on both task and process. Team building is a process of teaching group members how to fix themselves.

The Ideal Team

To work with teams, the consultant needs a model of the characteristics of a good team. Generally, the ideal team has the following characteristics:

- Efficient
- Productive
- Cohesive
- Produces work superior in quality and quantity
- Composed of team members who are competent to carry out their duties
- Problems and conflicts within the team quickly and professionally addressed
- High-quality decisions made
- Sense of satisfaction in the work accomplished shared by all members
- Team constantly learning and growing and adapting to change

Of course, how these qualities will manifest depends on the nature of the team and the tasks they have been formed to accomplish. For example, a ballet team needs to feel a stronger sense of cohesion than a gymnastics team.

Elements of an Empowered Team

When appropriate (depending on the nature and purpose of the team), the consultant can discuss the important elements of an empowered team, and ask critical questions about how to foster each element:

Respect: There is respect when people expect the best from each other and assume that others have constructive motivations. Each person has personal needs, agenda, and preferences that must be negotiated. What are some of the ways you can create mutual respect with your team members?

Information: People who work together need complete information. The leader needs to inform people clearly and completely and then let them make conclusions. Information should flow freely and not be hoarded or hidden. What are some of the ways you can inform your team more fully?

Control and decision making: People want to make decisions about how they reach goals and the best way to get a job done. Empowering leaders don't assume they know but ask people to work with them to decide how to do things. This may take longer at the start, but it builds complete agreement and higher commitment to getting the best results. What are some of the ways you can share power with your team?

Responsibility: Empowerment means that responsibility is not all on the leader's shoulders. He or she can count on help and will share the rewards and credit with everyone. When this happens, the leader sleeps better and feels less helpless and deserted when there is a crisis. What are some of the ways you can share responsibility with your team?

Skills: People need new skills, and they need to keep learning to keep up with the team's needs. People need to have the opportunity to learn, so they can be true partners. What are some of the ways you can facilitate your team's learning?

When to Do Team Building

Teams are not always the best medium for accomplishing an organization's objectives, and should not be used simply because it has become popular to do so. However, for established or newly created teams, team building may be necessary to maintain or to rebuild a team's cohesion, morale, and productivity. Dyer (1987) discussed several factors that might lead a consultant to consider implementing team-building interventions:

- Loss of production or output
- Increased number of complaints within the staff
- Conflicts or hostility among staff members
- Confusion about assignments or unclear roles
- Decisions that are misunderstood or not carried through properly
- Apathy or lack of interest or involvement among staff members
- Ineffective staff meetings; low participation in group decisions
- Start-up of a new group that needs to develop quickly into a team
- High dependency on or negative reactions to the manager
- Complaints from customers (both internal and external) and the quality of service

CASE EXAMPLE

A consultant once received a call from a medical school asking him to help a department with considerable interpersonal conflict. The conflict was so severe that the school was placed on probation by their accrediting body.

This is a situation that had structural issues—the department chair usurped the authority of the division head, and there was considerable interpersonal conflict between these two major faculty members. There was also very poor organization within the department. In this case, the conflict was mainly between two or three key individuals, so team building was not an appropriate intervention. The consultant only worked directly with the key individuals.

When Not to Do Team Building

There are times when team building is not an appropriate intervention, such as when issues involve influences outside the control of the team members. Consultants must be aware that attempting team building at such times will often backfire, leading to further discontent and resentment among team members. Dyer (1987) discussed several factors that contraindicate team-building interventions:

- Technical difficulty
- A systems issue
- An issue between two individuals that does not affect other team members
- An administrative foul-up
- When the manager is using the intervention for some hidden purpose

STEPS IN TEAM BUILDING

S. L. Phillips and Elledge (1989) discuss phases involved in team building. Though they can be adapted depending on situational need, the following outline can serve as a guide for team-building interventions.

Phase I: Getting Started

In this stage, the consultant should attend to the following, discussing them with those who are involved in the team building project. This sets the foundation and tone for the rest of the intervention:

- The boundaries of the consultant's analysis
- The project's objectives
- The type of information the consultant will seek
- The consultant's role in the project
- The product the consultant will deliver
- The support and involvement the consultant will need from the client system

Phase II: Collecting Data

S. L. Phillips and Elledge (1989) recommend asking the following types of questions to gather information about the team's current situation. The questions the consultant asks will vary depending on the nature of the team and the problem:

- Tell me about your job. What are your responsibilities? How do you fit into the larger picture?
- In general, what is it like to work in your department?
- What challenges do you see for your department? For your unit? For you personally?
- What are the strengths and weaknesses of your team?
- Given those strengths and weaknesses, what do you perceive to be the team's problems and opportunities?
- What do you expect of your manager?
- How could your manager make your job easier?
- What can you tell me about the relationships between people that would help me facilitate the session? In other words, how do the people in your unit get along?
- What would make you feel that the team-building session had been successful? What do you want to carry away from the session?
- What else can you tell me that would help me to make the team building valuable?

If time and resources permit, consultants can also gather data through questionnaires or through assessment instruments (such as personality and values measures).

Phase III: Analyzing the Data

Once the data have been gathered, the consultant can look through the information for themes and patterns. If formal assessments were given, the individual responses can be scored and compared with national norms as well as with the prevailing norms of the team, to see how each person "fits in."

Phase IV: Giving Feedback

Feedback is then given to the team, based on the patterns found in the data. Frequently, giving feedback can serve as an intervention in and of itself, as people may discover that they have different styles of communicating, different interpersonal needs, or different life values. Individuals should have the opportunity to give input on the feedback they receive, so that adjustments can be made in the interpretation of the data.

Sometimes recontracting is necessary after giving feedback. If the assessment and feedback reveal that the actual problem is of a different nature, then team building may take on a different form, or may not be needed at all.

Phase V: Implementation

Once the assessment and feedback sessions have clarified what needs to be done to build the team, the consultant can facilitate the activities necessary to accomplish the established goals.

The team-building process may include goal setting, interpersonal relationship development, role analysis and clarification, and an analysis of the team's process dynamics. The nature and scope of the intervention will depend on the nature and purpose of the team, but will generally involve fostering trust and openness among team members (Robbins, 2001). Sometimes this involves performing group exercises (Dyer, 1987; Pfeiffer & Jones, 1978; S. L. Phillips & Elledge, 1989).

When conducting a team-building session, the consultant should be clear about the objective of the intervention, which is to improve how the members work together as a team. The consultant should emphasize that the focus should be on looking at the process of team functioning rather than the content of team functioning.

A good way to begin a team-building intervention is to discuss the characteristics of an effective team, since team members may have differing ideas about this. To spark discussion, the consultant can provide a list or description of how an effective team might manifest itself, such as that given by McGregor (1960). The consultant can then ask members of the group how they differ from the ideal and work with them to create a plan to close that gap.

- The "atmosphere" tends to be informal, comfortable, relaxed. There are no obvious tensions. It is a working atmosphere in which people are involved and interested.
- There is a lot of discussion in which virtually everyone participates, but it remains pertinent to the task of the group. If the discussion gets off the subject, someone will bring it back in short order.

- The task or the objective of the group is well understood and accepted by the members. There will have been free discussion of the objective at some point, until it was formulated in such a way that the members of the group could commit themselves to it.
- The members listen to each other! The discussion does not have the quality of jumping from one idea to another unrelated one. Every idea is given a hearing.
- There is disagreement. The group is comfortable with this and shows no signs of having to avoid conflict or to keep everything on the plane of sweetness and light. Disagreements are not suppressed or overridden by premature group action.
- On the other hand, there is no "tyranny of the minority." Individuals who disagree do not appear to be trying to dominate the group or to express hostility. Their disagreement is an expression of a genuine difference of opinion, and they expect a hearing in order that a solution may be found. Sometimes there are basic disagreements that cannot be resolved. The group finds it possible to live with them, accepting them but not permitting them to block its efforts.
- Most decisions are reached by a kind of consensus in which it is clear that everybody is in general agreement and willing to go along. However, there is little tendency for individuals who oppose the action to keep their opposition private and thus let an apparent consensus mask real disagreement. Formal voting is at a minimum; the group does not accept a simple majority as a proper basis for action.
- Criticism is frequent, frank, and relatively comfortable. There is little evidence of personal attack, either openly or in a hidden fashion.
- People are free in expressing their feelings as well as their ideas both on the problem and on the group's operation. There is little pussyfooting, there are few "hidden agendas."
- When action is taken, clear assignments are made and accepted.
- The chairperson of the group is not dominated, nor on the contrary, does the group defer unduly to him or her. In fact, as one observes the activity, it is clear that the leadership shifts from time to time, depending on the circumstances. Different members, because of their knowledge or experience, are in a position at various times to act as "resources" for the group.
- The group is self-conscious about its own operations. Frequently, it will stop to examine how well it is doing or what may be interfering with its operation (McGregor, 1960, pp. 232–235).

For ease of discussion, the consultant could also use a shorter list such as the following (Dyer, 1987; Varney, 1989):

Characteristics of Effective Teams

- Goals are clear and understood and accepted by all team members. Goals must be specific and challenging.
- There is a climate of trust and support.
- Differences among people are identified and worked through rather than ignored.
- People understand and accept their roles in the work unit and how they fit into the overall framework of both the team and the organization.
- Communication is open.
- There is a low level of conflict.
- Formal and informal organizations are of high quality.
- Control within the team is satisfactory.
- Decisions are made that solve problems in precise and clear terms.
- The team produces results and achieves a high level of satisfaction.

A discussion of the characteristics of ineffective teams may also stimulate ideas about dysfunctional process occurring in the team (Likert, 1976; McGregor, 1960).

Characteristics of Ineffective Teams

- Domination by the leader
- Warring cliques or subgroups
- Unequal participation and uneven use of group resources
- Rigid or dysfunctional group norms and procedures
- A climate of defensiveness or fear
- Uncreative alternatives to problems
- Restricted communications
- Avoidance of differences or potential conflicts

To foster a support structure that facilitates the team's productive processes, the consultant can also help the team create a set of ground rules that all team members agree to abide by. Consultants can also set some ground rules for the team-building intervention, which can serve as a model for the group's later functioning. Following is an example set of ground rules.

Ground Rules

- Keep the time boundaries
- Be willing to participate fully
- Be open and honest with yourself and each other
- Be prepared to work
- Be willing to have fun

The consultant could also do a preassessment of team functioning (Dyer, 1987). Before the team-building session, each team member is asked to come prepared to share his or her perception of the following: (1) What keeps this team from functioning at its maximum potential? (2) What keeps you, personally, from doing the kind of job you would like to do? (3) What things do you like in this team that you want to have maintained? (4) What changes would you like to see made that would help you and the whole team?

During the session, team members each take a turn sharing their information. The responses are listed on a flip chart or posted on the wall, and common themes are identified. The most important issues are listed in order of priority, and they become the items for group discussion. The consultant should help team members sort the problems into (1) those problems we can work on here; (2) those problems someone else must handle (and identify who that is); and (3) those problems we must live with since they appear to be beyond our ability to change.

Another approach to team building is simply to ask and process the following three questions:

1. What are the biggest problems our team is currently facing?
2. What keeps our team from being as effective as it could be?
3. What actions do we need to take to solve our problems and improve our team expectations?

The "critical incident" approach involves asking and processing the following questions:

- When did the team work well and when did it fail—why?
- How and what can we learn from our successes and failures?
- How do we improve our functioning?

Role clarification is another important team-building tool. Sometimes difficulties arise in teams simply because members are unclear about their role and/or the precise roles of other members of the group.

In addition to looking at group process, the consultant can focus on improving individual functioning on the team. The confirmation-disconfirmation process involves having group members summarize how they view themselves and their own work performance on the team, including their strengths and areas that they believe they need to improve. Other members are asked to confirm or disconfirm the person's diagnosis.

Before ending the team-building session, the consultant should help the team develop a list of concrete action items to achieve the goals they have created. Such items should include a description of what needs to be done, the main person or persons responsible for the item, and a time frame for getting it done. The team members should also agree to report back on any future learning or discoveries that may be relevant to the whole group.

Phase VI: Follow-Up

Proper follow-up is crucial to the success of any project. The consultant must remember that team building is an ongoing activity. The consultant can perform a spectacular team-building activity, but it is crucial that steps be put into place to ensure that the team will implement the necessary action steps. The consultant can later assess the effectiveness of the intervention and make "course corrections" along the way as needed. Ideally, the consultant's intervention will have positive repercussions throughout the entire client organization.

CASE EXAMPLE: TEAM-BUILDING DESIGN FOR A NEW TEAM

The following case example makes use of an intervention designed to help new teams function effectively. It comprises seven steps:

1. Introduction
2. Mission-and-Purpose Statement
3. Building an Ideal Team Model
4. Role Clarification
5. Data Feedback
6. Action Plans
7. Follow-up Planning

Case Background

The consultant was called in to work with a company when the company was about to fall apart due to a conflict between the owner and the president of the company. The consultant started the intervention by working with the individuals and the dyad, and was able to help them resolve their problems. The coaching had been viewed as so helpful that the owner and president asked the consultant to do some coaching with each member of the executive team.

During the years preceding the resolution of their problems, the executive team had aligned with either the owner or the president and had created a divisive, destructive team atmosphere. The consultant was asked to do team building in this context. The following extract is an outline of the presentation given to the company:

Team Building
Sam's Electronics

Introduction: My name is John Rudisill, and I am an organizational psychologist who has consulted with Sam's Electronics and other companies regarding team building.

Model:
—*Goals (reason, values for existence):* What is the primary reason for this team?
—*Roles (definitions):* What does each team member do?
—*Procedures (structure):* What policies/procedures support your activities?
—*Relationships (communication):* What are the communication/relationships between team members? (Place these things on a pyramid, using a flip chart.)

Goals: (1) Improve the effectiveness of your group in which you must work together to achieve results and (2) provide an opportunity for your group as a whole to analyze its functioning, performance, strengths, and weaknesses. So, we will be trying to better understand the way you interact and to improve your effectiveness.

Ground rules: Be on time, be willing to participate fully, be open and honest with yourself and each other, be prepared to work, be willing to have fun. Any ground rules that you want to add?

Attitudes: Company perspective, accountability, team focus.

Comments by the leader: Executive X.

Data gathering: We need to start by discussing your concerns about the team. What are issues this team needs to work on? List two to three issues.

Voting and discussion of the issues: Select 2 items that are the most important to discuss. Let's discuss them in turn.

Individual feedback: Take a few moments, and for each person in the room, write down what you would like them to do more of, less of, and keep doing the same. After you finish writing these down, exchange them with each other.

Closing: What do you want to talk about that hasn't come up?
   Remember that team building is an ongoing process. It must be continuous.

The first team-building meeting was viewed as highly successful and helpful, so the president wanted to hold another meeting to begin to deal better with the performance problems and relationship problems on the team. Specifically, one team member was not performing well and was seen as being protected by the owner, while another team member (the only woman) was viewed as harsh and controlling, and was seen as being protected by the president. The following extract outlines the next presentation, in which team members were rated and given anonymous feedback on a particular exercise.

Team Development
Sam's Electronics

Purpose: Improve teamwork as well as individual managerial competency through the feedback process and through action planning.

Ground rules: Be as open as you can be (including presenting actual scores if you are comfortable), try to be positive and supportive but honest and straight, and keep the information discussed in the room. Any other ground rules?

Rules about giving feedback: Avoid personal attacks; focus on specific behaviors (not attitudes, characterizations, or personalities). For example, it is better to say, "When you cut me off in last week's meeting, I felt powerless" instead of "You're really rude." Connect behaviors to results. For example, say "When you don't follow through on your commitment to be at meetings on time, I get behind in my own work and have to work overtime to catch up. That makes me less efficient in my work." Avoid hearsay, accusations, and exaggerations. Relate only what you have personally experienced. Let others speak for themselves. Provide constructive information: "If you had acknowledged that you received those improvement ideas I left in your in-basket, I would have felt that I was being listened to." Include positive as well as negative feedback. People need to know what they are doing well if they are to believe that they can improve. They also need to know what success looks like in order to have goals.

Rules about receiving feedback: Approach feedback as a partnership process, not a debate. Focus energy on understanding the behavior being discussed, not fixing it right then and there. You might need time to consider alternatives, gather more information, check facts, and so on. Don't be reluctant to ask questions to gain a better understanding of the feedback. To confirm your understanding, request specific examples so that you will know which behaviors people are referring to: "If I understand correctly, you're saying . . ." Take feedback seriously. Bring a notepad and take notes. Seek a balance between positive and negative feedback. If you receive only positive feedback, ask about practices or behaviors in which you could improve. If you receive only negative feedback, ask about practices or behaviors in which you're strong.

Confidentiality: With the exception of your manager, the people who gave you feedback assumed that their individual scores would remain anonymous. So under no circumstances should you ask people to disclose who gave you what scores. If people volunteer their scores, that's another matter; then it's their choice.

Process: Who would like to go first? (Each team member begins one at a time.)

- Begin by discussing how you feel about the feedback you received.
- Talk about your strengths from the feedback (highest scores). Give specific examples about how you have carried out the item. Ask people to share their examples of how you have demonstrated the item. Then ask them how you can become even better.
- Talk about your opportunities for improvement (lowest scores). Describe your understanding and perception of the feedback about areas for improvement. Give examples of times when you may not have done as well as you could. Ask people for their examples, too, and then get feedback on how you can improve.
- Discuss the items with the largest gap between your self-ratings and the observer ratings. Ask people to help you understand why there's such a difference between your perceptions of yourself and their perceptions of you.

- Encourage people to speak up and contribute other feedback and suggestions. Let them know that they can go beyond the feedback items if they want.
- Share your action plans. Give people specifics about what you plan to do over the next few weeks to improve. Ask them not only to hold you accountable, but also to give you positive reinforcement when they see that you're doing what you said you would do.
- Express your appreciation to people for giving you feedback and discussing your results.
- Follow-up in 6 months on the results of your action items.

Chapter 9

DIVERSITY ISSUES IN CONSULTATION

As mental health professionals, we know that matters of diversity affect all areas of our lives. Our specialized training equips us particularly well to deal with these issues in the workplace, since we have learned that there is a wide variety of perspectives on mental and physical health (Spector, 2000). It is important to continually update our knowledge and explore our own ignorance and biases when engaging in this type of work. In working with groups of people, it is particularly important to balance important issues with a particular individual's experience and sense of identity in relation to that larger group.

Issues of diversity can arise during consultation in one of three ways: directly, indirectly, and peripherally.

Sometimes a consultant is directly asked about issues of diversity. Clinicians sometimes need to better understand a client with whom they are working. Executives may want to create a safer environment for all employees, may be responding to employee reports of being treated unfairly, or may need to meet a legal requirement for fairness in the workplace. The consultant may choose to work directly with individuals on these issues, refer the individual to appropriate educational materials, or deliver a workshop on diversity to a group.

Sometimes diversity issues arise indirectly. The consultant may be asked to "fix" a problem with a clinical client or with an organization, but may discover that the problem is caused by lack of sensitivity to diversity on the consultee's part, or by institutional policies that perpetuate unfair treatment of certain individuals.

The previous two scenarios are fairly clear-cut, because the consultee is specifically asking for help with a particular situation. However, diversity issues also can arise peripherally. In the course of consulting, the consultant may discover a lack of sensitivity to diversity issues in the consultee's attitudes or in an organization's policies. This can present a consultant with an ethical dilemma, as the consultant has been hired only to do the job requested by the consultee. Yet, as mental health professionals, we feel an obligation to our society to root out injustices whenever we can. In such cases, the consultant may be able to find subtle ways of bringing up these important issues, perhaps framing them as potential legal liabilities to bring them to the consultees' attention. Most mental health professionals have developed skills for bringing difficult-to-hear information to clients who at first appear as though they are not ready to listen.

WHY DOES DIVERSITY IN THE WORKPLACE MATTER?

Mental health professionals are increasingly receiving in-depth training in diversity issues. Unconscious biases and even overt discrimination continue to affect large numbers of individuals. Organizations are paying greater attention to matters of diversity. One would like to think that leaders are becoming more enlightened; however, it is more realistic to think that diversity is becoming more important because of practical legal and financial concerns (Jackson, 1992; Jackson & Ruderman, 1995; Norton & Fox, 1997).

Increasingly, developed societies are becoming based more on service and information economies, in which interactions between people are key. The customer bases of organizations are becoming more diverse, and recognition of similarities and differences between people ease the process of doing business.

The globalization of business has also become important in recent decades. Modern technologies allow organizations to more easily do business with people from around the world. When doing business internationally, knowledge of various cultures is crucial for the survival of the business. A common danger in international work situations is to attribute personality deficiencies to people from another culture that are really attributable to cultural differences.

The changing labor market is also putting pressure on organizations to pay closer attention to matters of diversity. Serious problems can develop in company mergers and buyouts when incompatibilities in corporate cultures are ignored.

Because workplace diversity is crucial to the survival of organizations, it has become a strategic imperative in many companies across the country (Griggs & Louw, 1999). One cannot deny the continuing presence of discrimination when 97% of top business executives are white males (Carr-Ruffino, 2002; Lublin, 1996). The numbers have been changing dramatically in the past 2 or 3 years, but the numbers of women and minorities are still small. Over and above the moral imperative to change society's mistreatment of certain groups of individuals, the increasing diversity of the workforce demands that companies and people within companies develop greater cultural sensitivity. Companies are developing more flexible benefits packages (e.g., offering more flexible hours, the option of working from home, the possibility of taking leaves of absence) to accommodate the diversity they must manage (Education and Training Committee of the Society for Industrial and Organizational Psychology, 2005).

Origins of Stereotypes

As mental health professionals have learned from their training, stereotypes are shortcuts people use to quickly identify and make sense of complex phenomena. Consultants can help client systems understand the roots of stereotyping to reduce discrimination and prejudice. In Box 9.1, Carr-Ruffino (2002) provides an overview of the stereotyping process.

TYPES OF DIVERSITY

Gender Diversity

There are more women in the workforce today than ever, and they are better educated than ever. By the year 2000, the workforce became half male and half female. Women

=== **Box 9.1** ===

Making Complex Reality Manageable

When we stereotype, we form large classes and clusters for guiding our daily adjustments. We must deal with too much complexity in our environment to be completely open-minded. We don't have time to learn all about every new person or situation we encounter. Of necessity, we associate them with old categories in our mind in order to make some sense of the world.

Shortcutting with Categories

We tend to place as much as we can into each class and cluster. Our minds tend to categorize events in the *grossest* manner compatible with the need for action. We like to solve problems as easily as possible, so we try to fit them rapidly into a satisfactory category and use this category as a means of prejudging the solution.

Quickly Identifying Things

A stereotype enables us to readily identify a related object. Stereotypes have a close and immediate tie with what we see, how we judge, and what actions we take. In fact, their whole purpose is to help us make responses and adjustments to life in a speedy, smooth, and consistent manner.

Incorporating Multisensory Experiences

For each of our mental categories, we have a thinking and feeling tone or flavor. Everything in that category takes on that flavor. For example, we not only know what the term *Southern belle* means, we also have a feeling tone of favor or disfavor that goes along with that concept. When we meet someone that we decide is a Southern belle, that feeling tone determines whether we like her more or less than we would if we got to know her on her own merits.

Being Rational—Or Not

Stereotypes may be more or less rational. A rational stereotype starts to grow from a kernel of truth and enlarges and solidifies with each new relevant experience. A rational stereotype can give us information that can help us to predict how someone will behave or what might happen in a situation. An irrational stereotype is one we've formed without adequate evidence or because it met an emotional need. We notice behavior that "proves" the stereotype is true, reinforcing it. As for behavior that refutes the stereotype, we either don't notice it at all, or we classify it as a rare exception.

Adding the Emotional Whammy

Our minds are able to form irrational stereotypes as easily as rational ones, and to link intense emotions to them. An irrational idea that is engulfed by an overpowering emotion is more likely to conform to the emotion than to objective evidence. Therefore, once we develop an irrational stereotype that we feel strongly about, it's difficult for us to change that stereotype based on facts alone.

Justifying Dislike

Sometimes we form a stereotype linked to an emotion related to fear—such as hostility, suspicion, dislike, disgust—and set up a framework for prejudice toward an entire group of people based on our experience with one or a few.

Source: From *Managing Diversity: People Skills for a Multicultural Workplace,* fourth edition (pp. 76–77), Boston: Pearson Custom Publishing.

now earn 31% of master's degrees, 39% of law degrees, 13% of engineering degrees, and half of all undergraduate degrees.

However, stereotypes about women's performance in the workplace still remain, such as the idea that women tend to benefit more from a company focus on being "family friendly." Lublin (1996, p. B1) lists sexist stereotypes about a businessman versus a businesswoman:

Man	Woman
A businessman is aggressive.	A businesswoman is pushy.
He is careful about details.	She's picky.
He loses his temper because he's so involved in his job.	She's bitchy.
He's depressed (or hung over), so everyone tiptoes past his office.	She's moody, so it must be her time of the month.
He follows through.	She doesn't know when to quit.
He's firm.	She's stubborn.
He makes wise judgments.	She reveals her prejudices.
He is a man of the world.	She's been around.
He isn't afraid to say what he thinks.	She's opinionated.
He exercises authority.	She's tyrannical.
He's discreet.	She's secretive.
He's a stern taskmaster.	She's difficult to work for.

There also still remains a "glass ceiling" (Morrison et al., 1987; D. Smith, 2000). Despite all the changes that have occurred in the past few decades, with organizations stating that women can achieve any position to which they aspire, subtle discouragement and sometimes flagrant efforts by men prevent women from reaching higher job positions (Harrison, 2004; Morrison, 1992). For example, 95% of senior-level managers in the largest U.S. organizations are men, and less than 7% of the members of the boards of the top 1,000 U.S. organizations are women (Gilbert, Stead, & Ivancevich, 1999).

Sexual Harassment in the Workplace

Sexual harassment in the workplace continues to be a concern for both men and women (L. F. Fitzgerald, Drasgow, Hulin, Gelfand, & Magley, 1997; L. F. Fitzgerald, Hulin, & Drasgow, 1995; K. T. Schneider, Swan, & Fitzgerald, 1997). Consultants can educate the client system about these issues and help organizational leadership promote an environment free of sexual harassment (Stockdale, 1996). Carr-Ruffino (2002) provides the following suggestions for men, women, and organizational leaders (making the assumption that most situations involve heterosexual males harassing heterosexual females):

What Can Men Do to Avoid Problems?
- *Raise your awareness.* Sexual harassment is a rather complex issue, but you can learn enough to stay out of trouble.
- *Respect the word "No."* When you're at work, it's best to forget the old idea that a woman's "no" may not really mean "no" or that it merely makes the conquest more challenging and exciting.

- *Align your attitude.* Are you still harboring the belief that women are inferior? That men should be in control? If so, work on shifting your beliefs to align with current reality.
- *Support clear policies* and training that spell out what harassment is and how the organization will handle it. If you understand sexual harassment, and your company has clear policies about its definition and consequences, you can relax and be yourself (assuming your attitude is in line).
- *Be a role model.* Now that you're savvy about sexual harassment, help other men get it by treating coworkers with respect. For example, refer to women as women, not as "girls," "chicks," "ladies," or similar names. Don't participate in storytelling and jokes that demean women as a group. Let others know you don't want to hear or see women being referred to as sex objects.

What Can Women Do to Avoid Problems?
- *Avoid the sexual stereotype trap.* Women don't need to automatically and unthinkingly fall into others' expectations about their role. *Sex object* is one of the age-old stereotypes that women can avoid by dressing and acting in a businesslike, professional way. Check flirtatious and femme fatale tendencies of the office door.
- *Avoid sexual liaisons at work.* The objective of the office sex game is to increase the man's status with other men. This is one of the ways a man becomes "one of the boys" who make decisions about promotions and salaries. A woman may therefore increase the status of any man she has sex with and at the same time decrease her own status.
- *Say no tactfully but clearly.* Women can let men know if they don't like being called "honey," "babe," and similar names. Women can send I-messages when they say no to requests for a drink, lunch, dinner, or date: "I like you but I don't go out socially with business friends," "I like you but I never go out with married men," "I value our relationship but my husband would be hurt if he couldn't share the occasion," "I like you but I'm not comfortable with going beyond a business relationship." The underlying message is you're not interested in sexual involvement and will always say no to such overtures.

What Can Organizations and Leaders Do?
- Management establishes and publicizes a strong policy that specifically describes the kinds of actions that constitute sexual harassment and sets out the consequences for offenders.
- Management suggests that if a manager-subordinate relationship becomes "serious," one party should change jobs, out of fairness to other subordinates.
- Management regularly signals that it is committed to fighting harassment.
- The firm provides training seminars designed to sensitize employees to the issue.
- The firm sets up complaint procedures and mechanisms that encourage private complaints of harassment and that bypass immediate supervisors, who are often the source of the problem. (pp. 160–161)

Age Diversity

As the population ages, particularly those from the "baby boom" generation, more older workers are available to work. Increasingly, employees are not retiring at or before the age of 65, whether from a desire to stay active or due to financial necessity. Many older individuals find they can no longer maintain a comfortable lifestyle, particularly with the rising cost of health care, and are returning from retirement, even if they already had what they hoped would have been a sufficient pension.

Middle-aged women have also been returning to work in greater numbers, as historical family pressures for them to "stay at home with the children" have lessened, and as it has become more difficult to earn a living on only one salary.

Professional internships have also become popular as a way to introduce young students to the skills and demands of specialized positions in the workplace. Hence, managers must learn to effectively work with the needs of a wide age range of employees.

Cultural Diversity

The cultural background of employees affects their sense of values and how they view the world, and these values affect their attitudes toward work. More than 40% of new entrants into the U.S. workforce come from non-"majority" groups, with about 22% consisting of new immigrants, and about 20% consisting of African American or Hispanic employees (Loden & Rosener, 1991).

There has also been growth in international business, requiring businesses to hire individuals of different cultural backgrounds to work in an environment that may have been designed in another country. Employees tend to maintain ties to their national and cultural heritages, and employers must be aware of this. Significant overt and covert racism still exists. Prejudice and discrimination must be actively sought out and dealt with directly (Shuler, 1998).

Rosinski (2003) described seven categories of cultural aspects that are important for consultants to know and to teach to organizational leadership: sense of power and responsibility, time management approaches, definitions of identity and purpose, organizational arrangements, notions of territory and boundaries, communication patterns, and modes of thinking. Each category contains dimensions that the consultant must assess and address when working with individuals and organizations from diverse backgrounds.

Sense of Power and Responsibility

- *Control:* Some cultures value the idea that people must be in control of their internal and external environment at all times. Such cultures tend to value the idea of "conquering nature," and expect individuals to take responsibility for creating the life they desire.

- *Harmony:* Harmony can be seen as achieving a balance between control and humility. Such cultures see these opposite poles as necessary and inevitable aspects of nature, and individuals attempt to not allow any one particular aspect to dominate.

- *Humility:* An orientation of humility involves recognizing that human beings cannot fully control nature, that the external forces of luck, fate, or divine intervention play a large role in one's daily life. Success is seen as a combination of both effort and good fortune. Such a viewpoint stresses acceptance of that which is beyond an individual's control.

Time Management Approaches

- *Scarce:* Some cultures view time as scarce and treat it like a precious commodity that must be carefully saved and spent. Such cultures strive for efficiency and organization to make the most of what they perceive to be a very limited resource.

- *Plentiful:* Cultures that view time as plentiful tend to take things slowly. Such individuals may prefer to follow natural rhythms rather than artificially designed tight schedules. This viewpoint stresses that "there is time for everything."

- *Monochronic:* In cultures with a monochronic orientation (Hall, 1983), individuals prefer to fully attend to one thing at a time. Tasks are done in a sequential manner, and the individual is devoted to one person, activity, or project at a time.

- *Polychronic:* A polychronic orientation (Hall, 1983) stresses a preference for parallel processing. Individuals balance multiple tasks and relationships, or jump from one person or task to another as needs and importance levels change.
- *Past:* Some cultures, particularly those with a long history, place great value on the past. Individuals from such cultures often prefer to place their present actions and future goals within the context of where they have come from, and take into consideration the values and lessons from important persons in their history.
- *Present:* Cultures that value the present orientation adopt a "here-and-now" approach to living. The present moment is considered the true eternal reality, and things are generally taken as they come. In some forms of this orientation, this viewpoint can take on a desire for "instant gratification" and short-term benefits.
- *Future:* A future orientation takes into consideration that which will be happening in the long-term. Short-term profits are not considered as important as long-term growth. New relationships are carefully cultivated, as they are likely to grow into deep and rich relationships.

Definitions of Identity and Purpose

- *Being:* Cultures that value a sense of being stress the importance of personal growth. Value is placed on living a "good life." That which is intrinsically rewarding, such as personal development and relationships, is preferred over extrinsic rewards, such as money and material goods.
- *Doing:* Cultures with a doing orientation tend to stress the importance of achievements that are visible and measurable by external standards. What an individual "does for a living" forms a large part of the individual's sense of identity.
- *Individualistic:* Cultures with an individualistic orientation see the smallest unit of survival to be the individual. Persons from such cultures identify primarily with self, and the needs of the individual are satisfied before those of the group. The well-being of the group is assumed to happen when individuals are self-sufficient. This type of culture values independence and personal freedom (Storti, 1999).
- *Collectivistic:* Collectivistic cultures tend to see the smallest unit of survival to be the primary group (such as the family). The individual's role or function in the group (whether family or work) forms a large part of the individual's identity and sense of purpose. Taking care of the group assures the well-being of the individual. Such cultures stress and value the harmony and interdependence of group members (Storti, 1999).

Organizational Arrangements

- *Hierarchy:* Cultures with a hierarchy orientation tend to believe that society and organizations need to be stratified to operate in the best way. Certain individuals tend to hold most of the power and are expected to use that power responsibly. Subordinates are expected to perform their duties and are not expected to take initiative.
- *Equality:* The equality orientation stresses that people are generally equal, but simply must play different roles at times within society. Those in power tend to deemphasize their roles, and try to involve everyone in decision making. Subordinates are encouraged to take initiative, and tend to feel uncomfortable if they are supervised too closely.

- *Universalist:* A universalist orientation emphasizes that there are proper ways to do things and approach situations and these should be applied in a universal manner. Fairness is viewed as treating everyone equally by the same set of rules.
- *Particularist:* The particularist viewpoint emphasizes that circumstances and context must be considered for each case. This approach stresses that people must consider their relationships and the unique variables involved in any given situation.
- *Stability:* Though everyone recognizes that change is inevitable, cultures high on the stability orientation prefer to avoid drastic changes. Any changes that need to be made should be incremental, and should fit within the current paradigm. Whenever possible, rules and guidelines are used to make change orderly and predictable (Hofstede, Pederson, & Hofstede, 2002).
- *Change:* Cultures that value change tend to see it with curiosity and excitement rather than anxiety. Change presents opportunities for things to be made better. Such cultures tend to value unusual or innovative ideas and flexibility (Hofstede, Pederson, & Hofstede, 2002).
- *Competitive:* In cultures that value competition, individuals and teams perpetually strive to do better than their competitors. The workplace becomes an environment where individuals engage in a contest that has both "winners" and "losers." One's victories may come at the expense of others.
- *Collaborative:* Cultures with a collaborative orientation tend to stress the importance of working together to achieve goals. Individuals come together, inspired by the good of the entire group, sharing information and effort so that everyone succeeds.

Notions of Territory and Boundaries

- *Protective:* In cultures with a protective orientation, individuals erect mental and physical boundaries around themselves. Their thoughts, feelings, and personal life are considered private, and attempts at intimate exchanges in the workplace tend to be seen as unwelcome intrusions. People may feel vulnerable if others know too much about them.
- *Sharing:* In sharing cultures, open communication about all aspects of one's life is considered important and desirable so that people feel comfortable working together. Boundaries and distance are seen as threatening, since these make it difficult for others to get to know someone.

Communication Patterns

- *High context:* In cultures that emphasize high context communication patterns, individuals pay close attention to more than just the words being used. Such things as speech patterns, tone of voice, silence, body language, facial expressions, and eye contact are also important contextual considerations (Rosinski, 2003).
- *Low context:* Cultures with low context communication patterns use an explicit communication code (Hall & Hall, 1990). Such cultures tend to emphasize the importance of using words that are direct and unambiguous. In business transactions, things are not generally taken seriously unless they are in writing.
- *Direct:* In cultures with a direct orientation, individuals tend to speak their mind in a blunt manner. They tend to get directly to the point and do not leave their meaning ambiguous. Individuals from such cultures tend not to be offended by such directness, as forthrightness and clarity are valued.

- *Indirect:* Cultures that value an indirect orientation tend to say things in a round-about way. Saying something directly may cause another person to lose face, or may disrupt the harmony of the team. The preservation of the relationship is a high priority. Individuals may make subtle suggestions, use metaphors, or communicate through another person.
- *Affective:* An affect of culture values emotions and warmth to establish and maintain interpersonal relationships. Emotions and passion in one's arguments are respected and considered valuable.
- *Neutral:* Cultures with a neutral orientation tend to devalue emotions. Logic and objectivity are considered crucial when making one's arguments. Emotions are felt to get in the way of clarity of thinking.
- *Formal:* In formal cultures, one is expected to follow the rules of conduct. One must determine the degree of formality required for a given situation and comply with the need for formal language or behavior. Individuals must adhere to protocols, rituals, and rules of etiquette (Brake, Walker, & Walker, 1995).
- *Informal:* Cultures that prefer informality tend to believe that formality gets in the way of open and authentic communication. Individuals from such cultures generally feel uncomfortable with deference, and usually treat people the same. Social conventions and customs are seen as unnecessary, and individuals tend to prefer casual, relaxed, and spontaneous conduct (Schmitz, 2000).

Modes of Thinking

- *Deductive:* The deductive style of thinking emphasizes concepts and theories, which are then applied to particular cases. Individuals with this thinking style prefer to generalize from one concept to another, placing their trust in the power of thought (Stewart & Bennett, 1991).
- *Inductive:* The inductive style of thinking emphasizes collecting data before reaching conclusions. Such cultures tend to distrust theory and generalizations, concerned that they might be impractical, unrealistic, or too abstract (Althen, 2002). Once the facts are gathered, the individual must also rely on intuition to see the larger picture that integrates all of the data.
- *Analytical:* An analytical style of thinking breaks problems down into pieces in order to solve them. Analytical thinking tends to be linear or sequential, investigating the chain of cause and effect.
- *Systemic:* A systemic style of thinking involves bringing together all of the parts to look at a coherent whole. The emphasis of this style of thinking is to see the connections between the parts, and how the parts and the whole are interrelated.

Obviously, cultures and individuals do not fit neatly into these dimensions, and any given culture or individual will contain aspects of many dimensions. What matters is that the consultant should be aware of these dimensions and how they interact with each other.

Rosinski (2003) stresses that coaches or consultants must do a thorough self-assessment of their own ideas and values before working with diverse cultural groups. Knowledge of these dimensions can also help managers and employees function more effectively together by fostering awareness and understanding. These dimensions play out in many ways within any given culture, and individuals within a culture show considerable variation in the ways they choose to internalize these values. Individuals from other countries who are working in the United States may assimilate the values of the workplace environment they are in, but may continue to hold on to traditional values in their private lives. Others may have felt pressure to abandon all traditional values and be "American." Awareness of such issues can be helpful to consultants in conceptualizing problems and designing intervention plans.

Family Situations

Strict workplace policies can cause significant hardships for single mothers (e.g., needing to care for a sick child and missing work, being overlooked for travel opportunities because of family demands). However, single employees have increasingly become subject to what might be termed "reverse discrimination." Single employees (without children or spouses to "worry about") are often pressured by employers to shoulder a disproportionate share of the travel, overtime, and other special requests (Education and Training Committee of the Society for Industrial and Organizational Psychology, 2005).

Physical and Psychological Disabilities

The Americans with Disabilities Act placed needed attention on the extra accommodations employers must make to integrate the skills and contributions of persons with disabilities into the workplace. However, the special treatment received by these employees can often create tension in the workplace that a manager must learn to actively manage (Education and Training Committee of the Society for Industrial and Organizational Psychology, 2005).

Many times, managers and employees simply do not know what to do, or if they should do anything different at all, when working with individuals with disabilities. As with all matters of diversity, one of the consultant's primary goals is to help individuals feel more comfortable dealing directly with the issues involved. Comfort levels can be increased simply by fostering an atmosphere in which individuals can speak freely about these matters, and through offering direct psychoeducational information. Carr-Ruffino (2002) provides an excellent overview of frequently asked questions about working with individuals with motor, visual, and communication disabilities.

Frequently Asked Questions about Disabilities

FAQs about Persons with Mobility Impairments

Q: How do I offer help to a person with a disability? Or should I?
- Offer help: it's never the wrong thing to do. It can always be declined if not wanted, but always ask *first* if the person wants you to help and take *no* for an answer.
- If help is wanted, ask specifically what you can do and how to do it, or suggest something and get agreement.
- If you assist another helper, remember the person with the disability is in charge.
- Handle the helping situation as unobtrusively as possible; avoid a "circus."

Q: How do I help persons using wheelchairs, crutches, and so on?
- Never grab their appliances except in cases of obvious immediate physical danger.
- After helping, stay a moment and make sure matters are in hand before leaving. Let the person know you are leaving.

Q: Should I open doors for persons with mobility impairments?
- Everyone can use help with doors at times.
- Hold the door itself—rather than their arm or wheelchair—until the person is completely inside.

Q: How can I be considerate of people who use wheelchairs?

- Avoid blocking aisles and other spaces that a wheelchair user needs to access—don't block them with briefcases, wastebaskets, and so on; push chairs under tables or desks; be aware.
- When having a conversation with a wheelchair user, try to seat yourself in front of the person, so you can talk eye to eye. If you must stand, step back so the person isn't required to look up to you.
- Reaching elevator buttons may be impossible for a wheelchair user; offer to help.
- Users of nonmotorized wheelchairs may need help getting up inclines or around barriers, but never begin pushing a wheelchair without asking permission.
- Never release the chair without warning, so the wheelchair user is always in control.
- Be sure you know exactly where the person wants to go.
- Begin pushing a wheelchair cautiously if you are not familiar with it. Go slowly at first; wheelchairs can gain surprising momentum.
- Note the size and protrusion of the chair, such as protruding foot plates. Pay attention to the terrain, such as step-downs, and watch where you're going.
- When entering a crosswalk in a street, remember the wheelchair user's feet may be further out than you think and may be dangerously close to passing traffic.
- Going up steps, lean the chair back to raise the front wheels and push the chair up frontwards.
- Going down steps, ask if the person prefers going down frontwards or backwards. Either way, raise the front wheels and keep them up until the entire chair is down the step. The occupant should always be tilted toward the back against the backrest instead of toward the front where there is no support.

Q: How do I show consideration for persons who walk with difficulty?

- When approaching steps, walk alongside them and offer your arm, which they can grasp, giving them control and support. Grabbing their arm can upset their balance.
- If more help is needed, put your arm around their waist.
- Any time a person falls, ask how you can assist, or offer your arm for the fallen person to take if he or she needs it. Don't grab the person.

Q: What should I consider when I'm planning activities that require mobility-impaired persons to go to unfamiliar places?

- Mobility-impaired persons need to know in advance whether they will encounter a difficult barrier—such as inadequate parking places, ramps, and restrooms.
- Find out what kinds of parking arrangements they need.
- Wheelchair users need access to restrooms with hallways and doors wide enough for the chair, enough space inside the stall, and perhaps a handbar by the commode.
- Never insist on simply carrying a disabled person over, around, and through obstacles. They may find it demeaning, unpleasant, or even scary—and it could be dangerous for both of you. All of us prefer to be independent and self-possessed.
- When in doubt, ask the disabled person for some tips on places that are accessible and comfortable.

FAQs about Persons with Visual Impairments

Q: What should I consider when giving directions to visually impaired coworkers?

- The single most useful thing you may be able to do is to furnish relevant information about the immediate surroundings. Often just a few words will do.
- Furnish simple information without hesitation, anytime it seems appropriate.
- When giving directions, be sure you really know where the target location is.
- Find out what types of directions are most helpful; this will depend on what the person can see or not see. Use numbers, where possible. Ask yourself, how many blocks down the street? How many doors down the hall?

- Give directions that are as specific as possible. Describe turns or curves as *left, right, clockwise,* and so on. Terms such as *north* or *south* will probably be irrelevant.
- Describe anything out of the ordinary along the way, such as possible safety hazards.
- Tell persons with some vision about large, noticeable landmarks.
- Be as complete as necessary without overloading the person with information.
- If you think the place is simply too hard to find, offer to take them there.

Q: What should I do when I'm walking with a visually impaired person?
- City streets pose one of the biggest hazards for visually impaired persons. Offer your arm, but do not clutch the person's arm. Be sure you understand which street the person wants to cross.
- Don't leave the person until she or he is safely up the opposite curb.
- If the person does not take your arm, walk closely enough for her or him to reach over and touch you. Avoid getting separated in crowds.
- If the person takes your arm, walk slightly ahead to guide the way and proceed normally. Never push the person ahead of you.
- Avoid sudden turns or jerky movements.
- Tell the person when it's time to step up, step down, or step around some obstacle.
- Watch for overhead obstacles, especially with a taller companion.
- When approaching steps, elevators, or other possible barriers, pause and briefly describe what's ahead.

Q: What should I know about helping persons who use canes?
- If a person touches your foot with a cane, step aside and let her or him pass.
- Don't touch a cane without permission.
- When walking with a person who uses a cane, offer your arm.

Q: What should I know about helping persons with guide dogs?
- Guide dogs and service dogs are used by a minority of visually impaired persons to help them get around and by mobility impaired persons to perform certain tasks.
- A guide dog is on duty anytime it's wearing a harness.
- Take care to do nothing that will interfere with the dog's performance. Have faith in the dog and do not interfere unless there is a genuine emergency.
- Don't disrupt the routine and training by touching, feeding, petting, playing with, speaking to, or commanding the dog unless you're encouraged to do so.
- If you have a dog, keep it away from the guide dog.
- When walking with someone who is using a dog, offer your arm.

Q: What should I consider when communicating with visually impaired persons?
- Be aware that they rely on sound and touch to know what's going on.
- When you first meet a visually impaired person, feel free to shake hands. You might say, "May I shake your hand?" to cue them that you're extending your hand.
- When you meet the person thereafter, identify yourself, and any others you are with.
- When you would normally hand a business associate a business card, brochure, or other written material, give the visually impaired person the option to accept. You might offer to stay a moment and help interpret the material.
- When you enter the presence of visually impaired persons, speak to them and let them know you're there. Otherwise they may be unduly jolted when they hear you make some noise. Also, let them know when you're leaving.
- When leaving in a public place, say how long you'll be gone. Consider whether you need to offer to guide the person to a place where he or she can wait comfortably.
- When visually impaired persons hear your voice, they may be unsure whether you are talking to them or to someone else. They may remain silent rather than respond to comments they think might be meant for someone else.

- Address them by name when you're in a group or in public. If you don't know their name, stand directly in front of them and begin speaking. You may also gently touch their arm or repeat yourself to be sure they understand.
- Don't yell.
- Offer to describe visual sites.
- Speak up tactfully when some aspect of their grooming seems unpremeditated.

Q: When making plans that include visually impaired persons, what should I keep in mind?
- If you're planning to meet outside the office, the key issue is likely to be transportation. Give some advance notice so they can arrange for a ride.
- If you're not sure whether a visually impaired person would be able to attend an event, ask. Invite them and allow them to make the decision; then respect their wishes.
- At restaurants, remember to offer help in reading the menu and calling the server.

FAQs about Persons with Hearing or Speaking Impairments

Q: What do I need to know generally about working with persons with hearing or speaking impairments?
- Most people with speaking impairments have normal hearing, and many hearing-impaired persons have excellent speech skills, particularly those whose hearing impairment is not longstanding or is not severe.
- When you initiate a direct conversation with communication-impaired persons, begin by asking, orally or in writing, how best to communicate.
- When introducing communication-impaired persons to others, make every effort to introduce only one or two persons at a time. Try to find a quiet spot and pronounce names slowly and distinctly.
- If you're asked to make a telephone call for a communication-impaired person, get the key information first, perhaps asking the person to write it.
- Before you hang up, check to be sure the message is complete, and after you hang up, give a complete report.

Q: What do I need to remember about lip-reading?
- When talking to persons who use lip-reading, position yourself about three or four feet directly in front of them with adequate light on your face so they can see your lips.
- Face them squarely without looking down or turning your head.
- Keep your hands away from your mouth and avoid eating, smoking, or chewing gum.
- Be aware that lip-reading is tiring, so avoid long monologues. Use a give-and-take format. Take a break during longer conversations.

Q: What do I need to remember about communicating nonverbally?
- Your eyes are especially expressive, so remove dark glasses, hats, and so on. Maintain a natural and relaxed manner without straining to exaggerate.
- If nonverbal communication is inadequate, find other methods.
- When both speaking and using gestures, be sure the gestures correlate with the speech. Random motions throw the listener off balance, trying to sift them from the real clues.

Q: How about writing out messages?
- Writing out messages is slow but is sometimes used. Be creative when you communicate in writing. Often a simple diagram, picture, or map is most effective.
- Watch the person's face as he or she reads your message, just as you would do if you were speaking, so you can gauge the understanding and reaction.

- When persons begin writing to you, don't talk or otherwise distract them until they finish. Allow them to finish writing before you try to read the message, and read the entire message before you begin to answer.
- In a group, offer to read the person's written message aloud to others.

Q: How should I communicate when a professional interpreter is used?

- Professional interpreters who use sign language may be used by people with severe impairments. When you speak through an interpreter, your key goal should be to respect the dignity and autonomy of the impaired person who is the "listener." The interpreter is merely a device in this situation, a tool.
- Face the hearing-impaired person and speak as though no interpreter were present.
- Direct all your comments to the listener, the person with whom you have business, saying, for example, "Your project is being reviewed." The interpreter will relay these exact words to the person.
- Never direct comments intended for the listener to the interpreter, saying "His project is being reviewed." This has the effect of excluding the listener, implying that he is a helpless bystander.
- Remember to look at the listener, not the translator, and to speak to her or him in directed address, using *you,* not *he* or *she.*
- Avoid engaging an interpreter in side conversations that exclude the other person.
- Remember that any translation process is difficult. Choose simple, specific words to be as clear and direct as possible, avoiding slang.

Q: How about communicating by telephone?

- A telecommunication device for the deaf (TDD) is used by many people with speaking or hearing impairments for communicating by telephone. If you don't have a TDD, you can still communicate through the device by going through a voice exchange system, available in most cities.
- Regular telephone communication with a hearing-impaired person is often possible without translator equipment, if the person has enough hearing ability.
- Organize your message ahead of time so you can convey it in a concise, direct manner.
- Try to quiet the noise at your end.
- Talk directly into the receiver clearly and firmly. Speak moderately, slowly, and pause at the end of a sentence.
- Be prepared to spell, rephrase, or use more creative ways to get your message across.
- If you have trouble hearing or understanding, ask for clarification as soon as you start getting lost.
- Keep the conversation short unless you are encouraged to extend it.

Q: How do I plan and conduct meetings that include communication-impaired persons?

- Select a room with good acoustics and a minimum of extraneous noise.
- Check ahead of time to determine what devices, such as interpreters, are needed.
- Offer the people with impairments preferential seating, where they will have a good view of speakers. Ask what they prefer.
- Ask speakers to stay in one spot rather than pacing the floor, for lip-readers.
- Pay special attention to the use of visual aids, handouts, charts, illustrations, and other communication aids.
- Write down new words or terms as you introduce them; it is almost impossible to lip-read an unknown word.
- Write down important facts.
- Repeat all comments or questions from other people in the room before you respond to them.
- If you sit next to a hearing-impaired person in a meeting, be as quiet as possible. If you must communicate with the person during the meeting, write a brief note.

- Allow the hearing-impaired person to observe any notes you're taking.
- Afterwards, offer to answer questions.
- Make occasional eye contact with speaking-impaired persons, to see if they have anything to contribute to the discussion.
- If they can't speak up quickly, you can create a break in the conversation and encourage them to participate.
- If you sit next to a speaking-impaired person, offer to ask questions for him or her during the meeting.

Q: How do I work effectively with persons with hearing impairments?
- The first step is getting their attention without startling them. Stand in front of them and say their name loudly, but don't shout. If you don't know their name, stand directly in front of them and begin speaking. You may also gently touch their arm or repeat yourself to be sure they understand.
- If they don't respond, tap them lightly on the arm or shoulder. If you're not in touching range, wave your hand and try to make visual contact. You may also get attention by knocking on the desk or rapping on a nearby wall, as many are sensitive to such vibrations. Flipping the light switch will get the attention of everyone in the room, so use this method with greater selectivity.
- Effort and concentration are needed by hearing impaired persons in order to understand the speech of others. Conversing at length while walking down a hall or street may be exhausting or impossible.
- You may be able to help as an interpreter when a hearing-impaired person is trying to understand someone with a foreign accent or a child with a high-pitched voice.
- Giving needed information is one of the most helpful things you can do—especially about any sound that may spell danger, such as honking horns, sirens, and alarms—but also information that comes over public address systems, radio, and other sources where lip-reading is impossible. (pp. 364–369)

It is important to differentiate individuals who have lost their hearing and become hearing impaired from those who are deaf and belong to the Deaf culture. Members of the Deaf culture generally do not feel that they are impaired or have any kind of disability, they simply communicate differently than hearing persons.

Sexual Orientation

Although one would think that in an enlightened society issues of sexual orientation would not arise in the workplace, significant discrimination and misunderstanding still exist. Tensions among employees can rise if managers handle these issues inappropriately, particularly in teams with employees who believe that orientations other than heterosexual are wrong (Education and Training Committee of the Society for Industrial and Organizational Psychology, 2005).

The Link between Sexual Orientation and Performance

When managers send signals or messages that it is not okay to be gay in the workplace, whether intentionally or not, they negatively impact work performance. Negative messages or signals force many employees to hide their sexual identity. This hiding takes a tremendous amount of psychological and physical energy. These employees divert their energies away from work performance to protect themselves by covering up facts, keeping low profiles, lying, changing pronouns, and so forth. When people feel excluded, as sexual minorities often do, they are much less inclined to devote energy toward making the organization successful.

Powers and Ellis (1995) believe that although everyone possesses some homophobia, most managers are not blatantly homophobic. However, they have found that managers usually lack the skills, knowledge, and resources to treat all employees fairly, and so tend to ignore issues and situations about which they are ignorant or uncomfortable. Powers relates the following all-too-common anecdotes:

> For years, I have consulted with a small group at one of America's largest firms. It is a group that celebrates weddings, birthdays, anniversary, engagements and other similar events. It operates in a very collegial fashion. I do not believe there are many people in this group with a blatantly homophobic bone in their body. Yet, 6 months ago, the group hired a new staff member. He is a 30-year-old man who has a rainbow flag on his computer. He has been in a loving relationship for 4 years. Yet in this highly social organization, not one person has asked him about his personal life, inquired whether he might be in a relationship, or even remotely broached the subject of his sexual orientation. Neither he nor I believe this stems from homophobia as much as it does from simply not knowing how to talk about these things in a way that does not embarrass him or the person asking. I also believe that if someone were to ask, "What is it like to be a gay man in this group?" or "Are you in a relationship?" or any of hundreds of other questions that would open up discussion in this area, he would be delighted to respond and their working relationship would be strengthened.
>
> But people are afraid, and not just about gay issues. The fear is about differences. I recently attended a professional conference of an organization dedicated to improving work performance. At the opening event, I spotted, among two thousand participants, a very striking woman. Probably in her mid-forties, she was dressed professionally, *and* she had bright purple hair. I immediately walked over to her and said, "You have purple hair, what's it like?" She beamed and proceeded to tell me how much she enjoyed it. She also said most people in the business world acted as if she didn't have purple hair. We both laughed at the extent of people's denial. I discovered that she was a highly successful management consultant from London, England.
>
> The next day, I addressed a group of 150 or so people and I asked, "How many of you saw the woman with purple hair at the reception last night?" Every hand went up. I then asked, "How many of you were curious about her?" Again, every hand went up. I then asked, "How many of you talked to her?"
>
> Not a single hand was raised.
>
> When asked why, they all basically said the same thing—they were afraid they might embarrass her or themselves, so they did nothing. (Powers & Ellis, 1995, pp. 8–9)

Powers and Ellis (1995) go on to say that the fear of saying or doing the wrong thing is often paralyzing. Work relationships and productivity will continue to suffer until the issues of sexual orientation and other matters of diversity are openly addressed. Consultants can help facilitate such communication within organizations.

Personal Idiosyncrasies

In addition to the types of diversity commonly thought of, consultants must also help consultees deal with the personal idiosyncrasies of their clients or employees, as they can have a significant impact on how they function in their lives or in the workplace. These can include political views, personality characteristics, and behavior quirks.

A MODEL DIVERSITY POLICY

The National Society for Performance and Instruction (NSPI; now known as the International Society for Performance Improvement, 2005; Powers & Ellis, 1995) developed a diversity policy that is a model for other organizations to follow because it is so all-inclusive. The policy can be easily adapted to fit a particular organization.

> NSPI is an all-inclusive Society. It values differences in people and diversity within our organization and our profession. It recognizes the different perspectives and contributions an all-inclusive people can make to improving human performance. It is NSPI's policy to welcome and reach out to people of different ages, races, nationalities, ethnic groups, genders, physical abilities/qualities, sexual orientations, health status, recovery status, religions, backgrounds and educational experiences, incomes, material status, marital or parental status, class, military experiences, and geographic locations, as well as any others, who may from time to time experience discrimination or abuse. NSPI does not discriminate against any group or individual. In fact, the organization will actively oppose any and all forms of discrimination. It is also NSPI's desire to help others (clients, customers, constituents, and colleagues) to develop similar policies and support diversity and performance improvements within the workplace. (Powers & Ellis, 1995, p. 125)

TECHNIQUES FOR MANAGERS

Consultants can help managers take a closer look at their company's diversity and selection policies. Most diversity policies speak to providing an inclusive workplace, and thus employees are also responsible for embracing the organization's diversity policies and values. Managers can try to select employees who are aligned with company diversity policies and organizational values, by doing such things as asking for examples of working successfully with people of varying backgrounds during the employment interview (Powers & Ellis, 1995). Consultants can also help managers set performance expectations for all employees.

The following list of workplace performance expectations, written specifically for issues regarding sexual orientation, can serve as a model for many different areas of diversity (Carr-Ruffino, 2002; Griggs & Louw, 1999; Powers & Ellis, 1995):

- Champion an all-inclusive workforce. Do ask! Do tell!
- When interviewing candidates for jobs, let them know that your organization is all-inclusive including gays, lesbians, and bisexuals.
- Welcome newly hired sexual minorities into the workplace.
- Let employees know what their responsibilities and expectations are when it comes to diversity, particularly as it relates to gays, lesbians, and bisexuals.
- Provide feedback that reinforces and develops behaviors that contribute to making the workplace more inclusive.
- Recognize and reward employees who are contributing to making the workplace more inclusive.
- Encourage employees to participate in workshops, classes, and other developmental experiences related to this area of diversity.

- Respond to criticism by referring to your desire to create an all-inclusive workplace.
- Stand firm in the face of criticism.
- Let the message ring loud and clear that you will not tolerate even subtle forms of discrimination.
- Encourage lesbian and gay employees to point out training and business policies and practices that discriminate based on sexual orientation of employees and customers.
- Review on a regular basis employee responsibility not to discriminate.
- Respond to homophobic jokes and statements by saying, "That's not okay in this organization."
- Encourage employees to bring harassment or discrimination complaints to you.
- Refer employees experiencing harassment or discrimination to the proper authorities within the organization.
- Follow up to ensure that harassment or discrimination cases are being vigorously and fairly pursued.
- Add a "domestic partnership" option to the usual "married/single" choice.
- Use examples of same-sex couples in business exercises, training role-plays and so forth.
- Be sure to specifically invite same-sex partners to company events, travel, and so forth where spouses are traditionally included.
- Order and display gay publications, like *10%*, the *Advocate, Out,* or *Victory* where other magazines are displayed.
- Bring gay, lesbian, and bisexual speakers into the workplace to talk about workplace and/or social issues.
- Publicize upcoming gay-related events.
- Ensure that gays and lesbians receive bereavement leave after the death of a same-sex partner.

CHALLENGES OF DIVERSITY

As mental health professionals, we have learned that attention to diversity issues is simply the just and proper thing to do. However, as consultants to organizations, we may need to address such issues as "challenges" to motivate consultees to take action.

The *availability challenge* refers to the fact that in the past, employers were often able to control diversity, because there were more people than there were jobs. In recent years, however, qualified employees have become more scarce, forcing employers to become more flexible. Employers must realize that "different does not mean deficient."

The *fairness challenge* refers to the need to treat everyone fairly. In the past, this was typically viewed as equal treatment, as symbolized by the expression "Equal Employment Opportunity." In practice, this meant that everyone was treated as a member of the mainstream culture. Now employers must embrace a new awareness of diversity, essentially focusing on and valuing differences.

The *synergy challenge* seeks to reframe the prejudiced view that minority employees needed to be "accommodated," fostering the goal of using every individual's unique talents to strengthen the organization. Today's work environment requires more and more group-based work. Diversity in an organization can create positive and negative conflict: it can facilitate creative problem solving; can close down communication; and can derail group processes. Group leaders must minimize destructive conflict and maximize diversity of input.

THE GREAT PROBLEM OF DIFFERENCE

Any comparison of two things, whether it is two events, two people, or two objects, presents the observer with a choice between emphasizing the similarities or the differences. While there is value in looking for similarities among different people, overemphasizing this can result in loss of respect for the very real differences between people. In diversity or multicultural training (or just individual differences training), the basic task is to help people perceive differences and not only tolerate them, but prize them. The organizational benefit from diversity training is based on the idea that more creative solutions are based on more heterogeneous input and perceptions. Just as has been argued in the study of evolution, the organization has a greater potential of adapting to new challenges that require new responses if there is a range of potential responses, options, and solutions. Sometimes conflict is increased, but this conflict can also increase creativity. The other focus of diversity training is to help people come to an awareness that certain concepts (such as race) or qualities such as color have been assigned excess meaning and do not predict behavior as mainstream cultural once thought (such as intelligence, potential for violence, initiative; Campbell, Draper, & Huffington, 1991).

INSTITUTIONAL STAGES IN THE DIVERSITY PROCESS

The long history of prejudice and discrimination in the workplace is not easily undone. Initially, organizations may pay attention to diversity issues simply to be in *legal compliance* (e.g., minimum percentages of minority employees hired as required by law). The next stage consists of *climate change,* as a critical mass of underrepresented populations begins to build in the organization, and their differences and needs cannot be ignored by members of the dominant group. Eventually, a *change in the restrictive policies and structures* develops in the organization. This is an institutional change that generally takes a lot of time and effort to achieve.

Consultants can help manage diversity by working with both managers and employees. One can provide managers with training in how to recruit and hire diverse employees as well as in how to orient and integrate new employees. Employees can receive training in realizing the differences that exist, in learning how differences affect the working environment, and in maximizing productivity without ignoring employee differences. Box 9.2 provides reasons for adopting a diversity program.

Stages of Identity Development

Mental health professionals can bring their knowledge of identity formation into the workplace and adapt it for organizational settings. One of the strengths of mental health professionals is their ability to raise awareness of diversity issues in the workplace. Of course, the consultant should not be so naive as to expect that simply bringing up issues in a psychoeducational way will immediately enlighten the client system. Issues of diversity bring up many emotions in people, and mental health professionals must bring to bear all of their training in handling emotions in clients and in handling

=== **Box 9.2** ===

Why Adopt a Diversity Program?

Warrick (2005) stressed the importance of adopting the organization's point of view in helping them to understand how crucial it is to take diversity issues seriously. He stressed prevention as the key to human resource management for modern organizations. He gave three basic business reasons for organizations to adopt a Diversity Program:

1. Employment Law Prevention

Adopting a diversity awareness and diversity education program eliminates many misconceptions that eventually lead to legal actions, public relations problems, and client loss. Employment lawsuits make up 66% of all the lawsuits filed in the United States, suggesting that an organization has a greater chance of being sued by employees than by anyone else. Employers win over 85% of these lawsuits, which suggests that employees sue out of anger, not because they have a good case. Employees are using the courts as a forum to have their complaints heard. Even if the employer wins the lawsuit, consider the legal costs:

Trial Costs

Jury Trial:	$100,000 to $150,000
Appellate Court:	$250,000 to $500,000
Supreme Court:	$500,000 to $1,000,000

2. Public Relations Promotion

Beyond the costs of lawsuits, organizations want to avoid the public relations cost of being seen as having diversity problems. (Many Denny's restaurants refused to seat blacks . . . or seated whites before blacks. Denny's stock dropped from $11 per share in 1998 to $.67 per share in March 2003.)

3. Personal Career Protection

If an executive is terminated for illegal harassment (i.e., Race, Age, Sex, Sexual Orientation), it is the end of that executive's career. No organization wants to encounter these legal or public relations issues, and organizations will certainly not hire an individual with such a history (Carr-Ruffino, 2002; Griggs & Louw, 1999; Warrick, 2005).

issues of diversity in appropriate ways. The consultant should be especially aware of the different stages individuals will be in regarding their acceptance of and ability to process diversity issues.

Helms (1994a, 1994b, 1994c, 1995) and others (Casas & Pytluk, 1995; Hardiman, 1982; Helms & Piper, 1994; Sodowsky, Kwan, & Pannu, 1995; Sue & Sue, 1999) have done extensive research on the stages of formation of racial identity. Consultants should carefully review these stages and be prepared to quickly assess and handle individuals at various stages when they work with the client system in organizations. Box 9.3 describes a model of the stages of white racial identity, along with the information-processing strategies that White people use within each stage

===== **Box 9.3** =====

White Racial Identity Ego Statuses and Information Processing Strategies (IPS)

Contact status: Satisfaction with racial status quo, obliviousness to racism and one's participation in it. If racial factors influence life decisions, they do so in a simplistic fashion. IPS: Obliviousness.

Example: "I'm a White woman. When my grandfather came to this country, he was discriminated against, too. But he didn't blame Black people for his misfortune. He educated himself and got a job; that's what Blacks ought to do."

Disintegration status: Disorientation and anxiety-provoked by unresolvable racial moral dilemmas that force one to choose between own-group loyalty and humanism. May be stymied by life situations that arouse racial dilemmas. IPS: Suppression and ambivalence.

Example: "I myself tried to set a nonracist example [for other Whites] by speaking up when someone said something blatantly prejudiced—how to do this without alienating people so that they would no longer take me seriously was always tricky . . ." (Blauner, 1993, p. 8).

Reintegration status: Idealization of one's socioracial group, denigration and intolerance for other groups. Racial factors may strongly influence life decisions. IPS: Selective perception and negative out-group distortion.

Example: "So, what if my great-grandfather owned slaves. He didn't mistreat them and besides, I wasn't even there then . . . So, I don't know why Blacks expect me to feel guilty for something that happened before I was born. Nowadays, reverse racism hurts Whites more than slavery hurt Blacks."

Pseudoindependence status: Intellectualized commitment to one's own socioracial group and deceptive tolerance of other groups. May make life decisions to "help" other racial groups. IPS: Reshaping reality and selective perception.

Example: "Was I the only person left in America who believed that the sexual mingling of the races was a good thing, that it would erase cultural barriers and leave us all a lovely shade of tan? . . ." (Allen, 1994, p. C4).

Immersion/emersion status: Search for an understanding of the personal meaning of racism and the ways by which one benefits and a redefinition of whiteness. Life choices may incorporate racial activism. IPS: Hypervigilance and reshaping.

Example: "It's true that I personally did not participate in the horror of slavery . . . But I know that because I'm White, I continue to benefit from a racist system which stems from the slavery era. . . . White people . . . must begin to ask ourselves some hard questions and be willing to consider our role in maintaining a hurtful system. Then, we must try to do something to change it."

> **Box 9.3 (continued)**
>
> *Autonomy status:* Informed positive socioracial-group commitment, use of internal standards for self-definition, capacity to relinquish the privileges of racism. May avoid life options that require participation in racial oppression. IPS: Flexibility and complexity.
>
> *Example:* "I live in an integrated [Black-White] neighborhood and I read Black literature and popular magazines. So, I understand that the media presents a very stereotypic view of Black culture. I believe that if more of us White people made more than a superficial effort to obtain accurate information about racial groups other than our own, then we could help make this country a better place for all peoples."
>
> *Source:* From "An Update of Helms' White and People of Color Racial Identity Models" (p. 185), by J. E. Helms, in *Handbook of Multicultural Counseling,* J. M. Pontoretto, J. Casas, L. A. Suzuki, and C. M. Alexander (Eds.), 1995, Thousand Oaks, CA: Sage.

to deal with the data they perceive about racism in the world around them (Helms, 1995).

Helms (1995) also developed a model for the development of racial identity for people of color (see Box 9.4) along with information-processes strategies for dealing with racism.

Cass (1979) also described stages for gay and lesbian identity development. The first stage is identity confusion, in which a sense of incongruence develops between a perception of being heterosexual and having gay or lesbian thoughts and feelings. The next stage is identity comparison, in which the person moves toward accepting gay or lesbian thoughts and feelings, but maintains a façade of heterosexuality to avoid social alienation. The next stage is identity tolerance, in which the person begins to admit to him- or herself that he or she is gay or lesbian. The person begins to seek out friends in the gay and lesbian community, and may make contact with positive role models. The next stage is identity acceptance. The individual increases contact with other gay and lesbian individuals, and selectively discloses his or her sexual identity. Some individuals successfully remain at this stage for most of their lives. The next stage is identity pride, in which the individual no longer wishes to hide his or her sexual identity, but the individual harbors anger toward heterosexual nonacceptance and rejects heterosexual values and institutions. The final stage is identity synthesis, in which the individual takes pride in being gay or lesbian, no longer wishes to hide his or her sexual identity, and integrates a public and personal view of self. As the dichotomy between the gay world and the straight world begins to seem less clear-cut, sexual identity is integrated into all other aspects of self.

PRINCIPLES FOR TREATING HUMAN DIFFERENCES

Just as mental health professionals have a code of ethical conduct to provide guidance on their behaviors in the therapy setting, managers can adopt a set of principles for

=== **Box 9.4** ===

People of Color Racial Identity Ego Statuses and Information-Processing Strategies (IPS)

Conformity (pre-encounter) status: External self-definition that implies devaluing of own group and allegiance to White standards of merit. Probably is oblivious to socioracial groups' sociopolitical histories. IPS: Selective perception and obliviousness to socioracial concerns.

Example: "I think we ought to have a 'multiethnic' racial category because I think it's unfair that Black people force you to be Black. I have a Black father and a White mother. So, what does that make me? I think racial tensions in this country would be a lot less if Black people didn't try to force people like me to be one of them."

Dissonance (encounter) status: Ambivalence and confusion concerning own socioracial group commitment and ambivalent socioracial self-definition. May be ambivalent about life decisions. IPS: Repression of the anxiety-provoking racial information.

Example: "I talked 'White,' moved 'White,' most of my friends were White . . . but I never really felt accepted by or truly identified with the White kids. At some point, I stopped laughing when they would imitate Black people dancing. I distanced myself from the White kids, but I hadn't made an active effort to make Black friends because I was never comfortable enough in my 'Blackness' to associate with them. That left me in sort of a gray area" (Wenger, 1993, p. 4).

Immersion/emersion status: Idealization of one's socioracial group and denigration of that which is perceived as White. Use of own-group external standards to self-define, and own-group commitment and loyalty is valued. May make life decisions for the benefit of the group. IPS: Hypervigilance toward racial stimuli and dichotomous thinking.

Example: "So there I was, strutting around with my semi-Afro, studiously garbling the English language because I thought that 'real' Black people didn't speak standard English, . . . contemplating changing my name to Malika, or something authentically Black" (J. Nelson, 1993, p. 18).

Internalization status: Positive commitment to one's own socioracial group, internally defined racial attributes, and capacity to assess and respond objectively to members of the dominant group. Can make life decisions by assessing and integrating socioracial group requirements and self-assessment. IPS: Flexibility and analytic thinking.

Example: "By claiming myself as African American and Black, I also inherit a right to ask questions about what this identity means. And chances are this identity will never be static, which is fine with me" (Jones, 1994, p. 78).

==================== **Box 9.4 (continued)** ====================

Integrative awareness status: Capacity to value one's own collective identities as well as empathize and collaborate with members of other oppressed groups. Life decisions may be motivated by globally humanistic self-expression. IPS: Flexibility and complexity.

Example: "[I think of difference not] as something feared or exotic, but . . . as one of the rich facts of one's life, a truism that gives you more data, more power and more flavor . . . [You need a variety of peoples in your life] . . . so you won't lapse into thinking you're God's gift to all knowledge as North American Negro" (Jones, 1994, p. 80).

Source: From "An Update of Helms' White and People of Color Racial Identity Models" (p. 186), by J. E. Helms, in *Handbook of Multicultural Counseling,* J. M. Pontoretto, J. Casas, L. A. Suzuki, and C. M. Alexander (Eds.), 1995, Thousand Oaks, CA: Sage.

---

guiding them in treating human differences. Hankins (2000) provides the following suggested set of principles:

- All organizational personnel deserve to be treated with respect and dignity.
- Individual differences can be visible and invisible. Addressing invisible differences is as important as addressing visible ones.
- People should treat each other fairly and equitably.
- Talent, intelligence, skills, and abilities are distributed among all groups.
- No one should be advantaged or disadvantaged relative to others by virtue of his or her membership in a particular group.
- Prejudice and discrimination are deterrents to productive, healthy organizations and must be sought out and driven from the organization.
- People should be treated as individuals—not just as members of a group.
- It is not appropriate to prejudge, stereotype or discriminate against others for reasons that include race, gender, ethnicity, age, religion, or physical condition.
- Prejudice and discrimination are problems. Every person, by his or her attitudes or behavior, is either part of the solution or part of the problem.
- If people have the right information, and believe it to be true, they will generally be moved to action.
- All diversity issues should be addressed, including those pertaining to women, minority men, and white men.
- All organizational members have a responsibility to help create the cultures in which they wish to work.
- It should be assumed that all employees want to succeed and are capable of doing so, and treated accordingly.
- A full appreciation for human diversity can be reached when people no longer define (or judge) each other based on cultural or physical attributes, but on the content of their character. (pp. 15–16)

GOALS OF DIVERSITY TRAINING

Just as mental health professionals develop treatment plans when intervening in psychotherapeutic settings, the consultant should clarify his or her goals with the organization when intervening in matters of diversity:

Transcultural skills training: One goal is to educate about differences to increase understanding, reduce conflict, and enhance mutual appreciation. For example, a consultant may wish to educate people on the cultural aspects of Vietnamese immigrants versus Thai immigrants.

Awareness programs: Another goal of diversity training is to create awareness and sensitivity to unconscious beliefs and attitudes of bias and prejudice. For example, the consultant may share a story about an individual, and only later reveal the gender of the person being described. The consultant can demonstrate that alternative ways of perceiving, based on experience, enrich our view of reality rather than threaten or detract from it. To make this point, the consultant may wish to use the classic gestalt woman illusion, in which one can see either a young woman or an old woman in the same drawing.

Organizational development and transformation: This goal entails developing an understanding that certain concepts or qualities have been assigned excess meaning that interferes with understanding and effectiveness, limits human potential, and squanders human resources. The consultant may bring this about through breaking down barriers, letting people get to know each other, and having people find similarities in each other.

DOING DIVERSITY PROGRAMS

The consultant can make use of several "canned" programs on the market, such as those available from University Associates (www.universityassociates.com). Videotapes also provide a useful way to stimulate conversations. The diversity trainer has to have the ability to draw people out and not be judgmental, because most of the material that comes up in the seminars involves long-standing patterns of beliefs of the participants, heavily influenced by the way they were raised by their parents and their surrounding culture. Diversity issues tend to raise a lot of emotions within everyone involved.

There are also several exercises for groups, some of which include questionnaires to assess ability to take another person's perspective (M. H. Davis, 1983; Pedersen, 2004). Leader-Member Exchange Theory (LMX), discussed in Chapter 4, posits that leaders and members high on the following aspects are likely to have better working relationships (Graen & Uhl-Bien, 1995):

- Accurate in ability to perceive how others understand and respond to world
- Can view situations from many perspectives
- Able to perceive other's perspective in depth

ASSESSING DIVERSITY ISSUES WITHIN AN ORGANIZATION

Before intervening to help organizations become more sensitive and responsive to diversity issues, consultants should carefully assess the current organizational culture with the consultee. Carr-Ruffino (2002) lists important questions to ask managers about diversity issues in their organization:

1. Have you ever had employees from the (Asian American, Gay, Disabled, etc.) group on your work team? If so, what did you learn about meeting the needs and desires of people from this group? The unique kinds of contributions they can

make? How to help them make that contribution? Unique problems? Ways of solving those problems?

2. Does the organization have any policies or strategies for *attracting* and *hiring* diverse employees in general? Specifically, for certain groups?
3. Does the organization have any policies or strategies for *retaining* people from these groups?
4. Does the organization have any policies for promoting people from these groups?
5. Has the organization adopted any specific plans or programs designed to help minorities and/or women to
   —Identify their values, priorities, and thus their career goals?
   —Identify corporate career paths that might fit their career goals?
   —Gain experience and training needed to be promoted along chosen career paths?
6. Does the organization provide *training opportunities* specially targeted for these groups?
7. Does the organization have some system to *monitor* whether diverse employees have equal or *fair access to training opportunities* at all levels?
8. Has the organization adopted any *plan or strategy to prepare and move* diverse employees *into the highest levels*?
9. Does the organization provide *training programs* specifically designed to help people deal effectively with a culturally diverse work environment?
10. How would you describe the *corporate culture* here? How does it relate to typical values and priorities of key diverse groups?
11. What do you perceive to be the *greatest barriers* to developing and using (within the organization) the *full potential* of members of these groups?
12. What do you think are the *most important problems* that diverse employees face in adapting to the organizational culture here? General problems? Problems specific to each group?
13. Does the organization focus on *work teams*? If so,
    —Are these self-directed teams?
    —Are minorities and women often part of the teams?
    —Is creativity and innovation encouraged?
    —Do you think people are more productive when they work in teams?
    —How successful are the teams in the organization?
14. When these teams are successful, what are the chief factors? In other words, what makes a successful team click? (pp. 67–68)

Consultants may wish to conduct a full "diversity audit" to learn more about an organizations culture. Carr-Ruffino (2002) presents the following outline to serve as a guide for conducting a diversity audit.

Step 1: Investigate

Visit the organization and observe or ask questions as follows:

1. Observe the physical setting.
   • What's your initial impression?
   • What does the physical layout seem to communicate?
   • Is the image consistent in all divisions? facilities?
2. Collect and analyze written materials, such as annual reports, newsletters, news releases, manuals.
   • What does the company say about itself?
   • What type of culture do written materials reflect?
   • Do you see signs of diversity at all levels in the materials?

3. Observe reception area procedures.
   - Formal or informal?
   - Relaxed or busy?
   - Elegant or plain?
   - What is the receptionist doing? How does she or he interact with visitors?
   - What procedures or processes are used with visitors?
   - Do visitors wait?
   - Do you see signs of diversity so far?
4. Ask employees questions, such as these:
   - Tell about the history of the company. (Notice what facts seem accurate, what myths surface.)
   - What has made the company successful? (Look for company values. Do people generally agree on which company values are most important?)
   - What kind of people work here? Who gets ahead? (Look for signs of diverse role models, descriptions of role models; look for clear agreement about how to succeed. Are role models constructive, serve the company well? Do women and minorities often succeed?)
   - What's it like to work here? How do things get done? (Look for important rites, rituals, meetings, or bureaucratic procedures; do all departmental or team subcultures have some unifying values? Do rites, rules, and procedures encompass or respect the diversity found within the organization?)
5. Observe and ask, how do people (really) spend their time?
6. Ask about career paths:
   - Who gets ahead? What departments were top people once in? What positions did they hold? Do people from diverse groups get ahead?
   - What do people have to do to get promoted?
   - What does the company reward? Competence in key skills? Performance against objective criteria? Seniority? Loyalty? Good team player? Other?
7. Find out how long people usually stay in jobs. (Short terms usually mean people are motivated to make their mark quickly and to steer clear of longer-term, slower payback activities. They also can mean people from diverse groups became discouraged, felt they couldn't reach their career goals, and left.)
8. Find out what people are talking about and writing about.
   - What are memos and reports about—actual content?
   - What are meetings about? What is actually discussed, who talks to whom?

Step 2: Review and Analysis

Go over the results of your survey to determine how strong or weak, how conformist or flexible, you think the company is. Use it to help identify companies that are in danger of failing. Look for:

1. *Patterns and themes:* Think about patterns that emerged from the stories and anecdotes that people volunteered. What are the key points? Do most stories revolve around customers? Political infighting? Individual initiative that was rewarded or punished?
2. *Inward focus:* People don't pay much attention to what's going on outside the company with customers, competitors, new trends. They focus on placating the boss, looking good, getting one up on the people around them. They seem to over-emphasize budgets, financial analysis, or sales quotas.
3. *Short-term focus:* If people spend most of their time and energy meeting short-term goals, then sustainable business receives no support and the company is headed for problems.
4. *Is turnover high or trending upward?* Look at the whole company and at subcultures within the company. Look at the track records of employees from diverse groups,

such as minorities. Poor morale often begins with a lackadaisical attitude, moving on to loud complaints, and finally people start leaving.

5. *Weak culture:* When a culture is weak or in trouble, people get frightened and anxious. This fright shows up in emotional outbursts in the workplace, such as condemning company policy at a meeting or getting angry with coworkers or bosses. Did you hear any stories that indicate that stress, anger, or other emotions are building up? If so, did you get any clues about the causes?

6. *Fragmentation or inconsistency:* When a division is unhappy about how headquarters is handing things or tells jokes about what goes on there, it's usually a sign that the parts of the culture are not integrated into a coherent whole. Signs that normal variations in different functions of the firm are becoming a problem:

   - Subcultures (within departments, or sometimes within ethnic groups) are becoming ingrown. Regular interaction among subcultures is declining.
   - Subcultures are clashing, publicly trying to undermine each other. The healthy tension among two subcultures has become destructive.
   - Subcultures are becoming exclusive. One or more subculture is acting like an exclusive club. People are feeling left out and resentful, not pulling together toward company goals.
   - Subcultures act as if their values are more important than company values, not giving key overriding company values top priority. (pp. 68–70)

PART THREE

CONSULTING TO
LARGE SYSTEMS

Chapter 10

THE NATURE OF ORGANIZATIONS

A large textile company asks Charlie Watson, a newly licensed clinical psychologist, to help their organization run better. Knowing that this is a rather vague goal, Charlie asks for specific details on what the organization wishes to achieve. The consultee responds that the organization seems to have reached a plateau in terms of growth and profitability. The board of directors has asked for an outside, objective consultant to bring a new perspective on the situation. Charlie agrees to meet with the consultees to find out more about the organization. Charlie then telephones his colleague, Dana Moore, who had previously agreed to provide Charlie with support and consultation in his new organizational consulting career.

ORGANIZATIONAL STRUCTURE

How a business or nonprofit agency is organized has a major impact on daily operations (Angelica & Hyman, 1997; Drucker, 1990; DuBrin, 2000; Wilbur, 2000). It is important for a consultant to understand a particular organization's structure in order to efficiently gather data and design effective interventions.

Weisbord proposed an organizational model composed of six interdependent parts (Marvin, 1978; Weisbord, 1976, 1992; Weisbord & Janoff, 1995; see Figure 10.1). This model can help a consultant remember to address important areas that affect an organization. Addressing *purpose* is to focus the company on the business it is in, so it does not get off track. An organization must also pay attention to its *relationships,* since people (both external customers and internal employees) are vital to any business operation. An organization's *structure* determines how the work is divided and includes procedures and policies for running the organization efficiently. *Helpful mechanisms* involve the supportive technologies that must be coordinated for successful operation. An organization must also be sure that *rewards* are in place so that there are incentives for the crucial operations to get done. In the center of Figure 10.1 is *leadership,* which works to balance the other components so that they are in the right proportions to accomplish the organization's goals. Underlying the six areas is the external environment, which has a potential impact on all six areas, since organizations do not operate in a vacuum.

At their initial meeting, the consultee shows Charlie the company's table of organization. The consultee informs Charlie about the details of the division of labor and the

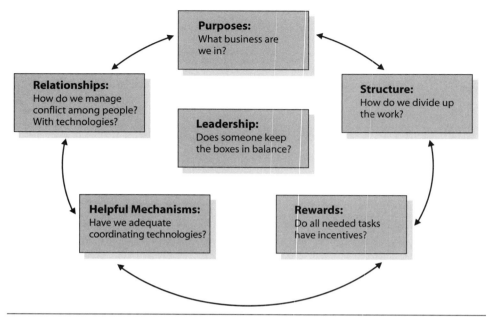

Figure 10.1   Weisbord's six-box model.

chain of command. Like any reputable consultant, Charlie refrains from giving the consultee immediate feedback before understanding the big picture. At the end of the meeting, Charlie offers to call the consultee later in the week to set up the next appointment. When Charlie gets back to his home office, he writes down the content of the meeting in detail. Charlie then does research on organizational structure and calls Dana for guidance.

Important Terms and Concepts

A large part of developing comfort as a consultant in organizational settings is gaining a familiarity with daily business concerns and basic vocabulary used within organizations. Consultants should learn the following general terms and concepts before working with specific organizations and their unique structures (Robbins, 2001; Schermerhorn et al., 2000; Steers, 1981).

Centralization refers to the degree to which decisions are made centrally, that is, by one person or a small group of persons.

The chain of command (also called the *scalar chain*) refers to the unbroken line of authority and responsibility extending from the top of the organization to the lowest levels, and makes clear who reports to whom (Robbins, 2001, p. 623).

Departmentalization involves creating separate departments within an organization. Departments can be created on a functional basis (grouping activities by functions performed), or they can be based on the specific product being produced (activities are grouped by product line, placing more focus on the customer).

Division of labor refers to how jobs are broken down into simple, routine, and well-defined tasks. A clear-cut division of labor contributes to productivity because it allows employees to become experts and more efficient at specific tasks. It reduces job satisfaction, however, as employees may become bored and may not appreciate the "bigger picture" in terms of the value of the work they are performing.

Equity or fairness is the concept that managers should be kind and fair to their subordinates.

Espirit de Corps involves promoting team spirit to build harmony and unity within the organization.

Impersonality refers to the concept that rules and controls are applied uniformly, avoiding involvement with the personalities and personal preferences of employees.

Initiative refers to an employee's ability to take immediate action for emergent, unusual circumstances without first seeking specific approval. Employees who are allowed to originate and carry out plans will exert high levels of effort. If employees are afraid to act without permission, they are likely to miss crucial business opportunities, and will not speak up when they see new, more efficient ways of doing things.

Line authority refers to a position with authority to direct the work of a subordinate in performing an operational function.

Locality refers to the fact that employees closest to the work are most likely to have sound suggestions for improvements in doing the work.

Order involves making sure that people and materials are in the right place at the right time.

Remuneration involves the perception that workers are paid a fair wage for their services.

Span of control refers to the number of subordinates a manager can efficiently and effectively direct. There have been recent trends to increase span of control (6 used to be considered the maximum number that could be effectively supervised) and to reduce the number of layers. Sears Roebuck historically had 12 layers, whereas Wal-Mart was a 3-layer company (Walton & Huey, 1993).

Stability of tenure of employees is important to an organization's bottom line, as high employee turnover is inefficient.

Staff authority refers to positions that support, assist, and advise line managers.

Subordination refers to the concept that individual interests must be subordinated to the general interests of the organization and its members.

The table of organization is a graphic representation of an agency's structure.

Unity of command refers to the concept that a subordinate should have only one superior to whom he or she is responsible.

Unity of direction means that each group of organizational activities that have the same objective should be directed by one manager using one plan.

ORGANIZATIONAL CULTURE

Every organization tends to develop its own unique culture, whether intentionally or unintentionally. Culture is the pattern of shared beliefs and values that gives the members of a company meaning and provides the rules for behavior in their organization (Schein, 2000).

Organizational leaders often attempt to build the culture they feel will be most useful in achieving the organization's long-term goals. For example, Sam Walton was well known for his work in developing Wal-Mart's culture. After a 1975 trip to Japan, where he was deeply impressed by factory workers doing group calisthenics and company cheers, he decided to create a cheer for his own employees. "Gimme a W!" he would shout. The workers would shout back, and Walton went through each letter of the Wal-Mart name. At the hyphen, Walton would shout "Gimme a squiggly!" while squatting and twisting his hips, which the workers would also do. Walton was attempting to create a unique corporate culture through symbolism (Ortega, 1995, 1998; Peters & Waterman, 1982; Walton & Huey, 1993).

Consultants should have a good understanding of the principles of organizational culture. Such information is important when consultants are asked to work directly on changing the organization's present culture, but they must also make certain that any individual or organizational intervention plan considers the cultural context in which it will be carried out. Ignoring the organization's cultural context when consulting is akin to ignoring a client's family and systems context when providing psychotherapeutic interventions in clinical settings.

The Purposes of Cultures

Cultures serve many purposes, whether it is an organizational culture or any other type. One purpose is to serve as a *boundary-defining role* that creates distinctions between one organization and others. It also conveys a sense of identity for organization members. A culture facilitates the generation of commitment to something larger than individual self-interests, and it enhances social system stability. Culture is the social glue that holds an organization to the standards it considers valuable.

Culture serves as a sense-making and control mechanism that guides and shapes the attitudes and behaviors of employees. It defines the rules of the game, and therefore defines who progresses in the organization. Because culture is so crucial to an organization's performance and therefore to its success, a consultant must be able to help an organization foster a culture that is most conducive to the achievement of its goals. Of course, before designing any intervention, the consultant must first assess what is currently happening and how things got that way.

Assessment of Culture

Culture is assessed by looking at behavior (since actual behavior reveals true culture) and inferring the rules (written and unwritten) or norms by which a group operates. The culture may or may not be what is written or espoused. Individuals who are new to the organization often run into cultural violations unknowingly, and are counseled, educated, or sanctioned by the more senior organization members.

Culture often uses symbols (like McDonald's golden arches) or slogans. It is gestural, and may be manifested by how people dress or whether there are executive parking places. Folklore or stories that teach culture often arise within organizations. For example, Thomas Watson, the chief executive officer (CEO) of IBM, supposedly had an interaction with a young manager who had bungled a project costing thousands of dollars, and when he was called into Watson's office, he asked if he was fired. Watson was reputed to have replied in the negative, stating that he had just paid thousands of dollars training the young manager (Watson, 2003). The Iams Company is known for its focus on people, and for their love of animals. The stories that get told both inside and outside the organization define its culture (Sellers, 2004).

One way to get in touch with culture is to ask a team, "Tell me how this place really operates. What are the rules for this organization?" Make sure you ask how it handles leadership, power, relationships, diversity, risk, and protocol. Then ask how this is different from the way things are supposed to operate. What does the consultee want the culture to be? Given that the organization can pretty well create whatever work environment culture they choose, what is keeping them from having the culture they want? Collaborate with the consultee to develop a workable plan for achieving the desired culture.

CHARACTERISTICS OF ORGANIZATIONAL CULTURE

Cultures within organizations have several characteristics. Consultants who want to assess or change an organization's culture should be aware of these multiple aspects (Robbins, 2001; Schermerhorn et al., 2000; Steers, 1981):

Member identity: The degree to which employees identify with the organization as a whole rather than with their type of job or field of professional expertise. Faculty members at Harvard University feel a kinship with the history of the institution and do not generally see themselves as simply holding down a teaching job.

Group emphasis: The degree to which work activities are organized around groups rather than individuals. This varies depending on the nature of the organization. There is more group emphasis in field hockey teams, where players must cooperate to win, than in wrestling teams, in which individuals take turns competing.

People focus: The degree to which management decisions take into consideration the effect of outcomes on people within the organization.

Unit integration: The degree to which units within the organization are encouraged to operate in a coordinated or interdependent manner.

Control: The degree to which rules, regulations, and direct supervision are used to oversee and control employee behavior.

Risk tolerance: The degree to which employees are encouraged to be aggressive, innovative, and risk-seeking.

Reward criteria: The degree to which rewards such as salary increases and promotions are allocated according to employee performance rather than seniority, favoritism, or other nonperformance factors.

Conflict tolerance: The degree to which employees are encouraged to air conflicts and criticisms openly.

Means-ends orientation: The degree to which management focuses on results or outcomes rather than on the techniques and processes used to achieve those outcomes.

Open-system focus: The degree to which the organization monitors and responds to changes in the external environment.

An organization's *dominant culture* expresses the core values that are shared by a majority of the organization's members. Typically, however, there are *subcultures,* or minicultures within an organization, usually defined by department designations and geographic separation.

FINDING THE ORGANIZATIONAL CULTURE THAT BEST FITS THE INDIVIDUAL

Every individual is likely to have unique preferences in terms of the characteristics of the work culture. Assessment instruments can be used to determine how easily an individual will fit in with a particular work environment. This information can be used to assist individuals in career assessments or to identify and intervene in potential problem areas.

ORGANIZATIONAL CHANGE AND RESISTANCE

Organizational change is as old as organizations themselves. The pharaohs of ancient Egypt probably struggled with a need to change the organizations that built their pyramids. One can only imagine the degree of organization needed, with continual modifications, to successfully construct the Great Wall of China. What we call reengineering today was probably practiced in some form back then.

In any case, changing organizations is not exactly new. What is new is the scientific study of the processes involved in organization change (Conner, 1992).

Ways to Describe Organizational Change

Change can occur in many ways, and consultants should be aware of how they play out in organizations (Robbins, 2001; Schein, 2000; Schermerhorn et al., 2000).

Revolutionary versus evolutionary: Revolutionary change tends to be rapid and dramatic. Evolutionary change tends to be slow and gradual.

Discontinuous versus continuous: Discontinuous change does not occur all at once, tending to start and stop as time goes on. Continuous change is steady and observable.

Episodic versus continuing flow: Episodic change is marked and punctuated. Continuing flow describes change that tends to be slow and steady.

Transformational versus transactional: Transformational change tends to involve paradigm shifts and inspiring visions. Transactional change involves pursuing clearly established objectives.

Strategic versus operational: Strategic change describes the long-term movement of an organization. Operational change involves daily or short-term functioning of an organization.

Total system versus local option: Total systems change involves the entire organization. Local option change involves only subcomponents of the organization.

Environmental Pressures for Change

Situations in the external environment often create problems for organizations. These events often prompt consultation requests. The following subsections view four environmental factors in light of the four frames of leadership: structural, human resource, political, and symbolic (Bolman & Deal, 2003).

Globalization

Organizations can no longer ignore that they are affected by processes and events around the world. They can no longer isolate themselves in small regional areas (Friedman, 2000). From the structural perspective, globalization represents a size, complexity, and communications problem. From the human resource perspective, globalization presents a challenge for dealing with wide differences in attitudes, needs, and skills. From the political perspective, globalization creates the potential conflict between different regions and between the central office and regional offices. From the symbolic perspective, the challenge of globalization is in figuring out how to build cohesiveness and common purpose in the face of cultural differences (Bolman & Deal, 2003).

Information Technology

In the early days of computers and information technology (IT), staying on the cutting edge gave an organization a competitive advantage. Today, however, keeping up with IT only allows an organization to remain competitive (Applegate et al., 2003). From the structural perspective, increases in efficiency due to advances in IT have allowed for decentralization and downsizing. From the human resource perspective, advances in IT allow people to develop new skills to do things better. The political perspective sees advances in IT as responsible for power shifts, with operating units gaining more control functions. The symbolic perspective sees the advances in IT as providing meaning and excitement for work in high-technology environments (Bolman & Deal, 2003).

(De)regulation

Laws give organizations predictable environmental structure. When new laws are created (regulation) or when old laws are removed (deregulation), organizations must respond to these changes (Beatty & Samuelson, 2001; McAdams, Neslund, & Neslund, 2004). From the structural perspective, structural shifts are needed to respond to these environmental changes. From the human resource perspective, the organization must actively respond to the changes in needed attitudes and skills. The political perspective calls on the organization to monitor the internal and external power shifts (e.g., deregulation often suggests that the consumer is becoming more important, and the government is becoming less important). From the symbolic perspective, these environmental changes may require a redefinition of organization's culture and mission (Bolman & Deal, 2003).

Demographic Changes

This refers to changes in the workforce, such as an increase in minorities and women, and the approaching retirement of the baby boomers (Mathis & Jackson, 2003). From the structural perspective, organizational units need to respond to changing populations concretely, such as with training and affirmative action programs. The human resource perspective sees the changing workforce as having more varied needs and new training requirements. The political perspective looks at the possibility of conflict between newcomers and old-timers as the workforce changes. From the symbolic perspective, old-timers may feel a sense of loss, and newcomers may feel a sense of alienation when the old vision for the company is fading and the new vision has not yet fully formed (Bolman & Deal, 2003).

Other Environmental Pressures for Change

Product obsolescence: Sometimes an organization's products or services are simply no longer needed, due to improvements in technology. With the invention of the transistor, there was simply no need for manufacturers to improve on the ability to make a better vacuum tube.

New sources of competition: Sometimes an organization may be doing everything perfectly, but may face new and more powerful competition. Local grocery stores have had to be creative to survive against the national superstore chains.

Changes in consumer demands: Frequently, consumers' tastes simply change. At one time, Citizen's Band (CB) radios were very popular, but interest in them faded. An organization must choose to either refoster interest in the product or service (which is very difficult to do), find new uses for the old product or service, modify the product or service, or develop newer, more interesting products or services.

Economic shocks: Sometimes changes in the economy can have a major impact on an organization. When Silicon Valley faced some challenges, the world prices for high-tech computer chips greatly affected many businesses.

Social trends: Social tendencies can also affect how an organization does business. Saturday night at the movies was a major event for many families before the invention of television.

World politics: Acts of war, trade policies, and terrorist acts can all influence how organizations do business.

Charlie is excited about the brilliance of his intervention plan. He expected to see immediate results, and to be showered with appreciation. However, despite its simplicity and brilliance, the plan does not quite go as well as it should. Charlie meets with Dana, and describes the situation. Dana normalizes Charlie's experience, and discusses with him the concept of resistance.

RESISTANCE

Despite the best intentions of all parties, pressure for change is often met with individual and organizational resistance (Wallace & Hall, 1996). This can cause consultants a great deal of frustration—the very individuals who invited the consultant in to make changes sometimes strongly resist the consultant's attempts at change. There are many causes of individual resistance; they are best addressed directly when designing intervention plans:

- Habit (we reduce complexity through habit)
- Security (safety)
- Economic factors (changes in pay)
- Fear of the unknown (change creates ambiguity and uncertainty for the known)
- Selective information processing (hear what we want to hear)

Employee resistance might manifest itself in several different ways (Bolman & Deal, 2003):

- They might withdraw from the organization by quitting or being chronically absent.
- They might remain on the job, but withdraw psychologically or emotionally, becoming indifferent, passive, and apathetic.
- They might resist the organization by reducing their productivity, or by using deception or sabotage.

- They might try to climb the hierarchy to get better jobs, though the pyramidal structure of most organizations means that there are far more jobs at the bottom than at the top.
- They may pass on to their children the myth that work is unrewarding with slim hopes for advancement.
- They might create groups and organizations (such as labor unions) that try to redress the power imbalance between person and system.

Most managers dread the idea of a union moving into their workspace and making demands. Most often, this occurs when employees feel that they are not being listened to or treated fairly. Consultants should know that it is illegal to fire employees for trying to organize a union. Yet, the AFL-CIO estimates that ten thousand workers a year are fired for participating in union-organizing drives, and these firings are usually justified in terms of unrelated minor infractions. Wal-Mart employees who have bucked the company by getting involved in a unionization drive or by suing the company for failure to pay overtime have reportedly been fired for breaking the company rule against using profanity (Beatty & Samuelson, 2001; McAdams et al., 2004; Ortega, 1998). Consultants with a mental health background can help managers work with employee resistance more productively by helping managers do things that ensure the employees feel heard (active listening skills, open forum to discuss concerns, etc.).

Causes of Organizational Resistance

Consultants also often meet resistance on the organizational level (Wallace & Hall, 1996). The following are some of the causes of organizational resistance that must be monitored and addressed before any system level intervention can be successfully implemented:

Structural inertia: Sometimes change is difficult for an organization because of its structure. In the selection and hiring process, people are chosen who fit the organization's culture. New hires also receive training that reinforces the way things have always been done. The employees' roles are formalized in specified job descriptions, rules, and procedures.

Limited focus of change: As we know from systems theory, subsystems are interdependent. Limited changes in subsystems tend to get nullified by the larger system.

Group inertia: Group norms also tend to constrain change. If senior employees like things the way they are, they may put pressure on others to not "rock the boat."

Threat to expertise: Any type of change, especially that involving new technology, may pose a threat to a worker's self-esteem and sense of worth, especially if the person has gained great skill or knowledge in a technology that is becoming obsolete. In the past, blacksmiths spent a great deal of time and energy learning their craft, so they naturally resisted the mass production of the automobile.

Threat to established power relationships: Any redistribution of decision-making authority can threaten power relationships. Power and political alliances take a great deal of time and energy to create and are not easily given up.

Threat to established resource allocations: Individuals naturally want to hold on to hard-earned resources for themselves or for their departments. People may be concerned that changes will mean a reduction in resources.

People tend to work toward their own goals and gains in organizations. A consultant needs to figure out what those agendas are and try to fit them into the larger goals of the organization.

Tactics for Overcoming Resistance to Change

Just as mental health professionals learn to recognize and to expect resistance in the psychotherapy process, consultants have learned to recognize and prepare for resistance during the consultation process. These techniques can be used directly by the consultant, and can also be taught to organizational leadership to facilitate change throughout the organization:

Education and communication: Sometimes resistance to change stems from a fear of the unknown. Educating and communicating with employees about the problems involved in doing things the old way and the reasons and benefits for doing things the new way can help people see the logic of change. Sometimes organizational members have legitimate questions and concerns that need to be addressed before the change process can continue.

Participation: Encouraging employee involvement in the change process fosters ownership of the ideas that are produced. Involved organizational members may come to see the complications and multiple factors involved in making complex change decisions, and will have a chance to make suggestions and voice their objections before change begins. It is more difficult for people to resist plans for change that they have participated in.

Facilitation and support: Change involves the loss of old, familiar, comfortable ideas and ways of doing things, and the introduction of new, different, sometimes frightening steps into unknown territory. Consultants and organizational leaders should help facilitate this transition for employees. This may involve providing a formal or informal forum to "grieve" the loss, depending on the nature of the change involved. Formal forums could include the provision of individual counseling sessions or group discussions. Informal forums could include "farewell" parties or a light-hearted memorial display to the old way of doing things. Consultants and organizational leaders should also facilitate the transition into the new way of doing things by providing in-depth skills training and opportunities to experiment with the new technology so that individuals can become comfortable and familiar with the new way of doing things.

Negotiation: Sometimes change involves employees making tangible or psychological concessions in the adoption of new methods. New high-tech computerized machinery may greatly increase productivity and hence benefit the entire organization, but may require much more mental and physical energy from the employees who operate them. Negotiation involves offering something of value in exchange for employee acceptance of the desired change, such as increased wages, increased vacation time, or remodeling the employee lounge.

Manipulation and co-optation: This method involves subtly and surreptitiously manipulating the organizational environment and its employees into accepting the change process, perhaps through fostering a sense of inevitability. This could even involve planting confederates among the employees to extol the virtues of the proposed changes, or spreading rumors about the potentially disastrous results of not changing. Consultants should discourage organizational leaders from adopting these methods, as they can severely backfire if they are discovered by the employees, destroying trust and building resentment.

Coercion: Sometimes managers simply force the proposed changes, regardless of expressed resistance on the part of the employees, doling out consequences up to and including termination for those who do not adopt the desired changes. While this may sometimes be necessary, this method should generally be avoided, as it tends to increase employee resistance.

Wallace and Hall (1996) suggest the proven methods for overcoming resistance shown in Box 10.1.

The How and Why of Change

Block (2000) believes that individuals get stuck by asking the wrong kinds of questions about change. He warns that consultants must watch out for "how" questions. Though these questions are important, the consultant should look for the deeper meanings and feelings behind them:

- *How long will it take?* We want to make good time regardless of where we are going.
- *How do we get them to change?* If only they would change, we would be better off. The top thinks the bottom is the problem, the bottom thinks the top is the problem, and when they get together, they both agree the middle is the problem.
- *What are the steps needed for . . . ?* Life can be reduced to a step-by-step plan. A Day-Timer notebook is the icon, lists with milestones are the drug, and more discipline is the prescription that never cures.
- *How do we measure the effect?* There is no value in the invisible world. It is the measure of reality that becomes the point. Alan Watts once said that we have reached the

---

=== **Box 10.1** ===

Methods to Reduce Resistance

- Early focus on relationship-building skills
- Working toward egalitarian relations
- Being approachable, available, and helpful to all who request assistance
- Clarifying the goals of the consultation process
- Informing both consultees and concerned staff of the consultant's commitment to confidentiality
- Observing the organization's written (and unwritten) behavioral norms
- Avoiding all judgmental remarks, whether positive or negative, about specific consultees, staff members, and clients
- Modeling a rational problem-solving approach
- Recommending small steps and a gradual pace for change interventions
- Holding to an unwavering belief in both the efficacy and value of the consultation process

---

Source: From *Psychological Consultation: Perspectives and Applications* (p. 120) by W. A. Wallace and D. L. Hall, 1996, Pacific Grove, CA: Brooks/Cole.

point at which we go to our restaurants and eat the menu. We have become more interested in the definition and measurement of life than in living it.

- *How do we communicate this?* The problem is they do not understand us. "A problem in communication" is the ultimate empty diagnosis. It denies real conflict and raises spin to the level of purpose. Our finest example of this is Washington, DC, where their only work is to manage image and the news. Questions of communication are most often the easy way out of questions of will, courage, and commitment.
- *What are other organizations doing or where has this worked?* We want to lead and wish to go second at the same time. There is some value in discovering what others are doing: It gives us hope. More often, though, the question is a wish for safety, for when we hear where it has worked, we then talk of how unique our situation is. (p. 322)

Block (2000) believes that "how" questions tend to result in an organization simply trying harder to do what it is already doing. "Why" and "where" questions help an organization to think about deeper, more systemic changes. Block gives the following examples:

- *What is the point of what we are doing?* We live in a world measured by wealth and scale. Are we here to make money, to meet budgets, to grow the operation? Is this enough? And who is the beneficiary of this? Who are we here to serve, and what price are we willing to pay to stay true to our answer?
- *What has to die before we can move to something new?* We want change but do not want to pay for it. We are always required to put aside what got us here to really move on. Where do we find the courage to do this?
- *What is the real value of our product and service?* And in whose eyes? How valid is our promise and what are the side effects of our delivery? Are our advertising and the way we present ourselves a picture we even believe is true?
- *What personal meaning do people find in what we are doing?* What intrinsic rewards exist for us? Do we show up voluntarily, or have we indentured ourselves simply to sustain our life outside of work? Many people think work is just that, work, and to expect more is to be a fool.
- *What would happen if we did nothing?* When is change for its own sake? Maybe we should just get better at what we do now.
- *What are the capacities and strengths that we are not using fully?* Give up on fixing weaknesses; find out what more is possible. Sometimes we do not even know our strengths, as individuals and as institutions. What strengths do others see in us? Years ago in our consulting firm, we asked clients why they hired us. They said that what they found attractive was our seeming disinterest and reluctance in working with them. We were shocked. We thought that if we seemed aloof, it was because we were disorganized and sloppy; they saw it as a sign of integrity.
- *And what are we learning for the next generation?* This question is for the second half of life, but it is still a useful focusing exercise. Our materialistic culture consumes its resources and bets on science or miracles to cope with what we leave for those after us. What will our legacy be? (pp. 333–334)

Driving and Restraining Forces

Lewin's (1951) force field analysis of planned organizational change looks at driving (or facilitating) forces and restraining (or constraining) forces. In any organization in need of change, there will be forces pushing to drive the change, and forces attempting to restrain the change. These forces may take the form of habit, resistance to change, attitudes, structure, or finances. The consultant should help consultees focus on attacking the forces that they can control, and minimizing the effects of the forces over which they have little control.

One of the consultees approaches Charlie, and asks for a private meeting with him. She expresses her frustration at the organization's inability to agree to provide health insurance for same-sex partners. The consultee feels that for an organization as large and with as many resources as hers, to provide health insurance for spouses but not for same-sex partners is blatantly discriminatory. After discussing this with her, Charlie asks her to help him list the driving and restraining forces for the implementation of such a policy. Under driving forces, they list desire for fairness, desire of current employees with same-sex partners to be treated equally, possibility of attracting more employees, image of the organization as progressive and modern. Under restraining forces, they list: discriminatory attitudes among management and employees, societal prejudice, and budgetary considerations. Charlie works with the consultees to further develop the list, and then helps to develop a plan for nurturing the driving forces and combating the restraining forces over which they have the most control. As the next step, they plan to develop, distribute, and analyze a survey to assess current attitudes of the employees regarding this issue. Charlie also discusses with the consultee that although this is a major issue that should continually be fought for, equal health benefits for same-sex partners may realistically be a long-term project.

Three Steps in Organization Change

Lewin (1951) posited that rather than immediately attempting to move an organization toward change, three steps were needed to make lasting changes:

1. *Unfreezing* occurs when the need for change is recognized and steps are taken to make members of the organization receptive to change.
2. *Moving* involves moving the organization in the new direction and includes helping employees acquire new behaviors, values, and attitudes.
3. *Refreezing* entails reinforcing the changes that have been made to help stabilize the organization at a new state of equilibrium.

During another meeting with Charlie, the consultees express their exasperation with the information technology (IT) department. Despite their high rate of pay, the IT workers are not very responsive. They tend to be aloof and cliquish, remaining isolated because the department is housed in a separate building.

What Can Change Agents Change?

A consultant can work to change three main elements: *structure, technology,* and *people.* Structure can be changed by altering policies and procedures, as well as through the organization's chain of command and power structure. Technology can be improved by providing new computer systems or simply by helping organizations learn different ways of doing things. People are often the most crucial variable. People can adapt to new incentives and can benefit from customized educational programs, as long as they feel informed, feel they are being heard, and feel that their concerns are being addressed.

In most situations, all three areas need to be addressed to achieve lasting change.

Charlie brainstorms with the consultees on ways to improve the situation with the IT department. After briefly discussing structure, technology, and people, he lists the three areas on the board and asks for initial ideas about how change could come about through each one. Under structure, the following suggestions are made: housing the IT department within the main building to reduce isolation, having all employees wear more prominent name badges, and requiring IT workers to personally follow up after each repair to make sure a problem has been resolved. Under technology, the following suggestions are made: beginning a series of computer training courses for employees to reduce dependence on the IT department personnel, purchasing and installing new software that would allow IT workers to quickly resolve computer problems remotely, and consulting with other organizations about how best to interact with the IT department. Under people, the following suggestions are made: replacing some of the members of the IT team, implementing an incentive program to reward IT workers for friendly behavior, and offering training courses to the IT team in active listening skills.

Eight Steps That Lead to Successful Change

One of the first tasks of the consultant is to ensure that the process of change being implemented is sensitive to individual needs for cultural fit, leadership, integration, communication, meaning, clarity, and hope. Such a change process has been suggested by Kotter (1996b).

1. Establish the Need for Change

Any effective change effort begins with a thorough understanding of the current situation (Moran & Brightman, 2000). Effective change must make sense in terms of higher order goals for the company. The consultant can help companies understand change by examining trends in the environment (e.g., technology, competition), identifying and discussing company weaknesses, addressing potential crises, or taking advantage of major opportunities. High levels of distress have been related to a reliance on informal sources of information (Terry & Callan, 1997).

Several studies have revealed the importance of company explanations of how and why change decisions were made in assisting individuals with change. Bardwick (1991) discusses the high need for information among employees in periods of organizational change. She suggests that when anxiety is high, rumors multiply if solid information is unavailable. Once the rumors start, they have a life cycle of their own and it becomes harder and harder to kill them. Marks and Mirvis (1992) also comment that constricted communication during an organizational transition creates anger, distrust, and cynicism that tends to linger on afterward.

Many organizations undergoing downsizing efforts do not provide good communications (Smeltzer & Zener, 1992). Brockner and Grover (1994) speculated about why organizations often fail to explain the reasons their layoffs were necessary and how they made termination decisions. He suggested that organizations may believe that providing information reduces their power over the employees and that employees might use the information against them (e.g., in lawsuits).

Results by Wanberg, Bunce, and Gavin (1999) found just the opposite. Explanation was associated with higher perceived fairness of the layoff, higher willingness to endorse the terminating organization, and less desire to sue that organization, even after reemployment.

2. Create a Delta (Change) Team

Many companies use some form of transition structure to help direct organizational change (Marks & Mirvis, 2000). This step involves putting together a group with sufficient authority to lead the change and getting that group to work together like a team (e.g., a common purpose, trust). The more the change strategies fit the coping strategies used by employees, the more likely change will occur in a positive manner.

3. Develop a Vision and Strategy

If leaders have a clear vision of the changed organization's destiny, employees are more likely to achieve a sense of control over the event (Yukl, 1998). Consultants can help companies create a transformation vision to help direct the change effort and to develop strategies for achieving that vision. Enlisting others to develop a critical mass to support change is a key step (Moran & Brightman, 2000).

4. Communicate the Change Vision

Kotter (1996b) discusses constantly communicating the vision and strategies through multiple media. Communication before and after organizational change is a key step (Nikandrou, Papalexandris, & Bourantas, 2000). Cunningham et al. (1989) have suggested the use of imagery to facilitate organizational change. Change workshops (Greenly & Carnall, 2001) have been used to help employees increase their level of ownership and commitment to a change process. The use of metaphors as tools of organizational change has been discussed in the literature (Akin & Palmer, 2000). Lastly, have the Delta Team role-model the behavior expected of others.

5. Facilitate Action

Consultants can assist companies in eliminating implementation obstacles and change systems or structures that undermine the change vision. They can encourage risk-taking and creative ideas, activities, or action.

6. Make Something Happen (Soon)

Kotter (1996b) says to plan for visible improvements in performance, or "wins." Create short-term wins. Visibly recognize and reward people who made the wins possible.

7. Standardize Improvements to Generate More Change

Use increased credibility to change all systems, structures, policies, and procedures that don't fit together or don't fit the transformation vision. Hire, promote, and develop people who can implement the change vision. Revitalize the process with new projects, themes, and change agents.

8. Make Change Process Part of the Organizational Culture

Articulate the connections between new behaviors and organizational success.

Develop means to ensure a broader base of leaders through development and succession. Encourage enhanced performance through emphasis on process and stakeholder focus.

The consultant can help individuals cope by helping management attend to the human dimensions of structural and technological change as suggested by sociotechnical system design interventions (Greenwood, 2002; Trist, Higgin, Murray, & Pollack, 1963) or a structural design intervention (Galbraith, 1973).

STRATEGIES FOR INDUCING ORGANIZATION CHANGE

Chin and Benne (1976) described three strategies for inducing change in organizations: the rational empirical strategy, the power-coercive strategy, and the normative-reeducative strategy. The consultant can use any combination of these strategies, depending on the change needs of the organization (Bennis, Benne, Chin, & Corey, 1976; Bennis & Goldsmith, 1997).

The Rational-Empirical Strategy

This strategy is based on the assumption that people are basically rational and will act in accord with their self-interest once they have been provided with the necessary information. Providing information to facilitate change is most effective when resistance to change is due to a lack of knowledge.

The Power-Coercive Strategy

This strategy involves using power, in the form of either rewards or punishment, to coerce employees to comply with plans for change.

The Normative-Reeducative Strategy

This strategy is based on the assumption that peer pressure and social norms are potent forces of change. Research indicates that group discussion about the best way to make changes is an effective means for overcoming resistance to change and maximizing productivity after the change is instituted (Coch & French, 1948).

REFRAMING ORGANIZATIONAL CHANGE

Bolman and Deal (2003) wrote extensively on four ways of framing organizations and leadership, which are known as structural, human resource, political, and symbolic (see Chapter 4). Let us now look at how they applied these frames to organizational change.

The Human Resource Approach to Change

How People Are Affected by Change

Change causes people to feel incompetent, needy, and powerless. Developing new skills, creating opportunities for involvement, and providing psychological support are essential.

What the Leader Should Do

Human resource leaders believe in people and communicate that belief. Effective human resource leaders empower: They increase participation, provide support, share information, and move decision making as far down the organization as possible.

The Structural Approach to Change

How People Are Affected by Change

Change alters the clarity and stability of roles and relationships, creating confusion and chaos. This requires attention to realigning and renegotiating formal patterns and policies.

What the Leader Should Do

Structural leaders do their homework. Structural leaders develop a new model of the relationship of structure, strategy, and environment for their organization. Effective structural leaders continually experiment, evaluate, and adapt.

The Political Approach to Change

How People Are Affected by Change

Change generates conflict and creates winners and losers. Avoiding or smoothing over those issues drives conflict underground. Managing change effectively requires the creation of arenas where issues can be negotiated.

What the Leader Should Do

Political leaders clarify what they want and what they can get. Political leaders assess the distribution of power and interests. Political leaders build linkages to other stakeholders. Political leaders persuade first, use negotiation second, and use coercion only if necessary.

The Symbolic Approach to Change

How People Are Affected by Change

Change creates loss of meaning and purpose. People form attachments to symbols and symbolic activity. When the attachments are severed, they experience difficulty in letting go. Existential wounds require symbolic healing.

What the Leader Should Do

Symbolic leaders frame experience. Symbolic leaders discover and communicate a vision. Symbolic leaders tell stories.

Armed with background knowledge of the nature of organizations, consultants will be better prepared to assess the current functioning of organizations, which is the topic of the next chapter. Thorough background knowledge and a comprehensive assessment is crucial before designing organizational interventions.

Chapter 11

ASSESSMENT OF ORGANIZATIONS

As in psychotherapy, consultants should always do a thorough assessment before attempting an intervention. The presenting problem is usually only a small part of the diagnostic picture. Even if the consultee requests only a small, specific intervention (such as a diversity training workshop), the consultant should still attempt to assess the organization's current and desired state, if only informally through discussions with the consultee and observation of organizational activities.

At times, the consultant is specifically asked to do a complete assessment of an organization. This may be for the purpose of defining organizational challenges or for monitoring progress toward organizational goals. This chapter will address the many facets of conducting a thorough organizational assessment.

Before discussing how to find dysfunctional activities within an organization, it may be helpful to consider what a healthy workplace looks like.

A HEALTHY WORKPLACE

A healthy workplace is characterized by a work environment that allows an organization to fulfill its mission while attending to the needs of its most important resource—its employees. To help consultees create better organizational environments, consultants should know the characteristics of a healthy workplace listed in Box 11.1.

Unhealthy workplaces have cultures that don't allow employees a sense of meaning, support, participation, autonomy, safety, equity, empowerment, services, respect, and success. They often show the typical signs of a dysfunctional organization, such as low employee morale, communication problems, high rates of turnover and absenteeism, divisiveness and unresolved conflicts, and diversion from the primary purposes of the organization.

ORIGINS OF THE HEALTHY WORKPLACE CONCEPT

The fields of industrial psychology and organizational psychology have been around for many years. The fields have combined to form industrial-organizational or I/O

===== Box 11.1 =====

Ten Characteristics of a Healthy Workplace

A healthy workplace allows employees to have a sense of

1. *Meaning* in their work, often based on a noble vision the organization is pursuing.
2. *Support* based on caring and thoughtful relationships with superiors, peers, and subordinates in the organization.
3. *Participation* in decision making so that input is sought and those closest to decisions help shape the final outcomes.
4. *Autonomy* to be able to have decisional latitude within the constraints of their job role.
5. *Safety,* so that appropriate safeguards to health and welfare are in place.
6. *Equity,* so that appropriate procedures are in place to justly distribute resources and rewards.
7. *Empowerment* to openly share ideas and fully devote themselves to the work of the organization.
8. *Services* that provide life support for employees such as health care and retirement benefits, family leave, seminars and training, EAP (Employee Assistance Program), and exercise equipment.
9. *Respect* for diversity and the individual personhood of each employee.
10. *Success* in their chosen enterprise allowing for the stability and progression of the organization and its employees.

psychology (Warr, 1996). Other fields in psychology such as social, clinical, and counseling psychology have also taken an increased interest in aspects of the healthy organization. More recently, health psychology has focused on the influence of the workplace on health outcomes forming new specializations of psychology such as occupational health psychology. Consultants rely on knowledge of these behavioral sciences to work with organizations to help them balance concerns over profitability with concern for their employees. The American Psychological Association (2005) has worked to promote the concept of a psychologically healthy workplace by encouraging state psychological associations to set up programs for organizations to compete for the state's Psychologically Healthy Workplace Award and ultimately National Award, chosen by APA.

WHY MAINTAINING A HEALTHY WORKPLACE IS IMPORTANT

Unhealthy workplaces tend to be unsuccessful workplaces because they do not inspire the motivation, loyalty, and dedication of employees. Attendant costs of the unhealthy workplace include turnover, absenteeism, and the increased health, disability, and workers' compensation costs often associated with worker stress and burnout. Increased costs and lowered worker productivity should get the attention of even the most bottom-line oriented business owner.

Normal Organizational Activities

Organizations must perform certain tasks to survive, and these activities ideally should also serve to solve problems as they arise. Levinson (2002b, pp. 284–285) developed a list of activities typically performed by organizations, and divided them into those having to do with product or organization and those having to do with people:

Having to Do with Product or Organization
- Processing materials
- Rendering services
- Periodic reports
- Quality control revision of tasks and processes
- Changes in space and schedules
- Expansion and acquisition
- Acquaintance with competitors' products and response thereto
- Acquaintance with changes in consumer's wishes and response thereto
- Responsiveness to social changes
- Research: basic, product, market, economic
- Pilot efforts
- Proving grounds
- Testing products
- Organization planning
- Projections of future trends
- Sales promotion and indoctrination
- Self-laudatory advertising
- Image-creating efforts
- Symbolization
- Publicity statements by key figures regarding organization's worth

Having to Do with People
- Building attractive surroundings
- Functional physical facilities
- Morale-building activities
- Encouraging socialization off the job to foster cohesion
- Company parties and conversational coffee breaks
- Background music
- Encouraging shared fantasies of organizational achievement
- Providing uniforms and other efforts to foster organization
- *Espirit de corps*
- Personnel selection, training, benefit, and caring functions
- Management-connected directly with major work goals
- Participation in professional and trade associations and community activities
- Seeking support from community and other organizations
- Exhorting (internal and to the community)
- Mild pressure
- Nagging
- Expressing overtly internal feelings in advertising ("we like to serve")
- Complaints of management in public service messages or message seeking public support
- Protection from arbitrary authority
- Protection from industrial hazards
- Care for accidental results
- Spontaneous and unplanned postponement of tasks (relief)
- Organizational moratorium periods (minimal activity or productivity to repair, recover, reorganize)

- Operation of Parkinson's Law (work expands to fill the time for its completion)
- Occasional absenteeism, breakage, flare-up of hostility in reaction to inadequate problem-solving or because of frustration

Activities of a Dysfunctional Organization

Organizations that are dysfunctional attempt to make changes in the organization, but do so in a misguided way. Levinson (2002b) divides dysfunctional organizational activities into first-order, second-order, third-order, and fourth-order.

First-order activities are simply exaggerations of normal adaptive activities. All organizations make efforts to adapt to changing circumstances, but when an organization is dysfunctional, it sometimes does so in inappropriate ways. In terms of product organization, the company may decide to do spot audits and time studies of individual employees (Ilgen & Hulin, 2000). Rather than seeking out root causes of the problem, individual employees are made to feel the pressure of improving performance, and begin to build resentment. In terms of people, the organization may continually give pep talks and may chronically complain about things.

Second-order activities are disruptive activities that have a high cost in terms of money, stress for individuals, and organizational survival potential. As the situation escalates, the organization becomes more desperate, and begins to take more drastic measures. In terms of product organization, the company may make arbitrary changes, or may suddenly eliminate established departments, which destroys employee morale. In terms of people, the organization may withdraw into itself, giving up ties to the surrounding community, which harms both the organization and the community in the long run. In an attempt to find blame for the problems in the organization, members may scapegoat certain individuals or parts of the organization.

Third-order activities are maladaptive and disruptive activities characterized by episodic blatant expressions of hostility. At this point, organizational leaders and members no longer abide by ethical or legal standards, having reached a point of high feelings of desperation and hurt. In terms of product organization, wanton damage to property of others or reputations may take place, blatantly manipulative practices may occur (such as lying to customers to gain business in the marketing department), and motivation and legal relationships may be destroyed. In terms of people, there may be open violations in labor relations (such as refusing to pay for vacation time), and apathy is likely to develop among employees.

Fourth-order activities are self-destructive activities resulting in the demise of the organization, and may involve a forced merger, bankruptcy reorganization, or going out of business. At this point, the organization feels like a sinking ship, and members may try to get anything they can out of it.

These activities should be seen as warning signs for troubled organizations. Diagnosis and intervention attempts should look to see how organizations have coped with problems currently and in the past, and investigate which interventions have worked and which have not.

TARGETS FOR ORGANIZATIONAL DIAGNOSIS AND INTERVENTION

As consultants begin to try to diagnose where the problems are occurring in an organization, they can quickly become overwhelmed by the complexities involved. Sperry

(1996), Blake and Mouton (1983), and Goodstein (1978) have written about five major areas of organizational functioning where problems arise. These five areas, which are often interdependent, can serve as targets for consultants to focus their diagnosis and intervention efforts.

1. *Power/authority:* Power refers to the capability of having an effect, and authority refers to the right to exercise power. *Power/authority issues* revolve around whether power and authority are used effectively in both formal and informal matters within an organization. *Power/authority issues* can arise over the ways power and authority are in fact used or over the ways their use is perceived by those who are not in positions of power. *Power/authority issues* are the most common focal targets, outnumbering others by a frequency of about three to one (Blake & Mouton, 1983).

2. *Morale/cohesion:* Morale is a state of high, positive mental energy among members of an organization. Cohesion refers to the degree to which members of the group experience a positive sense of togetherness and unity. *Morale/cohesion issues* concern how members perceive the organization and its direction as well as the degree to which members see themselves as part of a team.

3. *Norms/standards:* Norms are the rules that govern appropriate behavior by members of all, or some, part of the organization. Standards are the criteria organizations use for measuring quality. *Norms/standards issues* are frequently raised when an organization is forced to cope with internal and/or external changes, and both are usually difficult to change.

4. *Goals/objectives:* Goals are the aims and purposes of an organization, and objectives are those things that are accomplished when goals are met. *Goals/objectives issues* are frequently related to norms and standards issues and typically arise when goals and objectives are either poorly defined or have not been achieved. *Goals/objectives issues* frequently surface during investigation of norms/standards issues.

5. *Roles/communication:* Roles are expected behavior patterns attributed to a particular position in an organization. The structure of an organization specifies the reporting relationship of all roles within a given organization. Roles, along with the policies and procedures for communication, are essential in achieving the organization's tasks and goals. Communication is the transmission of information and understanding among individuals in various roles and the organization. *Roles/communication issues* arise as roles become less clear and boundaries blur, particularly with the roles of manager and subordinate (Sperry, 1996, pp. 80–81).

GOALS OF ORGANIZATIONAL ASSESSMENT

Rather than randomly exploring the organization, the consultant should work toward five specific goals when conducting an organizational assessment.

The first goal is to *determine how the organization came to be the way it is.* This will involve research on how the organization was formed, how things have changed over time, what the current organizational structure is and how it has changed over time. This also involves exploring the recent past, and contributing factors to the organization's current situation (e.g., the state of the economy, recent changes in policy, recent layoffs).

The second goal is to *determine what kind of information to gather* to assess the problem, issue, or desired change. This will be determined by the urgency of the problems, the scope of the problems, the size of the organization, the organization's consulting budget, and the time available. For example, technical issues (e.g., how to implement a new record-keeping software program most effectively) will require gathering different kinds of information than interpersonal issues (e.g., two department heads who are expressing open hostility toward each other).

The third goal is to *determine what parts of the client system should be explored.* Should only the problem area be explored, or should other areas be included? If the sales department is experiencing lowered numbers, does the problem lie there, or have the manufacturing and shipping departments begun sending out lower quality products?

The fourth goal is to *determine what levels of the client system should be explored.* Does the issue involve an individual, a department, the entire organization, or the external environment? From the perspective of the organization, the consultant can explore patterns of accountability, communication flow, decision-making structures, and policies and procedures. From the perspective of larger, external systems, the consultant can explore the impact of international corporations, societal environments, communities, and external relationships (e.g., customers and vendors).

The fifth goal is to *determine what data-gathering method and tools to use.* Based on the determination of what information needs to be gathered, the consultant may want to use a particular assessment tool or a specific combination (observations, questionnaires, interviews, analysis of documents, etc.) to most effectively gather the needed data.

When evaluating the current state of an organization, the consultant should consider the advantages and disadvantages of doing the assessment independently, or of involving members of the organization. Davidson (2002) makes several suggestions for choosing the best approach:

> An independent approach to a valuation is best pursued when (1) there is extreme time pressure to get information quickly, (2) the organization cannot afford to take employees away from their regular work to participate in an evaluation project, (3) accuracy of evaluation is critical, or (4) the political climate is such that questions are likely to be raised about conflict of interest if the evaluation has heavy internal involvement. Resistance to independent evaluations can be reduced if they make a deliberate point of gathering opinions from all relevant stakeholder groups (as all good evaluations should). The difference between this and a collaborative approach is that organizational members do not have input into decisions about evaluation methodology.
>
> Participative and collaborative approaches (such as evaluative inquiry) are appropriate when (1) there is a need to increase the capacity of individuals and teams to learn about what works in their own organizations, (2) the potential for resistance to findings (or changes arising from those findings) is high, or (3) organizational unlearning is important. In the latter case, organizational stakeholders might be working with faulty assumptions, which they are unlikely to change without directly participating in a joint inquiry and seeing the truth with their own eyes. (pp. 365–366)

Although organizations sometimes need an independent assessment of their functioning, most cases will involve a collaborative effort in which the consultant and the organization members work together to both diagnose and intervene to correct problems within the organization. The consultant should always consider how to involve the client system in this process. This is especially helpful in determining the kinds of data needed to understand the problem, determining how to acquire the information, and in determining how best to analyze and summarize the data. Involvement of the client system is also important for deriving the most significant implications for a change effort.

Considerations for Assessment Questions

When formulating how to proceed with the assessment, a number of factors should be considered. The consultant: (1) must get people to open up and question their assumptions about the causes of their problems; (2) must get them to accept the need for objective fact finding to supplement their own data assumptions; (3) must obtain their appropriate understanding and commitment of the time and energy that will be required of them, and (4) must involve them enough in the diagnostic data-collection process for them to feel ownership of the data and accept its validity. Research and consultant creativity will be needed to address these factors.

Types of Assessment

Just as in clinical practice, there are a number of ways to gather data for an assessment. One of the simplest ways is through observation. Informal observation involves paying attention to what is happening whenever the consultant interacts with the organization. With formal observation, the consultant looks for something specific. A consultant may be asked to sit in on a managerial meeting to look for the underlying dynamics of why the meetings are never very productive.

The consultant may also make use of unobtrusive data. This type of data is gathered without imposing on individuals or invading their space. It provides information about past patterns, and may take the form of reports (e.g., work done by past consultants, marketing plans, strategic planning reports), descriptive data (e.g., employee absenteeism statistics, financial balance sheets, number of industrial accidents by year), and environmental indicators (e.g., trends in the stock market, consumer spending data, changes in the prime interest rate).

Another common assessment instrument is surveys, which come in a variety of forms. Surveys with *standardized closed responses* can be purchased off the shelf from organizations and researchers who spend time creating and testing them. "Closed response" means that all of the answers are provided to the respondents, and they choose what they consider to be the best response. One example of such an instrument is the Survey of Organizations (SOO; J. C. Taylor & Bowers, 1972). Taylor and Bowers have identified supervisory leadership, peer relationships, and organizational climate as the critical factors in identifying the key elements of an effective organization.

Surveys can also have *customized closed responses*. The consultant writes a survey to provide specific information and creates the response choices, taking care to make the choices clearly and easily differentiable and measurable (e.g., with a Likert scale).

Surveys with *customized open responses* involve the consultant developing questions that address specific assessment questions, but allow all the respondents freedom to choose how to respond. Question stems may begin with "Tell me more about . . ." or "What if . . ." The question may ask the respondents to rate some aspect of the organization on a scale from 1 to 10, then ask them why they chose that number, and what it will take to get to a higher number. This forces respondents to "own" the number they pick, by asking them to back it up with data and with suggestions for change (this helps prevent mere complaining). Downsides of this type of survey include that the amount of data gathered can be cumbersome, and the qualitative nature of the data can be difficult to analyze.

Another assessment instrument, familiar to mental health professionals, is the interview. *Unstructured* interviews involve presenting the interviewee with only a general topic (e.g., "I'd like to talk with you about how responsive you feel management is to the needs of employees."). Interviews with *structured open responses* involve asking the interviewees a set of preformed questions, and allowing them to respond however they like (e.g., "Tell me about the best and worst experiences you have ever had with the Human Resources department."). Interviews with *structured closed responses* involve asking interviewees preformed questions, and allowing them to choose from a set number of given responses (e.g., "In regard to management's responsiveness to employee needs, in comparison to how they were last year, would you say that management is (1) more responsive, (2) less responsive, or (3) about the same as they were last year?"). This method is frequently used for telephone surveys.

The Assessment Interview

While interviews are a rich source of information, they can also be time consuming for both the consultant and for the organization's employees. As a general rule of thumb, when the number of interviews per consultant gets over 20, consultants should consider using a standardized assessment instrument.

The Consultant's Preparation

Although things will always come up for which you cannot plan, preparing yourself ahead of time will make it easier to deal with the inevitable ambiguities that arise.

With the goals of the assessment in mind, think through the questions that will be most useful. It is generally best to ask about six questions. Try not to ask too many questions, as it is usually preferable to have key questions answered in depth than to assault the interviewee with a barrage of questions. Prepare for note taking by using 5×7 note cards—one card for each question for each person. This will facilitate later tracking of the data.

Usually, the questions are not given to the interviewees in advance, allowing the consultant to receive spontaneous responses. You should, however, discuss the interview plans with the consultee (often the head of the organization or a senior manager) ahead of time to be certain that your questions will gather the data you will need to answer the referral question. During the orientation meeting, wherein you learn more about the company and its concerns, you should also discuss where and how the interviews will be held. Preferably, the interviewees should come to you in a private, comfortable setting.

Preparing the Interviewee

As in clinical practice, consultants should first clarify the purpose of any interview and should present their background and qualifications. Of crucial importance is to distinguish between anonymity and confidentiality. Consultants should explain that they cannot promise confidentiality, as the data that is gathered will be aggregated and presented in a report. However, the consultant should work to preserve anonymity (not attaching the individual's name to the data that is gathered), with the caveat that some bits of data may make it difficult to preserve anonymity (e.g., if the interviewee continually raises child-care issues, and is the only one in the organization with children, management is likely to realize who is raising this concern).

Consultants with a mental health background should also emphasize that the interview is not therapy. If sensitive personal issues begin to arise, the consultant should remind the interviewee that the purpose of the interview is only to collect information and should suggest following up with the human resources department.

To allow for open communication, interviewers should not disagree with the interviewees' opinions, though the consultant may wish to point out incongruencies in the information being presented, or may wish to bring up inconsistencies with data gathered elsewhere in the organization.

Consultants should allow enough time for the interview to gather all the needed information, and for the interviewees to express the things that concern them. Normally, sessions last 45 minutes to one hour.

Opening the Interview

When beginning the actual interview, the consultant should stress the need and the expectation for open communication. The consultant should also describe the interview process (e.g., "I am going to ask you a few standard questions, but I also would like you to bring up things that you feel are important"), and specify any particular rules (e.g., whether it is appropriate to mention people by name).

Working on Data Generation

Listen carefully to the interviewees, and openly jot down the important points. Be certain to feed back and clarify items as needed. Explain that items that are written down are likely to be on the report. At the end of the interview, allow interviewees to look over the card and to cross out any items that they don't feel comfortable having reported.

Do not allow an interviewee to personally attack other members of the organization. If you get a general comment about another person's personality or attitude, ask the interviewee to break it down into specific behaviors, and ask how those behaviors specifically influence the organization in a positive or negative way.

Given the limited time you will have with any one individual, you may need to work to keep people on track so that you can ask all of the prepared questions. If the interviewee's response at first appears not to follow from your question, accept what is said and try to determine the relationship of their answer to your question.

Mental health professionals can use their interviewing skills to actively solicit further information ("And what else?"), to observe body language, to listen to intonation, and to get a sense of the interviewee's emotional reactions to questions and situations.

As interviewees describe typical situations or important incidents, ask about others and their own reactions and behaviors regarding the event. Ask them how they would do things differently, or how they would work to perpetuate positive situations.

Finally, encourage them to share something that you didn't necessarily come to talk about, and ask if they have any questions for you.

Closing the Interview

When closing the interview, be sure to thank the person. Summarize the data you have gathered, ask for any additional comments or questions, and remind the interviewee of the next step in the process (e.g., "After I finish interviewing other members of the organization, I will write a report for your supervisor, who has told me she will post it onto the local intranet site.").

Feedback Meeting

Feedback meetings can be potentially anxiety-provoking for consultants and consultees alike. Although everyone involved would generally like to see things improved, change is often frightening, and individuals may fear being personally criticized. A consultant may begin to feel defensive if things are not kept in perspective.

When giving feedback to the management team, set up ground rules for working together, fitting your style with the audience as appropriate. Maintain the rule about not naming names (except perhaps that of the manager) and not personally attacking individuals, but emphasize that your loyalty is to the contract and not necessarily to being positive.

Quickly squelch any generalized, vague statements. If someone is criticized as not being very supportive, ask specifically what that person is doing that is not supportive. Vague statements tend to ignite reactions and defensiveness in others.

When presenting the items to be discussed, number them for easy reference. Ask for items that can be influenced, impacted, or controlled, and steer away from those that cannot (e.g., the national economy). Then ask people to pick out themes or clues within the data, especially those that contribute to accomplishing the organization's stated objective. One way to do this would be to write each individual item on a sticky note, and then have the group put the items together in groups. You can then give the participants a break to walk around with a pad of paper and come up with eight themes that they are proud of, surprised by, or confused by. Start individually, then go to the group for reactions.

The participants should then rate the themes on both urgency and importance, prioritizing them through the nominal group technique. Problem-solving techniques can then be used to work on each theme (e.g., brainstorming). Concrete, specific action plans should be developed, along with the individuals responsible and the timelines for implementation.

Remember that the raw data is only useful in getting the themes, and should be thrown away. The consultant needs to be very directive around the process, and not necessarily the content.

The overall process of the meeting should start with specifics (looking at the specific data that was gathered), expand to a more general focus (looking for the themes in the data), then return to specifics (looking at precise action steps that can be taken to create change).

Sources of Ambiguity in Organizations

Ambiguity occurs often in organizations and is a major factor in leadership's decision to call on a consultant in the first place (Hatch & Ehrlich, 1993; Meyerson, 1990). McCaskey (1982) noted that there are seven areas that are often sources of ambiguity in organizations: (1) uncertainty about what the problem really is; (2) uncertainty about what is really happening; (3) uncertainty about what the organization really wants; (4) uncertainty about the resources that the organization needs; (5) uncertainty about who is supposed to do what; (6) uncertainty about how to get what the organization wants; and (7) uncertainty about how to determine if the organization has succeeded. These seven sources of ambiguity should be considered when the consultant is formulating the questions to ask, in order to seek out the organization's sources of ambiguity when conducting an assessment.

SYSTEMS MODEL INTERVIEW QUESTIONS

Following is a list of questions that consultants can draw on when making an organizational assessment. They relate to Structure, Mission/Goals/Values, Technology, People, Leadership Procedures, Environment, and General (Levinson, 2002b; Tobias, 1990; Wallace & Hall, 1996).

Structure

How would you describe the reporting relationships in your organization?

How would you describe the use of power in the organization?

How clearly defined is your job? Jobs of others?

How well are tasks, jobs, and activities integrated in your organization? Can you give some examples?

Generally speaking, are policies and procedures carefully explained to people in your organization? How would you explain your answer?

Describe the methods for quality control in your organization.

From your position in the organization, would you say that the way you are organized is working effectively to accomplish the mission? What are the present strengths or limitations?

Are the existing structures useful for the attainment of the goals and tasks?

How do people adapt to or cope with these structures?

Are the structures supportive of the needs and capabilities of the leadership (management) and the workforce?

Do the structures encourage cooperation and collaboration?

Do the structures facilitate a rational use of resources and technologies?

What major strengths and weaknesses result from the structures' interaction with other elements in the system?

Mission/Goals/Values

How clearly defined are the goals of your organization?

What factors within the system most influence goals attainment (positively/negatively)?

What does your organization do to shape its future?

How does your organization define success for its products or services?

How do individuals achieve their personal goals in your organization?

What values does your organization seek to enhance and reinforce?

How is conflict managed in your organization?

Is there a difference between what the organization says and what it does? Describe this.

How well do people in your organization get along?

Describe how people in your organization work together.

How would you describe the opportunities in your organization for growth and development?

What would this company be like if it were highly successful in its various missions?

Technology

How would you describe the training you received to do your job? How about others?

How would you describe the understanding people have of the requirements of their jobs?

To what degree do people have the necessary skills to do what is expected of them? Please explain your answer.

Generally speaking, are the tools and the equipment adequate for the tasks of people in your organization?

How is work space allocated in your organization?

How is information processed in your organization?

Are the facilities in your organization adequate for the work requirements? Describe your view of this.

When technological changes occur, are the structures and processes adapted or modified accordingly?

Do changes produce resistance?

Is there a timely attempt to prepare people for technological and organizational changes, for example, through personnel management, training, or participatory decision making?

What and where are the most important strengths and weaknesses between technology (including processes and procedures and the other elements of the system)?

How do changes in procedures and support systems affect people and structures in the organization?

People

How are people treated in your organization?

How are people managed in your organization?

How are people in this organization rewarded?

Every organization has informal groups. How would you describe the informal groups in your organization?

How are individuals motivated in your organization?

In what ways in your organization are people involved in decision making?

In what ways in your organization are people involved in problem solving?

In what ways in your organization are people involved in planning and goal setting?

What generally happens when a person takes a position that differs from the "party line" in your organization?

What is the basic attitude of various employee groups toward the organization?

What are the effects of these attitudes on performance and teamwork?

How do mangers and their subordinates adapt to the existing structures?

Do the employees feel that the structures, technologies, and procedures serve as an incentive to full involvement (motivational effectiveness)?

What are the biggest obstacles, problem areas, and sources of conflict?

Leadership Procedures

Are the existing leadership procedures and processes focused on the specific goals/objectives and tasks?

Do these leadership procedures fit the organization's specific social and technical realities (technologies, other procedures, composition of workforce, etc.)? Are managers sufficiently trained in using the procedures (e.g., performance valuation)?

What is the leadership style most predominant in your organization? What is your reaction to this style?

Describe the processes used by managers to convey other kinds of information and decisions, and to what extent are managers concerned about the long-term success of the organization?

What are the most significant strengths and weaknesses in the leadership procedures and their application?

Environment

How would you describe the appropriateness of the resources coming into your organization?

How are opportunities for your organization identified?

What constraints does the environment place on your organization?

Generally speaking, are the users/customers of your organization satisfied with your product or service?

What are the major factors in the organization's environment that influence the work?

What characteristic environmental problems arise?

In which elements of the system are the interactions with the environment most visible?

What is the organization's greatest strength vis-à-vis the environment (competitive advantage, labor market, productivity, etc.)?

What is the organization's most obvious weakness vis-à-vis the environment?

General

What do you see as interfering with getting the job done the way you would like see it get done?

What things are going well now? What are the strengths?

What things are impeding or blocking your being as successful as you want?

Other assessment questions can be developed for specific problems. For example, when trying to deal with two departments that are in conflict, the consultant can ask the following questions:

- What do we like about what _____ group is doing?
- What concerns us about the _____ group?
- What do we predict the _____ group will say about us?

Chapter 12

ORGANIZATIONAL INTERVENTION

Rumiko Suzuki, a licensed mental health counselor with a business background, receives an e-mail from John Simpson, the executive director of a local nonprofit agency that serves the needs of the chronically mentally ill. He had received her name, with a strong recommendation, from a consultant they had used in the past who was now retired. The e-mail states that the organization has been expanding and needs to revise its strategic planning. Rumiko replies that she would be interested in meeting to discuss the situation further, and arrangements are made for Rumiko to visit the executive director at the agency.

For a mental health professional accustomed only to intervening at the individual level, attempting an intervention for an entire organization may seem overwhelming. However, as we know from the *Butterfly Effect* (the concept that complex systems may have a sensitive dependence on initial conditions, Gleick, 1987), small interventions can have major impacts.

STEPS IN ACTION LEARNING OR PROCESS CONSULTATION

In many ways, the processes involved in organizational interventions mirror that of clinical interventions with individuals. First, contact is made and rapport is established; second, an agreement is made as to the goals and methods of the intervention; third, data is collected and an accurate diagnosis of the problem is made; fourth, feedback is given so that the problem can be specifically defined; fifth, an intervention plan is created; sixth, the intervention is implemented; seventh, the effectiveness of the intervention is evaluated and the plan is adjusted as needed; and eighth, a decision is made as to whether the consultation relationship needs to be extended, redeveloped, or terminated (Schein, 2000; Wallace & Hall, 1996).

Phase 1: Entry

The entry phase consists of making the initial contacts with the organization. The consultant must identify the consultee and clients and make an initial determination as to the potential fit between them and the consultant. The factors determining fit may be as subtle as personality style or may involve the consultant's competency and ability to perform the requested services. This will also be a time for credential testing, when the consultee tries to determine if the consultant is truly qualified or experienced enough to handle the presenting issue. An appropriate referral may be needed if the consultant does not feel able to serve the consultee for the particular situation.

Another important goal in this phase is the clarification of the consultee's expectations. What does the consultee wish to see happen? What does the organization see as the consultant's role? How do they envision the process of getting where they want to go?

This phase is also the time to begin to establish relationship norms (getting a feel for what the relationship will be like, which will involve setting boundaries and determining the consultee's readiness for change). This phase is also a time for building rapport and developing trust, which will be needed before interventions can be implemented effectively.

Weiss (2004) highlights the importance of dealing with the true decision maker in the organization (rather than speaking only to the gatekeeper), which means that the consultant should always try to work at the highest possible level in the organization. The consultant should also inquire about the organization's and the consultee's previous experiences with consultation, including what has been done so far on the presenting issue and what the results have been of previous intervention attempts.

Potential ethical issues also need to be addressed early on. The consultant should openly discuss any potential conflicts of interest, such as a history of consulting with a competing organization. Issues of confidentiality also need to be addressed (e.g., who will own the raw assessment data, what steps will be taken to preserve anonymity, and who will be permitted to see the final report).

Of major importance in this first phase is determining the true nature of the problem at hand. What is the consultee really asking for? Why has the organization decided to take action now by seeking out a consultant? Why have they chosen you?

The presenting problem is often not the real reason for the consultation request. The consultee may simply be too embarrassed to discuss the actual reason, may be going through the motions only because a supervisor ordered the action, or may be consciously deceiving the consultant for some ulterior motive (e.g., hoping the consultant will take the initiative to suggest firing someone). Likewise, the consultee may lack an understanding of what makes the consulting process work, or may simply be unaware to the nature and scope of the true problem. The consultant must work to conceptualize the problem on multiple levels, determining how it affects the entire organization.

As in therapy settings, empathy and support are among the most important tools for the consultant in this first phase of developing a relationship with the consultee system.

Once a relationship has been established, the problem initially defined, and a determination made that the consultant can be of help, the contracting phase begins.

Rumiko arrives at the agency and is given a tour by the executive director. After settling down in John's office, they begin with some small talk about the pictures on the walls of exotic trips that John has taken through Europe. John then asks about Rumiko's experience and background before proceeding to give a history of his agency and the events leading up to their current situation. Since John has made use of consultants before, he is clear about what he wants and expects from Rumiko. Her primary task would be to facilitate a strategic planning session with all of the agency's key personnel. He would also like her to help him prepare for the meeting, including the financial implications of deciding whether to purchase a new building. Rumiko states that she is very interested in the project, and John states that he thinks he would enjoy working with her. John gives Rumiko some written material about the agency and asks her to submit a written proposal.

Phase 2: Contracting

Contracting is the process of making an agreement between the consultant and the consultee. This process can be formal, as in writing up a detailed document, or informal, as in making a verbal agreement. The contract may be legally binding, or may be a "psychological" contract, which refers to implicit expectations between the parties. It is crucial for consultants to have a basic knowledge of contract law, since even simple verbal statements can be legally enforceable (Beatty & Samuelson, 2001).

The goal of this phase is to determine if a work contract will be struck, and to determine precisely what that contract will be. This will include defining the desired project outcomes, specifying the roles of the parties involved, and setting the parameters for the activities that will be performed.

There are many elements to consider in the contracting phase. To begin with, the primary consultee must be identified. Consultants will likely work with a number of people in any organization and need to be clear about the person to whom they are responsible. Similarly, there must be clarity about the confidentiality limits of the consultants' service. Will the consultants give feedback to the entire organization or only to the hiring consultee? What if consultants discover unethical practices in the organization? Consultants should also discuss issues of access and support needed to facilitate an effective intervention. What sources and types of information will be available? With whom can consultants speak? What is off limits? Any physical resources should also be negotiated, such as provision of office space and a computer within the organization for interviewing employees and analyzing data. Consultants should discuss their values or operating principles, such as the ethical obligation to give testing feedback to individuals unless it is made explicitly clear in advance that no feedback will be given.

The goals or intended outcomes of the consultation should be discussed, defining the consultants' "deliverables," that is, what the consultants will provide to the organization in exchange for money. Examples include such things as provision of a 2-day seminar, creation of an employee mental health tracking system, or a detailed written report of the consultants' assessment and intervention recommendations.

The consultation objective should be specific, with measurable outcomes. If a university psychology department requested a consultant to help it become a stronger research organization, the consultant should first ask the department more about what exactly this would entail. Do they want the professors to actively publish more research? Do they want to build laboratories? Do they want their professors or students to receive more in-depth training in research? Do they want to base more of their teachings on the research literature? Do they want more grant funding?

Winum, Nielson, and Bradford (2002) noted that the basic dimensions of the desired outcomes of every organization can be categorized as *mission, people, structure,* and *systems,* and they give examples of the desired states for each dimension:

Mission Dimension
- All members of the organization are clear and aligned about the mission and strategy of the organization.
- The strategy of the organization co-evolves with conditions in the external environment.
- The desired values and culture of the organization are behaviorally evidenced throughout the organization.

People Dimension
- The selection of people into the organization results in a highly competent workforce.
- Talented individuals are retained by the organization.
- New employees of the organization are well oriented, trained, and integrated into the organization such that they rapidly reach high levels of productivity.

Structure Dimension
- There is efficiency and minimal redundancy in the use of resources.
- Departments operate with the resources and authority they need to execute their tasks well.
- Assignments and responsibilities change to keep up with changes in the size of the organization.

Systems Dimension
- Employees are informed in a timely manner about what they need to know to do their jobs effectively.
- The compensation system enables the organization to offer salary and benefits that effectively reinforce desired job performance.
- The accounts payable process results in just-in-time payments. (pp. 648–649)

The time frame for the consulting process should also be explicitly discussed, including how long the service will be provided to the organization and to the individual consultee. Does the organization have a set deadline for the accomplishment of the goals? Availability of the consultant should also be negotiated. Does the organization have 24-hour access to the consultant if necessary? Is there an additional fee associated with added availability? How should the consultant be contacted?

Fees and costs should be explicitly discussed. Will the consultant charge a flat rate for the service, or charge by the hour? Will the fee include all expenses, or will ancillary expenses be billed to the organization? Will there be an approval process for unforeseen expenses?

The evaluation process should also be considered. How will the effectiveness of the intervention be determined? What if the consultees do not feel that they "got their money's worth"? The possibility of contract renegotiation, if needed, should also be considered.

At times, a formal contract will not be drawn up. Contracting will take the form of a discussion between the consultant and a representative of the organization. Though verbal agreements are legally binding in most states, consultants should still write a letter that summarizes their understanding of the agreement to avoid confusion.

Once a clear agreement has been made, the consultant should begin gathering data and formulating the issues at hand.

Rumiko submits to John a written proposal for the project. She explicitly writes down the goals and objectives for the project in terms of her expected role. She estimates the time she believes will be necessary for the project and sets her fee accordingly. After receiving the proposal, John asks if she can resubmit the proposal with a set fee for the entire project rather than with an hourly fee, which will make it easier for John to get budgetary approval for the project from the board of directors. Rumiko agrees, and the proposal is soon signed and returned to her.

Phase 3: Data Collection and Diagnosis

This phase entails assessing the organization and the issues involved, identifying the specific problems to be dealt with, and formulating the issues in the larger organizational context.

The first goal of this phase involves determining what to assess and how to do the assessments to best understand the problem, issue, or desired change. Determining what kind of information needs to be gathered will influence the consultant's choice of assessment procedure. The simplest form of assessment is observation, which can take place informally (e.g., walking through the organization to see how things are run) or formally (being assigned to "shadow" an employee for several days). The consultant also may want to read over written reports and other documents from the organization, and may decide to research environmental influences on the organization (such as economic trends and best practices).

Surveys and interviews are frequently used to gather data. Surveys can make use of standardized instruments or can be customized to a particular organization and its needs. Standardized instruments have the advantage of being field tested, often with norms for comparison with other organizations, but customized instruments have the advantage of directly addressing the specific issues at hand. A combination of instruments may be used whenever practicable. Survey instrument responses can be open ("tell us about your experience with the human resources department") or closed ("please mark your response on the scale below"). Likewise, interviews can be unstructured or structured.

The consultant will also need to determine what parts and what levels of the client system should be explored, since the initially identified issues often have larger effects on organizations. From the perspective of the individual, the consultant should consider issues concerning motivation, quality of work life, rewards, and attitudes. From the perspective of the group, the consultant should explore interpersonal relationships and group leadership. From the perspective of the organization, the consultant should assess patterns of accountability, communication flow, and the structure of decision-making processes (Cannon-Bowers & Salas, 1998; Salas & Fiore, 2004). From the perspective of larger systems, the consultant should consider the influences of international corporations, societal environments, and communities.

Levinson (2002a) organizes the assessment process into four steps, with the first three for gathering the data and the fourth as inferential:

1. Genetic data (identification and description of the organization, its history, and the reasons for the consultation)
2. Structural data (the formal organization, plant and equipment, finances, personnel demographics and policies, general policies and practices, and time cycles)
3. Process data (information and communications transmission)
4. Interpretative data (how the organization perceives itself and its environment, its basic knowledge and how it makes use of that knowledge, the emotional atmosphere of the organization and its capacity to act, and attitudes about and relationships with multiple stakeholders, things and ideas, the consultant, power, and itself) (p. 322)

All of the data should be considered in the context of the specific organization, its culture, and the issues facing all other organizations like it.

The consultant should carefully consider how to involve the client system in this phase, such as in determining the kinds of data needed to understand the problem being addressed, determining how to acquire the information, analyzing and summarizing the data, and deriving the most significant implications of the data for future change efforts.

One of the biggest compliments a consultant can receive is to be described as "someone who knows how to ask the right questions." Asking questions is crucial, because often people can solve their own problems once someone helps them ask the right questions.

Box 12.1 shows a work sheet that can serve as a framework for the consultant in this phase (Levinson, 2002b; Tobias, 1990; Wallace & Hall, 1996).

Once the assessment is completed, the results should be presented to the consultee to help further define the problem.

Rumiko begins doing research on best practices for agencies like John's, and investigates other external factors like availability of grant funding. She then meets with John and asks him about what the agency is doing and where it wants to go. She learns more about the past strategic planning done by the agency and gets copies of its financial statements to begin calculating the viability of purchasing another building. She later types up a summary of what she has learned, and distributes it (with John's approval) to those who will be attending the strategic planning session, along with a brief description of what will take place and how the participants can best prepare.

Phase 4: Feedback and Problem Definition

This stage involves presenting the data that the consultant has gathered to key personnel and then to the client system. Results of the surveys, interviews, reviews of histori-

---

=== **Box 12.1** ===

Initial Diagnostic Interview Work Sheet

1. What is the problem or the reason that you called me in?
2. What is the impact of this problem? (For whom is it a problem? Where is the problem occurring or not occurring? How big is the problem? What would be the consequences of not addressing the problem?)
3. What factors contribute to perpetuating the problem? (What are people doing or not doing that could be creating or sustaining the problem? How might such things as organizational reward systems, structures, rules, policies, and relationships contribute?)
4. What have you tried so far to address the problem? What have been the results? (What has worked? What has not worked? Why?)
5. Ideally, what would you like to happen? (What would it be like if the situation were the way you want it to be?)
6. What interventions might bring about this preferred solution? (Which do you see as most likely to succeed? Why?)
7. What forces support this intervention? (Key people, resources, time, outside events, and so on.)
8. What forces inhibit this intervention? (Key people, resources, time, outside events, and so on.)
9. What are you (the client) willing to invest in finding a solution? (Your time? The time of others? Money? Risk? Involvement? Commitment? Resources?)
10. What do you want from me (the consultant)? (Support? Active involvement? Resources? Type[s] of consulting services? Nature of the relationship?)
11. Is there anything else that I need to know in order to understand the situation?
12. What are the next steps we need to take? (Who? What? When? How? Where?)

cal data, and observations are first given to the consultee. The consultee is then prepared for the feedback meeting for the larger group of stakeholders.

There are several elements to consider during this phase. The consultant should reflect on the following questions:

Who should attend the feedback meeting?

How will those involved in the study find out the results?

How will the consultant convey the main purpose of the feedback meeting—which is to gain commitment to action?

How will the consultant manage the potential resistance to the data feedback?

How will the consultant show support for the consultee and the client system?

Honest feedback, along with open discussion with the consultee, will help define the problem. This leads to clear goals for the future. Once goals are established, the intervention steps needed to achieve those goals can be formulated.

At the strategic planning session, Rumiko facilitates the discussion of where the company currently is and where it plans to go. During the meeting, it becomes apparent to all that the agency is heading in an entirely new direction, though it will still be based on its mission of serving the chronically mentally ill. Though everyone is excited and "on board" about where the agency is going, there is a lot of uncertainty about how best to proceed. Each participant is assigned tasks to complete before the next meeting that will lay down the road to the agency's future desired state.

Phase 5: Planning the Intervention

Once the problem has been defined, and goals for the future have been set, designs for intervention can be made. The goal of this phase is to devise a sequence of steps toward solving the problem. To assure the efficacy of the intervention, the consultant should work with the consultee to identify criteria or evidence to verify that each step has been achieved as the intervention proceeds. Since the consultee will often have an idea of the best intervention strategy, the consultant may need to rely on experience and training to negotiate the most appropriate intervention strategy. Later, the consultant may want to write a letter of understanding for the consultee summarizing the steps of the intervention, or may want to develop a formal agreement for complex situations.

To set meaningful goals, both the consultee and the consultant need a detailed picture of a preferred and feasible future. The consultant should consider who should be involved for a plan of action to have the best probability of success, and formulate ideas for how best to involve them in the implementation.

Rumiko works closely with John and other members of the agency to develop a plan of action. Research is done to find examples of similar things done by other agencies, and various courses of action are assessed for their potential risks and payoffs. At the next meeting, these plans are debated and altered until a consensus is reached about the best way to proceed.

Phase 6: Implementing the Intervention through Others

Only rarely can a consultant single-handedly implement an intervention. Decrying the perfect intervention plan to the client system and expecting them to implement it on their own is also not likely to be efficacious. A common error among consultants is to offer intervention plans prematurely, and to provide advice rather than helping the consultee to participate in the development of intervention plans.

The goals of this phase are to help the client system to develop the skills necessary to increase their chances of achieving success in the actions they take, and to work with the client system to coordinate multiple skill development activities. The consultant can help do this by initiating sessions designed to examine progress and to review progress issues as they arise.

Consultants should remember that the client system's motivation for the continuing effort comes from frequent experiences of successful movement on a defined path that leads somewhere. By understanding why an organization has been operating the way that it has, the consultant can minimize resistance and channel the organizational energy onto a more efficacious path.

Consultants tend to neglect helping the client system prepare for anticipated action. Too often, consultees understand intervention plans intellectually, but may have difficulty putting them into practice. Rehearsal and simulation exercises may be needed by the client group, though they may be reluctant to formally request assistance.

As always, the consultant should provide encouragement and support to the organization throughout the intervention process. It is important to help the client system celebrate milestones.

Consultants often blame organizations for not following their recommendations. However, part of the skill of the consultant is to frame recommendations in ways that the consultee can accept, as challenging as this may be at times. As in therapy, mental health professionals should remember that all positive change should be attributed to the consultee. When failure occurs, the consultant should engage in introspection and try to determine how better to deal with resistance in the future.

Once the agency decided on a firm plan, Rumiko helped the members outline it in a document with definable actions and goals. Individual agency members were chosen to be responsible for each goal, with specific dates for each subgoal being discussed and agreed on by the responsible person.

Phase 7: Evaluation

As the intervention proceeds, continuous evaluations should be made of how things are going. The consultant should work with the consultees to determine and use appropriate procedures to elicit feedback about progress. They should also decide who should be involved in the assessment of this feedback. The feedback should be used for reexamining goals, revising action strategies, prompting decisions concerning mobilizing needed but unused resources, and for changing assignments and roles as needed.

The consultant should work with the consultee to prepare for early warning signs that action is off course in order to make corrections as soon as possible. The consultant should be especially vigilant for blockages and resistance to effective action so that it can be adequately addressed.

Rumiko assisted John in developing a plan to monitor each agency member's progress on achieving the subgoals. She also made herself available to assist in the remediation of any strategies that were not working to achieve the goals on time and on budget.

Phase 8: Extension, Recycle, or Termination

The final phase involves determining the future of the intervention. This may involve starting over with a new problem, extending the length of (or recontracting) the current intervention, or terminating the consultant's involvement.

Goals for this phase might include the development of a plan for follow-up support or provisions for gradual termination of the consultant's help, as well as the development of a plan for a continuing review of milestones. This might simply mean establishing a minimal periodic maintenance plan, such as an annual review session. It will also be important to document any successes made during the change process, which will provide inspiration to both internal and external stakeholders. This phase is also the time for consultants to receive feedback on their performance, to better serve the consultee as well as other consultees in the future.

Consultants should bear in mind that many positive changes achieved often succumb to habitual negative influences. Changes tend to last for a short while, and then there is regression to old patterns. Organizational counterreactions to the change tend to grow over time, and must be handled quickly by organizational leadership to guarantee the continuity of the change.

John quickly found that as the agency began to change, many unforeseen consequences needed his attention. He contracted with Rumiko to use her services on an as-needed basis as the agency began operating in its new endeavors.

CASE EXAMPLE: EMPLOYEE STRESS

A clinician in private practice wants to expand her consultation activities, and so is delighted when a local company executive telephones her to ask if she can help the company "do something about employee stress." The executive rattles off a list of statistics of absenteeism, sick leave, insurance benefits, and recent layoffs as evidence that the problem is real, and says they need some help right away. Just then, the clinician's next patient arrives, and she promises to call the executive back. How should our clinician-consultant handle this situation?

Box 12.2 lists potential questions to ask the consultee.

=== **Box 12.2** ===

Questions to Ask Potential Consultees

- What is the nature of the employee stress, and what do the statistics cited earlier mean to your company?
- What type of consultation do you believe I could provide that would be helpful in solving this problem?
- What efforts have you made so far to deal with this problem on your own?
- Why have these efforts not worked as well as you would like them to?
- What made you decide to seek consulting assistance at this particular time?
- In what context does this problem exist: In your organization? In the larger environment?
- If we were to start working together, what would be the first steps as far as you are concerned?

ORGANIZATIONAL CHANGE AND DEVELOPMENT

Organizational development (OD) refers to a set of behavioral science-based theories, values, strategies, and techniques aimed at the planned change of the organizational work setting for the purpose of enhancing individual development and improving organizational performance, through the alteration of organization members' on-the-job behaviors (Porras & Robertson, 1987, 1992).

Organizational development entails a wide range of diverse techniques and approaches that share the following characteristics:

- The involvement of the entire organization
- The adoption of a systems approach and a humanistic philosophy
- The commitment and support of top management
- A focus on individuals and relationships between individuals
- The use of a change-agent (catalyst) who guides the change process
- A view of OD as an ongoing and long-term process

The Managerial Grid

The Managerial Grid (Blake & Mouton, 1964), as discussed in Chapter 4, can be used as a comprehensive OD strategy that targets the formal organization (e.g., policies, goals), the informal organization (e.g., work groups, communication processes), and the employees themselves (e.g., their values and attitudes). The strategies include the use of seminars, team building, interpersonal development, goal and structural change, and program evaluation. The consultant's goal is to train the organization's personnel to conduct these intervention strategies. Hence, the intervention begins with management and works its way down through the organization.

The Managerial Grid describes the behavior of managers and the climate of the organization in two dimensions: concern for production and concern for people. The goal is to develop managers and organizations that are high in both dimensions.

Quality

One of the trends that consultants should be aware of when working with organizations is the push toward quality (Peters & Austin, 1985). In the last decades of the twentieth century, businesses began paying more attention to the quality of the products they produced. Even a rejection rate of 5% adds up to a lot of lost profit when a company is mass-producing products. Hence, the management philosophy of *total quality management* (TQM) was developed, which strives to continuously improve all organizational processes for the constant attainment of customer satisfaction (Hackman & Wageman, 1995; Robbins, 2001; Sashkin & Kiser, 1993).

W. Edwards Deming was the founder of the TQM movement (Schermerhorn et al., 2000). Deming built a series of fourteen points for managers to implement (Deming, 1982a, 1982b; Schermerhorn et al., 2000):

1. Create a consistency of purpose in the company to
   a. Innovate.
   b. Put resources into research and education.
   c. Put resources into maintaining equipment and new production aids.

2. Learn a new philosophy of quality to improve every system in the organization.
3. Require statistical evidence of process control and eliminate financial controls on production.
4. Require statistical evidence of control in purchasing parts; this will allow the organization to reduce the number of suppliers.
5. Use statistical methods to isolate the problem areas.
6. Institute modern on-the-job training.
7. Improve supervision to develop inspired leaders.
8. Drive out fear and instill learning throughout the organization.
9. Break down barriers between departments.
10. Eliminate numerical goals and slogans.
11. Constantly revamp work methods.
12. Educate all employees in statistical methods.
13. Retrain people in new skills.
14. Create a structure that will push, every day, on the preceding thirteen points (Schermerhorn, 2000, p. 224).

Robbins (2001) describes five aspects of total quality management:

1. *Intense focus on the customer:* The customer includes not only outsiders who buy the organization's products or services but also internal customers (such as shipping or accounts payable personnel) who interact with and serve others in the organization.
2. *Concern for continuous improvement:* TQM is a commitment to never being satisfied. "Very good" is not good enough. Quality can always be improved.
3. *Improvement in the quality of everything the organization does:* TQM uses a very broad definition of quality. It relates not only to the final product but also to how the organization handles deliveries, how rapidly it responds to complaints, how politely the phones are answered, and the like.
4. *Accurate measurement:* TQM uses statistical techniques to measure every critical performance variable in the organization's operations. These performance variables are then compared against standards or benchmarks to identify problems, the problems are traced to their roots, and the causes are eliminated.
5. *Empowerment of employees:* TQM involves the people on the line in the improvement process. Teams are widely used in TQM programs as empowerment vehicles for finding and solving problems. (p. 15)

Several types of quality management systems have been developed. The International Organization for Standardization (ISO), an international federation of national standards bodies from some 100 countries, promotes quality by setting certification standards for its ISO 9000 series. Firms seeking this certification must obtain a third-party assessment and undergo periodic audits to let vendors and customers know that they meet this standard of quality (Schermerhorn et al., 2000).

Another quality standard, known as *six sigma,* was developed by Motorola and popularized by Jack Welch at GE. This quality standard only allows 3.4 errors per one million opportunities, which translates into 99.999997% error-free work (DuBrin, 2000).

Quality of Work Life Intervention and Quality Circles

Quality of work life (QWL) interventions are designed to humanize work and the work environment. The emphasis of this approach is on worker participation and involvement at all stages of decision making. This idea makes use of autonomous work groups, flexible work schedules and compensation plans, in-house training and education programs, and union-management cooperation.

Quality circles (QCs) are widely used in Japan, and they are increasing in popularity in the United States. They involve worker participation and are included in QWL interventions.

The main goal of quality circles is to improve productivity, as well as to increase employee satisfaction, morale, and personal growth and development. Each QC consists of a small group of employees who work closely together on a particular job and meet regularly to discuss production problems. Although research has not shown significant effects on worker attitudes, QCs appear to increase productivity and decrease absenteeism.

Quality circles are most successful when workers are adequately trained in problem-solving skills, are assured that their suggestions will not cause them to be penalized in any way, and when they feel their efforts are strongly supported by management (Steers, 1981; Ungson & Steers, 1984).

Process Consultation

Schein (1969, 2000, 2001) has written extensively about process consultation, which is a popular approach to organization development. Mental health professionals will find process consultation to be similar to the principles of group therapy.

Process consultation refers to activities designed to help members of an organization perceive, understand, and then alter processes that are undermining their interactions with one another. A process consultant observes individuals interacting during meetings or other usual activities, and then shares the information gathered about the process with the individuals and helps them identify actions that will improve their interactions. The focus is on behaviors rather than attitudes, and the target behaviors are typically related to communication, leadership, decision making, conflict resolution, and members' roles in groups.

A process consultant focuses on helping the consultees fix their own problems by asking clarifying questions and teaching them how to learn about themselves and create their own interventions. This viewpoint postulates that if consultees are always spoon-fed solutions, they will become dependent on consultants, or may not be able to effectively implement solutions given by an outsider.

The Sociotechnical Approach

The sociotechnical approach focuses on the social and technological aspects of the organization, and posits that both must be addressed adequately to create effective organizational change (Cooper & Foster, 1971; Emery & Trist, 1978; Johnson et al., 2002; Pasmore, 1988).

This approach is associated with the Tavistock Model (Johnson et al., 2002). Tavistock studied the coal-mining industry in the 1940s. Results of the research indicated that absenteeism, hostility between workers, and other problems were directly related to changes in social patterns that resulted from new technological conditions (Diamond & Allcorn, 1987). Too often, organizations implement a new technology and expect workers to adjust automatically. The sociotechnical approach involves trying to jointly optimize both key issues of physical products and social/psychological outcomes. The assumption in this approach is that technological change must be accompanied by planned changes in social patterns to guarantee organizational effectiveness.

Structural Design Approach

The structural design approach focuses on structure and technology, and assumes that organizational problems are related to suboptimal organizational structures. In designing an intervention, the consultant first divides the organization's tasks into specific groups or units. These units are then coordinated to achieve overall effectiveness through implementing an organizational structure that considers the environment, size, technology, and goals of an organization.

Rewards System Approach

The rewards system approach focuses on performance management and feedback systems by rewarding desired behaviors and work outcomes. Example rewards would be pay, opportunity (promotions, increased learning, wider job experiences), and fringe benefits.

High-Involvement Organizational Approach

The high-involvement organizational approach focuses on the organization's culture as well as on design components. This approach emphasizes a shift from a control-oriented organization to one based on commitment. It seeks to diffuse decision making, power, knowledge, information, and rewards throughout the organization. Hence, it emphasizes interventions that reinforce employee involvement.

CONSULTING STYLES

Even mental health professionals with minimal consulting experience will likely have an idea of their preferred consulting style, perhaps through interactions with parents, teachers, or other professionals when dealing with clients.

R. Lippitt and G. Lippitt (1975a, 1975b; G. Lippitt & R. Lippitt 1986) investigated the multiple roles that consultants fulfill and developed the Consulting-Style Inventory. They placed the multiple roles on a continuum, with the locus for decision making moving from client centered at one end (Objective Observer) to consultant centered at the other end (Advocate). Client-centered roles (as used in psychotherapy) allow the client or consultee to be active and involved in all of the stages of the consulting process. A consultant-centered role is one in which the consultant must be active and directive on how things proceed.

Objective Observer (Facilitator)

The objective observer does not express personal beliefs or ideas and does not assume responsibility for the work or the result of that work. In this role, the consultant observes the client's behavior and provides feedback; the client alone is responsible for the direction that is ultimately chosen. The consultant asks questions that help the client clarify and confront a problem to make decisions.

Process Counselor (or Process Consultant/Facilitator)

The process counselor observes the client's problem-solving processes and offers suggestions for improvement. The consultant and the client jointly diagnose the client's process, and the consultant assists the client in acquiring whatever skills are necessary to continue diagnosing the process. In this role, the focus is on interpersonal and intergroup dynamics that affect the problem-solving process. The consultant observes and reports the data to the client to improve relationships and processes.

Fact Finder ("Seeing Eye Dog")

The fact finder serves as a researcher, collecting and interpreting information in areas of importance to the client, which includes developing criteria and guidelines for collecting, analyzing, and synthesizing data (using a variety of methods). Fact finding enables the consultant to develop an understanding of the client's processes and performance. As a result of the insights gained, the consultant and the client can evaluate the effectiveness of a change process in terms of solving the client's problem.

Resource Identifier and Linker to Resources (Alternative Linker)

In this role, the consultant identifies alternative solutions to a problem; establishes criteria for evaluating each alternative; determines the likely consequences of each alternative; and then links the client with resources that may help solve the problem. However, the consultant does not assist in selecting the final solution.

Joint Problem Solver (Detective)

The joint problem solver works actively with the client to identify and solve the problem at hand, often taking a major role in defining the results. This function consists of stimulating interpretations of the problem, helping to maintain objectivity, isolating the causes of the problem, generating alternative solutions, evaluating alternatives, choosing a solution, and developing an action plan. The consultant also may function as a third-party mediator when conflict arises during the problem-solving process.

Trainer/Educator (Teacher)

The trainer or educator provides instruction, information, or other kinds of directed learning opportunities for the client. The ability to train and educate is necessary in many helping situations, particularly when a specific learning process is essential if the client is to develop competence in certain areas. As a trainer/educator, the consultant must be able to assess training needs, write learning objectives, design learning experiences and educational events, employ a range of educational techniques and media, and function as a group facilitator.

Information Specialist (or Content Expert) (Fact-Finding Expert)

The information specialist serves as content expert for the client, often defining "right" and "wrong" approaches to a problem. The client is primarily responsible for defining the problem and the objectives of the consultation, and the consultant plays a directive role until the client is comfortable with the approach that has been recommended. Although the needs of both the consultant and the client may encourage this consulting role, the consultant should not adhere to this behavior pattern exclusively. The client may become increasingly and also inappropriately dependent on the consultant; also, the dependence may lead to poor problem solving because of limited consideration of alternatives.

Advocate (Magician)

The advocate consciously strives to have the client move in a direction desired by the consultant. In the most directive of the eight roles, the consultant uses power and influence to impose ideas and values about either content or process issues. As a content advocate, the consultant tries to influence the client's choice of goals and means; as a process advocate, the consultant tries to influence the methodology underlying the client's problem-solving behavior.

Though we each have our own preferred roles, a consultant must be flexible, depending on organizational and situational needs. Each of the eight roles is appropriate if it meets the following conditions: It is negotiated with the client and agreed to by the client; and it is needed in the current situation that the consultant and the client share. The ability of the client is a determining factor of what role the consultant should take. If the client is able and willing to be actively involved in the consulting process, the consultant should adopt one of the more client-centered roles. If the client is unable and unwilling to be actively involved, one of the more consultant-centered roles should be used.

This continuum can also be seen as one of responsibility allocation. More client-centered roles shift the majority of the responsibility for the outcome to the consultee. When the client takes responsibility, the intervention is more likely to be implemented. A more client-centered approach is generally used in actual practice, though there may be times, such as in an organization that lacks management sophistication, when more directive approaches are needed.

All consulting styles are valid, depending on the situation. To function effectively as a consultant, you want to achieve comfort in each of these roles. Think about how you would answer the following questions:

- Is your style more client centered or consultant centered?
- How flexible are you in your use of consulting roles? Do you move easily from one to another as the situation demands?
- Are any roles particularly dominant for you? How do they serve your clients?
- Are there any roles that you underutilize? How could the increased use of these roles benefit your clients?
- What could you do to lessen your reliance on favorite roles or to use all of the options with equal ease?

Dr. Weismann, a counseling psychologist who is just beginning to expand into consulting work, receives a request to help an organization with a transition from manual paperwork to an environment that is fully computerized. Management is having difficulty making the transition work. Dr. Weismann calls his mentor, Dr. Patel, to ask her about managing difficult transitions in organizations.

TRANSITION MANAGEMENT

Transitions tend to be difficult for human beings, yet they are becoming increasingly common in today's organizations. Consultants with a mental health background are especially suited to deal with the emotions and other issues that come up during periods of change, such as dealing with loss, uncertainty, hope, and the search for meaning.

Bridges (1980, 1991) wrote about three phases that people and organizations tend to go through during transitional periods. The first phase involves letting go of the old situation and the old identity with it. During this phase, people experience disengagement, disidentification, and disenchantment.

In the second phase, people feel themselves to be wandering in a "neutral zone" between the old reality and the new reality. However, people also begin to experience discovery.

In the third phase, people experience a new beginning that is more than the "new start" required in a change. People experience a new visioning.

Dr. Weismann is unhappy with how things are going so far with the organization that wanted help with its transition to becoming fully computerized. He telephones Dr. Patel to get some insights and perspectives on why the consultation does not seem to be progressing very well. She asks what the organization's vision and mission are, and Dr. Weismann replies that he has never seen those things written down in any of the materials he has been given. In fact, Dr. Weismann feels that one of the problems in the organization is that there is not a clear, cohesive sense of what the organization needs to be doing either now or in the future. Dr. Patel suggests talking to the consultee about setting up a strategic planning session.

STRATEGIC PLANNING

Another important consultation intervention and management skill is strategic planning. Strategic planning is a process by which an organization creates its future. It envisions its future by setting clear goals and objectives within time frames and develops the necessary procedures and operations to achieve that future. Knowledge of strategic planning is useful in consulting for other organizations, but it is also important to help assure that one's own organization or consulting business will succeed. Several books provide details on strategic planning (F. David, 2001; Pearce & Robinson, 1997; Wright, Kroll, & Parnell, 1998), but the following will serve as a general overview of the process.

As in many consulting applications, asking the right questions is extremely important. When facilitating a strategic planning session, the consultant will typically run down a list of questions, allowing the participants to come up with the answers or with further questions. In most cases, the consultant acts only as a facilitator and does not influence what the actual decisions will be. Often, a strategic planning session takes place in a retreat setting away from the distractions of the workplace and can take from one to several days, depending on the complexity of the organization.

There are eight areas to be considered: planning the planning, forecasting the future environment, formulating the vision and mission, exploring the current status of the organization, formulating the overall strategy, relating the strategy to the organization's capacity, developing a plan of action steps, and implementing the strategic plan.

Planning the Planning

As in any endeavor, good preparation is important to a successful outcome. The key question in this stage is "What do we need to think about regarding our planning process?" The following questions can be used to guide the organization through this process:

Why are we planning at this time?

How do we establish a mandate?

What is our time frame?

What is the readiness of the unit?

Who should be involved? What roles should they play?

What will the planning process be?

Is there member support for strategic planning?

Is the unit willing to dedicate the time and resources to planning?

Forecasting the Future Environment

The key question in this stage is "What are we going into?" Although it is impossible to accurately foretell the future, the members of the organization can make educated guesses about potential changes and trends. The following questions should be considered:

What macro changes (large-scale external changes, such as the economy) are predicted that will have an impact on our organization?

What trends do we see around the basic demographics affecting our membership?

How is the business environment likely to change in the next 3 to 5 years?

What is the regulatory environment likely to be?

What weak or distant forces are likely to come into play?

What changes in technology may affect our operations?

What changes are predicted in the availability of quality members to join the unit?

What do we anticipate in terms of members and clients leaving the unit?

Formulating the Vision and Mission

The key question in this stage is "Where are we going?" Typically, a vision statement encompasses the next 3 to 5 years of the organization's operations, and the mission statement focuses on what the organization will be doing in the coming year (Abrahams, 1995; F. David, 2001).

A vision statement expresses the long-term goals of the organization, and is based on the values held by the organization (F. David, 2001; Wright et al., 1998). The following questions should be considered in formulating the vision statement:

What are the core values and guiding principles? Individually and as a unit?

What aspects of current culture should be changed?

What about us is unique?

What is our source of energy and commitment?

How would we like to be known in the future?

What are the values of our stakeholders? Are our values consistent with these stakeholders?

The strategic planning committee next develops a statement of mission that should succinctly summarize what business the organization is in and should concisely declare the purpose or function that the unit is attempting to fulfill in society or the economy. In so doing, the following questions should be considered:

What is the core or primary reason we exist (function)?

What are the secondary reasons?

Who are our primary clients?

How does the unit go about servicing its clients?

What is different about our business from what it was 3 to 5 years ago?

What is the driving force: services offered? Profit?

What makes the difference between success and failure in this business?

Each unit or department head should develop a mission statement for each of the departments of the organization. These statements should be derived from the organization's overall mission statement. Each department head should present his or her mission statement to the strategic planning committee for critique, especially as to whether the goals are consistent with the organization's mission statement and the values of the division.

Current Status

The key question in this stage is "Where are we now?" Before developing a plan for the future, the organization must be clear in its knowledge of where it is starting from. A brief assessment should be made of the current status of the organization and each department, in consideration of the following questions:

What do we currently do? To what ends?

How do we operate? What is our structure?

What are our services?

What are our vital statistics (composition, size, finances—budget, assets, liabilities)?

What are our origins, purposes, values, and functions?

External Environment

It is important to develop an awareness of the larger context of which the organization and its departments is a part. Those attending the strategic planning meeting should consider both potential threats and potential opportunities in the external environment, and should discuss the following questions:

Who are our current allies, competitors, and adversaries?

What events or circumstances are likely to occur that threaten us or present us with unique opportunities?

What are the forces outside our unit that are likely to support or resist change?

What actions of ours can generate new options or opportunities?

What assumptions do we currently have that we could challenge about our environment?

Internal Environment

Likewise, an honest assessment should be made of the strengths and weaknesses of the internal context of the organization. The organizational members should discuss the following questions:

What are our principal services?

What is the quality of our services?

What forces exist for change and improvement?

What forces are restraining us from improving?

What untapped potential can we identify?

What is the status of relationships, rewards, procedures, structure, and leadership in our organization?

What currently drives this unit? Services offered, market needs, customer needs, technology, production capacity, size/growth, return/profits?

Overall Strategy

The key question in this stage is "What is most important to think about in terms of how we get where we want to be?" The overall strategy must be determined before the specific steps can be considered. In choosing an overall strategy, the following questions should be considered:

What are the key result areas that will determine our success?

What long-range objectives will best support our mission?

What operational moves are critical and possible?

Table 12.1 lists major strategies that organizations can adopt.

Table 12.1   Strategic Planning Initiatives in Organizations

Strategy	Definition
Forward integration	Gaining ownership or increased control over distributors or retailers
Backward integration	Seeking ownership or increased control of a firm's suppliers
Horizontal integration	Seeking ownership or increased control over competitors
Market penetration	Seeking increased market share for present products or services in present markets through greater marketing efforts
Market development	Introducing present products or services into new geographic area
Product development	Seeking increase sales by improving present products or services or developing new ones
Concentric diversification	Adding new, but related, products or services
Conglomerate diversification	Adding new, unrelated products or services
Horizontal diversification	Adding new, unrelated products or services for present customers
Joint venture	Two or more sponsoring firms forming a separate organization for cooperative purposes
Retrenchment	Regrouping through cost and asset reduction to reverse declining sales and profit
Divestiture	Selling a division or part of an organization
Liquidation	Selling all of a company's assets, in parts, for their tangible worth

Source: From *Strategic Management,* eighth edition, by F. David, 2001, Upper Saddle River, NJ: Prentice-Hall.

Relation of the Strategy to Our Capacity

The key question in this stage is "How can we avoid not getting there by being overwhelmed?" The organization must determine how it will implement its chosen strategy given its current capacity and resources, in consideration of the following questions:

Which of our goals and objectives are beyond our reach?

What would have to change to be realistic?

Where are the needed areas for creativity and invention?

What priorities and timing would help us achieve our objectives?

Plan of Action Steps

The key question in this stage is "How do we get there?" At this point, the organization members should establish the specific goals and business objectives it will need to fulfill the mission statement.

Each unit or department head should establish goals and business objectives for each subunit of the unit. These statements should be derived from the unit mission statement, in line with the organization's overall mission statement. Each unit head should present the unit's goals and business objectives to the strategic planning committee for critique, especially as to whether the goals and objectives are consistent with the unit mission statement and values of the unit.

All members in the unit should list action steps for the unit and their subunit that will accomplish the mission statements taking the unit from where it is now to where it should go. Each action step should be as specific as possible, and should attempt to make the outcomes measurable within a specific time frame. Organization members should try to take advantage of any current opportunities and guard against any potential threats.

Each person should then present the action steps to the strategic planning group, which critiques the plan, again making certain that the mission statement and values of the organization are served.

The team places in priority the action steps of the unit and subunit through the nominal group technique. The strategic planning team then reviews a draft of a compilation of the plan and makes appropriate revisions. The strategic planning committee should also develop appropriate contingency plans, since things rarely go the way we want them to in actual practice.

Important questions to consider in this stage are:

What is the best way to involve the entire organization in the change process?

What conflicts can be expected and how can they best be managed?

Implementation of the Strategic Plan

The key mission of this stage is actually "getting there." The best and most impressive plans are worthless if they are not properly implemented. Action steps should be assigned to specific organization members with due dates, and progress should be monitored by the managing members. The following questions should be considered in this stage:

What control systems are needed and what management reports will be required?

What are the criteria for success and for identifying needed corrective action?

Who needs to get feedback on the unit changes? Who should give it?

What parts of the external environment need to be informed or assessed?

What reward systems will ensure continuing motivation for improvement?

What contingency plans need to be made for efforts that do not meet expectations?

The strategic plan should be revisited periodically and modified to meet changing internal and external conditions. The time frames for these reviews should be agreed on before the end of the strategic planning session.

Whereas a strategic plan is a general short- and long-range plan for where the company is going, the business plan is a detailed document that encompasses the strategic plan and describes how the business will operate at all levels. There are many good sources for business planning (Abrams, 2003; B. Adams, 2002; S. Peterson & Jaret,

2001; Pinson, 2001), but detailed plans are meaningless before the organization has completed its strategic planning.

SWOT Analysis

Business schools continue to teach business leaders today a simple shorthand formula for conceptualizing business strategies (F. David, 2001; DuBrin, 2000; Whetten & Cameron, 2002). A SWOT analysis focuses on an organization's *strengths, weaknesses, opportunities,* and *threats.* The first two items are internal to the organization, and the second two items are external to the organization. Strengths are those things that the organization can build on and use to its advantage. Weaknesses within the organization should be acknowledged, and can either be tolerated, ignored, or fixed. Opportunities refer to situational factors in the external environment that can be exploited by the organization to its benefit. Threats are situational factors in the external environment that have a potential for negative impact on the organization. Threats must be anticipated to minimize the likelihood of their occurrence, and contingency plans should be made to deal with potential and inevitable problems.

This model can be used as a brief planning model. Strengths and weaknesses involve the current state of the organization. Opportunities and threats involve planning for the future. Comparing where the organization is now versus where it would like to be in the future is known as a "gap analysis." Possible new paradigms and visions of the future should be considered, along with the values of the organization. These should be compared with its present state, and action items should be created to reduce the gap between the present condition and the future desired condition of the organization.

Dr. Weismann approaches the consultee, excited about the potential benefits of conducting a strategic planning meeting. The consultee is a bit skeptical though about the value of taking the time to do this. He remembers reading about strategic planning in graduate school, but he had always felt that it was simply "common sense stuff," and not worth the time involved. However, given the current state of the organization, and the strength of the rapport that has been developed, the consultee is willing to give it a try.

With the support and assistance of Dr. Weismann, the managers of the organization compile an inclusive list of employees to attend the strategic planning session. A Friday afternoon is reserved at a local hotel conference room to begin the session. It soon becomes apparent to everyone involved that it is not at all clear why the organization is in existence and where it should be going. Almost every member seems to have a different idea of what the organization should be doing. Some members felt that profit alone was the only important goal, some felt that the most important thing was to provide a good living for the employees, some felt that providing services to the underserved was primary, and some felt that the organization should be committed to providing cutting-edge technologies. While all of these and the other goals were important, they sometimes work against each other when setting goals. Dr. Weismann skillfully uses his group process facilitation skills to keep the members communicating openly and honestly, but at the end of the session, the members cannot even agree on how exactly the mission statement should be formulated.

After the meeting, the consultee thanks Dr. Weismann for his help, acknowledging that it is no wonder that the organization is not doing well when no one agrees what exactly should be done. Plans are quickly made to set aside several days the following week to continue these meetings.

PART FOUR

SPECIAL TOPICS

Chapter 13

PRACTICE MANAGEMENT

This chapter investigates some of the practical issues in establishing a consulting practice, as well as some of the ethical issues involved in consultation. While there are many sources of information for the specific details of running a consulting business (Cohen, 2001; B. Nelson & Economy, 1997; Weiss, 2004; Yenney, 1994), this chapter will focus on an overview of issues most relevant to those with a mental health background.

GETTING STARTED

Potential clients working in both business and medical settings look more at experience and ability than credentials. For them, results are everything. Although it may be helpful to earn an MBA to appear competent to work with organizations, the best way to build a consulting business is to do a good job. When an opportunity presents itself, thoroughly prepare for the job and execute the assignment with quality. Though it may be slow to get started, business will likely increase through reputation spread by word-of-mouth.

To build a consultation business as a clinician, one typically starts with clinical work and only later moves into consultation. Having a clinical private practice may be more likely to provide a steady income. The clinician may then later decide to get involved in consultation to break the monotony of clinical work with the challenges of working in a new setting. The clinician may also feel a pull to do consultation work after developing a larger systemic understanding based on the contexts being presented by therapeutic clients. As an analogy, clinical work is usually trying to pull someone out of the stream downriver, and consultation is usually trying to deal with the person who is throwing the people into the stream.

If a clinician in a private psychotherapy practice gains several clients who all happen to work in the same section of a large hospital, the clinician should consider offering consultation to that hospital unit.

If a clinician working at a prison receives numerous questions and individual requests for supervision in dealing with difficult inmates, the clinician could offer to conduct a training session on that subject.

A clinician may notice that many executives are presenting with complaints of being lonely and isolated, with no one to confide in. The clinician might consider setting up a therapy or support group for CEOs, perhaps through the chamber of commerce.

For those mental health professionals who are serious about establishing a consulting practice, the guidelines in Chapter 12 on strategic planning should be useful in formulating a business plan.

Martin (1996) lists practical challenges faced by mental health professionals as they transition from private practice to organizational practice:

- Creating a consulting service and product line that meets the needs of the targeted corporate market while platforming and showcasing various clinical talents, specialties and successes.
- Learning the inner workings of the business world as well as various industry technologies in order to establish the credibility needed to secure consulting contracts.
- Adapting to the new language and rituals of the business world while simultaneously observing and dispelling its myths and illusions.
- Marketing oneself through the use of business cards, brochures, presentations and seminars.
- Protecting oneself legally and financially in a new career with different boundaries, ethical implications and professional liabilities than a clinical practice.
- Establishing contacts within corporations that lead to meeting with qualified decision makers who control management services budgets and authorize consultancy projects.
- Mastering a sales process which includes approaching the decision-maker, undertaking a needs analysis, designing the project proposal, closing the contract, and measuring results.
- Building a consulting practice distinguished from the competition based on a timeless positioning that can be communicated through a simple tag line. (pp. 7–8)

Martin (1996) also warns about the internal and interpersonal challenges of making such a transition:

- Coping with fantasies of failure that surface with a monumental change in career identity. These manifest somatically (the nausea accompanying the first sales call) or resigned as inner voices discouraging one from making any possible contribution to the business world at all.
- The initial terror of having to physically go onsite for a client visit. It's one thing to think about leaving one's office to do this new kind of work. An altogether different barrier exists when visiting a prospective client to make the pitch.
- Managing the grief of losing the "doctor knows best" image when consulting in a corporate environment; where "PhD" often means "mind reader" and the less said about a clinical background, the better.
- Proactively competing for business against aggressive management consultants who want to control the lion's share of the corporate consulting budget.
- Preparing the family for your entrance into the corporate world. This will include subscriptions to publications such as *Industry Week, Forbes, Fortune,* and the *Wall Street Journal* and an obsession with the daily activities of the world's financial markets. This entails a change in your image as well: trading in tweed blazers for Armani suits and Italian loafers.
- Being comfortable as an advisor to corporate clients, who are often amazed by the psychotherapist's ability to apply clinical principles to business operations and then devise viable solutions that work. (Executives are truly impressed by the lightning quick ability clinicians have in applying complex psychological concepts to a variety of everyday business problems.) (pp. 8–9)

Martin (1996) suggests some important do's and don'ts for consultants to consider when building a consulting practice. These are listed in Box 13.1.

===== **Box 13.1** =====

Do's and Don'ts for Building a Consulting Practice

- *Do* entertain your clients regularly. Lunches, dinners, sports events, and conferences are appropriate social occasions. Bonding must continue to deepen. Unlike private patients, corporate clients expect to be entertained, and social occasions are excellent update and strategy sessions.
- *Do* give appropriate gifts such as books, CDs, audiotapes, gift baskets, and videos. Make sure that you note birthdays and send cards [assuming the individual celebrates birthdays]. This nurturing is not expected and will be much appreciated.
- *Do* document your project weekly as well as any changes in its scope and direction. Start this process by preparing a contract and making sure it is signed before you begin work. All changes in scope require client sign-off as well.
- *Do* detail your payment terms and collect fees prior to delivering work. This starts with a preliminary retainer.
- *Do* give formal presentations of successes and project progress and barriers once or twice a month. The consulting process requires endless justification and salesmanship, as well as client direction and support to keep it effective.
- *Don't* ignore the client support personnel, like secretaries and administrative assistants. They can make or break your project. Include them in gifts and other forms of acknowledgment.
- *Don't* promise what you can't deliver or commit to unrealistic time frames. Clients detest consultants who oversell their contribution or can't deliver on time.
- *Don't* assume any client knowledge that you learn is in the public domain. Do not discuss your clients with anyone except your clinical supervisor. Many profitable relationships have been destroyed by "airplane socializing."
- *Don't* ask for referrals. Wait until sufficient reciprocity is built and they will come spontaneously. Give your corporate clients time to see the benefits in what you provide.
- *Don't* abuse your client relationship by becoming a broker of sorts. Other consultants will approach you for referrals to your top clients. If you believe their services are needed, then make an introduction. However, taking fees for this reduces you to being a "broker."

Source: From *Couch to Corporation: Becoming a Successful Corporate Therapist* (pp. 83–84), by I. Martin, 1996, New York: Wiley.

PRACTICE MANAGEMENT ISSUES

Record keeping is very important for mental health professionals, and some type of systemic method should be adopted for tracking one's consultation work (Rudisill & Archambault, 1988, 1999).

Clinicians are accustomed to maintaining patient charts that record the essential demographics of the patient or client, along with such things as treatment plans, progress notes, and correspondence. Although the specifics of such charting may vary from organization to organization, most clinicians are accustomed to and proficient in the demands of clinical record keeping.

Charting for Consultation

As clinicians attempt to play increasingly direct roles with employers and companies, ways to monitor the relationship between the clinician and company must be devised. The "Company Chart" is a method of record keeping that tracks the progress of the clinician's relationship with a company. The Company Chart is analogous to the clinical charts that are used with patients or clients.

When a clinician works directly with companies, it is important to track the assignments and obligations that develop along with the various company relationships. Remembering key contacts and following up on assignments and opportunities are important survival skills in corporate practice.

There are several other reasons for developing a corporate chart. Being able to review the entire relationship with a company allows consultants to plan and act strategically to maximize their contribution to a company. If the primary consultant needs assistance with the work or needs to transfer the assignment, the record will enable another consultant to rapidly learn the progress to date on a consulting project. New consultants can see what has been done thus far and get a feel for the culture and needs of an organization prior to entering the system.

Figure 13.1 presents a sample charting system for use by clinicians in their work with companies. This form can be used in solo or group practices to monitor relationships with company officials and can be modified to suit the consultant's needs. Mental health professionals will find the "DAP" (Data/Description, Assessment, Plan) format of the progress notes to be familiar. These organizational notes can easily be maintained within a word processing computer program (as a paperless chart) as well as by means of a physical chart (Rudisill & Archambault, 1988, 1999). If the consultant is also doing clinical work with members of a particular organization, separate clinical charts should be maintained for those patients or clients to maintain the confidentiality of their information.

Consultants may also choose to add other pieces of information to their charts including personality notes on key people such as their personal and business values (what is important to them), interpersonal style, conversational interests, and needs and motivators. Consultants could also include a table of organization, pre- and postevaluations, information about billing such as timeliness, or anything else the consultant finds valuable.

It is typically useful to review the charts on a periodic basis to pick up any loose ends and suggested leads. The consultant should use chart notes to place important dates (such as follow-up progress meetings) in their calendars. The consultant's top 10 accounts may perhaps be reviewed monthly, while inactive or smaller accounts can perhaps be reviewed every 6 months.

Billing

Billing arrangements should be made clear in the initial agreement between the consultant and the consultee. There are several ways to bill the client; the one best known to clinicians is *fee-for-service* based billing. In this arrangement, the client is billed for

EXAMPLE CONSULTING, INC.
Company Chart

Company Demographics

Company Name: XYZ Company

Address: 123 Brown Street, Dayton, Ohio 45424

Telephone: (937) 555-5555   Fax: (937) 555-5555

Product/Service: Office forms

Size of Company (gross sales): 50 million   No. of Employees: 250

Ownership Structure (*private or public*): Family owned

Referred by: Mary Smith, PhD

Original Contact Person: Mr. George Person, CEO, 555-5555, person@example.com

Original Referral Issue: Team building for the executive team

Additional Contract Stakeholders:

Ms. Linda Individual, HR Director, 555-5555, individual@example.com

EXAMPLE CONSULTING, INC.

Psychological Intervention Plan

Company Name: XYZ Company

Provider(s):   John R. Rudisill, PhD
               Richard Sears, PsyD, MBA

Date of Initial Plan: December 15, 2005

Date of Revised Plan:

Problem Analysis Summary (*includes concise statement of the referral problem and the consultant's analysis of the problem*): XYZ Company has been bought by ABC Corporation and Mr. George Person is the new CEO. He has replaced the existing management team and brought in his own group of executives. He wants to do team building to get his new team off to a good start.

Overall Intervention Goal(s): To improve the functioning of the executive team

Objective(s): To provide team building to the executive team

Intervention(s): Team building, including interviewing each manager at the company, holding a 2-day off-site team-building retreat, meeting for a follow-up on the action plans in 6 months

Contract for Services (*includes financial arrangement*): $5,000 for the project to be completed by March 15, 2006.

Additional Services to be Marketed (*here the consultant can note if additional services appear to be needed during the course of the project*): Team building for the executives' teams, strategic planning for the company, executive coaching.

(continued)

Figure 13.1   Sample charting system.

Organizational Progress Note

Date of contact and whether an actual or phone contact was made is entered with each contact with a company employee.

12/1/05 Phone call from Mr. Person

D (*Description of the contact*) = Mr. Person called today on referral from Mary Smith whom he had seen for marital counseling. Mr. Person wants to build a strong executive team and a common culture. He is particularly concerned about Mr. Human, the CFO, because he is a holdover from the old management team.

A (*Assessment of the contact*) = Mr. Person appears eager to build a team and is willing to commit resources to "front load" his team's functioning.

P (*Intervention plan*) = Meet with Mr. Person to discuss his goals and expectations for the team building and to begin to negotiate a process for accomplishment of his goals.

Signature and title of the consultant

John R. Rudisill, PhD
Director, Example Consulting, Inc.

12/7/05 Luncheon meeting with Mr. Person and Ms. Linda Individual, HR Director at Bingo Restaurant, Drs. Rudisill and Sears

D = Mr. Person is trying to implement a culture based upon four "P"s—Product, People, Partnerships, and Profit. He wants to make sure that all of his new managers are on board with his philosophy and intended culture. He also wants his team to develop an initial rapport and begin to understand their individual differences. He would like us to work with Ms. Individual regarding the arrangements for the team-building process.

A = Mr. Person seems to want to create a specific culture and to improve the likelihood of his team working together effectively. We will need to help the team understand, and where appropriate, grieve the old culture prior to moving forward with the new culture.

P = Send a thank-you note regarding the meeting (attachment 1) and one week later send a contract with a preliminary design for the team building process (attachment 2). The specific retreat will be designed after Richard and I meet with the managers.

Attachments

Attachments are exhibits (e.g., training programs, thank-you letters, contracts, surveys, project management outlines) that are referenced in the progress notes.

Figure 13.1 Continued.

December 7, 2005

Mr. George Person, CEO
XYZ Company
123 Brown Street
Dayton, Ohio 45424

Dear George:

Thank you for the opportunity to meet over lunch to discuss developing a "team-building" program for the Executive staff of XYZ Company. I am impressed by your commitment to developing a well-functioning team and your foresight in wanting to "front load" the team-building process. I will be sending you a proposal next week regarding the team-building project. I look forward to working with you.

Yours truly,

John R. Rudisill, PhD
Director, Example Consulting, Inc.

PROPOSAL

Team Building

This proposal outlines an individualized team-building process designed to improve communications among the executive team at the XYZ Company.

SCOPE OF THE PROJECT

The consultant will interview each manager at the company to assess the "state of the team." The consultant presents the results of these findings at a 2-day off-site retreat for the executive team. The themes resulting from the assessment process will form the agenda for the retreat. Six months following the retreat, a 1-day retreat will be held to follow-up on action items generated by the initial retreat.

The purpose of the initial interviews is to assess the current state of the team. The purpose of the team-building sessions is to develop the (a) interpersonal effectiveness of the newly consti-tuted team, (b) understand the previous culture, (c) formulate the new culture, (d) understand their own communication style (strengths and weaknesses), and (e) develop specific strate-gies to work effectively together in the future.

TIME ESTIMATE

The entire project (except for the 6-month follow-up meeting) will be completed by March 15, 2006. The individual interviews will occur during the last week of January and the retreat will be held during the last week of February.

Figure 13.1 Continued.

COST

$5,000 for the project.

CONFIDENTIALITY

Participants will be granted anonymity but not confidentiality. Information shared in the interviews will be aggregated and presented to the entire group.

CONSULTANTS

This proposal is presented by John R. Rudisill, PhD & Richard Sears, PsyD, MBA of Example Consulting, Inc. Dr. Rudisill and Dr. Sears are organizational consultants. Both Dr. Rudisill and Dr. Sears may be reached at (937) 555-5555.

Program Evaluation

Results of a program evaluation of your contact with the company are recorded here (e.g., customer satisfaction survey, etc.)

The evaluation of the team-building project would go in this section.

Closing Comments

The consultant would here include notes about the disposition of the case, e.g., if the case was transferred to another consultant.

Figure 13.1   Continued.

each hour that the consultant works on the project. Although this initially seems like an attractive way of doing things, when based on the average hourly rate for psychotherapy as well as extra expenses like travel time and traveling costs, the resulting hourly rate often sounds exorbitant to consultees. Additionally, business-minded executives may be worried about the consultant dragging certain jobs on to increase their pay.

Project-based billing involves setting a specified fee for the entire consulting service. Weiss (2004) recommends using this billing method exclusively. It allows the consultant to focus on accomplishing the project apart from counting hours. Consultees like this method, as the set fee is more easily incorporated into their budgets, and they do not have to worry about consultants prolonging their services unnecessarily. A danger with this method is that projects can sometimes be more complicated than first estimated, resulting in increased time and resource expenditure by the consultant. However, provision can be made for this in the initial agreement, and most consultees will be open to reasonable renegotiation.

Retainer-based billing involves receiving a set fee (usually on a monthly basis) from the consultee for the privilege of having access to the consultant when needed. This can provide a more steady income for the consultant, but may result in unpredictable time investment in the consultee's organization.

Value-based billing involves billing based on the value that the consultant believes has been provided to the organization. This is usually an add-on to what may have already been set through project-based billing or retainer based billing. This happens most often when the consultant has a long-term relationship with the consultee, and is somewhat subjective. A consultant who thinks that the service provided far exceeded expectations may simply ask the consultee to provide a higher payment for the service. Likewise, a consultant who feels that the project did not go very well, may reduce the fees charged to the consultee.

Setting billing fees can be challenging. Charging too much discourages clients from using the services, while charging too little appears unprofessional and makes it difficult and awkward to raise the fees at a later date. Researching what other consultants in the area charge can be helpful, as well as stressing in the proposal the end value of the consulting services to that organization. Charging different rates to different clients is not a good policy. It is best to charge the same rates for everyone, but to offer discounts for certain groups.

Marketing

Although word of mouth is helpful in sustaining an established consulting practice, it is imperative to develop a comprehensive marketing plan, especially for start-up enterprises. For more details on the specifics of developing marketing plans, consultants can reference business textbooks such as Lamb et al. (2003).

One way to develop a reputation in the community is to give away a few services per year to nonprofit institutions. These are known as *loss leaders,* because even though consultants lose time and money on these projects, they may lead to future business. Serving on the governing boards of nonprofit agencies is also helpful (J. Carver & Carver, 1997; Houle, 1997).

Another approach is to talk to as many groups of people as possible (e.g., clubs, universities, and the local chamber of commerce). Doing seminars on selected topics serves several beneficial functions. It helps consultants get exposure in the community, establishes their reputation as experts, and fosters confidence so that people get to know and feel comfortable with the consultants' services. By performing specialized seminars for specialized groups, a consultant can develop a reputation for being the only person in the area qualified to handle such issues. Seminars are also a good place to gather qualitative data. By informally conversing with attendees, consultants can gather a sense of the needs of the community and what potential barriers there may be to seeking their services. It is important to network as often as possible, even with other consultants or with individuals who are already using consultants. Conflicts of interest, lack of expertise, or too much business may arise, prompting referrals to or from these sources.

In terms of the market, there are many consultants, but very few with a mental health background. Hence, it is sensible to play up strengths, such as expertise in process, assessment, people skills, counseling skills, group dynamics, and systems awareness (assuming previous training in these areas).

When developing a marketing plan, it is essential to consider what consumers want. In general, they look for inexpensive, prompt, hassle-free service (effortless, flawless, and instantaneous performance); premium service (with consumers raising their standards continuously); and superior and innovative products. Although no single business can fulfill all of these desires, focusing on one or several of them may help distinguish the consultant from competitors.

There are two major types of marketing in consultation: that done to secure new contracts, and that done to extend existing contracts (e.g., a consultant who has done executive coaching for an organization may be asked to give regular seminars on mental health issues in the workplace). For established consultants, practice growth comes mainly from extending existing contracts, with existing clients creating new contracts through word of mouth.

An Internet presence can be an effective marketing tool, both for attracting new business and for providing information to current clients. A web site should describe the consultant's background and qualifications and should provide descriptions and examples of services offered. An added bonus, designed to attract new clients and to keep your past and current clients interested, would be to provide free information and tips for organizations on the web site. Consultants can create white papers that apply scientific thought to specific real-world organizational situations. The knowledge and skills of mental health professionals can be very valuable for organizational settings. Box 13.2 is an example of a white paper.

Business marketing texts extol the value of conceptualizing marketing using the "4Ps"—Product, Place, Promotion, Price—that together are known as the *marketing mix* (Lamb et al., 2003). Product refers to everything that is offered to the consultee. A consultant should carefully consider the types of consulting services to offer potential consultees. Will the consultant perform crisis consultation? Will a consultant offer seminars and workshops, and if so, on what topics? What about executive coaching and development? Knowing exactly what kinds of products will be offered helps the consultant develop a better plan to market those products.

Place refers to distribution strategies. Where will the consultant offer services? Will the consultant typically travel to the organization's facilities? How far is the consultant willing to travel for consultation services or for conducting seminars? Will services be conducted online, by telephone, or only in person?

Promotion refers to all of the strategies involved in getting the word out to potential customers. This could include advertising, press releases, promotional events, and personal selling.

Prices can be raised and lowered, and hence can be used as an important marketing tool. Offering reduced rates to first-time customers can sometimes entice them to use services they might not have otherwise seriously considered.

Segmenting and targeting specific populations for one's services is important to maximize the potential efficacy of one's marketing strategy. An undifferentiated approach, in which all members of organizations are lumped together to receive the same marketing message, is likely to be inefficient at best. Segmentation of the communities that the consultant wants to work with is likely to be far more effective. The consultant may then approach one (a concentrated strategy) or several (a multi-segment strategy) of these segments simultaneously or sequentially (Lamb et al., 2003). A consultant's potential clients have both shared and unique needs. Traditionally, clients may be divided into the categories of individual executives, nonprofit agencies, small businesses, and large corporations. However, within these are many subcategories. Within the nonprofit sector, there are mental health agencies, hospitals, and museums. The potential client community may also be segmented by geography (e.g., by city, county, state, or country; by urban or rural settings), demographics (e.g., age, gender, income, ethnicity), psychographics (e.g., personality, motives, lifestyles), benefits (e.g., increased well-being, improved relationships), and usage rate (e.g., those who frequently involve themselves in self-improvement activities; Lamb et al., 2003).

All of these factors should be considered when developing a marketing plan, which provides a systematic way to build the consulting business.

Box 13.2

Using Cognitive Dissonance Theory to Increase Market Share
Richard W. Sears, PsyD, MBA (www.psych-insights.com)

Many businesses cater their products, services, and advertising to the needs and wants of consumers. However, by skillfully applying the concept of cognitive dissonance (first used in social psychology), businesses can create demand for their products or services. Though the details of the theory are complex (and critical for successful implementation), once mastered, the concept opens the door to nearly limitless marketing opportunities. In this paper, I present a brief background and some general principles of the theory. I then suggest how it might be applied to marketing for use in strategic planning, in order to more consciously diversify and expand market share.

Using Cognitive Dissonance to Increase Market Share

In a free market, competitive pressures keep prices down to an equilibrium level. Yet certain companies have certain products that rise up into near-monopoly positions. This allows the company to charge higher prices. But why should consumers pay more when a basic, low-price product will likely fulfill the purpose for which the product was designed? After all, it could be argued that those with wealth have created or maintained it through intelligent financial management. Why should some consumers desire all the "bells and whistles?" There is a certain qualitative satisfaction in saying that this discrepancy is due to variations in consumer tastes and preferences, but this explanation does not give much predictive power. Though tastes and preferences may never be fully understood or fully predictable, applying the classical concept of "cognitive dissonance" from social psychology (Aronson, 1999; Festinger, 1957) may help to illuminate some deeper reasons for this phenomenon.

The theory of cognitive dissonance was first formulated by Leon Festinger (1957). In the 1950s, the field of psychology was dominated by the idea of behaviorism, which basically taught that all behavior is motivated by rewards and punishment. However, Festinger and Carlsmith (1959) performed an experiment that the behaviorists could not explain.

Festinger and Carlsmith randomly divided their subjects into two groups. Both were given the same repetitive, boring task to do. However, the members of one group were paid $1 each and the members of the other group were paid $20 for their participation. They were then asked to tell the next subject coming in that the task had been very interesting. The original subjects were later asked to rate how interesting the task actually was.

Behaviorists would have predicted that those who were paid more money (i.e., received more reinforcement) would rate the task as more interesting than those who were only paid $1. However, the opposite is what actually occurred.

The researchers explained that those who were paid $20 could rationalize to themselves that they had a good reason to lie to the incoming subjects (they were paid to do so). However, those who were only paid $1 had a hard time rationalizing away the reason that they were lying to other people. Psychic

(Continued)

============================= **Box 13.2 (continued)** =============================

tension, or "cognitive dissonance" was created in their minds between two conflicting thoughts: (1) I am a good person who does not lie, and (2) I lied to someone. In order to reduce this tension, the subjects actually came to believe that the task really had been more interesting than it was.

This psychic tension is often described as a drive that a person seeks to reduce, in the same way that one seeks to reduce the drive for hunger by eating something. Cognitive dissonance is reduced by changing one or both of the conflicting thoughts to be consistent with the person's actions and self-concept. If the tension is too little, no action will result. If it is too great, the person may indulge in denial of the presented message.

Another classical experiment in cognitive dissonance demonstrates an important concept (R. Miller, Brickman, & Bolen, 1975). One group of schoolchildren was told that they "should" do better in math, and another group was told that they "are" good in math. The latter group subsequently performed better in math. This suggests that rather than telling consumers that they should buy a product, it might be better to build them up as the kind of high-class, sophisticated consumer who demands only the best.

To effectively use cognitive dissonance, marketing professionals must create a two-pronged advertising campaign: (1) brand identity, and (2) an image to stir the consumer into action.

Without brand identity (clearly differentiating one's product from the competition), the cognitive dissonance created in consumers may drive them to purchase expensive products from competitors. The product must not only be perceived as superior in some way, but must be unique and different in some identifiable way from all of the products of the competitors.

Fostering an image to create just the right amount of cognitive dissonance is both subtle and tricky, to say the least. The targeted consumer must be able to identity with the image portrayed. In general, the business wants to create a sense in the consumer that (1) people who have good taste, are sophisticated, intelligent, and so on, own X brand product; and (2) I do not own X brand product. For many consumers, the dissonance created may be dissipated by dissociation with a thought such as "Those people are just snobs, I don't need those products," or "That company is obviously just trying to trick me into buying their product." But if the ad is thoughtfully and subtly done, the consumer will feel some tension and will seek to reduce the tension by purchasing the product. This will require segmenting and targeting the market appropriately, depending on the product being sold.

Conclusion

Effective use of cognitive dissonance in a marketing campaign can be an important factor in fostering brand loyalty. Used in the right amount (the major trick), the consumer will feel driven to purchase a particular product. The theory of cognitive dissonance is much more subtle and complex than could be presented here. The important thing for businesses to realize, however, is that this concept can be a powerful tool for creative marketing professionals to diversify and/or expand market share.

=== **Box 13.2 (continued)** ===

References

Aronson, E. (1999). *The social animal* (8th ed.). New York: Worth Publishers.

Festinger, L. (1957). *A theory of cognitive dissonance.* Stanford, CA: Stanford University Press.

Festinger, L., & Carlsmith, J. (1959). Cognitive consequences of forced compliance. *Journal of Abnormal and Social Psychology, 58,* 203–210.

Miller, R., Brickman, P., & Bolen, D. (1975). Attribution versus persuasion as a means of modifying behavior. *Journal of Personality and Social Psychology, 31*(3), 100–119.

Finding a specialty niche is an important way to distinguish oneself. The marketing plan shown in Box 13.3 focuses on the promotion to become a "Diversity Trainer and Consultant."

The marketing plan should be updated every 6 months to 1 year, paying attention to where referrals come from during the period. Be sure to thank people for every referral. This lets them know that their efforts are appreciated and keeps the consultant's name in their minds. When it is necessary to give referrals to a physician or another consultant with more expertise in a specific area, make sure the referral source knows who provided it. If the person does not appreciate it or reciprocate, look for someone else to whom you can make referrals.

The consultant must create in the mind of the potential consultee the belief that the consultant has something of value to offer. When catering to businesses, it is important to emphasize the impact the service will have on the organization's bottom line. Working with a business executive improves the quality of life for that particular individual, but it also improves productivity through such things as improved communication and relationship skills. The increasing popularity of Employee Assistance Programs (EAPs) attests that businesses value the mental health of employees (Yenney, 1994).

Peters and Waterman (1982) discussed three models for customer value: *operational excellence, product leadership,* and *customer intimacy.* Operational excellence means that the consultant can do what others do, but can do it more efficiently and perhaps more inexpensively. Product leadership involves having the best and highest quality product (or service), attracting those who seek the premium niche. Customer intimacy involves having the best relationship with the client, individualizing one's product or service to meet the client's unique needs. Whenever possible, the consultant should try to do work on one or more of these models.

Marketing can be thought of as the process of selling oneself. Rackham and Ruff (1991) use the acronym "SPIN" to conceptualize the types of questions that can be helpful when making initial contact with a potential consultee.

S = Situation Questions

Questions should be initially asked about the client's present situation to establish a background. The consultant should make a personal acknowledgment of what he or she is hearing.

=== **Box 13.3** ===

Sample Marketing Plan

1. Speak to three organizations on the benefits of diversity training:
   a. Human Resource Directors Association
   b. Rotary Club
   c. Local American Society of Training Directors (ASTD)
   Be sure to stamp all materials, hand out cards, and ask people to sign a sheet if they would like more information about services. Follow the mailing of the information with a telephone call or a luncheon meeting.
2. Offer a free program for diversity training to the chamber of commerce. Following the program, contact each participant regarding the possibility of providing a diversity training in their company.
3. Apply to established organizations or speakers bureaus (e.g., the American Management Association) to become a diversity trainer in their course offerings.
4. Develop a telephone ad advertising diversity training services.
5. Put an announcement in various newspapers and local trade publications about the services offered.
6. Network with other diversity trainers about the services offered.
7. Target gatekeepers for such services and introduce yourself to them (e.g., company trainers).
8. Develop marketing materials (brochures, folders, etc.) that describe the program and your ability to consult in the local area.
9. Plan a diversity training workshop for general subscription:
   a. Develop a training announcement and send out selected mailings.
   b. Make high-quality arrangements.
10. Provide high-quality training and follow-up and continuously improve the offering by:
    a. Constant self and participant evaluation.
    b. Consider the development of audiovisual materials (e.g., cassette tapes) for purchase by other participants or in league with other companies to sell.
    c. Follow up on participants to see if you can meet additional needs or if they know of other companies that could use your services.

P = Problem Questions

Inquiries about the client's present situation should lead to questions that clarify the client's problems, difficulties, or dissatisfactions. The consultant should communicate an understanding of the problem.

I = Implication Questions

The client's concerns should be further clarified and developed by asking about the effects or consequences of the client's problems, which will give a shared understanding of the situation. The consultant should help the client verbally formulate needs and wants.

N = Need-Payoff Questions

Questions should then be asked about the value or usefulness of a proposed approach or solution. The consultant should then offer solutions and discuss an offer for services.

Research

Research is a major component in the professional training of most mental health professionals, and this training is important to apply to one's marketing strategy. Information gathered from simply asking "How did you hear about us?" when a new consultee calls the consultant unexpectedly can easily be used to track referral sources. If educational seminars or professional consultations, for which you receive payment, attract more clients than expensive newspaper or phonebook ads, then obviously you should invest your efforts and resources in the former strategies.

Consultants should take time to research the business aspects of running their consulting firms before beginning their practices. The best way to learn about something is to talk to people who are already doing what you want to do. If possible, an aspiring consultant should try to find a mentor, or at least interview another mental health professional who has become a consultant (preferably in another geographic region so that there will be no direct competition). Sindermann and Sawyer (1997) conducted a survey of scientists who had become consultants. Following is a summary of their findings:

- Most commonly, consultants started their businesses with personal funds or bank loans.
- Those who decided to form their businesses with a charter (e.g., incorporating), frequently used legal assistance.
- Early consulting contracts were most often secured through directly soliciting individuals and organizations or through word-of-mouth.
- Personal reputation is considered vital, as most consulting contracts come from referrals and from personal contacts.
- A well-developed, informative brochure about the consultant's services is considered essential.
- The majority of the clients of scientific consultants were through state or federal government, private industry, or other consultants (through subcontracting).
- Financial benefit is a primary reason for becoming a consultant, though many also desire freedom and independence and the opportunity to further develop their professional skills. Consultants find satisfaction in being able to creatively apply their expertise to help their clients.
- A large part of a consultant's time is spent doing research and writing reports and proposals, with relatively little time spent in meetings. The amount of travel for most consultants is very high, though this can fluctuate greatly.
- Charging hourly rates is very common, as well as using fixed costs. Some consultants use a cost-plus method. Some consultants use competitive bidding, though this requires some skill and knowledge of how competitors cost their services.
- Most employers require confidentiality agreements, and consultants feel that their work should be kept confidential.

- Consultants who work for consulting firms do not usually have a proprietary interest in the projects of the company, and most employers of consultants do not provide royalties or profit sharing (except perhaps in retirement plans).
- Almost all consultants who work for a consulting firm are involved in a wide variety of consulting projects and activities.
- Most consultants assume primary responsibility for their consulting work, whether they are independent or work for a consulting firm.
- Consultants are sometimes required to make statements or suggestions that are contrary to their personal feelings, and must sometimes accept decisions with which they do not agree.
- Many consultants reported that their findings were misrepresented by their clients when used to make decisions. This was thought of as a problem by half of the survey respondents.
- Rejection of findings for political reasons was reported by 65% of the survey respondents, suggesting that consultants should not take this too personally.
- Work performed by consultants does not always satisfy the client, especially when dealing with controversial issues.
- Consulting projects often make use of subcontracting to ensure success.
- Consultants have difficulty maintaining a steady flow of work (it is often "feast or famine").
- Getting paid on time is a major concern to consultants, especially when they have high expenses and low cash reserves.
- Survey respondents noted a wide range of stress in various projects, from very high to very little. Stress most often comes from meeting deadlines, excessive travel, and facing difficult and complex consulting problems.
- International consulting can be difficult due to communication challenges and philosophical or cultural differences.
- Consultants often find that clients feel they have become experts on a subject simply because of the expertise purchased from the consultant, and sometimes overstate their expertise to others after receiving the consultant's report.

MANAGING DIFFICULT CONSULTEES

Early on in their careers, consultants may be happy to receive any business at all. However, they must also be on guard against certain clients who can create problems. Sindermann and Sawyer (1997) call these "clients from hell," and caution consultants to avoid them whenever possible:

- The make-believe client who has no intention of ever hiring the consultant. Such a client invites the consultant in to talk about the situation in order to get free information or ideas, but does not follow-through with a contract or any payment.
- The would-be client who solicits proposals from many consultants, but has already decided to use a particular one. The consultant wastes a great deal of time gathering data and writing a proposal that may not even get read. This sometimes happens because a company has a policy that requires a manager to get several bids before hiring a consultant.

- The would-be client who wants to award a contract to a personal friend or relative. Such a person may ask for proposals from other consultants, and then give them to the friend or relative so that they can copy the best information for their own proposal.
- The client who, after hiring the consultant, continually asks the consultant to do additional work without wanting to give additional pay.
- The client who continually tries to micromanage the daily activities of the consultant.
- The client who is suspicious about every expense item, requiring overly detailed explanations for every expenditure.
- The client who always pays late, or who does not pay at all unless taken to court, later claiming that the consultant's work was unsatisfactory.
- The client who has a hidden agenda, unknown to the consultant who provided information in good faith.
- The client who asks the consultant to change the findings in the consultant's report to better suit the client's needs or agenda.

Sindermann and Sawyer (1997) provide consultants with the following suggestions for defending themselves against the clients from hell:

- Conduct a preliminary screening of the client or organization. Talk to colleagues or other consultants who may have had past interactions with the organization.
- Provide a standard credit form as part of the early interaction with the company, and ask for (and check) references.
- Check local and state tax records to find out about the organization's length of existence and financial health.
- Research the organization through the local chamber of commerce, better business bureau, or trade associations.

ETHICAL ISSUES IN CONSULTATION

Ethics is concerned with a consensual agreement on standards of professional care, based on scientific principles. Research in consulting does not yet exist to any great degree, so the field is learning by doing. As mental health professionals, we have received a great deal of training and supervision concerning ethical issues (Koocher et al., 1995; Lowman, 2002a, 2002b). Each mental health profession has its own code of ethics, consisting of aspirational principles and enforceable guidelines. The general aspirational principles (meaning they are aspired to but not enforceable) from the American Psychological Association (2002) apply to consulting:

- Competence
- Integrity
- Professional and scientific responsibility
- Concern for others' welfare
- Social responsibility

Consulting ethics are less clear than clinical ethics at this point. Only the most recent revisions in the APA Ethical Principles (American Psychological Association, 2002) have paid more attention to consulting.

Having a code of ethics is important because consultation is often an ambiguous activity. Consultants must cope with often unrealistic ideas consultees have about the process. Consultants are often identified with some familiar aspect of the consultant's role (e.g., university professor is seen as a teacher and a clinician as a therapist). Having a code of ethics helps the consultant to think through the ethical implications of activities before problems arise. Ethics, especially in this area, are context-dependent. There is no set of rules that if blindly followed, will result in ethical behavior. The eth-

---

Box 13.4

Business Ethics Case Analytic Framework: R^2C^2

1. What are the relevant moral facts and prioritized ethical issue(s) in this case?
2. Who are the stakeholders involved and how severely are they impacted?
3. *Results:* To what extent do (should) the results of the action produce more benefits than costs to stakeholders in the short and long range? (Current/Desired)
4. *Rules:* To what extent do (should) the rules followed to achieve results respect the *rights* of others and adhere to standards of *justice* and *fairness*? Are appropriate duties and obligations fulfilled and properly prioritized? (Current/Desired)
   a. To what extent does the action respect the positive or negative rights of key stakeholders?
   b. To what extent does the outcome of the action unjustifiably and disproportionately harm some stakeholders over others?
   c. To what extent does the procedure followed treat key stakeholders equally and fairly?
5. *Character:* To what extent does (should) this action enhance the character of affected stakeholders? Are intellectual, moral, social, emotional, and political virtues (readiness to act ethically) being cultivated or corrupted? Are individuals becoming better persons through this transaction/relationship? (Current/Desired)
6. *Context:* To what extent are (should) the intraorganizational and extraorganizational contexts (barrels) supportive of ethical conduct? (Current/Desired)
7. Is there justification for improving the inclusiveness and balance of the current judgment?
8. What are two alternative resolutions for the case, with their advantages and disadvantages?
9. What is your proposed resolution? What are your moral justifications for the resolution? To what extent will it enhance judgment integrity capacity?
10. How will your resolution be implemented, evaluated, and improved over time?

ical practitioner applies a set of principles to specific situations with results often unique to that situation.

Business professionals, however, do not have the same codified ethical standards as mental health professionals. With the public outrage at corporate scandals within the past few years (e.g., Enron and WorldCom), business schools have been placing more emphasis on ethics. Since there is no universal business ethics code, and since ethical codes cannot cover every situation, it is important to have a framework for making ethical decisions.

The most obvious way to alert consultees to ethical concerns is to tie it to the "bottom line" (profits). Even if firing an individual without warning after 10 years of loyal service is legal, remaining employees will likely feel insecure and begin looking for work elsewhere, reducing productivity.

There are other ways of conceptualizing ethical issues for organizational contexts, such as the R^2C^2 model (rules, results, character, and context; Petrick, 1997, 2005). Box 13.4 explores this model.

Petrick (2005) presents a consulting case study that details the steps involved in thinking through all of the relevant ethical issues. Such an ethics framework serves as a useful tool for consultants to analyze ethical dilemmas, and can be taught to consultees to assist in dealing with future ethical issues.

CASE EXAMPLE: ETHICS CASE ANALYSIS AND PROPOSED RESOLUTION

Mary Trustworthy and Glen Weasel are two new clinical health care professionals undergoing their 6-month probationary period of performance evaluation at Business Success, Inc. (BSI), a large private organizational development consulting firm. At noon, one of Mary's former consultees, Mrs. Innocent, comes to the office and asks for assistance, but since Mary is at lunch, Glen offers to provide assistance. Mrs. Innocent wants to purchase the latest online package for executive selection and development, with 6-month follow-up consulting services to be provided by BSI.

Glen sees an opportunity for a huge sale and, since generating revenue ("making the numbers" in office lingo) was stressed as the prime factor in determining new health care professional retention and promotion, he sells Mrs. Innocent a 1999 package with services, saying that this is the latest available package. He knows full well, however, that there is a 2005 package available but not in stock at BSI; getting rid of an old 1999 package would make him look good to top management as being cost conscious and thereby reducing inventory costs. When Mary returns from lunch, Glen tells her about the transaction and Mary is furious. Glen says that if Mrs. Innocent comes back he will direct her only to Mary. But Mary retorts that deceived consultees are unlikely to generate repeat business.

Mary stops by the office of a more senior clinical health care professional, Roger Bandwagon, and asks him whether she should report this dishonest exchange between Glen and Mrs. Innocence to the Division Manager, Victoria Ambition. Roger advises her that if she goes to Victoria complaining about Glen's misconduct before her formal performance evaluation it will look as if she is simply trying to make excuses for her lack of competitive initiative in generating revenue. Besides, Victoria has never made a public statement about acceptable and unacceptable means of generating revenue and there are no organizational "whistleblower protection" policies in place at BS Inc., so she would be reporting unethical conduct at her own risk.

1. What are the central ethical issue(s) and the relevant facts in this case?
    a. *Central ethical issue(s):* (1) *interpersonal dishonesty in client sales transaction*; (2) unfair advantage taken by one clinical mental health care professional over others; (3) risking loss of employee, managerial, and company reputation for professional integrity and future business; (4) lack of ethical infrastructure in the company to support ethical conduct from inadequate performance evaluation measures to a nonexistent whistleblower protection policy.
    b. *Relevant facts:* (1) Glen lied to client to generate revenue and look better than Mary on their performance evaluations; (2) Glen's lying hurt the client and Mary, and risked the loss of reputation and future business for the company; (3) the ethical infrastructure processes for reporting unethical conduct in the company did not appear to exist or to be routinely used.
2. Who are the stakeholders involved and how severely are they impacted?
    a. *Extraorganizational stakeholders:* (1) *client:* dishonest treatment is likely to result in anger, loss of trust, and likely loss of future business along with bad word-of-mouth publicity (high impact); (2) *organizational consulting industry:* further tarnishes industry image if dishonest sales practices are tolerated and become the norm (medium impact); (3) *competitors:* once competitors find out about this dishonest practice, they can use it against BSI (medium impact); (4) *government:* possible legal grounds for fraud inviting litigation and/or government regulation (medium impact); (5) *professional association:* exposes lack of emphasis in mental health professional association standards for adequate ethical infrastructures in organizations that hire clinical mental health professionals (medium impact); (6) *society:* erodes trust in consulting service sales transactions in general (medium impact); (7) *community:* increases distrust and local vulnerability to dishonest BS Inc. tactics by local community members (medium impact).
    b. *Intraorganizational stakeholders:* (1) *Glen:* chose to lie to client to generate revenue, gain comparative advantage over Mary, and hurt his character, Mary, and the company (high impact); (2) *Mary:* unfairly treated by Glen and the company for being honest (high impact); (3) *Victoria:* absent as a role model for honesty and apparently did not institute or enforce an ethics development system at work (high impact); (4) *Roger and other BSI mental health care professionals:* are influenced by tacit norms of accepted sales dishonesty, the narrow measure of generating revenue as the key performance indicator for retention and promotion, and the absence of any adequate ethical development system in the company to support whistle-blowers (moderate impact); (5) *owners/investors:* concern about jeopardizing long-term financial returns by legally risky behavior that indirectly displaces more financial risk on investors without their input (moderate impact).
3. *Results:* To what extent do (should) the results of the action produce more benefits than costs to stakeholders in the short and long term?
    a. Glen's lying results in some short-term benefits for him, but more short-term and long-term costs for Mary, other mental health professionals, the company, and other stakeholders. He is acting selfishly, and by doing so, he

offends clients, generates dysfunctional competition and distrust between fellow professionals, and risks the loss of future return business.

b. The full extent of the costs to other more remote stakeholders could be substantial if sales dishonesty provokes litigation for fraud, professional association censure, increased government regulatory intervention, and industry condemnation, domestically and globally.

4. *Rules:* To what extent do (should) the rules followed to achieve results respect the *rights* of others and adhere to standards of *justice* and *fairness*? Are appropriate duties and obligations fulfilled and properly prioritized?

   a. *Rights:* The act of lying by Glen was inherently wrong. It violated the client's right to the truth and the duty to treat clients with equal respect rather than manipulative disregard. It insults the dignity of clients by unilaterally depriving them of accurate information needed to make free, informed purchasing decisions. Without the truth, their freedom to intelligently use their purchasing power is taken (stolen) from them, and stealing is also inherently wrong. By lying, Glen also violates the mental health professional ethics code by not putting the client/consultee interest above his self-interests.

   b. *Justice:* The act of lying by Glen was unjust to Mary and other mental health professionals. The outcome disproportionately benefited Glen while displacing the bulk of the burdens of lost sales, future disgruntled clients, untrustworthy colleague relations and future negative performance appraisals on Mary, other mental health professionals, and Victoria. By lying, Glen procured benefits that he did not justly deserve or merit.

   c. *Fairness:* Lying was also procedurally unfair to the client who was deprived of her purchasing power and procedurally unfair to other mental health professionals who have told and continue to tell the truth to clients, even if they lose some sales. Deceived clients and honest mental health professionals were both victimized and treated unequally and adversely from others in the same categories. Glen did not "fairly earn" his sales but took advantage of client ignorance by misrepresenting a product and took advantage of colleague trust by engaging in suboptimization behavior patterns, that is, patterns that benefited him but hurt others and the company.

5. *Character:* To what extent does (should) the action enhance the character of affected stakeholders? Are intellectual, moral, social, emotional, and political virtues (readiness to act ethically) being cultivated or corrupted? Are individuals becoming better persons through this transaction/relationship?

   a. *Personal character:* By lying, Glen is weakening his character; he will be less willing to act ethically in the future. He is becoming a worse (vicious) person and professional rather than a better (virtuous) one. By lying, he betrays the *intellectual virtue* of respect for the truth; he indulges the *moral vices* of cowardice and imprudence because he is afraid to lose sales telling the truth; and he is downplaying the hurtful long-term consequences of his action. By lying, he erodes the *social virtues* of trust and cooperation, while fomenting the *emotional vices* of hatred and resentment among and between stakeholders. Finally, by lying Glen is violating the *political virtues* of workplace citizenship and civility by unilaterally abusing information power to take advantage of others.

b. *Group character:* Not only is Glen's character diminished but his bad example adversely impacts the collective readiness of others to act ethically at work. If Glen's misconduct is overlooked, condoned, or praised, it sends a message about the kind of selfish, dishonest person who will succeed at that company. Collective character corruption could then exacerbate client distrust, hateful resentment among coworkers, the rapid loss of workplace community, and the lack of readiness to act ethically in other transactions in the future.

c. *Leadership character:* The notable lack of Victoria's strong voice in support of honest client relationships, her absence in serving as a positive moral role model, and her inability or unwillingness to manage the organizational ethical climate of the company through responsible moral infrastructure processes indicates a lack of strong leadership character in the workplace.

6. *Context:* To what extent do (should) the intraorganizational and extraorganizational contexts (barrels) support ethical conduct?

a. *Intra-organizational context:* The implicit condoning of Glen's lying to generate revenue indicates that either a company *compliance* or *ethics development system* (with regular reporting of unethical acts without retaliation, a code of ethics, and an ethics audit) does not exist or is not routinely used. Nor is there any indication that performance appraisal and reward subsystems factor in ethical ways to achieve results so that unethical practices are penalized and ethical practices are commended. This lack of an ethically supportive company infrastructure indicates that the workplace moral context is poorly designed and risks the loss of company reputation.

b. *Extraorganizational context:* The extraorganizational context provides domestic, legal, and regulatory enforcement of fraud statutes in the United States to externally support honest sales transaction practices and related ethical conduct. Sanctioned sales dishonesty also exposes the company to other legal and financial risks under U.S. consumer protection laws, the U.S. Federal Sentencing Guidelines for Organizations (USFSGO) and/or the Sarbanes-Oxley Act (SOX). If family and friends found out, they would probably feel ashamed of Glen's lying and exert some social pressure to stop his lying. Shameful, socially irresponsible acts risk the loss of extra-organizational friendships, external industry and community reputation, and future business, so they should be condemned and avoided whenever possible.

7. (Judgment Integrity Capacity Decision) Is there justification for improving the inclusiveness and balance of the current judgment? There is justification for improving the inclusiveness and balance of the current judgment.

8. What are two alternative resolutions for the case, with their advantages and disadvantages?

a. *Resolution A: (Immediately Fire Glen)* Resolution A is to fire Glen. The *upside* would be it would remove a negative role model from the office and eliminate the risk of future client complaints and lost business due to sales dishonesty. The *downside* is that it would not be fair to Glen who assumed—in the absence of formal sales training emphasizing sustained customer relations, an explicit and enforced ethics development system, and managerial positive role modeling—that "getting his sales numbers" and "generating revenue" anyway he could (including lying) would be acceptable. Nor does it fix the corrupt system (intraorganizational context or barrel) that tacitly allowed the lying to occur. Without an ethics development system in place to retrain Glen and set future standards of sales honesty for all mental health professionals, a new hire with Glen's lying style would jeopardize the company again in the future.

b. *Resolution B: (Comprehensive Resolution to Rebuild Integrity Capacity)* Resolution B is to comprehensively address results, rules, character, and context (use the R^2C^2 method) to restore and rebuild professional and organizational integrity capacity with regard to standards for honest sales transactions. The *upside* would be that a comprehensive ethics development system—with strong managerial leadership to provide a supportive infrastructure through ethics training on positive client relations practices and the importance of character development at work, explicit and enforced standards of sales honesty, whistle-blowing protection policies even during probationary periods, an ethics audit with public accountability, a process for in-house ethics commendations, and visible managerial moral role modeling of integrity building sales practices—would retrain Glen and other mental health care professionals to develop "sales with integrity" practices that sustained client trust relationships and professional code compliance through truth telling. To avoid unfairly firing him, he would have to change his sales tactics so that they would adhere to explicit standards of honesty and fairness. In the process, not only Glen, but others in the company as well, would be strengthening their characters, that is, their readiness to act ethically in the future as a cooperative, workplace community. Finally, by incorporating a broader range of results than mere sales revenues, such as number of return clients, level of coworker perceived cooperation and teamwork, and number of client complaints, to be considered in performance appraisal and rewards, the company will be rewarding rather than penalizing those employees who generate sales revenues by safeguarding the reputation of the company. The *downside* is that this resolution takes time and is more complex than Resolution A, but addressing moral complexity in a simple-minded way, that is, taking the quick, decisive easy way out by firing, won't build professional and organizational integrity capacity fairly. If Glen does not respond appropriately to the ethics training, however, the manager should fire him.

9. What is your proposed resolution? What are your moral justifications for the resolution? To what extent will it enhance professional and company judgment integrity capacity?

Resolution B, is the preferred and proposed resolution.

a. *Comprehensive moral justification:* The moral justifications for the resolution are the following: (1) *Results:* there are more benefits than costs to Resolution B in the long run because it comprehensively counters selfish impulses to lie to clients by expanding the results expected for appraisal and reward to include benefits to multiple stakeholders; (2) *Rules:* Resolution B requires an explicit statement of company standards for sales honesty and provides a whistle-blowing policy for reporting unfair practices with impunity, thereby clarifying explicit rules and improving the chances of honest and fair sales transactions in the future; (3) *Character:* Resolution B takes the step to heal the wounds to group character inflicted by lying through community building, character development training that commends virtuous, trustworthy conduct and raises the level of rewarded cooperation between and among employees; (4) *Context:* Through the ethics audit and ethics commendations, the company can measure and motivate its system moral progress and signal that moral integrity capacity is important to protect the reputation of the firm. The whistle-blowing policy will signal that unethical business practices, for example, dishonesty in sales transactions, are to be reported and action will be taken. These practices would be investigated and swiftly, fairly adjudicated so that mental health professionals at all levels in the company would know that unethical conduct is penalized and ethical conduct is commended and expected. In addition, Resolution B serves notice to competitors, the public, and other stakeholders that they can expect high standards of honesty in sales practice from BSI and to factor that in their choice of places to do business. The improved company reputation can be used to "win back," attract, and retain future clients.

b. *Benefits of resolution:* Resolution B will directly enhance professional and organizational judgment integrity capacity by comprehensively, simultaneously, and realistically addressing moral results, rules, character, and context to protect the company's reputational capital for sustained competitive advantage now and in the future.

10. How will the resolution be implemented, evaluated and improved over time?

a. *Resolution implementation* and *evaluation processes:* Resolution B could be implemented either through internal managerial initiative with mental health professional inputs or external organizational ethics consultant intervention— or both. They would design a comprehensive ethics development system, beginning with an organizational ethics needs assessment to identify and prioritize perceived ethics needs and a structured ethics training program to address the prioritized issues. Resolution B would be evaluated by monitoring progress in ethics needs assessments, results of ethics training, and results of ethics audits over time, and eventual moral benchmarking. Sharing the success of the approach with industry, professional associations, as well as community and customer audiences would further invite feedback for ongoing evaluation and progress in consulting firm ethical standards.

b. *Resolution improvement processes:* Resolution B will be improved through regular structured feedback, corrective actions taken when warranted, and continual openness shown to incremental and/or breakthrough progress recommendations. Suggestions for improvement would be regularly so- licited from stakeholders and incorporated as warranted. Resolution B impacts will be coordinated with other organizational assessment and im- provement efforts to promote ongoing professional and organizational moral progress.

While such a detailed framework can provide structure to make difficult ethical de- cisions in complex situations, Wallace and Hall (1996) present a succinct set of steps for dealing with ethical issues in consultation:

1. Check personal values and motives carefully.
2. Review relevant sections of related professional associations' ethical codes.
3. Search the literature for reports of similar and related cases, noting decisions and recommended actions.

4. Seek the advice of colleagues, particularly those who work in the same settings and may have encountered the same or a similar ethical dilemma.
5. Contact the chairperson of the professional association's committee on ethical standards.
6. Project possible outcomes and consequences for alternative decisions on the issue.
7. Make a decision and act on it.
8. Document reasons for all choices and actions. (p. 272)

In discussing ethics, Haas and his colleagues (Haas & Fennimore, 1983; Haas & Malouf, 2002) explore major issues, practical issues, and legal issues.

Under major issues, Haas and Malouf (2002) discuss responsibility, integrity, and competence. Responsibility means that the consultant accepts that no one else is in charge of the consultant's behaviors. One must also be mindful of the impact of one's interventions. Consultants should also be active in the decisions to use and the implementation of consultation interventions. For example, the consultant should not train a manager to conduct therapy groups, as this has the potential to harm employees.

Petrick and Quinn (1997), speaking in a managerial context, define integrity as "the individual and collective process of repeated alignment of moral awareness, judgment, character, and conduct that demonstrates balanced judgment and promote sustained moral development" (p. 61). They put forth the idea that integrity involves three components: judgment, process, and developmental dimensions.

Haas and Malouf (2002) describe integrity as involving a clear awareness of one's values and their impact on the consulting process. This involves honesty with oneself and with consultees, identifying one's values explicitly and allowing consultees to freely choose whether to be influenced by them. The overriding concern of the consultant should be the enhancement of the client's well-being.

It is the responsibility of the consultant to assure the appropriate level of competence for the given assignment. Informed consent, a concern of mental health professionals, is also important when engaging in consultation activities (e.g., disclosing one's background and qualifications). The consultant should not overpromise or underpromise. Building in evaluation points along the way helps to assure that both consultant and consultee are getting what they desire. Knowing what one does not know, and seeking additional consultation from colleagues (or referring the project to someone more qualified), is another mark of competence.

Haas and Malouf (2002) also discuss practical issues. First, it is crucial to identify who the actual consultee is. It is also important to become familiar with the organizational context in which the services are being provided. In addition to the issue of competency, informed consent involves disclosing personal values and theories of change. The consultant should share an estimation regarding how much time, money, and effort the proposed intervention will require, along with any potential risks. Alternatives to consultation should also be discussed. A verbal or written contract should be created to state these understandings.

Clarification of information boundaries is also a critical practical issue. One of the consultant's primary resources is information. Knowing who is going to provide information, what information will be provided, and who is permitted access to the information should be clarified up front. The consultant should also be aware of what will be done with the information after the assignment is completed.

Haas and Malouf (2002) also warn the consultant to be aware of power issues to avoid becoming embroiled in the organization's internal struggles. Remember that the consultee has the power to terminate the consultation. Higher echelons of the organization have power over the lower ones. Independent power can be possessed by particular units in the organization. Power is used in organizations to accomplish things, and the consultant, as a source of power, may sometimes be manipulated by members of the organization.

Haas and Malouf (2002) also advise consultants to become aware of any potential legal issues that could affect a consulting practice. This could include laws affecting one's profession (e.g., psychologist) as well as general laws that affect how one does business (contract law).

A Mental Health Professional Consultant's Code of Ethics

Because there is no universally accepted code of ethics for consultants with mental health backgrounds, Gallessich (1982) created a set of principles based on information culled from the consultation literature (American Psychological Association, 1972; Benne, 1969; Division of Managerial Consultation of the Academy of Management, 1978; G. Lippit & Lippit, 1978; NTL Institute, 1980; Pfeiffer & Jones, 1977). It addresses the most important core issues in consultation, and is submitted for the reader's consideration.

> *Principle 1:* Consultants' clients are the agencies that hire them. Consultants place their clients' interest above their own.
>
> *Principle 2:* Consultants are responsible for safeguarding the welfare of their consultees and client organizations. Consultants inform consultees of any potential risks in consultation activities and help consultees make informed decisions on whether or not to use any service.
>
> *Principle 3:* Consultants present their professional qualifications and limitations accurately in order to avoid misinterpretation. They immediately correct any misunderstandings about their credentials and experience. They also inform consultees of any professional or personal relationships, biases, or values that are likely to affect their work.
>
> *Principle 4:* Consultants are careful to present their knowledge accurately.
>
> *Principle 5:* When consultants perceive a consultee to behave in an unethical manner, they express their observations and the reasons for their concern to the person involved.
>
> *Principle 6:* Consultants avoid involvement in multiple roles and relationships that might create conflicts of interest and thus jeopardize their effectiveness in the consultant role.
>
> *Principle 7:* Consultants avoid manipulating consultees.
>
> *Principle 8:* Consultants accept contracts only if they are reasonably sure that the client agency will benefit from their services.
>
> *Principle 9:* Consultants establish clear contracts with well-defined parameters. They ascertain that they are sanctioned to enter an agency through the express permission of its executive officer.
>
> *Principle 10:* Consultants fulfill their contracts and remain within contractual boundaries.
>
> *Principle 11:* Consultants strive to evaluate the outcomes of their services.
>
> *Principle 12:* Consultants assume responsibility for assisting administrators in establishing confidentiality policies to govern consultation and communicating these policies to the staff members involved in consultation activities.
>
> *Principle 13:* Consultants acquire the basic body of knowledge and skills of their profession.

Principle 14: Consultants know their professional strengths, weaknesses, and biases.

Principle 15: Consultants are aware of personal characteristics that predispose them to systematic biases.

Principle 16: Consultants are alert to differences between their own social and political values and interests and those of client organizations.

Principle 17: Consultants regularly assess their strengths and weaknesses in relation to current and future work.

Principle 18: When advertising or otherwise promoting their services, consultants are careful to describe them accurately and to avoid fraudulent information or claims.

Principle 19: Consultants serve public interests through offering a proportion of their time to agencies that are financially unable to pay for consultation services.

Principle 20: Consultants contribute to the growth of knowledge through their own research and experimentation.

Principle 21: Consultants are alert to the public's welfare.

Principle 22: Consultants contribute to the training of less experienced consultants.

Principle 23: Consultants behave so as to protect the reputation of their profession.

Principle 24: Consultants cooperate with other consultants and with members of other professions.

Principle 25: Consultants acquaint themselves with the current fee standards in their area of expertise and in the agency's geographic location.

Principle 26: When a consultant observes another professional to behave in an apparently unethical way, the consultant goes to that person to discuss these perceptions.

Principle 27: Consultants contribute to their profession by participating in the activities of peer associations and supporting their standards.

Principle 28: Consultants take active steps to maintain and increase their effectiveness.

Boundary Issues in Consulting

Mental health professionals are taught the importance of maintaining clear boundaries in counseling settings, such as the importance of avoiding dual relationships. In consultation work, sometimes the lines become blurred as to where consultation ends and therapy begins. In the important work on boundary issues in counseling by Herlihy and Corey (1997), A. Michael Dougherty discusses dual role conflicts in consultation.

Dual Role Conflicts in Consultation

Professional dual relationships are best avoided whenever possible when consulting. They make a complex process and relationship even more complex.

First, the complexity of the consultation process has contributed to disagreement among authorities in the field as to the boundaries of the consultant's role. This disagreement makes it difficult to ascertain what is ethical or unethical in many situations surrounding consultation, including dual relationships.

Second, there is disagreement in the field concerning the definition of consultation, which makes it difficult to define the appropriate roles the consultant can assume during the consultation relationship. An additional professional role only complicates these difficulties.

Third, counselors, when they consult, should be wary of multiple roles that might create conflicts of interest that could in turn reduce the efficacy of the consultant role. Consultants should decline to take on additional roles when these roles reduce freedom of expression or objectivity, or limit the consultant's commitment to the consultee organization.

Fourth, consultants need to guard against putting the consultee in interrole conflict in which two roles cause contradictory expectations about a given behavior. For example, consultation focuses on work-related concerns, and counseling focuses on personal concerns. Because it is difficult to differentiate these two foci, it is best to keep the expectations as simple as possible so that the consultee will not confuse the two relationships and bring up personal issues during consultation and work-related ones during counseling.

Fifth, the training of counselors conditions them to move naturally toward affective concerns and personal problems, and it is hard to turn off this tendency in other types of relationships such as consultation. This tendency can be particularly dangerous if the counselor, when consulting, determines that the locus of the work-related concern lies more in the personal issues of the consultee than in the client system itself. Counselors might, therefore, have a tendency to want to offer counseling services to a consultee based on the perception that the consultee will benefit both personally and professionally from such an additional relationship. Focusing on the emotional needs and concerns of consultees, however, breaks the peer relationship inherent in consultation and should therefore be avoided. Consultants should remember that referring that consultee for counseling is typically an option.

Sixth, the consultee may have an obligation to his or her organization not to use consultation for personal purposes because the organization has provided consultation services for professional, not personal, growth. Further, if the consultant agrees to provide counseling and this is kept private, the consultee might wonder later what other kinds of "cheating" the consultant might do (e.g., breaking confidentiality).

Seventh, if the consultant simultaneously engages in consulting and counseling roles with a consultee, word may get out that the consultant is "a great counselor." Many prospective consultees who have work-related concerns may avoid seeking consultation because they are concerned that the consultant will try to counsel them on a personal level (adapted from Herlihy & Corey, 1997, pp. 80–82).

Following are two consulting case examples involving potential ethical problems. Since the examples involve a licensed clinical psychologist, reference is made to the American Psychological Association's Ethical Principles of Psychologists and Code of Conduct (2002), which serves as an important guide for making decisions in these cases.

Ethics Case Example 1

Joseph Kowalski, a clinical psychologist who is just beginning a private consulting practice, receives a phone call from the district manager of a large retailer asking for assistance in the development of an organizational code of ethics. The manager knew Joseph from previous work done with the company and felt very comfortable working with him. Joseph briefly gathers more information, and then tells the caller that he would like to think about it and will call back later in the afternoon. Joseph has never before participated in the creation of an organizational ethics code, but would like to branch out into new areas to help him develop his consulting practice. He reads through his profession's ethical code as he tries to determine if he should undertake this assignment. He first takes notice of the standard of avoiding harm.

Ethical Standard 3.04 Avoiding Harm

> Psychologists take reasonable steps to avoid harming their clients/patients, students, supervisees, research participants, organizational clients, and others with whom they work, and to minimize harm where it is foreseeable and unavoidable. (American Psychological Association, 2002, p. 6)

Joseph reasons that assisting with the development of an organizational ethics code is not likely to be extremely harmful, particularly if he seeks consultation with colleagues. He then reviews the standard concerning competence.

Ethical Standard 2.01 Boundaries of Competence

> (a) Psychologists provide services, teach, and conduct research with populations and in areas only within the boundaries of their competence, based on their education, training, supervised experience, consultation, study, or professional experience.
>
> (b) Where scientific or professional knowledge in the discipline of psychology establishes that an understanding of factors associated with age, gender, gender identity, race, ethnicity, culture, national origin, religion, sexual orientation, disability, language, or socioeconomic status is essential for effective implementation of their services or research, psychologists have or obtain the training, experience, consultation, or supervision necessary to ensure the competence of their services, or they make appropriate referrals, except as provided in Standard 2.02, Providing Services in Emergencies.
>
> (c) Psychologists planning to provide services, teach, or conduct research involving populations, areas, techniques, or technologies new to them undertake relevant education, training, supervised experience, consultation, or study.
>
> (d) When psychologists are asked to provide services to individuals for whom appropriate mental health services are not available and for which psychologists have not obtained the competence necessary, psychologists with closely related prior training or experience may provide such services in order to ensure that services are not denied if they make a reasonable effort to obtain the competence required by using relevant research, training, consultation, or study.
>
> (e) In those emerging areas in which generally recognized standards for preparatory training do not yet exist, psychologists nevertheless take reasonable steps to ensure the competence of their work and to protect clients/patients, students, supervisees, research participants, organizational clients, and others from harm.
>
> (f) When assuming forensic roles, psychologists are or become reasonably familiar with the judicial or administrative rules governing their roles. (American Psychological Association, 2002, pp. 4–5)

Although Joseph has had limited training in ethics and in business, he feels that he would enjoy taking the time to do more research in these areas. He calls an acquaintance, a university business ethics professor, to discuss the situation. Joseph suggests that perhaps the professor would be more qualified to take on this consulting assignment, but the professor says that she will not have the time to take on any extra work for at least 3 months. However, if Joseph takes the job, she would be happy to talk with him about it over the telephone, and to review any documents they create.

Joseph calls the manager back and expresses his desire to take the assignment, but speaks honestly about his background and his lack of actual experience writing organizational ethics codes. Joseph lets the manager know that he will begin background research on his own time, and will consult with a professor colleague with expertise in this area at his own expense. Joseph lets the manager know that he can refer this professor to the organization, though she will not be available for another 3 months. Joseph also offers to assist the manager in finding a more qualified consultant if so desired. The manager responds that the organization would like to hire Joseph due to the excellent work he has done in the past with other matters, and asks Joseph to write up a proposal.

Ethics Case Example 2

A consultant is hired by the ABC Gum Company to assist in the selection of the new president. The consultant is a licensed clinical psychologist, and is asked to assess the remaining five candidates for the position. She carefully chooses the appropriate assessment instruments, meets with each candidate and explains her role in the selection process, and completes her assessments. She writes a detailed report on each candidate, and submits them to the organization's human resource department.

Two months later, one of the candidates leaves a message on the consultant's voice mail, having remembered her name from the assessments. The candidate states that he was not hired by the organization, and demands to know the results of the assessment done by the consultant. The man says that he has a friend in the mental health field who told him that anyone giving psychological assessments must give feedback to the person who took the test. Although the consultant feels this is a fairly clear-cut case, she quickly reviews her code of ethics before calling the man back.

3.11 Psychological Services Delivered to or through Organizations

(a) Psychologists delivering services to or through organizations provide information beforehand to clients and when appropriate those directly affected by the services about (1) the nature and objectives of the services, (2) the intended recipients, (3) which of the individuals are clients, (4) the relationship the psychologist will have with each person and the organization, (5) the probable uses of services provided and information obtained, (6) who will have access to the information, and (7) limits of confidentiality. As soon as feasible, they provide information about the results and conclusions of such services to appropriate persons.

(b) If psychologists will be precluded by law or by organizational roles from providing such information to particular individuals or groups, they so inform those individuals or groups at the outset of the service. (p. 7)

9.10 Explaining Assessment Results

Regardless of whether the scoring and interpretation are done by psychologists, by employees or assistants, or by automated or other outside services, psychologists take reasonable steps to ensure that explanations of results are given to the individual or designated representative unless the nature of the relationship precludes provision of an explanation of results (such as in some organizational consulting, preemployment or security screenings, and forensic evaluations), and this fact has been clearly explained to the person being assessed in advance. (p. 14)

The consultant calls the man back and informs him that she was very clear in their first meeting that her client is the ABC Gum Company, and that the man would not be permitted to see the results of the testing. The reports belong to the ABC Gum Company, and the consultant cannot release the information to the man.

Knowledge is an important way of avoiding legal and ethical difficulties in consultation. Here is a summary of the most important things a consultant needs to know:

- Who the client is
- What the law states
- The code of ethics for the consultant's profession
- The consultant's own values
- How to develop a clear contract
- When to consult with colleagues

When in doubt about the ethics of a particular decision, Whetton and Cameron (2002) suggest thinking about the ramifications of the decision in accordance with the following standards:

- *Front page test:* Would I be embarrassed if my decision became a headline in the local newspaper? Would I feel comfortable describing my actions or decisions to a customer or stockholder?
- *Golden rule test:* Would I be willing to be treated in the same manner?
- *Dignity and liberty test:* Are the dignity and liberty of others preserved by this decision? Is the basic humanity of the affected parties enhanced? Are their opportunities expanded or curtailed?
- *Equal treatment test:* Are the rights, welfare, and betterment of minorities and lower-status people given full consideration? Does this decision benefit those with privilege but without merit?
- *Personal gain test:* Is an opportunity for personal gain clouding my judgment? Would I make the same decision if the outcome did not benefit me in any way?
- *Congruence test:* Is this decision or action consistent with my espoused personal principles? Does it violate the spirit of any organizational policies or laws?
- *Procedural justice test:* Can the procedures used to make this decision stand up to scrutiny by those affected?
- *Cost-benefit test:* Does a benefit for some cause unacceptable harm to others? How critical is the benefit? Can the harmful effects be mitigated?
- *Good night's sleep test:* Whether or not anyone else knows about my action, will it produce a good night's sleep? (p. 70)

Chapter 14 ——————————————————————

CLINICAL CONSULTATION

Most mental health professionals become interested in the field of human service because they want to make a positive impact on the lives of others. We set out to master the myriad of information that plays a part in how people become who they are in order to assist them in becoming who they would like to be. During our clinical education and training, we gradually build a knowledge base of the many factors that create and affect the human experience. The fascinating elements of brain function, cognitive and learning processes, physiological and sensory development combine in innumerable scenarios emerging into the uniqueness of each individual. With these inherent ingredients composing a basic foundation, we must then layer on life experiences to the recipe of each developing person. Culture, home and community environment, relationships, and emotional and behavioral reactions to the world all blend together in a seemingly endless array of variables. What a formidable undertaking for any of us to seek complete understanding of all the elemental forces that drive the human condition! Acknowledging the whole person as a blend of strengths and weaknesses within the dynamics of settings in which they work, live, and play creates a deeper level of intervention. It becomes a logical conclusion that to make the most powerful impact on the well-being of the individuals we serve; we must be prepared to collaborate and team with other professionals.

Having chosen this vocation, mental health providers devote their abilities to figuring out why people do what they do, helping others overcome challenges, and supporting individuals to discover solutions for coping with mental illness. While our fields of study may vary in scope and focus as social workers, psychologists, and counselors, we are united in goal and vision. We continue to expand our grasp of the factors that affect adaptive, emotional, behavioral, and physiological functioning with varying orientations and use of different intervention strategies. Perhaps all in all, we are exploring multiple approaches at meeting people where they are in order to put tools into practice that best address the concerns they bring to us. As we move forward, separate yet together, it is with the mission of creating better outcomes for the people we serve. Thus, we must all combine knowledge with experience to offer the community viable pathways for emotional wellness. By developing effective methods of mental health consultation that embrace these principles, a new and wider level of expertise will become available.

What we offer as effective mental health providers has to also match the community's needs, attitudes, and resources. When current services are no longer effective or sufficient, it is up to innovative and motivated mental health professionals to work toward the development of new methods of assistance. The impetus for change emerges from a sense of dissonance between what people need and what is available. It is then that we find ourselves rising up to meet the challenges of creating improved and alternative ways of offering support.

In the late 1800s, people with mental illness were banished, abused, or left to their own devices as unclean, unfit, or even evil. Attitudes began to change in the 1900s when the benefits of humane care and efforts at rehabilitation contributed to the discovery that mental illness was treatable. The introduction of mental institutions as a therapeutic residential option was seen as both revolutionary and beneficent during those times. Yet when it became clear that this environment continued to propagate inequality and infringement of individual rights, we evolved into a powerful movement of deinstitutionalization and growth of community mental health services.

Again we are faced with the need to evolve. Providers in the community are asked to support individuals with a wide variety of mental heath needs. Clients often have limited access to resources resulting in the outpatient therapist having to play a case management role as well. The increased demand for services for clients with multiple concerns has had a huge impact on the community's ability to develop adequate services: too few programs, ever-declining dollars, and scarcity of adequately trained mental health professionals. People with medical and developmental challenges or cultural differences often have difficulty finding providers who have the necessary background to offer adequate care. Our clients have time-limited access to treatment that is controlled by managed care—our solutions now must be much tighter and more focused. What we were taught as models of best practice assessment, we are asked to squeeze into an initial diagnostic session to meet the demands of the insurance companies for drive-through diagnoses. And many of the tasks that would maximize our knowledge and treatment of our clients (e.g., observing client in the home or community, attending school meetings, participation in psychiatric appointments), are simply not deemed to be billable services.

This is not to say that mental health services delivered in a more traditional approach are not valuable and effective to those who are able to obtain them. Critical examination of the effectiveness of psychotherapy outcomes in the 1950s and 1960s (Eysenck, 1952; Hobbs, 1963) inspired an increased focus on seeking demonstrably efficacious interventions. Over the past 20 years, we have become more cautious and critical in our selected interventions via outcome studies and dedication to evidence-based practice. We have begun to identify those treatment approaches that have the most successful impact on specific diagnoses. Science may be slow to transform theory into practice, but we are providing a much richer array of successful treatment techniques than ever before. Still there is often not a high correlation between what is valued and what is valuable. For even as we clarify the merit of mental health prevention and intervention to people's welfare, less and less money is allocated within the community to pay for it.

Research in the field of human service has also begun to acknowledge the impact of prevention, behavioral health in recovery from medical illness, stress management and relaxation, and a plethora of self-directed pursuits of wellness-oriented lifestyles to promote positive mental health. Although we have acknowledged the mind-body connection for centuries, more and more research studies in the past 20 years are identifying the significant role that psychological variables play on health and illness (Brown et al., 2002). In fact, by the 1990s, the United States Public Health Service had publicized that people's lifestyles and behavioral choices make up seven of the top health-risk factors in the United States (VandenBos, De Leon, & Belar, 1991). Our new insights about the power of prevention and methods of coping with stress are not easily accessible to the mainstream public. Many people continue to struggle with overwhelming threats to their mental wellness rather than seek assistance or may be unable to afford or access care. Even after seeking help, one-on-one clinic based psychotherapy is not always sufficient to address the concerns of a person in the community due to costs, scarcity of providers, or the need for more collaborative or educational services. The possible contributions of mental health providers through behavioral health intervention, pain management, coping with chronic illness, and many other avenues loudly advocate for our need to expand in scope and in flexible access to the community.

Innovative approaches are being introduced through employee assistance programs, antibullying curriculum in schools, and crisis intervention to prevent the long-term damaging effects of trauma. The contributions of mental health professionals within medical and psychiatric circles have begun to revolutionize the comprehensive care of children and adults with developmental and chronic health concerns. An increased focus on the development of community-based programs has emerged out of the growing recognition of the limitations of traditional outpatient clinic services in meeting peoples' needs. Mental health programming in schools has found federal support due to the rapidly growing concerns in children and youth. Much of this progress has been driven by the flexibility and further-reaching efforts of clinical consultative approaches working to move viable efficacious treatment services into the community.

CONSULTATION SKILL DEVELOPMENT AS A THERAPIST

The purpose of this chapter is to guide mental health professionals in exploring consultation as an extension of primary treatment efforts as well as an alternative to the traditional therapeutic approach. A main premise being that the additional skills necessary to provide effective consultation are built upon a professional's solid foundation of clinical knowledge and expertise.

As a mental health provider, you may intend to expand your current practice to offer additional services or plan to develop a new program to address the concerns in your community. Others may simply wish to hone their existing skills in working with those providers with whom they already collaborate regarding ongoing clients. It is likely that most mental health professionals have already been involved in consultation without necessarily having any formal training or instruction specific to that area. These situations are likely to have been brief sidebars or "hallway consults" as a professional courtesy to colleagues in your clinic or via a telephone call for advice from another provider in the community. Such clinical consultation opportunities are most likely to arise when a mental health professional, through additional training and experience, is requested to share his or her more advanced understanding of particular diagnoses or disabilities, stages of development, specialized treatment methods, alternative lifestyles, and so on.

The demands for alternative or specialized services are increasing such that it is time for the creation of more structured systematic training in consultation for mental health professionals. While many graduate programs in school psychology offer specific training on the skills needed for consultation, there continue to be few courses in other areas of psychology and human service fields. In a survey exploring the adequacy of preservice training, Constenbader, Swartz, and Petrix (1992) found that 61% of school psychologists who responded received one semester or less of formal training in consultation. School psychologists are the most likely to have consultation as a major part of their professional expectations, yet as much as 25% had no training on any model of consultation. The amount of training in most graduate school programs specifically addressing consultation skills that is available to other psychologists, social workers, and counselors is likely to be much less.

Before reviewing the foundations of independent consultation as a different approach to meeting mental health needs, we explore how a therapist may incorporate consultative skills to their treatment repertoire. The steps in which a clinician becomes a consultant is most likely to occur through a process of experiences which are not often addressed in other resources on mental health consultation. Since we have established that limited coursework is available to train providers formally on general mental health consultation, much of the necessary professional development must be guided by the mental health provider's personal efforts. For those who are seeking a career in a specialized field of consultation (e.g., pediatric psychology, behavioral health), there are opportunities at pre- and postdoctoral levels to pursue formal clinical training. In any case, experience is always the education most crucial in fostering the emergence of a well-rounded and confident consultative perspective.

Presuming that times really have changed, mental health providers can no longer offer therapeutic services in a vacuum addressing isolated aspects of the individual who presents with mental health concerns. Because of the intensity and diversity of client needs and the growing evidence-based links between health, rehabilitation, and mental health, our scope of practice is already evolving. More professional programs are offering courses and training opportunities in psychopharmacology, developmental disabilities and autism, and psychological aspects of health issues; preparing the mental health provider with the knowledge base needed for effective collaboration with other experts in human services. Psychologists, social workers, and counselors are developing conceptually integrated ties with other professional disciplines. It has become much more typical in the past 20 to 30 years to find mental health professionals playing a vital role on a wide variety of inpatient and outpatient medical treatment teams and leading primary intervention programs in pediatric or behavioral health care centers. Thus, it follows that our therapeutic approach toward assessment, diagnosis, treatment, and connection with community supports in all settings, should demonstrate our acceptance and pursuit of a holistic perspective.

At its core, "Consultation involves sharing information and ideas; coordinating and comparing observations, providing a sounding board; and developing tentative hypotheses for action. The emphasis is on equal relationships developed through collaboration and joint planning" (Dinkmeyer & Carlson, 2001, p. 13). As mental health professionals, we have information about the general psychological dynamics that apply to individuals in a wide variety of situations. To make this information more useful to other professionals and benefit the client, it is beneficial to be broadly informed about the realm of services of different disciplines. As the previous definition suggests, the consultative relationship is intended to be collegial. Part of the art of consultation is creating a workable rapport in which consultants present themselves as knowledgeable and confident while not coming across as all knowing or condescending.

Holistic Approach

To be prepared to consult with other professionals regarding a client, a thorough evaluation is often necessary to explore the interdependence of potential contributing concerns. The initial assessment of an individual referred for a client-centered consultation, as in treatment, will vary somewhat depending on the approach and background of the mental health clinician. The information gathered is then conceptualized through the particular orientation of the clinician to provide a diagnosis and approach to intervention. While theoretical differences exist among us, in recent years there has been growing recognition of the importance of a biopsychosocial approach in understanding the multiple contributory causal factors involved in the development of atypical behavior.

A biopsychosocial model maintains that psychological, sociological, and biological causes of behavior exert an interrelated effect on the mental health of individuals. This viewpoint is now the dominant perspective in health psychology and behavioral medicine (Brannon & Feist, 1997). Advances in clinical research have demonstrated that all of these aspects in an individual's life contribute to the variability in overall physical and emotional wellness. To develop an integrated intervention approach that considers those factors which may be impacting on current difficulties, it is critical to gather information about the whole person as part of a diagnostic evaluation. Most mental health settings have incorporated many of these elements into standard intake protocols. However, this information may not be readily available during the consultation process. Depending on the setting in which the referral takes place, the consultant may not evaluate the client directly and have to rely on the consultee as the primary source of information. If mental health consultation is occurring because the referring provider does not have a successful approach to the client, some critical variable may be missing. This may create the need to seek out a missing piece of the puzzle by obtaining records or interviewing caregivers. In some cases, a referral may be necessary to an outside provider to rule out an unidentified variable. For example, a medical evaluation, if not completed, may be suggested to explore physical issues prior to initiating toileting programming for an older child.

Knowledge about Other Disciplines

Many mental health training programs offer opportunities for students to experience other areas of human service through observation, clinical practicum and short-term, clinic-based work experiences. Even within the rigor of a graduate training program, students may have access to medical or multidisciplinary treatment centers where they can observe other professionals at work. After spending time in a community as a provider, connections with other professionals are gradually built through brief consultations regarding clients, providing feedback on referrals, and learning about systems of care. Working with other disciplines contributes to the mental health professional's knowledge about when to seek a referral for their client as well as what the mental health perspective may have to offer other providers.

For example, working as a staff psychologist in a multidisciplinary diagnostic developmental center could provide the chance to explore the importance of all aspects of development and how different disciplines examine developmental progress. Working side by side with speech language pathologists, special educators, developmental pediatricians, social workers, nurses, and occupational and physical therapists provides the opportunity to learn about the content, tools, and approach of their individual disciplines. Having some understanding of how different professionals can assist clients makes it much more comfortable to contact providers in these fields to ask for specific information via consultation as an outpatient therapist. A consultation referral can be made to a speech pathologist to evaluate the auditory processing of a child with attention-deficit/hyperactivity disorder and learning disabilities; an occupational therapist may be asked to consult regarding the sensory defensiveness of an extremely anxious autistic client; a developmental pediatrician can be called to consult regarding the slowed growth and gain of a client with developmental delays. These consult requests for clients being served in outpatient psychotherapy can provide valuable information and resources for the client, and offer additional insight to the therapist. Making these consultation requests can demonstrate that the therapist values collaborative relationships and may lead to future consultation requests from those providers and their colleagues or generate requests to provide professional training workshops for their agencies (see Box 14.1).

As new clinicians, the most frequent opportunity to participate in consultation will be with the referring physician or psychiatrist who has sought input from a mental health professional in assisting the care of a patient. Historically, there is a sense of unspoken (and sometimes spoken) hierarchical structure between the physician and therapist with the physician tending to assume a superior role. Often the physician holds the primary responsibility for the patient and may even be in a supervisory role over the clinician. It may feel intimidating to offer differing opinions or suggest changes to a medical doctor, and the development of a respectful assertive style becomes crucial for success.

In most cases, the physician or psychiatrist has much less time available to spend with a client. Following an initial assessment, medical doctors' subsequent appointments are often brief (5 to 15 minutes) and typically focus on monitoring prescribed medications or dealing with acute care issues. Thus, they may not have the same access to a patient's time as a psychologist or therapist, who in a 50-minute hour may gradually glean much information that did not occur to the client to report to the doctor. Treatment in which the prescribing physician can rely on the psychotherapist to provide feedback and suggestions is much more effective than situations that lack collaboration between providers. Therefore, providing the physician with the benefit of the therapist's biopsychosocial perspective and additional insights into the client's concerns can greatly enhance the client's overall care. This should be addressed even when the

---

Box 14.1

Community Professionals Who May Request Consultation from the Outpatient Therapist

Pediatrician	Occupational or physical therapist
Physician	Nutritionist
Psychiatrist	Neurologist
School Team/Teachers	Case manager
Parent/Guardian/Relative	Group home/nursing home staff
Speech therapist	Inpatient unit social workers

issues or questions raised may cross over into areas of medical expertise, as noted in the following example.

CASE EXAMPLE: ASSESSING THE WHOLE CLIENT

Three children—two boys, ages 10 years and 7 years, and a girl, age 4—were referred for family counseling in an outpatient mental health center due to long-term sexual abuse by their biological father. By the time of the initial appointment in your office, 2 years had passed since the discovery of the abuse; the father was incarcerated; and the children had already been examined, interviewed, and treated by sexual abuse counselors. They all presented with worsening symptoms of inattention, hyperactivity, nightmares, and aggressive behaviors. The oldest child had begun acting out sexually against the younger children and reported having auditory and visual hallucinations. The 7-year-old boy had failing grades at school, was uncooperative with his mother and teachers, was aggressive toward others, and had significant fears of the dark with disrupted sleep patterns. The young girl was extremely physically active and talkative, struck other children at preschool, but at times would become withdrawn, sullen, and would refuse to leave her mother's side. All three children were diagnosed with attention-deficit/ hyperactivity disorder. The older two boys were also diagnosed with post traumatic stress disorder and had been on high doses of stimulant medication, antidepressants, and antipsychotics for the past 2 years. The referring psychiatrist requested family therapy to help the children cope with the sexual abuse as well as individual therapy with the oldest child to address reports of sexual acting out.

At first glance, the scenario seems tragic but clear-cut, and there was pressure for the therapist to quickly begin intensive therapeutic services. Review of the psychiatrist's intake showed minimal current information other than the presenting sexual abuse history 2 years earlier. After obtaining careful histories of the children's developmental, medical, academic, and social histories, a curious pattern became evident. All three children had shown a dramatic increase in agitated and out-of-control behavior in the past 4 months following the youngest child's third bout of a significant strep infection. All the children had experienced several illnesses related to strep infections and generally had marked waxing and waning of behavioral issues that had been interpreted as inconsistent response to former therapeutic interventions.

The psychologist consulted with the referring psychiatrist and the children's pediatrician regarding the unusual presenting pattern of psychological symptoms and recurring strep infections. The pediatrician's impressions from the history were consistent with the psychologist's observations and documentation. The pediatrician then ordered strep antibody titers for the children. The results suggested significantly elevated strep levels. All three children were subsequently diagnosed with PANDAS (pediatric autoimmune neuropsychiatric disorders) and were placed on strong antibiotics. The course of PANDAS typically follows a "relapsing-remitting pattern with significant psychiatric comorbidity accompanying the exacerbations; emotional lability, separation anxiety, nighttime fears and bedtime rituals, cognitive deficits, oppositional behaviors, and motoric hyperactivity" (Swedo et al., 2002, p. 320). Over the following weeks, the children were weaned off all other medications with the psychologist giving frequent feedback to the psychiatrist by carefully monitoring their reactions to drug tapers. The majority of the presenting symptoms remitted in all three children within 8 weeks. The children were then able to participate more fully in supportive family therapy sessions twice per month with significant improvements in coping skills and decreased aggressive behaviors.

Benefits to Patient Care

This example illustrates the importance of seeking consultation with other professionals to effectively meet the needs of people served in therapeutic settings. The psychologist was technically asked to consult with the psychiatrist when asked to offer treatment services and assist in providing more thorough care to the children. The feedback regarding the medical question was given respectfully to psychiatrist and pediatrician by sharing information observed that might have an impact on the overall progress of treatment. The consultant was able to offer additional objective perusal of the client's history and behavioral patterns. In many cases, the referring or cotreating provider may have missed potentially critical variables or simply not recognized them after a long involvement with the client. The contributions of the therapist can offer a fresh perspective on the client, serve to provide a well-rounded viewpoint, identify new hypotheses to remediate symptoms, or offer greater insight into the family dynamics. A collegial ongoing dialogue between the psychologist, pediatrician, and psychiatrist will continue as all providers work with the family, thus collaborating to develop a more effective treatment plan with multiple perspectives. As is evidenced from just one example, taking a holistic approach in conceptualizing the needs of others has immense value and can often prevent obstacles to better outcomes.

Broadness of mind leaves much more room for creative problem solving and incorporation of others' opinions. Consultation is, in that sense, born out of the recognition that a single vein of expertise is not always sufficient to meet a client's needs. This may extend from therapist to therapist regarding a referral that lies on the edges of their area of competency; from physician to mental health professional on the depression of a diabetic client; from teacher to school psychologist on the fears of a first-grade student.

Complicating Factors to Collateral Consults

It seems obvious to support and follow the best practices of well-rounded, collaborative treatment, especially in the age of the biopsychosocial model. Although seemingly a critical part of good client care and justifiably creating a basis for future opportunities, outpatient therapists must contend with other issues. As this is a time of managed care and tight budgets, practitioners must also think about reimbursement for their time. Whether self-employed or a part of a clinic setting, there are likely to be financial limitations on how much of one's schedule can be spent in non-reimbursable activities. Unless the provider is paid by a grant, contract, or alternative funding source, most insurance and managed care companies do not pay for consultation between providers. This may create complications for the mental health professional as well as those providers with whom collaborative consultation is needed. The proverbial "phone tag" that ensues back and forth in the free moments found between the cancellations of each provider can create much frustration in the attempt to discuss concerns about a mutual patient. The time spent by the other provider is also not likely to be billable time; thus they may have difficulty finding non-patient times in which to participate in a consultative communication.

Brief consultation by telephone is likely to be the primary method of consultation between two providers who independently see the same client. It is necessary to be clear and direct, build rapport quickly, and communicate at times with e-mail or voice mail to meet the client's needs in a timely fashion. Projecting a confident, open style that is cognizant of the other provider's point of view can take some experience to develop. Furthermore, rapport building can be much more difficult by telephone when contacting someone with whom there is not a pre-existing relationship. After spending time in a community and making connections, communication between different systems or providers becomes less cumbersome.

In some situations, the clients being treated in outpatient therapy are also seen by numerous other providers. There will be times when a collaborative meeting is needed in which multiple professionals can consult together as a team to develop a unified strategy or address an ongoing crisis. While these meetings can be difficult to coordinate between many different schedules, there are situations when it will be essential to have all involved parties present to develop an effective treatment plan. Naturally, this is much simpler if everyone involved is employed by a single agency that encourages a treatment team approach. Although a hassle in the planning, establishing team communication and relationships for clients who have complicated issues can have a major impact on their progress. This is the same premise as consultation—at least that the additive effect of the clinical expertise and a well-coordinated intervention plan contributes to a better outcome for the client. Thus, it is within the context of traditional psychotherapy and clinical intervention roles that the conscientious mental health professional begins skill building in consultation.

Becoming a Catalyst for Change

The scenario that follows is likely to be fairly familiar for mental health professionals involved in the treatment of children. However, one could easily adjust the details to find the example to be equally applicable for geriatric clients adjusting to a new nursing home placement, or for adults with intellectual disabilities or mental illness transitioning to a new residential placement. For most therapists who begin their careers in clinical practice, this situation is a typical introduction to the world of consultation. Many clinicians have not had specific or extensive training in consultation skills and thus must draw on their expertise in interpersonal skills, knowledge of characteristic sequelae of disorders, and philosophy of human behavior. The therapist's personal beliefs or theoretical orientation about why people act and feel certain ways is likely the foundation of their approach to any therapeutic intervention. It is, therefore, also the basis on which providers' mental health consultation abilities will be developed. Much like working with individuals in marital or family therapy, the task at hand is to gather an unbiased understanding of all parties, translate each side's point of view to the other, and develop an intervention that will address the identified conflicts. As a consultant, the mental health professional hopes to become the facilitator of objective, thorough analysis of the client's concerns and thus a catalyst for positive change in the community setting in question.

CASE EXAMPLE: USING INTERPERSONAL SKILLS

Your next client this afternoon is Michael, a 12-year-old boy with attention-deficit/hyperactivity disorder, anxiety disorder, and learning disabilities. He has been coming to see you off and on for the past 3 years with varying presenting concerns. Michael began sixth grade several months ago and is struggling to cope with the demands of junior high, both academically and socially. Both of his parents have learning challenges and mental illness. They are devoted to their son but have problems advocating for his needs at school. Michael's parents called for an appointment because their son made all Ds and Fs on his report card and has had multiple detentions during the first grading period. As you review the chart in preparation for the session, you recall that Michael had been an average student with the assistance of educational supports outlined in an Individualized Education Plan (IEP). He received speech and educational resources in the past with accommodations in place to provide additional supports for his attention and organizational difficulties.

In meeting with Michael and his family, you note that Michael is withdrawn and irritable. His parents complain that he refuses to complete work in school or at home. Michael has become argumentative about chores and bedtime and spends most of his time in his room. He has been staying up late at night and often refuses to go to school. Although you previously had a good rapport with Michael, he does not appear happy to have returned to therapy. The parents are afraid he is depressed or is doing drugs. They feel that nothing they try seems to help. Michael states that he hates school and does not want to go anymore. He feels that the teachers hate him and says that he has no friends.

You request that the parents bring in some examples of Michael's schoolwork and a copy of his current IEP to the next appointment. You also ask that they sign a release of information so that you can contact the guidance counselor at the school. A follow-up appointment is made for the next week.

After sending several voice-mail messages and faxing the release form, you are able to touch base with the guidance counselor. She does not know Michael and is not aware of the school's concerns. She agrees to contact each of his teachers to gather information about their concerns and will call you back.

The degree of detail illustrates how complicated this can be to even initiate. A great deal of time is needed for in-depth records review and for multiple contacts with the school to even begin to get information. However, the parents have an existing relationship with you, as the clinician, and you have knowledge of Michael over a long period. While you could have directed the parents themselves to the guidance counselor, you are aware that they are sometimes nervous connecting with others and have had difficulty advocating for Michael in the past. Michael trusts you also and is likely going to be able to share with you what is going on more easily or quickly than with a new person.

The guidance counselor calls the morning of your next appointment. She informs you that Michael's teachers see him as a lazy, ill-prepared student who rarely has his assignments and does not participate in class. He never takes notes, his papers are practically illegible, and he is often disruptive in class. The school has concerns that there is something going on in the home and states that the parents have not been cooperative. Many teachers had commented that Michael comes to school in dirty clothes, hungry, and tired. With a few additional questions, you discover that no attempts have been made to contact the parents, and the guidance counselor is not aware of any accommodations or supports in place for Michael through his IEP. She plans to contact the family to set up a parent conference.

You meet with Michael and his parents at their scheduled appointment. The family does not have a copy of the current IEP and a review of Michael's work indicates multiple concerns. One on one with Michael, you discover that he has been feeling completely overwhelmed at school. He can't always open his locker, loses his books, and has problems getting to classes on time now that he has eight different periods and no study hall. He says that most of the work is too hard and he isn't getting help like he did in elementary school. In addition, he shares that he has been having problems falling asleep at night and often skips breakfast and showers because of struggling to wake up in the morning.

Here's another layer of the dilemma. It seems pretty clear at this point that you are needed to support this child and his parents in determining what is going on at school. Michael is showing signs of depression although the school team's interpretation has created a negative perception of the parents' involvement in the home. Your time is not billable to the family's insurance, and they cannot afford to pay you out of pocket. The school has not asked for your consultation and potentially has not identified any problem aside from Michael's behavior and lack of motivation. Therefore, there is no established consultative relationship, although it is your hope to consult with the school to better support Michael's needs. The solution will lie in your ability as the mental health professional to connect positively with the school team and support your client in a time-efficient manner.

After your discussion with Michael and reviewing his schoolwork more closely, you make some initial hypotheses about how to proceed. You assist the parents in arranging an IEP meeting with the school team that you attend. Fortunately, the team is eager to hear your input. They recognize that most of the new teachers are unaware of the accommodations that Michael has had in place in the past. You request some organizational assistance with lockers, navigating the hallways, and keeping up with his work. You also request that an occupational therapy evaluation be completed due to the poor quality of Michael's handwriting. Michael's previous cooperation in school is identified as well as his current feelings of stress and depression. The school team is receptive and agrees that many of their observations were consistent with the mental health issues being described to them.

Several weeks later, the parents report a notable improvement in Michael's attitude and signs of more effort going into his schoolwork. The school team has made some modifications to assist Michael and is planning to update his IEP. They have dropped a class and added a study hall in which Michael can receive resource supports in completing his homework. The occupational therapist completed an evaluation and identified a significant deficit in handwriting, and has recommended a keyboard be made available while they work with Michael on a remediation plan. Within 6 weeks, Michael's symptoms of depression have faded and he has been able to adjust to school expectations with supports. There are no longer any significant negative behaviors in the home environment and Michael is attending school daily without complaint.

The outpatient therapist entering the school arena is conducting a type of school consultation although the actual client continues to be the child being treated in therapy. The psychologist in the case example was serving as an advocate for his client and sought to improve the client's functioning in the school environment. In the case of Michael, the therapist was able to facilitate a positive change in school by adding another perspective to the school team's understanding of the child's educational and emotional issues. In this type of situation, the school staff may or may not use the information and recommendations offered as they have not clearly accepted the role of the consultee. As will be discussed, clarifying the role of the consultee or "who is the client" is part of setting up an effective formal consultation. In developing meaningful recommendations for helping the child at school, the interpersonal skills of the psychologist in working with the school staff are as important as expertise in understanding human behavior. Regardless of the brilliance of the consultant's suggestions, the school has to work cooperatively and openly for the ideas to be incorporated.

The success of the therapist in consulting with the school team was enhanced by the mental health professional's effective interpersonal communication style. Although the school team had not asked for input, the therapist was able to present information in a nonthreatening manner that resulted in the joint development of strategies to benefit the student. The intervention with the school team was brief but was fostered by the psychologist's effective use of the core elements of a successful consultant. A channel of communication was opened that allowed the outpatient provider to become a part of the school team. The participants were able to share their perceptions of the child and integrate this information into developing hypotheses about the current problems and set tentative plans of action in place.

CORE ELEMENTS OF SUCCESSFUL CONSULTATION

Many of the core elements of consultation skills reflect just good common sense. In fact, they are the desired qualities that we would expect in responsible mental health clinicians. Naturally, we hope that those who choose human service careers are compassionate and sensitive people. In addition, confidence, competence, and a cooperative communication style allow a consultant to present with an approachable demeanor that respects what the consultee brings to the relationship. It is important to recognize and underscore the importance of the personal approach and attitude that add to the likelihood of a positive connection with others in a consultative relationship. While many of these qualities are critical in the therapeutic setting, they are perhaps more salient issues when they become the building blocks of a consultation plan that may include multiple consultees, agency teams, systems, and one or more clients.

Positive Caring Approach

Caring about others is often the initial impetus for individuals joining the field of mental health service and is a necessary, although not sufficient, element of consultation. Effective consultants have good interpersonal skills and feel comfortable initiating conversation and gathering information in a supportive manner. A friendly, non-critical attitude helps consultees feel that they will not be judged or made to feel incompetent. The individual, team, or system, that has taken the role of consultee, has accepted a somewhat vulnerable position by indicating that they are faced with a situation they cannot handle alone. By acknowledging this sensitively, the consultant is beginning to set the stage for others to be open to change. Even while establishing his ability to skillfully handle the request, the consultant should exude a nonthreatening expertise that communicates collegial respect for both the consultees and the clients involved. "Such consultants radiate concern for the people in the relationship, not only for the problem under discussion" (Conoley & Conoley, 1992, p. 19). Ultimately, the goal of consultation is to empower the consultees to maintain their learning to better handle future challenges independently.

Although not therapeutic, the working relationship is enhanced by the consultant's empathic efforts to grasp the other person's worldview (Dinkmeyer & Carlson, 2001). It takes time and patience to explore the group dynamics of the consultee's administrative team or agency, the motivation behind the primary consultee's reported concerns, as well as the perspective of the involved clients. It is in these initial joining moments of rapport building and holistic viewing of the situation in which the artfulness of consultation is most evident. These skills are not learned through coursework, but through a personal commitment to developing effective helping relationships with others.

Good Communication Skills

The ability to listen attentively to others in a manner that hears and validates what they are saying is the basis of any good cooperative relationship. Use of verbal and nonverbal strategies is part of communicating attentive listening and illustrates that the consultant is valuing the consultee's input. Communication about the presenting concerns will compose much of the interaction during the initial stages of any consultation process. Interviewing and information gathering should be done strategically to gather factual data while attempting to understand the consultee's feelings and perceptions about the consultation issues.

How and what is communicated to the consultee early in the relationship is likely to strongly bias the effectiveness of the consultation outcome. During the initial formation of the connection to the consultee, consultants need to resist the impulse to be overly directive or too quickly offer easy answers. Immediate solutions that are advice rather than assessment-driven for a situation that the consultee has defined as complex can create the impression of superiority or superficiality. It can be easy to fall into this trap (the situation sounds urgent and you are being paid to help). The consultant enters situations that are often presented as nearing or "in crisis" with the staff appearing to be desperate for your help; while you, as the consultant, do not want to present as an all-knowing expert. The consultees may repeatedly refer to you as the expert or press you for immediate impressions and recommendations. Some would-be consultees may defer the creation of all hypotheses to you and resist taking an active role in developing solutions. It then takes tactful interpersonal skills to communicate the relationship with consultees in a manner that can engage them in the process rather than offer the quick prescription they may be seeking.

Responsible Work Ethics

As an external consultant, you are entering a system on your own reputation or perhaps that of your agency. Your presentation and follow-through create part of the exterior packaging for the valuable problem solving and successful outcomes that you hope to facilitate. Flexibility and time efficiency will be needed as your introduce a new element into an ongoing system that has its own established agenda. Ethical behavior guarantees that the consultant will provide what is promised, follow up and offer modifications as needed, and interact with others respectfully in a manner that is culturally sensitive and nonauthoritarian (Conoley & Conoley, 1992).

Thorough Diagnostic Skills

There are differing opinions about the importance of direct client assessment as part of the consultative process. However, any method of developing a problem-solving approach will by definition require careful scrutiny of all the relevant variables with a discerning eye. Although the consultation model may vary, the focus should be on exploring the contributory factors in the situation to create an intervention approach that meets all the client's needs. Identification of the consultee-client relationship, consultee characteristics and problem-solving skills, and client behavioral responses to potential antecedents are all potential key elements in uncovering maladaptive patterns that may be impeding the client's success. The message is simply to approach a consultation request with a structured, well-planned evaluation or ongoing assessment process that is consistent with the consultation method being followed. Most importantly, the consultant should avoid making recommendations too hastily or run the risk of appearing careless, superficially invested, or noncollaborative.

Wealth of Content Knowledge

The mental health professional who desires to become a consultant must first have a firm grasp of human development theory. The American Psychological Association code of ethics states that psychologists should not practice outside their areas of competency as is true for other mental health professionals. As consultants, it is advisable to be selective about accepting referrals, choosing those that are within your range of expertise. While a provider may have an understanding of general mental health concerns about older adults or adolescents, this is likely not sufficient to consult to other providers about Alzheimer's or the self-cutting behaviors of teens. Knowledge about and experiential or postdoctoral training with special populations is valuable in the field of consultation. Often, individuals with mental health concerns that are specific to their unique situations (e.g., deafness, paralysis, cultural differences, homosexuality) have great difficulty finding providers who fully understand the context in which their problems occur. If the referral concerns are linked to dynamics that appear to be specific to an unfamiliar diagnosis, the consultant may wish to suggest another more appropriately trained consultant or seek out additional consultation themselves around the presenting concerns.

Many consultants have not had formal training in consultative methods but have unique clinical expertise needed by the requesting consultee. Even school psychologists, who often have consultative demands as part of their job descriptions, do not always have extensive training in particular models geared for intervention in the school system. Thus, it is not unusual to be faced with a situation in which the mental health professional has the necessary clinical experience to best address the consultee's referral but is not experienced in offering assistance to others through consultation. At the very least, it is important to have a systematic approach and a preplanned set of processes and procedures when consulting with others. This requires being extremely thoughtful from receiving the referral to the first contact with a potential consultee. Greater success and comfort with consultation emerges by developing an awareness of consultative models and problem-solving methods. Knowledge of more structured approaches provides a framework to guide consultants and increase their flexibility as the details of the presenting situation unfolds. If you are in the position where your unique expertise is needed, you may consider informing the consultee that you are working on your consultation format and appreciate their input and questions as you work together to assist the client.

System Savvy

It is essential to understand at least the basics of the organizational and political structure of the systems in which the consultation is taking place. The consultant runs the risk of sabotaging the outcome of the consultation if they aren't aware of the parameters within which the system is capable of change. When consulting within the schools, the consultant must be aware that teachers have only so much control over the classroom environment and have minimal time to allocate to one-on-one interventions with each student. Recommendations that are offered as part of the consultation intervention plan must not only consider the dynamics of the larger individual school environment (e.g., space constraints, backup support from other staff and principal, amount of resources) but also the state and district requirements that staff are expected to uphold (e.g., curriculum expectations, behavior plan guidelines). Consultants who work within different settings must consider all the system information to develop solutions that will be effective within the confines of the constraints and resources available. Likewise, consultants who address issues in health care settings, nursing homes, or group homes must understand the system boundaries to assure that the consultation plan has ecological value. Box 14.2 lists some succinct warnings for consultants.

Therapists providing mental health services will likely have opportunities to consult with other professionals when facilitating their clients' success in multiple environments (e.g., school, work, psychiatric, or medical inpatient units). This is differentiated from situations in which consultation is the primary service being offered. When consulting with other professionals for your client the consultee involved has not contracted for your services. You continue to be the mental health provider maintaining the primary responsibility for the care of the client and have not contracted with another party to seek an agreed-on outcome. Consultation that originates out of the therapeutic relationship is most likely to be a brief connection with another professional to share information and problem-solve immediate next steps for a mutual client. These situations are thus more spontaneous and less process oriented than formalized pur-

---

Box 14.2

Twelve Easy Steps for Failure as a Mental Health Consultant

1. Know it all.
2. Learn nothing about the consultee.
3. Be unaware of your own motives.
4. Be definite, dogmatic, unyielding.
5. Sulk when your advice is not taken.
6. Use ambiguity to your own advantage.
7. Avoid feedback mechanisms.
8. Keep professional status in the forefront.
9. Conspire to cause unwanted, unsanctioned change.
10. Form alliances with subgroups.
11. Pick a few consultees as therapy patients.
12. Interpret consultees' motives with all available jargon.

Adapted from "The Art of Being a Failure as a Consultant" (p. 37), by Q. Rae-Grant, in *Practical Aspects of Mental Health Consultation*, J. Zusman and D. L. Davidson (Eds.), 1972, Springfield, IL: Charles C Thomas; and quoted in *School Consultation: Practice and Training*, second edition, by J. C. Conoley and C. W. Conoley, 1992, Needham Heights, MA: Allyn & Bacon.

suits in consultation. There may be situations in which outside agencies contract with you as a therapist to work actively within their setting to support an individual who is your client in a client- or consultee-centered approach. In these situations, consultants must clarify their role with the consultee and establish who holds the responsibility for the implemented changes. The dynamics may be more complex in these situations because of the consultant's existing relationship with the client. However, handled appropriately, this type of consultation situation can offer positive benefits to the consultee as well as clinical insights for the client's future treatment.

As mental health providers offering clinical opinions in a professional capacity, it behooves us to be well prepared in our consultative skills and in creating a planned knowledge-based approach to helping others. In the rest of this chapter, we explore prevalent models of consultation that have been developed by professionals who have devoted their careers to this area of mental health services. As mental health professionals, you should consider your philosophical and theoretical orientation when selecting a model of consultation. The approach that you choose to follow and meaningfully implement will need to be consonant with your particular understanding of human behavior but also should be relevant to the referral situation and reflect evidence-based practice.

BRIEF HISTORY OF CONSULTATION

The impetus for mental health services to move beyond the clinic setting to improve treatment outcomes fueled movements to develop methods of consultation. These early efforts at consulting began as a means of offering an alternate response to meeting the community's mental health needs when scarce professional resources meant that many individuals would not have had access to care. In the late 1940s and 1950s, Gerald Caplan was a psychiatrist faced with this dilemma. He developed a process in which available professional resources could be used more efficiently, refining and assessing these efforts into what would become the first formalized model of consultation.

Caplan went into the community where thousands of adolescent immigrants were living in residential facilities. He focused the efforts of his staff on working with the caregivers there to initiate changes that would benefit a larger group of individuals more quickly (Caplan, 1970). Caplan conceptualized this process of mental health consultation as "the process of interaction between two professional persons- the consultant, who is a specialist, and the consultee, who invokes his help in regard to a current work problem with which the latter is having some difficulty, and which he has decided is within the former's area of specialized competence" (Caplan, 1963, p. 470). His approach acknowledged the importance of community-based care and demonstrated valuing the input and expertise of the professionals within the system requesting assistance. Caplan and subsequent providers recognized the importance of taking the expertise out of the clinic setting and translating it into functional guidance for direct caregivers who had more frequent contact with the clients. This movement acknowledged the greater likelihood of generalizability and prevention when presenting concerns could be evaluated and addressed within the community.

Caplan's continued work on this method of mental health services resulted in a wealth of insight into the basic features of effective consultative relationships. His intent was not only to indicate what elements were critical for establishing the consultation relationship but also to differentiate the consultative role from that of supervision, therapy, and teaching. In defining the underlying premises of consultation, Caplan's basic assertions established the guidelines for the development of multiple consultative approaches.

Foundational Assertions of Mental Health Consultation

- The consultative relationship is triadic between the consultant, consultee(s) and client(s).
- The consultant and consultee relate collegially rather than the consultee being subordinate to the consultant. The consultant and the consultee are seen as experts in their own areas.
- The content of discussions between the consultant and consultee is specific to the needs of the client or issue at hand and does not address personal problems of the consultee.
- Because the consultant is on equal footing and not in a supervisory or authoritative position over the consultee, the client's well-being and progress is the responsibility of the consultee.
- The consultee can choose whether or not to accept the recommendations or guidance of the consultant.
- The consultative relationship is bound by the guidelines of confidentiality.
- The purpose of the consultation is to assist the consultee with the challenges and needs of the presenting client and also to increase the consultee's skills for addressing future problems independently (Erschul & Martens, 2002).

DEVELOPING THE CONSULTANT-CONSULTEE RELATIONSHIP

Much of Caplan's contribution of outlining the essential elements of consultation involved clarifying the importance of carefully defining and building the consultant-consultee relationship. Developing a positive relationship with the consultee is a critical element in the art of consulting, one that potentially has the most impact on the client's outcome. At its most basic level, requesting consultation involves the consultee's setting aside ego and seeking guidance from an expert for the goal of improved services to others. Of course, some consultees may be directed by their supervisor or director to ask for a consultation. They may not yet be open to new approaches or may not even recognize that what they were doing was not fully effective. Thus, there can be tension and defensiveness in accepting the input of the consultant outsider. Consultants who honor the trust and vulnerability of those asking for help have a much better likelihood of opening an effective channel of positive change.

The length of the connection between the consultant and consultee is as varied as the types of consultations that may occur. Internal consultants who are both employees of the same organization may have a collegial relationship. They may have consulted about multiple individuals or difficult situations over a long period. Following up on the progress of a specific client or intervention is clearly easier under such circumstances. However, even for the external consultant, it may be helpful to plan ahead for the follow-along process from the beginning. This creates a sense of security for the consultee and may increase their comfort level in deciding to implement a new approach with the client. Confidence in achieving a positive outcome increases with the knowledge that the consultant is available to tweak the offered strategies and supplement them as needed. It is this comfort level and confidence that fosters the initial development of a trusting relationship between consultee and consultant.

There have been multiple points of dispute among those who have devoted their careers to establishing effective models of consultation. How does the relationship work? Who is in charge of the process? What should the role of the consultant be? What is the nature of the contact between the consultant, consultee, and the client? What model of consultation is the best? Many texts have reviewed the pros and cons of each side, and can offer research studies that support various points of view (Brown, Pryzwansky, & Schulte, 2001; Erschul & Martens, 2002). The effect can be to make consultation seem much more tedious and difficult to master to those seeking to understand basic consultation skills. A source of the confusion is that consultation refers to many kinds of professional activities, which can be delivered in multiple settings. Consequently, it has been difficult for research studies to be developed to adequately compare the impact of specific consultation methods on outcomes. The psychological or mental health consultant must be able to have an eclectic base of methods and approaches to adapt to the referral concern. Therefore, the exact nature of the role of the consultant is truly defined by the particular situation and the nature of the request of the consultees and their organization or system (Kurpius, 1978; Pryzwansky & White, 1983). No one theory has been defined as the best approach to consultation, any more than there is one theory that is most appropriate in psychotherapy. Thus, consultation, like mental health treatment in general, should be directed by the approach that the consultant has determined can most effectively facilitate change in the specific referral situation (Kurpius & Robinson, 1978).

Entering the System

To initiate a successful consultative situation, the consultant has to be confident in establishing her role and clarifying the expectations of the consultee who is requesting assistance. One of the potential dangers in initiating a consultative situation without a sense of underlying philosophy or theoretical approach is that faulty premises could be communicated that set the relationship off on the wrong foot. The frequent misconception of consultees is that they are sending the client to the consultant as a problem to be fixed. Those who are making the referral may come in a sense of crisis and be eager to find an expert who will quickly prescribe a solution to make everything better. At this point, the consultant must be able to sketch out the consultative relationship and the process that will take place. This clarifies that the consultee will maintain responsibility for the presenting problem and will be expected to play an active role in developing the solution. While the specifics of the actual consultative approach may differ depending on the situation, the consultants' grasp of varying methods of the process indicates that they have the skills to lead the intervention to a successful outcome.

Internal consultants have the advantage of prior knowledge regarding the agency and the political dynamics that must be considered to facilitate change. There may be underlying issues of staff allegiances, absenteeism, or pervasive negativity about clients that may color the information offered about the client or the environment. The internal consultant must gain the commitment of the staff in terms of modifying other expectations to afford time for a new request. Organizational philosophy may put additional pressure on the internal consultant by setting boundaries on the nature, cost, and time commitments that were recommended based on the plan analysis.

The following organizational issues, of which the internal consultant is already aware, should be considered at the outset of establishing a relationship as an external consultant entering into a particular system:

- What are the personal skills and history of efforts to change in the organization—before you agree to consultation terms, what's the likelihood that they are willing to integrate new ideas? Does the atmosphere and communicated philosophy of the agency suggest that they are willing to invest the time and resources generally needed to support the consultee in following through with the recommended intervention plan?

- Address the feasibility of a cost-effective plan: Consider the time, effort, and expense involved in completing a successful intervention—is the organization willing to allow ample time, staff support, and compensation to the consultant to facilitate a good outcome?

- Develop a contractual agreement with the consultee and involved agency that specifies the roles and responsibilities of involved parties. Include the logistics of the services including the number of hours each day that the consultant will be on site to avoid unwittingly setting up unrealistic expectations (see Chapter 6 for more information).

- Establish a long-term plan that looks at the sequential steps of the consultation process including preventing future problems. Identify the stages of assessment, intervention, evaluation, and follow-up to inform the agency of the time line of the consultant's and the consultee's commitment to the plan. Consider the underlying agenda of the consultee and organization (e.g., is this consultation request intended to be shown as a final effort before relinquishing responsibility of the client to another classroom/placement/unit/home?).

- Clarify the identified problem area and all the organizational levels in which changes may be needed. Identify the responsible consultee and the client. Be assured that all parties are in agreement and that any necessary client permission documentation has been obtained. Be clear on the consultee's expectations and attitude about receiving consultation.

- Be aware of the philosophy and structural limitations of the consultee and system involved. External consultants need to recognize any potential limitations or guidelines so that there is less likelihood of inadvertently breaking a rule in the system (e.g., clearing recommendations with an administrator prior to giving them to a designated consultee).

MODELS OF CONSULTATION—CAPLAN

Caplan's introduction of the idea of consultation emerged when the predominant model of intervention was through a psychodynamic perspective. Faced with an unusual request for services that exceeded his resources, he proposed an alternative method of meeting the needs of a large group that still reflected a belief in the force of internal emotional processes. Caplan asserted that the consultees had potentially developed an unconscious connection to a client that blocked their objectivity and effectiveness. Thus, a primary task of the consultant was to carefully identify the source of the interference that was preventing the consultee from being successful with the client. Then, through the use of discussion and problem solving, the consultant would work with the consultee to address other potential areas of difficulty: lack of skill, knowledge, self-esteem, or professional objectivity (Conoley & Conoley, 1992). Caplan (1970) recommended that this process be handled without direct confrontation through the use of stories and metaphors. Because consultation is held to be distinct from therapy, Caplan advised that consultants would have to be cautious that deeper concerns could emerge during the process and avoid responding therapeutically.

Variants of this model are recommended based on the presenting concern with the consultant having the flexibility to shift from one to the other as indicated. The assumption would be that the consultant would be continuously forming and assessing tentative hypotheses about the root of the problem in the consultee-client relationship.

- *Client-centered:* Most common type of consultation performed by mental health professionals. The consultant acts as a specialist who evaluates the client directly to develop recommendations for how the consultee can deal with the client's difficulties.
- *Consultee-centered:* Caplan's primary mode of consultation and main focus of his model. There is typically little or no direct assessment of the client; rather, the consultant discerns the need for intervention by gathering information from the consultee. The consultant develops a plan for improving the consultee's work performance by promoting gains in insight, information, and knowledge of what approach is needed to address the needs of a particular client.
- *Program-centered administrative:* The consultant works with an individual or group of consultees assessing current concerns related to ongoing or new programs and policies to develop recommendations for change.
- *Consultee-centered administrative:* The consultant's goal is to assess the consultee and administrative staff to develop more effective professional functioning of an individual, group, or entire organization.

CASE EXAMPLE: MENTAL HEALTH CONSULTATIVE APPROACH

A nursing home director contacts you about a resident at her facility who has become more withdrawn and resistant. At your initial meeting with the director, the resident is described as an 80-year-old woman, Ruby, who has been at the nursing home for 2 years. She was previously more involved with others and had a close relationship with her roommate. The director indicates that since Ruby's roommate moved out to live with her family several months ago, she has been more argumentative with staff and often refuses her medication. As you learn more about the nursing home program, you discover that there has been much staff turnover in the past year. The day charge nurse has been there 5 years and is primarily responsible for all the individuals during the day. This is the staff member who has shared the majority of the complaints regarding the client and requested that the administration assist her in coping with Ruby's situation. You schedule an appointment to meet with the charge nurse on the following day to gather more specific information about the presenting issues.

After the initial meeting, you review the information that you have gathered and contemplate how to proceed. You can already identify that there may be some issues to address with the overall nursing home program and consider taking a program-centered approach in which you could work with the director to look at more organizational changes and solutions to developing more effective programming for the patients. However, more information is needed to determine the role of the charge nurse and the uniqueness of Ruby's situation compared with other residents.

On meeting the charge nurse, you discover that she is initially somewhat defensive at the idea of talking with an outside consultant. She is made to feel at ease as you explain that the director felt the issue that was raised was important, beyond his ability to solve, and that the whole program could benefit from an outside consultation. As the charge nurse begins to share her concerns regarding Ruby, you note that she appears extremely frustrated and is negative about the other staff's actions. Ruby is described as a problem because she does not cooperate with the schedule, requires extra staff time to coax her to take medication, and affects the morale of the other residents when she refuses to eat with the group or attend activities. You inquire about the roommate loss and any other factors that the charge nurse thinks may be contributing to the situation. The nurse has questioned depression, health concerns, and new staff who are not yet fully trained as potential contributing issues.

As the consultant, you contemplate using a client-centered approach at this point. You certainly have indicators that depressive concerns or staffing issues may be contributing. However, these concerns do not sound particularly unusual for nursing home patients, and the nurse has already identified potential causal factors. There may be some reason why the nurse, who has years of experience in this facility, is not able to handle this situation or make necessary referrals on her own. Therefore, a consultee-centered approach is felt to be the best starting point to support the nurse in developing a plan to address the concerns.

During subsequent meetings with the charge nurse, you discover that she has assumed much personal responsibility for Ruby's difficulties. Several times, the nurse had voiced her concerns to the director that with all the new hires and scheduling changes, there were not enough fully trained staff members available to deal with patient issues. In the past, the director had not been able to offer any further administrative support and tended to reassure the nurse that she could handle the concern at hand. As the charge nurse, she has the responsibility for the staff and the residents and feels overwhelmed by the heightened demands of meeting Ruby's needs.

The goals of the intervention are developed by the charge nurse and the consultant. They identify together that the nurse has not been able to be objective because of the impact of Ruby's behaviors on others' potential views of her work performance. Feeling incompetent to address all the problems in the facility at once, the focus became shifted onto Ruby. The consultant and the nurse as consultee discuss possible strategies that could assist in supporting Ruby as well as elicit environmental changes for coping with staffing issues. New information regarding addressing depression in the elderly was obtained for the charge nurse who then trained her staff. Ruby was referred for a physical by the charge nurse and assigned an individual staff member with more experience. The client was identified by her physician as having worsening arthritis in her back and prescribed new medication. The staff was educated about the apparent signs of Ruby's depressive reaction to the loss of her roommate and recommended supports to offer her. The charge nurse developed a mentoring training method with senior staff training the newer staff with excellent results; administrative pay incentives supported this approach and the increased scheduling demands. The consultant's follow-up at 2 and 4 weeks later indicated that Ruby had shown significant improvement, and the charge nurse had continued to implement new staff training and mentoring programs.

Use of this model was effective because the consultee was empowered by the consultant's nonjudgmental support in seeking staff training information and implementing problem-solving skills (Conoley & Conoley, 1992). Through the facilitation of the consultant, the charge nurse was able to identify the interference of poor objectivity and esteem issues in meeting the client's needs. Her gain of new information, increased confidence, and problem-solving skills will benefit other clients in the nursing home now and in the future. The client was also able to improve as a result of the consultation efforts although there was little or no direct client contact (Brown et al., 2001). This was Caplan's original intent of the consultee-centered mental health consultation model, to improve the lives of clients through indirect assistance to a caregiver. Long-term gains of the consultee should also ensure that skills gleaned from the experience will continue to benefit others without further dependence on a consultative relationship.

BEHAVIORAL CONSULTATION—BERGAN

While behavioral consultation also seeks to develop a problem-solving process that benefits both the consultee and the client, the focus of the intervention is directed on the observable skills and knowledge of the consultee rather than on the interference of their internal issues (Bergan, 1977; Bergan & Kratochwill, 1990). The consultant acts in an instructive role and leads rather than collaborates, yet the intent is for cooperative interplay with the consultee throughout the process. Consultants who are strongly devoted to the use of this model tend to spend less energy developing a relationship with the consultant and are more focused on defining roles and constructing an effective intervention plan. Conflict can occur in the initiation of this relationship if the consultant garners too much control from the outset and overly directs the consultee without establishing a sense of mutual trust. Experienced consultants know the value of artfully directing the process while acknowledging the consultee's equally critical knowledge of the client and setting (Brown et al., 2001).

Behavioral consultation can be useful in a wide variety of settings and with people of all ages; however, it is most applicable in situations in which the environments are controlled by caretakers (e.g., schools, prisons, residential centers). The use of techniques such as token economies, positive reinforcement, or behavioral contracting requires that an authority figure or direct care provider contingently provide reinforcement of the client's behavior. The approach is based on the assumption that all behavior, both adaptive and maladaptive, is learned and maintained by environmental factors. Since human behavior is believed to be predictable, one can systematically assess the variables that maintain the behavior in order to manipulate and modify them. Behavioral consultants use their expertise in behavior management to gather detailed information and problem solve with the consultee to concretely identify problems and determine what strategies would best address them. The strategies themselves are based on proven learning principles; however, creating successful outcomes is also dependent on the appropriateness of a prescribed strategy in a given setting. For change to be achieved and maintained, the consultee must understand and accept his or her role in implementing the plan and the environment must be able to be controlled in the manner indicated (Piersel & Gutkin, 1983; Sugai & Tindel, 1993).

To achieve the desired outcome, it is critical that the consultee is able to effectively observe the client, communicate concerns, and carry out the intervention plan accurately. Consequently, much of the research related to this model has looked at the strategic interviewing and teaching skills of the consultant who must assist the consultee in learning each step of this process (Bergan & Kratochwill, 1990; Bergan & Tombari, 1975, 1976). The success of the consultation is dependent on the ability of the consultant and the consultee to come to a mutually agreed on concrete and measurable definition of the presenting problem(s). The necessary information that the consultant must obtain from the consultee falls into several subcategories: "(1) background—environment, (2) the setting in which the client's behavior occurs, (3) the parameters of the client's behavior, (4) special characteristics of the client, (5) the nature of the observations made, (6) plans that have been tried or might be tried, and (7) types of additional data needed to solve the problem" (Brown et al., 2001, p. 49).

Bergan and Kratochwill (1990) carefully outlined the steps of the behavioral consultation process with recommendations and guidelines for how each step could be addressed. Other variants of the behavioral consultation model are likely to follow similar processes, as the model is based on learning principles and general guidelines for effective consultation:

- *Problem formulation:* Successful problem identification involves taking into consideration the client's background, current behaviors, and clear details of the environmental setting and is highly related to effective plan implementation (Bergan & Tombari, 1975).
- *Plan generation:* Develop intervention strategies that are based on evidence from the analyzed data and its applicability with the consultee's style and environmental boundaries.
- *Implementation:* Consultees do best when they have frequent contact with the consultant during this phase for reassurance, tweaking of the plan, and reinforcement of their efforts (Fuchs & Fuchs, 1989).
- *Plan evaluation:* This step is often neglected as many consultees may decide it is not working and just stop rather than regroup, modify, and continue. Potential outcomes are lost when more careful evaluation could have generated some positive success. It is part of the consultant's responsibility in the initial planning stages to outline the need for refining the plan until it works.

CASE EXAMPLE: A BEHAVIORAL APPROACH

Your social work practice has just signed a contract with a residential program for chronically mentally ill adults. The goal is for the clinical staff to consult with group home managers regarding the behavioral concerns of the clients in the homes. You are chosen to provide the first consultation to the Smitty House because of your training in behavior management. Your first meeting is with the director of the residential program who informs you of his concerns about David, a 34-year-old man with schizoaffective disorder, who lives at Smitty House with three other men. The group home manager, Tom, has been complaining about David's recent increase in destructive behavior and cursing at staff and the other residents. David's outbursts make his roommates agitated and at times may throw off the whole evening routine. The director wants you to consult with Tom and work toward a solution.

Several days later, you meet with Tom at the Smitty House after all the residents have gone to work. Tom has been the group home manager for the past 5 years and knows David well. He shares that David has been stable on his medication for a long time and tends to keep to himself and follow his routine. Several months ago, David was promoted at the factory where he works and was given a more complicated task on the assembly line. David was positive about his raise and new job and told everyone at the house about his success. However, Tom reports that David has appeared to be nervous and agitated lately. He becomes angry at minor demands or shifts off the schedule and has been refusing to complete his chores around the house. David threw his dishes onto the kitchen floor 2 days ago and pushed his roommate's clean laundry off of the dryer. When David gets into these moods, he becomes loud and screams obscenities at whoever is around him.

As the consultant, you interview Tom in detail regarding David's history and past behavior in the home and gather more details about his recent behavior change. The primary behavioral concerns are identified as David's refusals to cooperate with daily expectations and destructive/aggressive outbursts. A data gathering plan is developed with data sheets prepared to record detailed occurrences of David's refusal and destructive behaviors, including the events occurring prior to and following any behavioral event. Tom is given the responsibility of creating the data form and training the other direct care staff on how to correctly complete it. Since the behaviors do not occur with high frequency, you plan on 3 to 4 weeks of data collection to get an adequate sample. You check in the following week to find that only half of the data collection forms have been completed. In addition to being concerned about getting an adequate data sample, you wonder about the staff's ability to implement the eventual intervention plan. A quick call to the director adds support to Tom's authority in requiring the direct care staff to complete the forms as he had requested.

Data collection over the following 2 weeks was much more successful. Analysis of the information gathered revealed a pattern in David's behavior. David exhibited significantly higher rates of refusal and aggressive reactions on days that he arrived home more than 60 minutes later than his old work schedule. His refusals and agitation occurred consistently when David had to miss a favorite television program to complete a chore in the home. An intervention plan was developed with the consultee, Tom, who will adjust David's schedule so that his chores can be completed at times other than when he desires television viewing. Tom also plans to discuss David's work schedule with David's case manager and explore the reasons behind the recent overtime. The consultant and consultee work together on a behavioral contract for David that explains the tasks necessary for him to complete each week to participate in all the weekend activities. David's input on the contract assists in negotiating times and schedules for chores. Tom and the staff will continue to take data to assess the effectiveness of the interventions.

You communicate with Tom every few days to follow up on David's cooperation with the behavior contract. By the 2nd week, there was a decrease in the aggressive behavior but not in his resistance to tasks. David appeared tired and irritable. You encouraged a team meeting with the case manager and group home staff. The team suggested supporting David in modifying his work schedule to cut back on overtime and worked with him to increase his leisure activities. Follow-up at 5 weeks found David to be successfully completing his behavioral contract; now earning trips to the recreation center as his reinforcement.

Behavioral models can be very effective at quickly isolating the factors that are contributing to a well-defined primary problem. In the example, cooperation and "buy in" from the consultee and his support staff was necessary to proceed with the problem identification. Tom's continued efforts as the consultee, even when the first interventions were not fully successful, were supported by frequent contact and problem solving with the consultant.

ECOLOGICAL MODELS—GUTKIN AND CURTIS

An ecological perspective combines the strengths of various models by addressing the interplay of each individual's unique characteristics within their specific environment. Just as successful consultants tend to be those who can be flexible within the situation to adjust the consultative focus, this model advocates that the consultant blend the core elements of various approaches to best meet the consultee's needs. Consultants should be aware of the internal forces impacting on the motivational states of consultees and use aspects of mental health consultation that may be needed to support professional growth and insight. Likewise, consultants must also carefully include a thorough examination of environmental conditions that may support or interfere with the client's functioning as emphasized in behavioral consultation models. Process consultation techniques can also be employed to support ongoing relationships between parties of the consultation as well as within the organizations that have requested assistance (Conoley & Conoley, 1992).

Therefore, the consultant's task is to consider individuals within their environments while contemplating potential areas for change to assist the client in adapting more successfully. The plan for intervention operates on the assumption that neither the client nor the consultee is necessarily identified as faulty but that the balance between them is askew. The consultant's goal is to effectively develop a collaborative relationship with the consultee, assess the client's needs, and develop strategies for minimizing the gaps between the consultee's expectations and the individual's ability.

The basic characteristics of the ecological consultation process vary somewhat among different practitioners; each describing a similar process in slightly different terminology. Gutkin and Curtis (1990) proposed a series of steps to direct the consultant through the process. Their generic problem-solving approach blends together elements of mental health and behavioral consultation models and outlines the steps commonly followed by most ecological models (Kampwirth, 1999).

- *Clearly identify and define the problem.* The consultant may need to assist the consultee in clarifying the core presenting concerns. Correctly identifying the problem is crucial to obtaining a successful outcome (e.g., "Johnny is driving me crazy" is not a well-identified problem).
- *Observe and assess all aspects of the situation to contribute to an accurate understanding of environmental and personal contributing variables.* All sources of influence should be examined: the environment, consultee, client, expectations placed on the client, client's family, and health issues.
- *Consultant and consultee engage in collaborative brainstorming about potentially successful strategies.*
- *Consultee selects a strategy felt to be appropriate to their setting and possible to effectively implement.*
- *Identify the ongoing responsibilities and tasks of the consultant and consultee.* Determining clearly how the team will collaborate and follow through eliminates confusion and maintains the flow of the process.

- *Implement the selected strategy.*
- *Assess the effectiveness of the outcome, modify the intervention as needed, recycle through the sequence if necessary until the desired outcomes are achieved.*

CASE EXAMPLE: AN ECOLOGICAL APPROACH

The school psychologist of a local elementary school contacts your office requesting a mental health consultation regarding Anna, an 11-year-old girl she suspects may have emotional problems. Anna's intensely emotional behaviors often interfere with her ability to complete her work and interact successfully with peers. The school psychologist would like you to consult with Anna's two primary teachers: Ms. Warm, a nurturing older teacher who has been quite distressed by the frequency of Anna's "meltdowns" in the classroom and Mr. Stiff, who feels that Anna overreacts on purpose to avoid difficult assignments. You are told that Anna is experiencing episodes of panic-like behavior in which she makes frequent erasures, often hides under her desk and rocks, has outbursts of crying, and engages in repetitive skin picking. She typically becomes so upset that the parents are called to take the child home, and the frequency of these events has been increasing. You are contracted by the school to consult with the child's team of teachers to assist in developing an intervention plan.

After establishing the rate and time line of the consultation, you arrange a meeting with Ms. Warm, Mr. Stiff, and Anna's parents to identify the specific problematic behaviors within the school setting. You discover that Anna has been diagnosed with an anxiety disorder by her pediatrician, although no medication has been prescribed. Her parents state that she has always been a sensitive, hard-working child who has recently become worried about grades and peer rejection. The group defines Anna's primary problems as panic reactions that may include crying, escape, and erasures or tearing up class work. The skin-picking behavior is more frequent and is identified as a separate primary concern. Information offered by the teachers and parents indicates that Anna has been struggling with her assignments and school work since entering the 5th grade. She is often upset by the comments of the other children in the class who tease her.

The consultant meets with the consultees several days later to collaborate on a plan to gather more specific information regarding the variables contributing to Anna's distress episodes at school. A data collection plan is established to record the panic reactions and skin picking in each class period to include the behavior observed, and its antecedents and consequences (what Anna does after the outburst as well as the reactions and responses of the teachers). The consultant is pleased with the collaborative efforts of the consultees who will create the data sheets and follow through with recording the data over the next 2 weeks.

Several weeks later, the consultant was able to review the results of this functional analysis of behavior. He noted that Anna's panic behaviors occurred more frequently and with greater intensity in Ms. Warm's classroom. The consultees and consultant hypothesized that the strong emotional reactions of this teacher could be reinforcing the behavior or increasing Anna's feeling of helplessness. The greater intensity of behavior in Ms. Warm's room corresponded to Anna's being sent to the office for a break or home from school; thus allowing her to escape the stress of the classroom. Anna's skin picking and destruction of her papers occurred more often in Mr. Stiff's room, typically during math class, a setting in which she received less support. As a result of the consultant-consultee brainstorming, multiple strategies for potential interventions were discussed. It was determined that several approaches would be used at the same time with both teachers (consultees) actively gathering data on Anna's responses. The intervention plan included tutoring in math and involving the school psychologist to teach coping strategies to the student (e.g., requesting help, self-regulation breathing, and establishing a safe place in the classroom for self-calming). Signs of escalation in the student were identified for the teachers who were coached on ways to prompt the child to self-calm. Both teachers agreed to respond caringly but without being overly emotional or judgmental about the behavior. Steps were identified within the behavior plan for successive levels of assistance: prompted self-calming, teacher-directed prompt to go the calming area, short break to the counselor's office, then call to parent if the child continues to be distressed. The behavior plan was modified with the creation of additional strategies over time as Anna began to share information about the source of her stressors in the classroom regarding peer relationships and fear of failure. The consultant continued weekly monitoring of the plan for several months as the teachers recorded the frequency of the concerning behaviors and the child's responses to intervention.

Use of the ecological approach in the consultation for Anna incorporated both a behavioral assessment of Anna's problem behaviors and also identified contributing factors from her relationships with the consultees. Maintaining a broader viewpoint and examining other related nontarget behaviors (e.g., declining math grades, reacting to peer teasing) allowed for the development of more effective and more in-depth interventions.

In the next chapter, we explore the use of consultation models with special populations, address the importance of understanding systems issues when consulting, and discuss the future of mental health consultation.

Chapter 15

CONSULTATION SERVICES FOR SPECIAL POPULATIONS

Many of the challenges that interfere with our overall sense of mental wellness arise out of the difficulties we face daily in dealing with our lives. When a predisposition to mental or physical illness exists, there is the added impact of psychopathology or atypical neurophysiology on a person's ability to cope. As research and clinical practice explores the characteristic stressors associated with particular conditions, disorders, or situations, mental health providers are afforded beneficial pathways of support and alternative interventions. In addition, the evolution of the field of mental health away from a reactive treatment of mental illness to the more positive focus on promotion of mental health has opened the door to a wealth of new service opportunities. Professional specializations in serving special populations have developed to implement more pertinent strategies for working to overcome obstacles and counteract deficits that can create barriers to success. This chapter reviews avenues for clinical consultation that have emerged in response to our growing understanding of the importance of collaborative methods in fostering improved mental health in the general population and for those with more complex needs.

As the study of human mental health has grown as a science, the boundaries between physiology and psychology have become less clearly defined. Even prior to this era of the mapping of the genome, we had begun to identify specific neurological structural and chemical differences in the brains of individuals with certain diagnoses. Schizophrenia has long been tagged as a psychiatric diagnosis with strong evidence of biological causality. Research has continued to unravel the genetic and neurochemistry pieces of the etiological puzzle in the occurrence of mood and anxiety disorders, autism, as well as brain changes as a result of experience. Consequently, the field of human services is no longer isolated to a list of diagnoses with regimented treatment prescriptions. We have reached an age of transition to a coordinated medical and social service system model as we look at the entangled impact of heritability versus life circumstance on risk and resilience. We have come a long way from the early debates of nature versus nurture, yet we are still working to blend our systemic efforts at generating better outcomes. So what does this have to do with mental health consultation? Everything.

There definitely has been a growth of collaborative systems rising to meet the burgeoning mental health needs of our community. Schools are incorporating on-site mental health services, pediatricians have begun to have psychologists on staff, and medical centers now almost routinely incorporate mental health providers on a wide variety of service teams. Not only have we begun to identify the medical aspects of psychological and developmental diagnoses, but we are also recognizing the psychological variables associated with medical conditions. As discipline-specific care becomes a less efficacious approach, there will be a more obvious demand for clinical consultation for specific populations.

For the mental health providers who sought specialization in their graduate or postgraduate training, the idea of consultation for special populations is a given. Many pre- and postdoctoral internships in clinical psychology are designed with the goal of contributing to the development of a professional who can offer specialized care to a specific population (e.g., behavioral health, genetic disorders, pediatric psychology, forensics, autism spectrum disorder, neuropsychology, sexual abuse victims and offenders, substance abuse, criminal justice) and participate in collaborative care within a wide variety of settings. According to the Association of Psychology Postdoctoral and Internship Centers (2005), 92% of predoctoral and 86% of postdoctoral internships in the United States and Canada incorporate participation in consultation/liaison work. Of those sites, one-third of all predoctoral and one-half of all postdoctoral sites provide training in health psychology. A focus on pediatric psychology and developmental disabilities are each emphasized in approximately one-third of all pre- and postdoctoral training programs. Within these categories, many providers then become focused on certain populations or subgroups (e.g., AIDS, cardiac health and stress, feeding disorders, Fragile X, autism). This continued development of the mental health professional hones the skills and abilities necessary to address the psychological needs of individuals who have a variety of factors influencing their mental well-being. Whether your expertise grew from a training program or was self-directed through career choices and opportunities to work with certain populations, this rich knowledge base creates the mental health consultants needed to address today's complex mental health challenges.

The following sections explore the roles and functions of a consultant in school, medical, and community settings. Within each of these settings are a wide range of opportunities to offer highly specialized consultation and services to populations of individuals with unique needs as well as innovative provision of prevention and wellness education. As each area is examined, relevant issues regarding the status of service needs are briefly discussed to provide the potential consultant with a basic grasp of the context within which consultation may occur. Standard or more frequent referral concerns are then discussed along with case scenarios.

SCHOOL CONSULTATION

School is the field of work presented to children to learn and develop cognitively, emotionally, and socially. This is where they spend the majority of their waking hours and are faced with both possibility and challenge. Over the past 50 years, there have been changing trends in our cultural expectations about children, including those with varying needs and ability levels. Since the days of the one-room schoolhouse, there has been considerable evolution in the opportunities available in the educational system. The passing of public law (PL) 94-142, Education for All Handicapped Children Act in 1975 and subsequent revisions to the Individuals with Disabilities Act (IDEA PL 102-

119) in 1990 and IDEA amendments in 1997 (PL 105-17) have established federally mandated guidelines requiring that all children between the ages of 3 and 21 receive free and appropriate public education.

Moving from complete exclusion of children with special education needs in the 1950s to the right for complete inclusion into regular education in the 1990s, the schools have been required to continually reinvent methods of assessment, support, and education of students (Erschul & Martens, 2002; Fagan & Wise, 2000). The role of the school psychologist has been that of diagnostician and gatekeeper into special education services as created by early educational reform. Psychologists and school staff must again evolve to meet the changing needs of students today. Children with significant physical, developmental, or emotional-behavioral challenges once considered to need placement in a separate facility because of the nature of their difficulties are now in special education classrooms within their district. Children with milder delays and challenges are out of the self-contained classrooms and are partially to fully included in regular education classrooms. This restructuring of classroom configuration has occurred fairly rapidly in many areas of the country creating a great emphasis on the need for consultative support to educators and school administrators (Hoff & Zirkel, 1999; Reschly, Tilly, & Grimes, 1999).

The state of education today in the United States is beyond the scope of this text and, frankly, is a somewhat overwhelming situation from the vantage point of many taxpayers, parents, and providers. Federal, state, and local funds that support school programming and services are comprised of fluctuating available resources based on tax levies, a district-specific tax base, and the schools' ability to meet state and federal educational guideline competency standards. The take-home message is at least to note that the school district's financial resources have a great deal of flux that is dependent on multiple funding strata. This translates down the line to the teachers and school staff having a wide range of requirements for mandatory grade-specific curricula, standardized testing, and development and implementation of individualized education plans for students with identified special needs. At the same time, educators are now being asked to include more students with significant needs into their classrooms. While this movement meets the goals of supporting the rights of individuals to have the least restrictive environment in which to receive their education, many educators are not prepared for the time demands or additional skills it may require to adequately serve these students.

In addition to the changing services to children with developmental concerns and learning challenges, there has been a strong movement of reform directed at addressing the mental health concerns of the school-age child within the school setting. According to the United States Public Health Service (2000), mental health care needs for children have reached the level of a public crisis. "Approximately 21% of children and adolescents between the ages of 9 and 17 have a diagnosable mental or addictive disorder that causes at least minimal functional impairment; almost half of these youth, or 11% of all youth, have significantly impaired functioning, and about one-quarter of youth with mental disorders, or 5% of all youth, experience extreme functional impairment" (Anglin, 2003, p. 89). The federal mandates of IDEA that support appropriate public education for children with special needs also apply to children with serious emotional disturbances as this is also considered a disability. The passage of this law has instigated new efforts on expanding school-based mental health services for children, however, there continues to be little information available regarding the planful systematic approaches in schools to lead these efforts (Rones & Hoagwood, 2000).

While the incidence of mental health needs in children has grown dramatically over the past decade, the availability of providers and the development of critical programming have not grown sufficiently to meet the needs of many communities. Burns and colleagues (1995) estimated that only one out of five children with a mental health disorder receives the appropriate level of mental health services to meet his or her needs. There are other obstacles to the provision of needed care to children that go beyond availability of adequately trained professionals: (1) inappropriate identification and referral; (2) no or limited insurance coverage of services; (3) family difficulty accessing timely services around work expectations; and (4) lack of family awareness and understanding of the need to seek treatment. For these reasons, there has been a national initiative exploring direct provision of mental health services to children in the school environment. In fact, because of issues of accessibility, opportunities for preventative health education, and the results of evidence-based prevention programs for drug and violence prevention programs (U.S. Department of Education, 2001), schools have been suggested to be the setting of choice for mental health services for children and adolescents (Burns et al., 1995; Rones & Hoagwood, 2000).

> The *Report of the Surgeon General's Conference on Children's Mental Health: A National Action Agenda* recognizes that the mental health needs of children and adolescents could be better met if our nation (1) enhanced schools' and educators' abilities to identify and respond proactively constructively to children with mental health needs; (2) promoted children's and adolescents' access to mental health services by co-locating them in schools and coordinating effort with community-based agencies; (3) developed a common language describing children's mental and behavioral issues that could be used across sectors; and (4) helped parents and school systems to work effectively together. (Anglin, 2003, pp. 100–101)

There is much work to do to improve community efforts to meet the emotional, behavioral, and academic needs of children. While the indicators of gaps in care and significant levels of difficulty are impossible to deny, the educational system is not fully prepared to meet these expectations. Further community and collaborative supports will be needed over time to develop efficient and effective models of service that fit into varied school environments. Continued monitoring of the successes achieved and the issues generated by ongoing efforts to meet these needs is important in the gradual creation of more effective solutions. Mental health/clinical consultation services provide opportunities to empower school faculty and staff with new knowledge and tools for supporting the children and adolescents in their care. Therefore, mental health professionals should be aware of systemic concerns in addressing mental health needs in the educational setting:

- Schools often under-identify children with significant emotional and behavioral problems. With the prevalence rates of mental illness in children growing, it becomes more critical to facilitate identification and prevent worsening problems.

- Programmatic supports that are available for children with mental health problems are often segregated and overemphasize behavioral control while neglecting academics and development of social skills. Children with difficulties in coping tend to be managed rather than treated or taught alternative, more appropriate behavior.

- Attitudes tend to be negative toward children's families, creating an adversarial rather than collaborative relationship. This further strains the unified family-school support connection that is crucial in supporting progress.
- Students with mental health problems are less likely to graduate and find a job and have an increased likelihood of engaging in delinquent behaviors (Knitzer, 1996).

Faced with the urgency of the substantial developmental and emotional needs within the school environment, there has been a growing awareness of the critical role of collaborative multidisciplinary consultation services. Widening this net to acknowledge children with special health care needs captures an additional 15% to 20% of children in the United States who have been identified as having an ongoing need for specialized attention within the school setting (Newacheck et al., 1998). Children with chronic illness, physical disabilities, and complex medical needs have a higher risk for difficulties with educational progress, overall poor adjustment to school, emotional problems, and more psychosocial difficulties than their same-age healthy peers (Boekaerts & Roeder, 1999; Lavigne & Faier-Routman, 1992). These children require individualized educational planning for learning issues and emotional or behavioral concerns that can also address any needs for specialized arrangements to deal with physical modifications, accommodations for support of medical issues, and potential periods of homebound education.

"School mental health providers, including nurses, counselors, school psychologists, school social workers, special educators, and their clinical partners—psychologists, psychiatrists, and psychiatric nurses—have a unique opportunity to address the mental health needs of students. . . . Professionals from different disciplines bring unique frames of reference, as well as different backgrounds, priorities, expectations, and clinical responsibilities. They may have different ways of conceptualizing students' strengths and difficulties, which, taken together, provide a comprehensive view to guide interventions" (Rappaport, Osher, Garrison, Anderson-Ketchmark, & Dwyer, 2003, pp. 107–108). Effective integration of the collective input of involved providers can be complicated at best, emphasizing the need for all parties to have clarified roles and mutually agreed-on outcomes if working within a team atmosphere.

In this arena, opportunities for beneficial mental health consultation are numerous. The school has become the hotbed of possibility for creation of integrated services for meeting the full gamut of children's needs. This transitional period is both exciting and stressful for the educational and mental health communities who are in new territory establishing a joint service philosophy. Potential requests for mental health consultation may occur at multiple levels: programmatically for classroom or school-based mental health clinic settings; client-centered diagnostic consultations from school-based mental health staff, educators, guidance counselors or school psychologists; or in-classroom consultee-centered consultation. The numbers of possible combinations are impressive and should serve to communicate the substantial growth indicated for the future of consultation services.

Enter the Consultant

As school team members cope with the continuing challenges and new demands of their changing educational system, internal school psychologists may frequently be approached with requests for consultation to teachers and staff. However, they are often overly taxed with the diagnostic and assessment requirements of educational placement and planning. Likewise, teachers have their plates full with system requirements and classrooms filled with children. Typically, the children who prompt the busy teacher to request a consultation are those who are disruptive or not thriving in the classroom. Generally, the child goes on a waiting list for review, followed by the necessary steps of data collection, testing, and observation needed by the school team to review the situation. Next, there is consultation with administrators and the school psychologist, and discussion with the parent. By the time this process has determined what intervention is needed, issues with the child may have worsened and teachers may be more frustrated.

Requests for consultative assistance may be fraught with underlying conflicts from the outset. If teachers make a referral for a consultation because they cannot manage the needs of the student with the time they have available, they are likely to be resistant to the consultant's introduction of time-intensive interventions to promote changes within the classroom (Wickstrom & Witt, 1993) or may have initiated the consultation request with the intent of having the child removed and placed elsewhere (Erschul & Martens, 2002). Consequently, with both the teacher and the internal school psychologist busy with other mandated tasks, potentially effective consultation efforts may never get initiated or fully implemented. It is not surprising that time constraints are the greatest obstacle to successful consultation services (Costenbader, Swartz, & Petrix, 1992). Understanding the situational context of the school as a system is critical for external consultants who enter into the school setting and need to modify their efforts relative to these dynamics.

The importance of understanding the concerns of the school system and educational guidelines cannot be overemphasized. This knowledge arms the consultant with a great deal of advanced empathic understanding with which to initiate a relationship with a classroom teacher. In addition, it provides the consultant with a beginning framework of understood limitations and boundaries of the school teams' availability, resources, and administrative support in terms of potential consultative recommendations. As indicated earlier, the consultee is ultimately responsible for conducting any recommended data collection and implementing the modifications for a particular client. While one can influence the likelihood of accepting valuable recommendations by demonstrating the plan's potential effectiveness (Von Brock & Elliott, 1987), "teachers are not passive recipients of consultant suggestions and often reject these suggestions because they involve too much time, contradict personal beliefs, or reduce personal freedom" (Erschul & Martens, 2002, p. 101). Consequently, the successful consultant not only must be able to implement models effectively to create meaningful recommendations specific to the child's profile but also must make them ergonomically sound, highly palatable, and user friendly.

The review of mental health consultation models in Chapter 14 outlined the use of different approaches on consultation that have all been successful in school environments. The concentrated discussion on that particular setting was included in this text because of the current high demand for school consultation. The following list of case scenarios outlines possibilities for mental health consultation in schools.

CASE EXAMPLES

- A 9-year-old boy with childhood onset bipolar disorder frequently crawls under his desk in class and begins screaming, crying, and banging his head. The classroom is typically cleared of students while multiple teachers try to calm the child. Although he was previously an honor roll student, the boy has been getting upset a lot lately, refuses to cooperate with classroom routines, and often tears up his work. The teacher feels that she can no longer manage the child's behavior problems and feels that he should be removed from her classroom.

- A principal requests assistance dealing with an upsurge of bullying and violence occurring before and after school at a local inner city high school. There has also been a growing incidence of outbursts of defiance and destructive behavior in multiple classrooms; lengthy out-of-school suspensions are at a record high.
- A 10-year-old girl in a local elementary school has recently been diagnosed with Juvenile Onset Diabetes. She missed multiple days of school because of medical appointments and has fallen behind academically. However, the child has been refusing to come to school because her peers have been teasing her about her insulin injections and trips to the nurse's office. Her parents called the school guidance counselor in distress because of these additional stressors on their daughter.

Resources for Consultants Working with Schools

Box 15.1 offers tips for consultants in their work with teachers. A few useful reference sources are included next.

SUGGESTED READING

- An excellent resource for specific intervention plans to address concerns related to a wide variety of developmental and emotional concerns within school settings can be found in the text, *Interventions for Academic and Behavior Problems II: Preventive and Remedial Approaches* (2002) edited by Mark R. Shinn, PhD; Hill M Walker, PhD; and Gary Stoner, PhD; National Association of School Psychologists, Bethesda, MD.
- *Functional Behavioral Assessment: A Systematic Process for Assessment and Intervention in General and Special Education Classrooms* by Mary E. McConnell (2001). Denver, CO: Love Publishing Company provides a user-friendly basic explanation of functional behavioral assessment with a wealth of reproducible forms for assessment, data collection, and behavior plan development.
- *Behavioral Assessment in Schools: Theory, Research and Clinical Foundations,* second edition, and its companion volume, *Conducting School-Based Assessment of Child and Adolescent Behavior.* The texts were developed together and edited by Edward S. Shapiro and Thomas R. Kratochwill (2000). New York: Guilford Press. They provide an excellent and detailed exploration of all aspects of school-based assessment.
- A thorough review of current information regarding advances in mental health program development in schools can be found in the *Handbook of School Mental Health: Advancing Practice and Research,* Weist, Evans, and Lever (Eds.) (2003). New York: Kluwer Academic/ Plenum Publishers.

PEDIATRIC PSYCHOLOGY

Pediatric psychology has emerged as a separate field of practice over the past 30 years, applying a developmental perspective to the exploration of the psychological, developmental, and physical health of children and adolescents. Its creation was the logical

===== **Box 15.1** =====

Tips for the Consultant to Help a Classroom Teacher

- *Be aware of the importance of the teacher's attitude toward the child.* The consultant could suggest a specific way in which the teacher might change their approach and indicate how this change, if it is done consistently, may influence the child. *The encouragement of this relationship is basic to the consultation process.*
- *Understand the efficacy of logical consequences, in contrast to punishment.*
- *Avoid rewarding misbehavior.*
- *Be aware of the nature of his or her relationship with the children.* Some teachers are too kind, and the children run all over them. Other teachers try to be too firm and too tough, and the children only rebel. The consultant can provide the teacher with a more objective observation of the nature of his or her relationships with the children.
- *Become aware of the power of the group and group discussion.*
- *Become aware of the way in which the child reveals lifestyle through interactions with others.* Observing nonverbal behavior (e.g., smiles, signals, and other facial expressions) may help to understand the child's personality and the way in which he or she seeks to become significant in the group. It is only as the teacher becomes aware of each child's unique lifestyle that the teacher has access to procedures for modifying his behavior.
- *Recognize that one of the most powerful tools for change is the proper utilization of responsibility.* Too often, teachers give responsibility to the child who has already demonstrated responsibility. It is much more useful therapeutically to give responsibility to a child who needs the responsibility to enhance development.
- *Be free from outmoded approaches for dealing with difficult children.* Teachers should be particularly cautious of using schoolwork or assignments as a punishment and should refuse to become involved in the client's attempts to manipulate the teacher. The teacher must become competent in understanding human behavior and motivation.
- *Recognize that talking at the child will not change the behavior.* It is often observed that teachers tend to talk too much and act too little. The consultant should help the teacher to see how a new relationship and logical consequences are more efficacious.
- *Develop a classroom council.* When there is considerable difficulty within a room, a classroom council can help set limits and rules that will be more acceptable to the total group.

Adapted from *Consultation: Creating School-Based Interventions,* second edition, by Don Dinkmeyer Jr. and Jon Carlson, 2001, Philadelphia, PA: Brunner-Routledge, pp. 82–84.

resolution of a common dilemma faced by both pediatricians and child clinical psychologists who were unable to meet the needs of many critical childhood problems independently. Problems that are addressed include the difficulties that may occur during a typical or atypical developmental course: behavior, education, and illness. Pediatric psychologists assume many roles to support the needs of children and their families who are faced with these concerns as well as the issues related to prevention, treatment, and coping with chronic illness and disease.

The multifaceted approach needed to care for the physical and psychological development of children requires a developmental perspective that incorporates families, schools, and health care systems. The field of pediatric psychology has in many ways forged a mediating role that acknowledges the importance of collaboration regarding the whole child across all involved systems. This area of specialization speaks to the importance of collaboration among professionals with a rapid expansion that has been supported by policy development and clinical research in medicine and psychology.

In practice, pediatric psychologists are likely to work with a broad range of presenting problems using skills that rely on an in-depth knowledge about the concomitant psychological factors associated with developmental concerns and physical difficulties. The role and practice of pediatric psychologists has evolved in recent years with opportunities increasing in community settings.

Primary Care/Outpatient Clinics

Pediatricians in primary care see children and adolescents throughout all phases of their development and are the most likely setting in which early identification of emotional and developmental problems can occur. With changes in managed care, there has been an ever-growing demand on pediatricians to diagnose and manage mental health concerns despite a lack of training and time to fully assess and treat them. Within primary care, pediatric psychologists have the opportunity to consult with the physician, provide direct clinical services of screening and assessment, and work with families in conjunction with the pediatrician in preventative approaches to developmental and behavioral concerns. Commonly occurring referral concerns include attention and school problems, aggression, noncompliance, and temper tantrums (Charlop, Parrish, Fenton, & Cataldo, 1987; Sobel, Roberts, Rayfield, & Barnard, 2001). Pediatric psychologists are also frequently presented with concerns regarding feeding/mealtime issues, toileting, sleep/bedtime difficulties and the full gamut of the expected conflicts that occur during development.

Inpatient Hospital Units

According to Thompson and Gustafson (1996), approximately 1 million children in the United States experience difficulties in their daily functioning because of some form of chronic illness, with another 10 million children experiencing lesser forms of chronic medical conditions. Many of these children have frequent or lengthy inpatient hospital stays and have been the inspiration for much of the rapid growth of pediatric psychology. Consultation/liaison services for acute and chronic illness units, such as neonatal/pediatric intensive care, oncology, and burns, are among the many special populations served by pediatric psychologists (Roberts, Mitchell, & McNeal, 2003). Interventions requested regarding mental health concerns on medical units may relate to depression or suicide attempts that instigated the hospitalization or issues which may be occurring as a concomitant factor of the medical condition being treated (e.g., behavioral acting out related to extended hospitalization or grief reactions to loss of functioning, separation from friends and family, or worsening of prognosis). Pediatric psychologists may also be asked to work with children and their families around adjustment to illness and symptom management. The psychologist or other mental health professional may often assist families in processing the information that they have received from medical staff about their children's chronic illnesses both to clarify questions as well as to provide support around the emotional impact on their families. Concerns about adherence to recommended treatment regimens and coping with the fear and pain associated with procedures are also common referrals to the pediatric psychology service.

Specialty Facilities and Clinics

Pediatric psychologists may also play a consultative or direct care role in centers outside of medical settings. They may assist in the promotion of healthy lifestyle changes, consult providers of rehabilitative services, teach education groups for parents of children with chronic illness, or offer supports to recreation programming for children with medical or developmental needs such as cancer, AIDS, or cerebral palsy (Roberts et al., 2003). Pediatric psychologists may also offer direct therapeutic services to children and their families in outpatient mental health clinics. The specialized nature of the pediatric psychologist's consultation and services to medical and health care providers, teachers, families, and a wide variety of professionals in human service professions emerges from their detailed background and understanding of the multiple challenges that impact children and their families.

Psychosocial and emotional issues are often an under-identified and grossly misunderstood aspect in supporting the overall well-being of children with special needs and their families. Children with chronic illness are at an increased risk for psychological adjustment problems and mental health disorders (Lavigne & Faier-Routman, 1992). The incidence of mental health disorders in children with mental retardation/developmental disabilities has been estimated to be 4 to 5 times higher than in children with typical cognitive development (Feinstein & Reiss, 1996). The realm of challenges that are present for individuals with disabilities and their families can be astounding. The accomplishment of tasks that we often take for granted: toileting, dressing, self-feeding, and learning to walk and talk are not automatic or possible for everyone. The impact of differing physical and cognitive abilities creates numerous consequences on the concurrent developmental process of emotional and social development, learning through play, and the establishment of relationships with family and community. Children with frequent exacerbations of illness or who require multiple procedures or hospitalizations experience lengthy separations from family and the normal progression of their developmental journey in their classrooms and communities. Many other factors experienced by children with chronic illness and developmental disabilities can contribute to an increased vulnerability to emotional problems: limited community inclusion, stigmatization, chronic stress, and peer rejection.

Methods of Consultation

The process of consultation in pediatric settings differs from other approaches to mental health consultation. Typically, it follows "a medical model in which the consultant's primary responsibilities involve assessment and communication to the physician about findings and advice concerning management" (Drotar, Spirito, & Stancin, 2003, p. 60). The details of the assessment process used depend on the nature of the referral question and could address anything from the developmental level of the child, the presence or absence of a mental health disorder, or input regarding the psychosocial interventions to assist the child in cooperating with the plan of care.

Roberts and Lyman (1990) review three models of consultation that can be selected by the mental health professional based on the consultation question or the preference of the referring physician.

Independent Functions Model

In this approach, the consultant and pediatrician each work independently of one another and do not actively collaborate on the treatment of the client. This model is often established for the purposes of the physician ordering the assessment of a specific diagnostic question. The appropriate protocol, unless clarified differently between the two professionals, is one in which the consultant receives information about the client and concern, completes the assessment, and communicates the findings back to the physician. The physician then uses the information in the treatment plan and shares any findings with the family. The consultative role does not fully tap into the skills of the mental health professional but is viewed similar to a medical consult for an x-ray or ultrasound; that is, the consultant as technician.

Indirect Consultation Model

This approach is similar to the consultee-centered mental health consultation model as the mental health provider consults to the physician who will then employ the new information with the patient/client. The consultant does not typically have contact with the client and operates based on the information provided by the physician. This method is likely to be used in teaching situations or in the support of pediatricians who are working to incorporate more behavioral interventions into their own practice. Examples of indirect consultation can include: phone consults about developmental or diagnostic questions or the appropriateness of a referral; provision of training seminars to pediatric staff; or consultation about the development of screening tools or protocols for frequently presenting problems in the physician's practice.

Collaborative Team Model

In a collaborative approach, the mental health professional and pediatrician work together as colleagues with mutual involvement in patient care. This is the most appropriate model for inpatient hospital settings or outpatient clinics in which the consultant serves as a collaborative team member with other providers whose common goal is providing comprehensive care to children with complex medical and psychosocial issues. Cohesive inpatient treatment teams regarding specific populations such as oncology, pediatric AIDS, cystic fibrosis, or sickle cell anemia may include the continued involvement of pediatric psychologists as well as clinical social workers on their teams, each with distinct contributions and roles.

Regardless of the parameters of the consultation, there are key elements to consider in achieving a successful consultation. Drotar (1995) notes that physicians look for thorough and concise written feedback in the form of a consultation report or chart note and often direct dialogue regarding the case. The feedback should include a history of the presenting concerns, procedures used, review of the child's primary concerns and recommendations for support and intervention with the patient. In addition to the effective summation of consultation findings, consultants need to exude a competent and positive approach to the development of the professional relationship. This includes dealing competently with different diagnostic or patient care philosophies, following appropriate referral protocol, rapid turn around from request to feedback, and maintaining an appropriate familiarity with medical terminology and abbreviations used.

The following list of case scenarios outlines consultations typical for pediatric psychologists and social workers.

CASE EXAMPLES

- A 4-year-old boy with 85% of his body covered with 2nd and 3rd degree burns is admitted through the emergency room. The burns resulted from the child being thrown in a tub of scalding water. The parents, fearing prosecution, abandoned the child at the hospital, and no other family members have been located. The burn unit staff calls for a consult as the child is in shock, is crying for his mother, and refuses to eat.

- You are asked to conduct an evaluation of a 6-year-old girl with Cystic Fibrosis during her visit to the outpatient follow-up clinic this afternoon. The team physician is concerned that the child has become depressed and is showing cognitive decline. Your results and recommendations will need to be reported to the physician within 24 hours.

- The pediatric unit on 4 south has requested a consult on a 13-year-old boy, Jamal, who has sickle cell anemia and has been admitted with severe abdominal pain, stomach distention, and constipation. He has minimal food and liquid intake. He seems to be withdrawn and afraid and is resisting the nurse's attempts to examine him. The child's mother is frustrated with her child's frequent admissions, is distressed that her son is being admitted to the hospital again, and is eager to return home to her two other children. The family is new to the area and has few community, medical, or family supports.

- In your role at Dr. Jones pediatric practice, you provide the nursing staff with training on newly developed screening tools for developmental delays and indicators of autism spectrum disorder.

SUGGESTED READING

- *Handbook of Pediatric Psychology in School Settings* (2004). Edited by Ronald T. Brown. Mahwah, New Jersey: Lawrence Erlbaum Associates, Publishers. This text provides a current examination of the needs of children with special health care concerns within the school environment, information of prevention and health promotion, and a review of developmental disorders and medical conditions that are likely to be encountered when consulting within school systems regarding pediatric issues.

- *Handbook of Pediatric Psychology,* third edition (2003). Edited by Michael C. Roberts. New York: Guilford Press. This text offers a thorough review of pediatric psychology with detailed chapters that include current information on the range of medical and psychological conditions affecting children today.

HEALTH PSYCHOLOGY/BEHAVIORAL MEDICINE

Research exploring the impact of psychological characteristics as contributing factors to physiological illness has been growing in the past several decades. We have long studied the effects of stress and lifestyle choices on prevention of and recovery from cancer, heart attacks, and gastroenterological conditions. The effect of interdisciplinary studies on these relationships has led to greater support of prevention programs, incorporation of stress management and relaxation into cardiac recovery programs, and the use of meditation in dealing with chronic pain. Many mental health professionals have become involved with the growing field of behavioral health, acting as consultants to physicians and clinics treating patients with a variety of disorders. As a field, we have identified the impact of illness on psychological well-being and established a clearer picture of the positive outcomes associated with specific interventions and treatment approaches (Kazdin, Bass, Ayers, & Rodgers, 1990).

Mental health professionals can utilize all of their previous training in therapy and assessment in a variety of health care settings, including hospitals, clinics, and private practice. Consultation skills are especially important in interacting and communicating with medical providers and patients, who may not always appreciate the value of the services provided by the mental health field. Several important areas of behavioral medicine are described next.

Pain Management

Pain is a natural process in the human body that provides important information about current functioning. Normally, even when significant physical damage has taken place, our brains adapt our pain thresholds. However, for some people, chronic pain is a constant stressor that makes each moment barely tolerable. Psychological states have a profound impact on the perception of pain, and mental health professionals can help patients cope with pain when medical interventions have not been fully successful. Consultants can education patients about the nature of pain, and work to help the patient understand the factors that contribute to and assuage pain. Psychotherapy can help patients find more meaning in life, foster greater social supports, reduce depression, and challenge dysfunctional thought patterns that work to maintain a patient's fixation on the sense that the pain is intolerable. The therapist can also use and teach the tools of biofeedback, hypnosis, meditation, and relaxation training.

Prevention, Health Education, and Support

Mental health professionals are often involved in the provision of psychoeducation about specific topics to patient populations, and this skill can be very useful in health-care settings. Such education can constitute *primary prevention* (providing general knowledge to everyone to prevent problems), *secondary prevention* (targeting groups who are most at risk for specific problems), or *tertiary prevention* (working to reduce the negative impact in populations who have already developed a specific problem or diagnosis). Examples of primary prevention would include educational groups about proper diet, the importance of exercise, and stress management. Examples of secondary prevention would be groups for smoking cessation and anger management. An example of tertiary prevention would be designing an intervention plan to help insure compliance to medication and other treatment regimes.

Mental health professionals can also leverage their group therapy expertise to develop support groups for individuals suffering from certain diagnoses, such as cancer, Alzheimer's disease, diabetes, and AIDS. Such groups can help patients adjust to the lifestyle changes concomitant with such diagnoses, can facilitate the development of healthy coping skills, and can provide an opportunity for patients to find social support and needed information about the progression of these conditions.

Assessments for Surgical Candidates

Even though surgical techniques and technology have improved greatly in recent years, surgery always entails some risks, and physicians take measures to ensure that the potentially irreversible step of undergoing surgery is not taken lightly. Mental health professionals can help medical teams determine the suitability of certain candidates for specific surgical procedures. Sex change operations are one example of a drastic surgical procedure for which candidates are required to undergo psychological evaluations (and a period of time assuming the role of a member of the desired gender). Individuals with chronic pain sometimes have the option of undergoing surgical procedures to decrease their pain, but if the pain is strongly related to depression and anxiety surgery will incur more risk than benefit. Bariatric surgery, in which portions of the gastrointestinal system are removed so that the individual's body cannot absorb calories as readily, is becoming increasingly popular as a radical attempt at weight loss. Behavioral and lifestyle changes are required after the surgery, and mental health professionals can help to assess the likelihood that surgery candidates will comply. Assessments of surgical candidates usually entail testing for psychopathology and personality issues (using an instrument such as the MMPI-2), a thorough clinical interview, and a detailed review of the patient's chart and history. Mental health professionals can make sure the candidates understand the nature and long-term consequences of the surgery and can help them through the emotional adjustments involved. In some cases, cognitive and neuropsychological testing may be necessary to assess the competence of the candidate to make important medical decisions.

The following list of case scenarios outlines consultations typical for health psychologists and other mental health professionals in behavioral medicine settings.

CASE EXAMPLES

- A 37-year-old woman with chronic back pain requests to have surgery to implant a device that will inject pain medication directly into her spine. The medical team asks for help in determining if this woman is an appropriate candidate for the surgery. Is this an appropriate intervention for this person for whom nothing else has been effective, or is a major component of her pain psychogenic? If her chronic pain is related to depression, personality variables, and poor compliance with treatment, the medical team does not want to risk the surgery.

- A 43-year-old man has been admitted to the hospital for severe abdominal pain. The patient is a wealthy business owner, and has been very impatient with all of the "stupid, overpaid doctors who can't figure out what's been wrong with me over the last couple of years." The attending physician has made a definitive diagnosis of cancer, and believes the patient's prognosis is poor. The physician would like help in knowing how to break the news to the patient, especially in light of the patient's angry, volatile moods.

- A gerontologist gives a 68-year-old man a diagnosis of Parkinson's disease. When the physician asks family members if they understand what this means, they respond affirmatively, but the family makes comments that indicate that they are confused about the ramifications of the diagnosis. The physician asks for a mental health professional to discuss the diagnosis with the family and process the emotional issues and the lifestyle changes that will need to be made.

- A 54-year-old man with diabetes has been hospitalized four times in the past 2 months with dangerously high blood glucose levels. His physicians feel that he is in danger of causing permanent damage to his bodily organs and limbs. They would like help in motivating the individual to adhere to his medication regimen. They also suspect that he may be abusing illicit substances.

Chapter 16

CRISIS CONSULTATION

Alice Johnson, a master's level social worker in private practice, has received a phone call from a major food manufacturing company. George, a machine operator and well-loved employee of the organization for over 10 years, was accidentally killed last evening when he tripped and fell into a large piece of machinery while working on the shop floor. The company president would like Alice to come over to the plant as soon as possible to assist in dealing with this tragedy.

Crises are inevitable in any organization. Robberies sometimes occur; tornadoes destroy buildings; accidents occur in the workplace; and employees and their loved ones get sick and die. Since the terrorist attacks of September 11, 2001, the need for preparation to respond to crises has become more salient in the minds of organizational leaders. Due to the highly charged, emotional nature of crises, organizations are increasingly looking for outside consultants to assist in working with those affected by a crisis, and new books and organizations have sprung into existence to help organizations plan for and manage crises (Blythe, 2002). Appropriately trained mental health professionals are ideally suited to prepare for crises, to process a crisis with organization members, and to help them move back toward "business as usual."

Mental health professionals who have been trained in individual crisis intervention may also find these techniques helpful in an organizational setting. Roberts' (1991, 2002) seven-stage model of crisis intervention can serve as a guide for intervening in organizational settings:

1. Plan and conduct a thorough assessment (including lethality, dangerousness to self or others, and immediate psychosocial needs).
2. Make psychological contacts, establish rapport, and rapidly establish the relationship (conveying genuine respect for the client, acceptance, reassurance, and a nonjudgmental attitude).
3. Examine the dimensions of the problem in order to define it (including the last straw or precipitating event).
4. Encourage an exploration of feelings and emotions.
5. Generate, explore, and assess past coping attempts.
6. Restore cognitive functioning through implementation of action plan.
7. Follow up and leave the door open for booster sessions 3 and/or 6 months later. (Roberts, 2002, pp. 15–16)

Blythe (2002) notes that there are four major areas of concern for senior management when a crisis strikes an organization:

1. *People:* No organization is better than its people. Human issues come first, especially when people are injured and deeply impacted. What should be done to address the needs of the people? How wide a circle of people is impacted? Who are they? Are they in continuing danger? What information do we need to give and receive from these individuals?

2. *Business disruption:* The organization's ability to continue normal productivity will undoubtedly be affected following a catastrophe. This may be due to loss of facilities and equipment, or disruption of employees' ability to work normally. Determine the damage that is irreversible and determine what remains functional. Assess what areas of the organization are inoperable or need to be shut down. Also, determine what work is appropriate to continue. In some cases, as in nuclear plants and other power generating facilities, work must go on. Beware, however, of outrage if you are perceived as putting productivity above the needs of traumatized people. As a general rule, you must address the people needs before the back-to-business needs.

3. *Reputation:* In the wake of workplace disasters, there is a tendency for faultfinding. Reporters, journalists, plaintiff attorneys, government regulators, employees, family members, financial analysts and community members may line up to assign blame for negligence. This is a time for honesty and integrity, and also a time to assure you get the best message out to involved publics. An early priority might be to contact a public relations firm or in-house PR counsel.

4. *Finances:* Catastrophe is not a typical budget item. In establishing priorities, you may attempt to consider the financial impact of a crisis not readily contained. (p. 28)

Sometimes an organization simply needs an outside, objective perspective, and a nudge to try something new. There is a tendency sometimes for people to believe that if they simply work hard enough, they will succeed. When a situation begins to worsen, organization members may become frustrated by their inability to make progress despite increasing efforts. J. Scott Fraser (1989) uses the analogy of a bird trapped inside a building. The bird flies up into the vestibule in an attempt to escape. When the bird runs into a glass window, it simply continues to fly higher and to strike the glass harder. However, the bird only succeeds at exhausting itself. It falls backward, seemingly away from the direction it intended to go, and finds itself on the floor of the building in front of an open doorway. When the bird flies forward at this point, it is able to escape the building. In a similar way, it can be difficult to convince organizational leaders to discontinue familiar ways of doing things and to try new approaches to situations.

In dealing with crises and change, Watzlawick, Weakland, and Fisch (1974) describe *first-order* and *second-order* change. First-order change refers to a change within the accepted premises and patterns of the system. These are changes in such things as intensity, frequency, and duration. Second-order change involves a change in the system's primary premise, rule, or pattern, usually yielding strikingly different or opposite patterns from that which occurred prior to the change. The bird's attempt to escape by trying to hit the window harder represents an attempt at first-order change. The bird's escape after falling backward and down represents a second-order change.

As Alice drives to the manufacturing plant, she tries to anticipate what types of situations she will encounter, and the tactics she will use when speaking with the employees of the organization.

J. Scott Fraser (1989, 1995, 2001), in researching interventions found to be useful with clinical crises, describes tactics that can also be useful in consulting for crises within organizations:

Normalizing: Normalizing involves placing the person's or group's responses in the context of normal response patterns, given the nature of the stressor. It helps in reducing shame, in increasing control, and in undercutting pathogenic labels.

When the employees tell Alice about their feelings, of sadness, rage, and fear, she listens attentively, and describes these feelings as normal responses to an abnormal event.

Positioning: In this tactic, the consultant deliberately adopts a stance or position with the client(s) which is most often the opposite of most helpful others. It places the clients in a position of being supported in their distress, and needing to explain their strength in the face of adversity.

Rather than telling the employees to "brace up" or "get over it," Alice expresses that this is a difficult situation to deal with, and acknowledges that it took a great deal of strength for the employees to even come to work today.

Go-slow messages: The consultant offers welcome cautions in the face of perceived needs to make anxiety-provoking changes. The consultant offers the clients a chance to discuss their need to make risky shifts and to discuss possible pitfalls without the pressure to actually act. This keeps the change impetus in the consultee's hands.

The president feels that she must make immediate changes throughout the organization. While she has shut down the machine responsible for the death, she feels pressure to fire the shift supervisor and make major modifications to how things are done. While Alice aggress that she should make employee safety a top priority, Alice encourages her to take more time in making these decisions, and to allow time for her and all of the other employees to process their feelings about what happened.

Restraints from change: This tactic is used to help amplify client motivation for change and to keep the responsibility and credit for it in the client's hands. Soft restraints are similar to "go-slow" tactics, while hard restraints marshal client oppositionality in the service of change. This is sometimes known as a "paradoxical intervention."

Demetrius, an employee who happened to be working on the shop floor on the evening when George was killed, expresses a great amount of fear and reluctance to return to work. He has accumulated several weeks of vacation time, but wonders if he should try to force himself to return to work. Alice suggests that he take the vacation time, perhaps all of it, advising him not to return to work until he feels ready. Alice judges that this will reduce Demetrius's anxiety level, and make it more likely for him to return to work sooner.

Predicting: Predicting is a variation of normalizing. This tactic uses generic pattern information on developmental or incidental crises to anticipate future phases, and serves to inoculate clients against overreaction. This tactic is frequently used at the termination of a crisis intervention. If a person knows that she will experience anxiety in the future, she will be less likely to feel anxiety about the anxiety she begins to feel.

Taquisha, another employee who was working on the shop floor when George was killed, tells Alice that she is doing fine and doesn't feel anything at all. Alice tells her that every individual responds differently to situations like this, but that most people will later experience grief reactions, fear about their own mortality, and perhaps even anger at the organization for not taking more active steps to prevent the death. These feelings can sometimes come on at unexpected times, and with surprising intensity.

Reframing: This tactic offers an alternate description of the current action, situation, person, or role that fits the "facts" as well or better than old frameworks. Reframing is used to initiate new patterns or block old ones. It is often used to make prescriptions or directives "make sense," and to increase compliance.

The company president begins telling Alice that she is becoming overwhelmed by the ramifications of the death of this employee. She expresses fears of the company's reputation being ruined, of the plant being shut down, and of her losing her job. Alice expresses that while those outcomes are possibilities, this is also an opportunity for the president and her company to show their responsiveness and concern by actively taking care of their employees and by restructuring plant operations to prevent further accidents.

Prescribing: This tactic involves directing clients to engage in new or current behavior patterns with some alteration in purpose, deliberateness, or manner of performance. This tactic is often used to undercut vicious cycles and problems created by attempted solutions. This tactic is sometimes used before successful terminations by prescribing "relapses" to consolidate control and gains. If people know that difficult times will occur in the future, they can prepare for them and not feel that they have lost all that they have worked for thus far when things temporarily appear worse. In many cases, prescribing the symptom, such as telling someone who cannot stop crying to only cry at designated times, lowers the felt pressure of the person to reduce the symptom, and the person no longer finds it necessary to cry at the designated time.

Alice works with the president just before she is about to meet with a representative from OSHA, who investigates work-related deaths. The president begins crying, overwhelmed by all the feelings she has about this incident. Alice expresses appreciation to her for having the strength to share her emotions with her, and underscores that it is important to not always hold them in, but notes that she will need to pull herself together to speak to the OSHA representative. Alice advises the president to choose a period every evening, say from 7:00 P.M. to 8:00 P.M., during which time she should allow herself to cry as much as she wants. If she feels her emotions becoming overwhelming during the workday at inopportune moments, she should remind herself to try to postpone those feelings until 7:00 P.M.

CRITICAL INCIDENT STRESS MANAGEMENT

One of the first comprehensive approaches developed to deal with crises and disasters is known as Critical Incident Stress Debriefing (CISD), which is an important factor of Critical Incident Stress Management (CISM; Everly, Lating, & Mitchell, 2000; Mitchell, 1983; Mitchell & Everly, 1993).

CISM is an integrated, multicomponent system that offers a full range of services spanning the full crisis spectrum from precrisis preparation and on-scene support through postcrisis intervention and referral for formal mental health assessment and treatment.

The formal CISD process is a seven-stage intervention designed to mitigate the psychological impact of a traumatic event, prevent the subsequent development of a post-traumatic syndrome, promote full recovery or further growth of the individual, and serve as an early identification mechanism for individuals who will require professional mental health follow-up subsequent to a traumatic event.

The debriefing process has both psychological and educational elements, but it should not be considered psychotherapy. Instead, it is a structured group meeting or discussion in which personnel who have been directly affected by a traumatic event are given the opportunity to discuss their thoughts and emotions about that event in a controlled, structured, and rational manner. They also get the chance to see that they are not alone in their reactions. Below are the seven core components of CISM (Harbert, 2000; Mitchell, 1983; Mitchell & Everly, 2000).

I. Preincident Preparedness Training

Before an incident ever occurs, it is important to be prepared. This is particularly important in occupations wherein there is a great likelihood that specific critical situations may develop. Knowing about the possibilities beforehand will help to desensitize individuals to the inevitable stress and anxiety that occur during a crisis, and will allow them to develop good coping patterns ahead of time. During the training of mental health trauma workers, they are shown photographs of serious injuries, are required to gain experience riding with qualified paramedics, and spend time observing in emergency rooms.

II. Individual One-on-One Psychological Support

Individual psychological counseling can be done on-scene shortly after a crisis using the SAFER model (Mitchell & Everly, 1994):

- Stabilization of the situation
- Acknowledgment of the crisis
- Facilitation of understanding
- Encouragement of adaptive coping
- Restoration of independent functioning or
- Referral for continued care

The model stresses that this intervention should only be done by a qualified mental health professional.

III. Demobilizations

Demobilization refers to a transition from the traumatic event to some form of normalization. It may involve simply providing a safe place and offering refreshments, comfort, and informal briefing about stress, trauma, and coping techniques. It is meant to provide psychological and psychophysiological "decompression" from the traumatic event.

IV. Critical Incident Stress Debriefing (CISD)

Critical incident stress debriefing is normally provided 24 to 48 hours after the incident. The team comprises a mental health professional and one or more peer support personnel who have received standardized training in CISM. The technique is basically a peer-managed and peer-driven process that uses mental health professionals for supervision and guidance. The meeting usually lasts 2 to 3 hours. Participants sit in a large circle and go through seven phases:

1. *Introduction phase:* In this phase, the facilitators introduce themselves and describe what the process will be like. The absolute importance of confidentiality regarding all things discussed is emphasized for all group members.
2. *Fact phase:* At this point, group members take turns describing who they are, what they witnessed, and what they did during the traumatic event.
3. *Thought phase:* In this phase, the participants are asked to express some of the personal thoughts they had during and immediately after the event.
4. *Reaction phase:* Participants are now asked to express some of their reactions and feelings surrounding the event.
5. *Symptom phase:* Group members are next asked if they experienced anything unusual during the event, if they are experiencing anything unusual presently, and how this event has affected them in their personal lives.
6. *Teaching phase:* In this phase, the facilitators present psychoeducational information on stress and on responses to traumatic events to normalize the experiences of the group members.
7. *Reentry phase:* Finally, the meeting is wrapped up, and plans are made for the future, including what to do if symptoms worsen.

V. Defusing

Defusing is something that usually occurs at the site of the traumatic event. It occurs immediately after disengagement from the activity, or within 12 hours. Defusing involves short group discussions about the incident for the purposes of debriefing, affirming the value of the personnel involved in the trauma, restoring cognitive processing of the event, establishing a safe place for group communication, and equalizing the fact-versus-fantasy information between members of the group involved in the event.

VI. Family Support

Frequently, there is a tendency for people involved in a traumatic incident to close off emotionally from family members, and this should be monitored by supervisors. Although family members do not need to know the gruesome details of the experience, the person must be careful not to shut out the family emotionally.

VII. Referral Mechanisms

Lastly, referrals and resources should be made available for everyone involved in the traumatic event for future follow-up.

Shalev (2000) writes that debriefing interventions should be viewed as stress management techniques rather than treatment for trauma. He makes the following arguments:

- That in the absence of immediate and measurable relief in distress there is no ground for assuming a long-term effect of debriefing;

- That the presence of short-term effect does not necessarily assure a long-term effect;
- That debriefing affects individuals by modulating their concrete and symbolic relationship with a larger group;
- That loneliness and isolation are particularly frequent among traumatized survivors, and are very harmful;
- That the traumatogenic elements of stress, that is, its being undesirable, intense, unpredictable, uncontrollable, and inescapable, continue to operate during that period in which debriefing is applied; and
- That, notwithstanding its exact protocol, debriefing should specifically address these elements. (p. 19)

Despite Shalev's warnings, practitioners often overrely on CISM for dealing with trauma. CISM, as it has classically been taught, has recently been criticized, with empirical studies showing mixed results in terms of its efficacy (Bledsoe, 2003; Macnab, Russel, Lowe, & Gagnon, 1999; Mayou, Ehlers, & Hobbs, 2000; National Institute of Mental Health, 2002; Rose, Brewin, Andrews, & Kirk, 1999; van Emmerik, Kamphuis, Hulsbosch, & Emmelkamp, 2002). The method was developed for use with emergency response workers, and practitioners have tended to attempt to apply it in many other settings. Also, the method's emphasis on a group approach, in which everyone is encouraged to talk about the incident, is potentially harmful to individuals who do not like to work in groups, and who are not yet ready to talk about or explore their emotions surrounding the event. In addition, use of the terms "debriefing" and "defusing" have been discouraged recently by crisis and disaster mental health professionals, due to the ambiguity and perhaps the military tone of these terms (National Institute of Mental Health, 2002).

Empirical research by Orner, King, Avery, Bretherton, Stolz, and Ormerod (2003) led to the development of five important components in crisis coping strategies: waiting and self-monitoring one's reactions, resting and relaxing, finding relief from somatosensory sequelae, reestablishing routines and a sense of control, and engaging in a graded confrontation with distressing reminders. These five components should be considered in every crisis intervention.

Disaster mental health professionals have more recently begun using the generic concept of "psychological first aid." (Everly & Flynn, in press; National Institute of Mental Health, 2002; Slaikeu, 1990). Similar to the concept of physical first aid, which is applied to medically stabilize patients before turning them over to a physician's long-term care, psychological first aid is intended to minimize the psychological impact of a crisis.

The Institute of Medicine (2003) notes that psychological first aid generally includes psychoeducation about normal responses to traumatic events; active listening skills; an emphasis on the importance of maintaining physical health, rest, and nutrition; and an understanding of when to seek further professional help. Slaikeu (1990) notes that psychological first aid has three functions: providing support, reducing lethality, and providing linkage to helping resources.

A promising, recent model of psychological first aid is known as the SACC model, based on the four steps on which it is built: Stabilize, Assess, Communicate, and Connect (Everly & Flynn, in press; Flynn & Schultz, 2004). The first step of Everly and Flynn's model is to stabilize. The goal of this step is to keep things from getting worse. This involves attempting to reduce the high levels of stress and arousal that people are experiencing, attempting to diminish the escalation of distress in those already present, and working to facilitate return to normal function. The crisis responder works to achieve these goals by providing basic needs (food, clothing, and shelter), by providing safety and security, by referring for needed medical care, and by reducing stressors to the degree that it is possible to do so.

The second step is to assess stabilized individuals using triage criteria that may predict posttraumatic stress disorder (PTSD). Everly and Flynn list the items in Box 16.1 as possible indicators of future difficulties with PTSD. The third step of the SACC model is to communicate a supportive and compassionate presence. This involves listening empathically and providing reassurance. It is important to provide credible and honest information, and not to give false hope (e.g., it is better to say "we will do everything we can to help," than to say "everything will be just fine"). The crisis responder should also provide psychoeducation about normal reactions to traumatic events, as well as psychoeducation about what to expect in the future (known as "anticipatory guidance"). Resilience should also be discussed. Levant (2003) discusses 10 ways to build resilience (see Box 16.2).

Mental health professionals should also use what they have learned about teaching stress management techniques. Box 16.3, from the U.S. Department of Health and Human Services (2002a), provides tips and should prove helpful for people who have recently experienced a traumatic event.

The fourth step in Everly & Flynn's model is to connect. The goal of this step is to connect the patient with a psychosocial support system of family, friends, and coworkers. This may also involve helping the individual connect with formal support systems, such as hospital-based counselors and clergy, community mental health programs, employee or student assistance programs, or faith-based resources. Everly & Flynn's model appears promising, as it is based on the experiences of disaster mental health workers, and on what has been found to work best in the literature. More research may be needed to test and refine the model, and to determine what modifications may be needed for different settings.

Box 16.1

Indicators for Posttraumatic Stress Disorder

- Dissociation
- Depersonalization
- Arousal of the sympathetic nervous system
- Panic or mania
- Psychotic processes
- Suicidality
- Homicidality
- Violent inclinations
- Inability to function
- Event-related belief that the individual was going to die
- Negative appraisal of acute symptoms
- Severe depression
- A significant psychiatric history
- Psychiatric medications
- Lack of adequate support system

═ Box 16.2 ═

Building Resilience

1. Make connections—develop a supportive network.
2. Avoid interpreting crises as overwhelming.
3. Accept that change is a part of living.
4. Move toward your goals.
5. Take decisive actions.
6. Look for opportunities for self-discovery.
7. Nurture a positive view of yourself.
8. Keep things in perspective.
9. Maintain a hopeful outlook.
10. Take care of yourself.

After what has seemed a long first workday after George's death, the president sits down with Alice and decompresses from the stress of the day. She asks Alice about how the business will continue to run, and about how long all of this will go on until things return to "normal."

MANAGEMENT CONTINUITY

Of high importance to managers of an organization experiencing a crisis is management continuity. This concept involves having plans in place to keep the organization running as well as possible after a crisis has occurred, such as bringing in temporary workers to give employees additional time off (strongly emphasizing to the employees that their jobs will still be there when they return).

═ Box 16.3 ═

After a Disaster: Self-Care Tips for Dealing with Stress

Things to Remember When Trying to Understand Disaster Events

- No one who sees a disaster is untouched by it.
- It is normal to feel anxious about you and your family's safety.
- Profound sadness, grief, and anger are normal reactions to an abnormal event.
- Acknowledging our feelings helps us recover.
- Focusing on our strengths and abilities will help you to heal.
- Accepting help from community programs and resources is healthy.
- We each have different needs and different ways of coping.
- It is common to want to strike back at people who have caused great pain. However, nothing good is accomplished by hateful language or actions.

===== **Box 16.3 (continued)** =====

Signs That Adults Need Stress Management Assistance

- Difficulty communicating thoughts
- Difficulty sleeping
- Difficulty maintaining balance
- Easily frustrated
- Increased use of drugs/alcohol
- Limited attention span
- Poor work performance
- Headaches/stomach problems
- Tunnel vision/muffled hearing
- Colds or flu-like symptoms
- Disorientation or confusion
- Difficulty concentrating
- Reluctance to leave home
- Depression, sadness
- Feelings of hopelessness
- Mood-swings
- Crying easily
- Overwhelming guilt and self-doubt
- Fear of crowds, strangers, or being alone

Ways to Ease the Stress

- Talk with someone about your feelings—anger, sorrow, and other emotions—even though it may be difficult.
- Don't hold yourself responsible for the disastrous event or be frustrated because you feel that you cannot help directly in the rescue work.
- Take steps to promote your own physical and emotional healing by staying active in your daily life patterns or by adjusting them. This healthy outlook will help yourself and your family (i.e., healthy eating, rest, exercise, relaxation, meditation).
- Maintain a normal household and daily routine, limiting demanding responsibilities of yourself and your family.
- Spend time with family and friends.
- Participate in memorials, rituals, and use of symbols as a way to express feelings.
- Use existing supports groups of family, friends, and church.
- Establish a family emergency plan. Feeling that there is something that you can do can be very comforting.

When to seek help: If self help strategies are not helping or you find that you are using drugs/alcohol in order to cope, you may wish to seek outside or professional assistance with your stress symptoms.

Source: From *After a Disaster: Self-Care Tips for Dealing with Stress,* by U.S. Department of Health and Human Services, 2002a, Washington, DC: Department of Health and Human Services, available from www.samhsa.gov.

It is also important to recognize that recovery from a traumatic event is an ongoing process. Organizations must do more than simply bring in grief counselors for a few days after an event. If a long-term perspective is not adopted, the organization may find decreased morale and increased absenteeism from months to years after the event. Box 16.4 provides information on the phases of a disaster that is important for consultants to know when consulting with organizations on a long-term basis (U.S. Department of Health and Human Services, 2000).

INDIVIDUAL RESPONSES TO A CRISIS

Individuals will respond very differently to any given crisis. A very common coping mechanism is to increase the use of substances. For example, increases in substance use have been found to occur following tornadoes (Godleski, 1997), and beer consumption rose 25% after Hurricane Hugo (Owens, 2004).

Traumatic events also tend to have psychological effects that last well beyond the event itself. The emotional effects of natural disasters and accidents tend to subside at

---

Box 16.4

Phases of Disaster

Both community and individual responses to a major disaster tend to progress according to phases. An interaction of psychological processes with external events shapes these phases. Examples of significant time-related external events are the closure of the emergency response phase, the damage assessment of one's personal residence, or receiving financial determinations. The following represents a compilation of phase lists developed by different disaster experts. These particular phases have been selected and described because of their relevance to disaster mental health planners and workers in providing ongoing disaster recovery assistance.

Warning or Threat Phase

Disasters vary in the amount of warning communities receive before they occur. For example, earthquakes typically hit with no warning, whereas, hurricanes and floods typically arrive within hours to days of warning. When there is no warning, survivors may feel more vulnerable, unsafe, and fearful of future unpredicted tragedies. The perception that they had no control over protecting themselves or their loved ones can be deeply distressing.

When people do not heed warnings and suffer losses as a result, they may experience guilt and self blame. While they may have specific plans for how they might protect themselves in the future, they can be left with a sense of guilt or responsibility for what has occurred.

Impact Phase

The impact period of a disaster can vary from the slow, low-threat buildup associated with some types of floods to the violent, dangerous, and destructive

Box 16.4 (continued)

outcomes associated with tornadoes and explosions. The greater the scope, community destruction, and personal losses associated with the disaster, the greater the psychosocial effects.

Depending on the characteristics of the incident, people's reactions range from constricted, stunned, shock-like responses to the less common overt expressions of panic or hysteria. Most typically, people respond initially with confusion and disbelief and focus on the survival and physical well-being of themselves and their loved ones. When families are in different geographic locations during the impact of a disaster (e.g., children at school, adults at work), survivors will experience considerable anxiety until they are reunited.

Rescue or Heroic Phase

In the immediate aftermath, survival, rescuing others, and promoting safety are priorities. Evacuation to shelters, motels, or other homes may be necessary. For some, postimpact disorientation gives way to adrenaline induced rescue behavior to save lives and protect property. While activity level may be high, actual productivity is often low. The capacity to assess risk may be impaired and injuries can result. Altruism is prominent among both survivors and emergency responders.

The conditions associated with evacuation and relocation have psychological significance. When there are physical hazards or family separations during the evacuation process, survivors often experience posttrauma reactions. When the family unit is not together due to shelter requirements or other factors, an anxious focus on the welfare of those not present may detract from the attention necessary for immediate problem solving.

Remedy or Honeymoon Phase

During the week to months following a disaster, formal governmental and volunteer assistance may be readily available. Community bonding occurs as a result of sharing the catastrophic experience and the giving and receiving of community support. Survivors may experience a short-lived sense of optimism that the help they will receive will make them whole again. When disaster mental health workers are visible and perceived as helpful during this phase, they are more readily accepted and have a foundation from which to provide assistance in the difficult phases ahead.

Inventory Phase

Over time, survivors begin to recognize the limits of available disaster assistance. They become physically exhausted due to enormous multiple demands, financial pressures, and the stress of relocation or living in a damaged home. The unrealistic optimism initially experienced can give way to discouragement and fatigue.

(Continued)

================= **Box 16.4 (continued)** =================

Disillusionment Phase

As disaster assistance agencies and volunteer groups begin to pull out, survivors may feel abandoned and resentful. The reality of losses and the limits and terms of the available assistance becomes apparent. Survivors calculate the gap between the assistance they have received and what they will require to regain their former living conditions and lifestyle. Stressors abound—family discord, financial losses, bureaucratic hassles, time constraints, home reconstruction, relocation, and lack of recreation or leisure time. Health problems and exacerbations of preexisting conditions emerge due to ongoing, unrelenting stress and fatigue.

The larger community less impacted by the disaster has often returned to business as usual, which is typically discouraging and alienating for survivors. Ill will and resentment may surface in neighborhoods as survivors receive unequal monetary amounts for what they perceive to be equal or similar damage. Divisiveness and hostility among neighbors undermine community cohesion and support.

Reconstruction or Recovery Phase

The reconstruction of physical property and recovery of emotional well-being may continue for years following the disaster. Survivors have realized that they will need to solve the problems of rebuilding their own homes, businesses, and lives largely by themselves and have gradually assumed the responsibility for doing so.

With the construction of new residences, buildings, and roads comes another level of recognition of losses. Survivors are faced with the need to readjust to and integrate new surroundings as they continue to grieve losses. Emotional resources within the family may be exhausted and social support from friends and family may be worn thin.

When people come to see meaning, personal growth, and opportunity from their disaster experience despite their losses and pain, they are well on the road to recovery. While disasters may bring profound life-changing losses, they also bring the opportunity to recognize personal strengths and to reexamine life priorities.

Individuals and communities progress through these phases at different rates depending on the type of disaster and the degree and nature of disaster exposure. This progression may not be linear or sequential, as each person and community brings unique elements to the recovery process. Individual variables such as psychological resilience, social support, and financial resources influence a survivor's capacity to move through the phases. While there is always a risk of aligning expectations too rigidly with a developmental sequence, having an appreciation of the unfolding of psychosocial reactions to disaster is valuable.

Source: From *Disaster Response and Recovery: A Handbook for Mental Health Professionals,* by U.S. Department of Health and Human Services, 1994, Washington, DC: Author, available from www.samhsa.gov.

about 16 months, but can persist for 3 years. However, the emotional effects associated with human-caused disasters tend to be longer lasting and tend to affect the entire community, and not just the individuals directly involved. A feeling of injustice will prolong the effects and negative feelings, and memories of traumatic events are especially strong on anniversary dates (Office of Alcoholism and Substance Abuse Services, 2001; Owens, 2004).

The tips listed in Box 16.5 are from the U.S. Department of Health and Human Services (1994). They are designed for mental health professionals and can be helpful for

---

Box 16.5

Key Concepts of Disaster Mental Health

The following guiding principles form the basis for disaster mental health intervention programs. Not only do these principles describe some departures and deviations from traditional mental health work; they also orient administrators and service providers to priority issues. The truth and wisdom reflected in these principles have been shown over and over again, from disaster to disaster. No one who sees a disaster is untouched by it.

- There are two types of disaster trauma—individual and community.
- Most people pull together and function during and after a disaster, but their effectiveness is diminished.
- Disaster stress and grief reactions are normal responses to an abnormal situation.
- Many emotional reactions of disaster survivors stem from problems of living brought about by the disaster.
- Disaster relief assistance may be confusing to disaster survivors. They may experience frustration, anger, and feelings of helplessness related to Federal, State, and nonprofit agencies' disaster assistance programs.
- Most people do not see themselves as needing mental health services following a disaster and will not seek such services.
- Survivors may reject disaster assistance of all types.
- Disaster mental health assistance is often more practical than psychological in nature.
- Disaster mental health services must be uniquely tailored to the communities they serve.
- Mental health workers need to set aside traditional methods, avoid the use of mental health labels, and use an active outreach approach to intervene successfully in disaster.
- Survivors respond to active, genuine interest, and concern.
- Interventions must be appropriate to the phase of disaster.
- Social support systems are crucial to recovery.

Source: From *Disaster Response and Recovery: A Handbook for Mental Health Professionals,* by U.S. Department of Health and Human Services, 1994, Washington, DC: Author, available from www.samhsa.gov.

dealing with disasters. Although these concepts were written specifically for major disasters, they can be applied to other crisis consultation situations as well.

Alice knew that it would not take long for news to reach the media about the death that occurred on the shop floor. Hoping to postpone the need to deal with the media, the president was not taking their phone calls, but the reporters have been very persistent. Alice suggests that she hold a press conference where she can deliver all of the information at one time, and begins to prepare the president for the conference.

COMMUNICATION WITH THE MEDIA

Managers often fear that a crisis in the workplace can lead to a public relations disaster. However, how the organization responds to the crisis may be the most critical component in public perception of the incident. Box 16.6 lists 10 tips for communicating about crisis situations, taken from the U.S. Department of Health and Human Services (2002b).

The president is forthright during the conference, and comes across as open, honest, and concerned. She responds to each of the reporter's questions thoughtfully and truthfully, not shying away from admitting her ignorance regarding some of the questions. Though not all of the later press reports were positive, the general image portrayed was one of a concerned company taking immediate, responsible action to prevent such tragedies in the future.

Box 16.6

Avoiding Communication Mistakes: Top Ten Tips for the Savvy Communicator

1. First do no harm. Your words have consequences—be sure they're the right ones.
2. Don't babble. Know what you want to say. Say it . . . then say it again.
3. If you don't know what you're talking about, stop talking.
4. Focus more on informing people than impressing them. Use everyday language.
5. Never say anything you're not willing to see printed on tomorrow's front page.
6. Never lie. You won't get away with it.
7. Don't make promises you can't keep.
8. Don't use "No comment." You'll look like you have something to hide.
9. Don't get angry. When you argue with the media, you always lose . . . and lose publicly.
10. Don't speculate, guess, or assume. When you don't know something, say so.

Source: From *Communication in a Crisis: Risk Communications Guidelines for Public Officials* (p. 86), by U.S. Department of Health and Human Services, 2002b, Washington, DC: Author, available from www.samhsa.gov.

CRISIS INTERVENTION FOR SCHOOL SETTINGS

Many of the preceding considerations for dealing with crises in organizations also apply in a school setting. Potential crisis situations include dealing with bereavement due to the death (whether caused by suicide, homicide, or accident) of a student or staff member, major environmental or terrorist disasters (floods, fires, tornadoes, earthquakes, hurricanes, bombings, chemical spills, etc.), and threats to physical safety (gunfire, stabbings, school bus accidents, hostage situations, etc.). It is also important to keep in mind that traumatic events in the community, region, or even elsewhere in the world can have significant impacts on the functioning of the students and staff of the school.

Of major importance to consultants and school staff is the prevention of further harm to students. Callahan (1996) found that intervention activities designed to help students after the school experienced a completed suicide actually made things worse. Students began to more freely talk about death and suicide, which may have contributed to a glorification or romanticization of death, resulting in a substantial increase in suicidal talk, threats, and attempts.

As in any setting, preparation is key for handling crises when they arise, and consultants can help schools put together a "crisis team." Schonfeld, Lichtenstein, Kline-Pruett, and Speese-Linehan (2002) suggest that the team consist of a crisis team chair, a crisis team assistant chair, a coordinator of counseling services, a media coordinator, a staff notification coordinator, a communications coordinator, and a crowd management coordinator.

Consultants can also help to develop a good crisis plan. Since every school will be different in terms of staff, policies, resources, and community connections, each school needs an individualized crisis response plan. Schonfeld et al. (2002) suggest the following guidelines for what to include in a school crisis plan, which should be reviewed and updated annually and discussed with all school staff:

- The name, physical address, and phone number of the school.
- Members of the school crisis team, including room numbers, telephone numbers (if applicable), and itinerant members' schedules. The best place for this information is the front page of the plan.
- A staff telephone tree that indicates who calls whom if a crisis occurs after school hours.
- An in-school crisis code to convene the team in an emergency. Specify the succession of crisis team members who are authorized to activate the code when the principal is out of the building.
- A description of the role of each team member.
- A list of alternates in case crisis team members are absent. For example, who covers the telephones if the secretary is absent.
- A list that assigns staff to cover classrooms of teachers who are involved in crisis management.
- A list of staff members who are knowledgeable in first aid and CPR.
- A list of the contents of the school crisis kit and its location.
- A neighborhood site to which school staff will evacuate students in the event of a natural disaster or extreme emergency. Specify a contact person and telephone number.
- Indicate the computer filenames of form letters to serve as notification to parents or guardians.
- An outline of expectations for all staff during a crisis event (e.g., custodians, teachers during planning periods). (pp. 69–70)

Newgass and Schonfeld (2000), of the National Center for Children Exposed to Violence, make a number of suggestions for managing crises in schools, and on mitigating their impacts on young people. The following is a suggested protocol for determining students' service needs in times of crisis (Schonfeld et al., 2002):

1. With certain students who are unaware of the crisis incident, it may be necessary to prepare them individually for classroom discussion because of their relationship with the victim. Examples of students who may benefit from preparation include close friends, fellow students with a special association (e.g., teammates), and relatives.
2. Because of their preexisting relationships with students, classroom teachers are the best persons to lead classroom discussions.
3. If classroom discussions prove to be inadequate in helping some students manage their emotional reactions to the incident, these students may benefit from services available through a support room.
4. Upon a student's arrival at the support room, the counselor should briefly evaluate him to rule out profound states of disorganization, anxiety, or depression. A student who is profoundly affected by his emotions might benefit from an expedited referral to a local mental health clinic or private practitioner. School staff should contact the student's parent or guardian to transport and accompany the student to these services.
5. Counselors should permit students they have determined to be appropriate for support room services to engage in casual, unstructured conversations with their peers and support room staff. A guiding principle is to achieve the greatest benefit to the students with the least intrusive intervention possible.
6. If casual, unstructured conversations prove to be inadequate to meet the student's needs, the counselor should consider structured, goal-directed groups as the next level of intervention. These groups should be sufficiently open to allow students to come and go as their needs are met.
7. Students who continue to exhibit needs following support room contacts on the first day of a crisis should be encouraged to return the following day. These students may also benefit from an ongoing support group.
8. Students who continue to exhibit considerable levels of need beyond those of the general student body (either in time or intensity) should receive individual attention from school support staff. Counselors should monitor these students for needs that may exceed the resources of the school.
9. Throughout the crisis period, school staff should inform parents of any exceptional responses their children make to the crisis. (pp. 55–56)

Consultants can also be helpful in training the teachers in how to intervene in potential crisis situations, such as in dealing with angry students. Callahan (1998) proposed a crisis intervention model for teachers, in which he posited that when a child reaches a crisis, he or she will vent hostility either verbally or physically. Callahan makes the following suggestions to a teacher who has encountered a verbally aggressive child, based on Greenstone and Leviton (1993):

• Determine what is troubling the student by engaging the student in a conversation about that which is going on.
• Discover specifically that which is leading the student into crisis right at this time.
• Determine the most pressing problem or need from the student's point of view.
• Outline those problems that can be immediately managed.

- Think through variables that might hinder the problem-solving process.
- Ask what can be done most effectively in the least amount of time to diffuse the crisis situation.
- Understand the similarities between the present situation and previous incidents.

The teacher must take care to notice if the child's verbal aggression begins to escalate to physical violence, and should try to ensure his or her own as well as the other students' safety (Hendricks, McKean, & Hendricks, 2003).

School staff may also not always be aware of the wide range of impact a dramatic event can have. Oftentimes, crises affect many more individuals than those who were directly involved. Newgass and Schonfeld (2000) list a number of risk factors for students, which consultants can discuss with school staff:

- *Group affiliation with the victim:* School staff should make themselves aware of the formal and informal social networks and the activities that the victim shared with other students: academic, shop, and special classes; after school clubs, teams, and extracurricular activities; community and social activities engaged in off-site; the victim's residential neighborhood.

   A staff member should consider following the victim's schedule of classes for the first day(s). The crisis team should reach out to the external sites to offer support and guidance to the nonprofessionals who might have regular contact with peers (e.g., the scout leader, Little League coach, or dance instructor).
- *Shared characteristics, interests, or attributes with the victim:* Students who perceive themselves as sharing characteristics, interests, or attributes with the victim may be more inclined to have increased anxiety and stress.

Students with Prior Demonstration of Poor Coping
- Social isolation
- History of suicidal ideation/attempts
- Prior history of arrests, acting-out behaviors, aggression, or drug/alcohol abuse

Students Exhibiting Extreme or Atypical Reactions
- Students with grief reactions surpassing those of the general student body that would not be explained by close affiliation with the victim
- Students with close relationships with the deceased that exhibit very little reaction to the news

Students with Personal History Related to the Trauma
- Former victims of crime or violence
- Students who have threatened or acted violently in the past

Students with Concurrent Adverse Personal Situations
- Family problems
- Health problems
- Psychiatric history
- Significant peer conflicts (p. 221)

As with other organizational or clinical consulting interventions, the consultant's goal for crisis intervention should be to connect the school or business to needed resources. This not only will involve making connections with external or community resources (such as the Red Cross), but will also involve fostering collaboration and encouraging further training of administrators, teachers, managers, and human resource personnel. In this way, the school or business can be better prepared to handle the effects of the long-term aftermaths, and will be better prepared to handle future crises. Consultants can leverage themselves to positively influence larger and larger numbers of people in the community, and perhaps even future generations.

Glossary

Ability   An individual's capacity to perform the various tasks in a job.

Absenteeism   Failure to report to work.

Accommodation   The willingness of one party in a conflict to place the opponent's interest above his or her own.

Achievement need   The drive to excel, to achieve in relation to a set of standards, to strive to succeed.

Action research   A change process based on systematic collection of data and then selection of a change action based on what the analyzed data indicate.

Active listening   Listening with intensity, empathy, acceptance, and a willingness to take responsibility for completeness.

Active practice   Providing trainees with opportunities to actively practice what they have learned to increase retention. Active practice is most effective when it is "spaced" rather than "massed."

Adhocracy   A structure characterized as low in complexity, formalization, and centralization.

Adjourning   The final stage in group development for temporary groups, characterized by concern with wrapping up activities rather than task performance.

Adverse impact   The result of discrimination against individuals protected by Title VII and related legislation due to the use of an employment practice (e.g., selection or placement test). When use of a selection or other employment procedure results in higher rejection rates for such individuals than for the majority group, adverse impact is said to exist. The "80% rule" can be used to determine if adverse impact is occurring.

Affective component of an attitude   The emotional or feeling segment of an attitude.

Affiliation need   The desire for friendly and close interpersonal relationships.

Arbitrator   A third party to a negotiation who has the authority to dictate an agreement.

Assessment center   (1) A set of performance simulation tests designed to evaluate a candidate's managerial potential. (2) Method of evaluating job applicants and current employees (usually management and administrative personnel); often used to determine promotability. Incorporates a variety of techniques including interviews, tests, and situational tests (e.g., in-basket).

Attitudes   Evaluative statements or judgments concerning objects, people, or events.

Attitude surveys   Eliciting responses from employees through questionnaires about how they feel about their jobs, work groups, supervisors, and/or the organization.

Attribution theory   Refers to the attempt by individuals to determine whether observed behavior is internally or externally caused.

Attribution theory of leadership   A theory that proposes that leadership is merely an attribution that people make about other individuals.

Authoritarianism   The belief that there should be status and power differences among people in organizations.

Authority   The rights inherent in a managerial position to give orders and expect the orders to be obeyed.

Autonomy   The degree to which the job provides substantial freedom and discretion to the individual in scheduling the work and in determining the procedures to be used in carrying it out.

Avoiding   The desire to withdraw from or suppress a conflict.

Base rate   Percentage of current employees who are considered successful or effective. Ranges from 0.0 to 100.0%. In determining a predictor incremental validity, a current base rate near 50% is preferred.

Bases of power   What power-holders control that allows them to manipulate the behavior of others.

Behavioral components of an attitude   An intention to behave in a certain way toward someone or something.

Behavioral consultation   One of the three major types of consultation. It attempts to assist consultees and their client systems through a systematic, problem-solving approach based on behavioral technology.

Behavioral symptoms of stress   Changes in an individual's behavior—including productivity, absence, and turnover—as a result of stress.

Behavioral theories of leadership   Theories proposing that specific behaviors differentiate leaders from nonleaders.

Behaviorally anchored rating scales (BARS)   (1) An evaluation method where actual job-related behaviors are rated along a continuum. (2) A method of performance appraisal in which dimensions of job performance are assessed in terms of behavioral anchors (critical incidents) arranged along a continuum (e.g., from very low to very high effectiveness).

Biographical characteristics   Personal characteristics—such as age, sex, and marital status—that are objective and easily obtained from personnel records.

Biographical information blank (BIB)   A form of self-report inventory used to obtain biographical data (biodata) about job applicants. BIBs use a multiple-choice format. When empirically derived, BIBs are associated with relatively high validity coefficients.

Bounded rationality   The theory that individuals make decisions by constructing simplified models that extract the essential features from problems without capturing all their complexity.

Brainstorming   (1) An idea-generation process that specifically encourages any and all alternatives, while withholding any criticism of those alternatives. (2) A method of generating creative ideas in which individuals or group members are encouraged to freely suggest any idea or thought without criticism, evaluation, or censorship.

Bureaucracy   Weber's organizational structure that is characterized by a division of labor, specialization of jobs, a hierarchy of authority, and a system of rules.

Capitation   An agreement with an organization to provide mental health services to a set number of employees, for a set fee, for a set period of time.

Career   A sequence of positions occupied by a person during the course of a lifetime.

Career anchors   Distinct patterns of self-perceived talents and abilities, motives and needs, and attitudes and values that guide and stabilize a person's career after several years of real-world experience and feedback.

Career stages   The four steps most people go through in their careers: exploration, establishment, midcareer, and late career.

Case study   An in-depth analysis of one setting.

Causality   The implication that the independent variable causes the dependent variable.

Central tendency bias   A rater bias in which ratees are assigned average or middle scores on all job performance dimensions.

Centralization   The degree to which decision making is concentrated at a single point in the organization.

Chain of command   The superior-subordinate authority chain that extends from the top of the organization to the lowest echelon.

Change   Making things different.

Change agents   Persons who act as catalysts and assume the responsibility for managing change activities.

Channel   The medium through which a communication message travels.

Channel richness   The amount of information that can be transmitted during a communication episode.

Charismatic leadership   Attributions of heroic or extraordinary leadership abilities made by followers when they observe certain behaviors.

Classical conditioning   A type of conditioning where an individual responds to some stimulants that would not invariably produce such a response.

Client   In some approaches to mental health and behavioral consultation, the person with whom the consultee is having a work-related or caretaking-related problem; in this instance, the client constitutes the client system (see below). One of the goals of consultation is to improve the functioning of the client.

Client system   The person, group, organization, or community with whom the consultee is having a work-related or caretaking-related problem. One of the goals of consultation is to improve the functioning of the client system.

Coalition   Two or more individuals who combine their power to push for or support their demands.

Coercive power   Power that is based on fear.

Cognitive component of an attitude   The opinion or belief segment of an attitude.

Cognitive dissonance   Any incompatibility between two or more attitudes or between behavior and attitudes.

Cognitive evaluation theory   The tendency that allocating extrinsic rewards for behavior that had been previously intrinsically rewarded will decrease the overall level of motivation.

Cognitive resource theory   A theory of leadership that states that a leader obtains effective group performance by, first, making effective plans, decisions, and strategies, and then communicating them through directive behavior.

Cohesiveness   Degree to which group members are attracted to each other and are motivated to stay in the group.

Cohorts   Individuals who, as part of a group, hold a common attribute.

Collaborating   A situation where the parties to a conflict each desire to satisfy fully the concerns of all parties.

Collaboration   The type of approach most consultants use when working with their consultees. This approach allows both parties to pool their strengths and resources in their efforts to solve the work-related or caretaking-related problem about which consultation is taking place. This approach minimizes the danger of too much dominance by the consultant.

Collectivism   A national culture attribute that describes a tight social framework in which people expect others in groups of which they are a part to look after them and protect them.

Command group   A manager and his or her immediate subordinates.

Communication   The transference and understanding of meaning.

Communication apprehension   Undue tension and anxiety about oral communication, written communication, or both.

Communication networks   (1) Channels by which information flows. (2) Communication networks, or the patterns of communication between people or departments in an organization, which are usually categorized as being either centralized or decentralized. Centralized networks are more effective for simple tasks and are associated with greater satisfaction for the central person only, while decentralized networks are better for more complex tasks and are associated with greater overall levels of satisfaction.

Communication process   The steps between a source and a receiver that result in the transference and understanding of meaning.

Comparable worth   A doctrine that holds that jobs equal in value to an organization should be equally compensated, whether or not the work content of those jobs is similar.

Competing   A desire to satisfy one's interest, regardless of the impact on the other party to the conflict.

Complexity   The degree of vertical, horizontal, and spatial differentiation in an organization.

Compressed workweek   A four-day week, with employees working 10 hours a day.

Compromising   A situation in which each party to a conflict is willing to give up something.

Conceptual skills   The mental ability to analyze and diagnose complex situations.

Conciliator   A trusted third party who provides an informal communication link between the negotiator and the opponent.

Conflict   A process that begins when one party perceives that another party has negatively affected, or is about to negatively affect, something that the first party cares about.

Conflict management   The use of resolution and stimulation techniques to achieve the desired level of conflict.

Conformity   Adjusting one's behavior to align with the norms of the group.

Conformity to group norms   Conformity to group norms is highest when the task is ambiguous or complex, when group consensus is high, and when members have participated in setting the group norms. Moreover, people high in authoritarianism and rigidity and who have low self-esteem are more likely to conform to group norms.

Consideration   The extent to which a leader is likely to have job relationships characterized by mutual trust, respect for subordinates' ideas, and regard for their feelings.

Constraints   Forces that prevent individuals from doing what they desire.

Construct validity   Validity based on expert judgment and the accumulation of evidence related to the extent to which a predictor measures a theoretical construct or trait (e.g., intelligence, verbal fluency, creativity). Evidence includes correlations with other tests, factor analysis, internal consistency, convergent and discriminant validity.

Consultant   A person, typically a human services professional, who delivers direct service to another person (consultee) who has a work-related or caretaking-related problem with a person, group, organization, or community (client system).

Consultant as negotiator   An impartial third party, skilled in conflict management, who attempts to facilitate creative problem solving through communication and analysis.

Consultation   A type of helping relationship in which a human services professional (consultant) assists another person (consultee) to solve a work-related or caretaking-related problem the consultee has with a client or client system.

Consultee The person, often a human services professional or a caretaker (e.g., a parent, teacher, or supervisor), to whom the consultant provides assistance with a work-related or care-taking-related problem. One of the goals of consultation is to improve the current and future functioning of the consultee.

Content validity Validity based on the extent to which a predictor reflects the job "universe" or requirements (activities, skills, responsibilities, etc.). Determined by "expert judgment."

Contingency theory Fiedler's theory of leadership effectiveness, which proposes that effectiveness is related to an interaction between the leader's style and the nature (favorableness) of the situation. Low LPC (least preferred coworker) leaders are most effective in unfavorable or very favorable situations; high LPC leaders are better in moderately favorable situations.

Contingency variables Those variables that moderate the relationship between the independent and dependent variables and improve the correlation.

Continuous reinforcement A desired behavior is reinforced each and every time it is demonstrated.

Contrast effects Evaluations of a person's characteristics that are affected by comparisons with other people recently encountered who rank higher or lower on the same characteristics.

Controlling Monitoring activities to ensure they are being accomplished as planned and correcting any significant deviations.

Core values The primary or dominant values that are accepted throughout the organization.

Correlation coefficient Indicates the strength of a relationship between two or more variables.

Cost-minimization strategy A strategy that emphasizes tight cost controls, avoidance of unnecessary innovation or marketing expenses, and price-cutting.

Criterion measure The test or other measure used to distinguish between acceptable and unacceptable levels of job performance.

Criterion-related validity Validity determined by correlating the predictor (e.g., selection test) with a measure of job performance (criterion). Can be concurrent or predictive.

Critical incident technique A method of job analysis and performance appraisal involving the identification of specific behaviors that are associated with outstanding and poor job performance.

Critical incidents Evaluating those behaviors that are key in making the difference between executing a job effectively and executing it ineffectively.

Cross-validation Process of determining predictor-criterion validity on a second sample independently drawn from the same population used in the original validation study. Usually associated with "shrinkage" (the cross-validation coefficient is lower than the original coefficient).

Culture shock Confusion, disorientation, and emotional upheaval caused by being immersed in a new culture.

Customer departmentalization Grouping activities on the basis of common customers.

Decisional roles Roles that include those of entrepreneur, disturbance handler, resource allocator, and negotiator.

Decoding Retranslating a sender's communication message.

Deep relaxation A state of physical relaxation, where the individual is somewhat detached from both the immediate environment and body sensations.

Defensive behaviors Reactive and protective behaviors to avoid action, blame, or change.

Delphi technique   A group decision method in which individual members, acting separately, pool their judgments in a systematic and independent fashion.

Demands   The loss of something desired.

Democratic leader   One who shares decision making with subordinates.

Dependency   B's relationship to A when A possesses something that B requires.

Dependent variable   A response that is affected by an independent variable.

Determinants of job satisfaction   High levels of satisfaction that are associated with certain worker and job characteristics (e.g., older employees, higher-level employees, and employees whose jobs allow them to use their skills and abilities tend to be most satisfied). The relationship between pay and satisfaction is complex and seems to be related more to the perception that one is being paid fairly than to the actual amount of pay.

Diagnosis   The second of the four stages of the consultation process. In this stage the problem to be solved in consultation is defined. Thus, in its simplest form, diagnosis is the equivalent of problem identification. In its more complex form, it is an ongoing process in which the target problem is continually redefined and worked on by gathering, analyzing, interpreting, and discussing data.

Differential validity   Exists when the validity coefficient of a predictor is significantly different for one subgroup than for another subgroup (e.g., lower for Black applicants than for White applicants).

Differentiation   The degree to which individuals in different functional departments vary in their goal and value orientations.

Disengagement   The last of the four stages in the consultation process. It typically involves the winding down of consultation, including evaluation of consultation, postconsultation planning, reduced contact, follow-up, and termination.

Dissatisfaction and turnover   One of the strongest correlates of satisfaction is turnover with high rates of dissatisfaction being associated with high rates of turnover. The average correlation is around $-.40$.

Distributive bargaining   Negotiation that seeks to divide up a fixed amount of resources; a win-lose situation.

Disturbed-reactive environment   An environment dominated by one or more large organizations.

Division of labor   Specialization; breaking jobs down into simple and repetitive tasks.

Divisional structure   A set of autonomous units coordinated by a central headquarters.

Dominant culture   Expresses the core values that are shared by a majority of the organization's members.

Driving forces   Forces that direct behavior away from the status quo.

Dysfunctional conflict   Conflict that hinders group performance.

Effectiveness   Achievement of goals.

Efficiency   The ratio of effective output to the input required to achieve it.

80% rule   A method for determining whether a selection or placement instrument is having an adverse impact. Involves dividing the hiring rate for the minority group by the hiring rate for the majority group: Adverse impact is suggested if the result is less than 80%.

Elasticity of power   The relative responsiveness of power to changes in available alternatives.

Employee-oriented leader   One who emphasizes interpersonal relations.

Empowerment   A process that increases employees' intrinsic task motivation.

Encoding   Converting a communication message to symbolic form.

Encounter stage   The stage in the socialization process in which a new employee sees what the organization is really like and confronts the possibility that expectations and reality may diverge.

Entry   The first of the four stages of the consultation process. It involves perceiving the presenting problem, formulating a contract, and physically and psychologically entering the system in which consultation is to occur.

Environment   Those institutions or forces outside the organization that potentially affect the organization's performance.

Equity theory   (1) The theory that individuals compare their job inputs and outcomes with those of others and then respond so as to eliminate any inequities. (2) The theory of motivation which proposes that an employee's motivation is related to her perception that her input/outcome ratio is similar to that of comparison others. A perception of overpayment is associated with higher levels of job motivation.

ERG theory   The three groups of core needs: existence, relatedness, and growth.

Ethnocentric views   The belief that one's cultural values and customs are superior to all others.

Exit   Dissatisfaction expressed through behavior directed toward leaving the organization.

Expectancy theory   (1) The theory that the strength of a tendency to act in a certain way depends on the strength of an expectation that the act will be followed by a given outcome and on the attractiveness of the outcome to the individual. (2) A motivational theory that regards job motivation as the result of three elements: expectancy, instrumentality, and valence. Highest levels of motivation occur when an employee perceives that high job effort results in high task success (high expectancy), that high success leads to the attainment of certain goals (high instrumentality), and that the outcomes are desirable (positive valence).

Expert power   Influence based on special skills or knowledge.

Externals   Individuals who believe that what happens to them is controlled by outside forces such as luck or change.

Extrinsic rewards   Rewards received from the environment surrounding the context of the work.

Feedback   The degree to which carrying out the work activities required by a job results in the individual obtaining direct and clear information about the effectiveness of his or her performance.

Feedback loop   The final link in the communication process; puts the message back into the system as a check against misunderstandings.

Felt conflict   Emotional involvement in a conflict creating anxiety, tenseness, frustration, or hostility.

Fiedler contingency model   The theory that effective groups depend on a proper match between a leader's style of interacting with subordinates and the degree to which the situation gives control and influence to the leader.

Field experiment   A controlled experiment conducted in a real organization.

Field survey   Questionnaire or interview responses that are collected from a sample and analyzed. Inferences are then made from the representative sample about the larger population.

Filtering   A sender's manipulation of information so that it will be seen more favorably by the receiver.

Fixed-interval schedule   Rewards that are spaced at uniform time intervals.

Fixed-ratio schedule   Rewards that are initiated after a fixed or constant number of responses.

Flexible benefits   A benefit program that employees tailor to meet their personal needs by picking and choosing from a menu of benefit options.

Flextime (1) An arrangement whereby employees work during a common core time period each day but have discretion in forming their total workdays from a flexible set of hours outside the core. (2) Job-scheduling technique in which employees are allowed to choose when to start and end work (within designated limits). Employees must work a full day and be present during certain "core" hours. Associated with high levels of motivation and satisfaction and decreased absenteeism.

Formal group A designated work group defined by the organization's structure.

Formal networks Task-related communications that follow the authority chain.

Formalization The degree to which jobs within the organization are standardized.

Forming The first stage in group development, characterized by much uncertainty.

Friendship group Those brought together because they share one or more common characteristics.

Functional conflict Conflict that supports the goals of the group and improves its performance.

Functional departmentalization Grouping activities by functions performed.

Fundamental attribution error The tendency to underestimate the influence of external factors and overestimate the influence of internal factors when making judgments about the behavior of others.

Generalizability The degree to which results of a research study are applicable to groups of individuals other than those who participate in the original study.

Genetic model of consultation A model of consultation that contains those characteristics common to the various types of consultation and the approaches to these types. It is what distinguishes consultation as a unique helping relationship from other helping relationships.

Geographic departmentalization Grouping activities on the basis of territory.

Goal-setting theory (1) The theory that specific and difficult goals lead to higher performance. (2) A theory of job motivation which proposes that individuals will be more willing to achieve goals when they have explicitly accepted those goals. Also proposes that assigning specific, difficult goals and providing employees with feedback about their achievement of those goals increases productivity.

Graphic rating scales An evaluation method where the evaluator rates performance factors on an incremental scale.

Group Two or more individuals, interacting and interdependent, who have come together to achieve particular objectives.

Group cohesion The feeling of solidarity among group members. Cohesiveness is high in smaller groups, when initiation or entry into the group is difficult, when members are relatively homogeneous, and when there is an external threat. High cohesiveness can lead to poorer decision making in some situations (e.g., groupthink).

Group demography The degree to which members of a group share a common demographic attribute, such as age, sex, race, educational level, or length of service in the organization, and the impact of this attribute on turnover.

Group order ranking An evaluation method that places employees into a particular classification such as quartiles.

Group polarization The tendency of groups to make more extreme decisions (either more conservative or more risky) than individual members would have made alone.

Groupshift A change in decision risk between the group's decision and the individual decision that members within the group would make; can be either toward conservatism or greater risk.

Groupthink (1) Phenomenon in which the norm for consensus overrides the realistic appraisal of alternative courses of action. (2) A mode of group thinking in which group members' desires for unanimity and cohesiveness override their ability to realistically appraise or determine alternative courses of action. Can be alleviated by encouraging dissent or having someone play devil's advocate.

Halo effect (1) Drawing a general impression about an individual based on a single characteristic. (2) Rater bias in which the rater allows his/her rating of an employee on one dimension to influence ratings of the employee on unrelated dimensions.

Hawthorne effect The concept that an intervention, regardless of its intent or content, produces a positive effect on worker motivation and/or performance when workers participate in a research study.

Hawthorne studies Series of studies originally designed to assess the effects of certain environmental factors (e.g., illumination, work break) on job morale and productivity. Results indicated the influence of the "informal organization" (e.g., group norms) and social relationships on productivity and attitudes.

Hierarchy of needs theory The theory that there is a hierarchy of five needs—physiological, safety, social, esteem, and self-actualization—and as each need is sequentially satisfied, the next need becomes dominant.

Higher-order needs Needs that are satisfied internally: social, esteem, and self-actualization.

Horizontal differentiation The degree of differentiation between units based on the orientation of members, the nature of the tasks they perform, and their education and training.

Human relations movement An approach to management that emphasizes social relationships and their role on productivity and morale. The Hawthorne studies were a major contributor to this approach.

Human relations view of conflict The belief that conflict is a natural and inevitable outcome in any group.

Human services organization A broad term describing an organization that as its major mission provides some form of contact with clients and has as its aim the improvement of the well-being of those clients, and therefore of society. Counseling centers, mental health centers, Head Start programs, homes for individuals with mental retardation, and social services departments are all examples of human services agencies.

Human skills The ability to work with, understand, and motivate other people, both individually and in groups.

Hygiene factors Those factors—such as company policy and administration, supervision, and salary—that, when adequate in a job, placate workers. When these factors are adequate, people will not be dissatisfied.

Hypothesis A tentative explanation of the relationship between two or more variables.

Idiosyncracy credits Positive sentiments within a group toward a member that allow him/her to occasionally deviate from group norms. A person accumulates idiosyncracy credits when he/she has a history of conforming to norms, has contributed in some special way to the group, or has served as the group leader.

Illegitimate political behavior Extreme political behavior that violates the implied rules of the game.

Imitation strategy A strategy that seeks to move into new products or new markets only after their viability has already been proven.

Implementation Third of the four stages of the consultation process. It is the "action" or "doing" stage, in which some action is taken on the problem. It begins with formulating and choosing a plan to solve the problem that has been diagnosed, and it includes implementing and evaluating that plan.

Implicit favorite model   A decision-making model where the decision maker implicitly selects a preferred alternative early in the decision process and biases the evaluation of all other choices.

Impression management   The process by which individuals attempt to control the impression others form of them.

In-basket   An assessment center job simulation technique in which participants respond to memoranda, letters, and so on typical of those they would encounter on the job. Used both as a selection technique and for management training.

Incremental validity   The increase in decision-making accuracy resulting from the use of a new predictor.

Independent variable   The presumed cause of some change in the dependent variable.

Indirect service   That type of service provided to the client system by the consultant. The consultant affects the well-being of the client system by helping the consultee help the client system more effectively. It is one of the characteristics of consultation that differentiates it from other helping relationships.

Individual ranking   An evaluation method that rank-orders employees from best to worst.

Individualism   A national culture attribute describing a loosely knit social framework in which people emphasize only the care of themselves and their immediate family.

Informal group   A group that is neither formally structured nor organizationally determined; appears in response to the need for social contact.

Informal network   The communication grapevine.

Informational roles   Roles that include monitoring, disseminating, and spokesperson activities.

Initiating structure   The extent to which a leader is likely to define and structure his or her role and those of subordinates in the search for goal attainment.

Innovation   A new idea applied to initiating or improving a product, process, or service.

Innovation strategy   A strategy that emphasizes the introduction of major new products and services.

Institutionalization   When an organization takes on a life of its own, apart from any of its members, and acquires immortality.

Instrumental values   Preferable modes of behavior or means of achieving one's terminal values.

Integration   The degree to which members of various departments achieve unity of effort.

Integrative bargaining   Negotiation that seeks one or more settlements that can create a win-win solution.

Intellectual ability   That which is required to do mental activities.

Intensive technology   A customized response to a diverse set of contingencies.

Intentions   Decisions to act in a given way in a conflict episode.

Interacting groups   Typical groups, where members interact with each other face-to-face.

Interactionist view of conflict   The belief that conflict is not only a positive force in a group but that it is absolutely necessary for a group to perform effectively.

Interest group   Those working together to attain a specific objective with which each is concerned.

Intergroup development   OD efforts to improve interactions between groups.

Interpersonal roles   Roles that include figurehead, leadership, and liaison activities.

Intermittent reinforcement A desired behavior is reinforced often enough to make the behavior worth repeating, but not every time it is demonstrated.

Internals Individuals who believe that they control what happens to them.

Intrinsic rewards The pleasure or value one receives from the content of a work task.

Intuition A feeling not necessarily supported by research.

Intuitive decision making An unconscious process created out of distilled experience.

I-O Psychology I-O (industrial/occupational) psychology entails the application of psychological concepts to work settings. I-O psychologists help employers deal with employees fairly; help make jobs more interesting and satisfying; help workers be more productive. See www.siop.org.

Japanese approach The Japanese approach to management is often contrasted to the traditional American approach and, in recent years, is becoming increasingly popular in the United States. Among other things, the Japanese approach emphasizes collective responsibility and decision making, a nonspecialized career path, lifetime employment, and implicit methods of control.

Job analysis (1) Developing a detailed description of the tasks involved in a job, determining the relationship of a given job to other jobs, and ascertaining the knowledge, skills, and abilities necessary for an employee to perform the job successfully. (2) Process of determining how a job differs from other jobs in terms of required responsibilities, activities, and skills. First step in the development of a predictor of criterion; also used for redesigning a job, identifying training needs, developing a job description or job specification, and determining the causes of accidents.

Job burnout A state brought on by the demands of the job often involving an inability to cope with continued stress and a feeling of constant psychological exhaustion. An early sign of burnout is often increased effort without an increase in productivity.

Job characteristics model Identifies five job characteristics and their relationship to personal and work outcomes.

Job description A written statement of what a jobholder does, how it is done, and why it is done.

Job design The way that tasks are combined to form complete jobs.

Job enlargement (1) The horizontal expansion of jobs. (2) A type of job redesign that involves increasing the number of tasks included in a job without increasing the worker's autonomy and responsibility.

Job enrichment Method of job redesign in which the job is made more challenging, rewarding, and so on, to increase job motivation and satisfaction. Based on Herzberg's two-factor theory.

Job evaluation A systematic analysis of job demands for the purpose of setting wages and salaries.

Job involvement The degree to which a person identifies with a job, actively participates in it, and considers his or her performance important to self-worth.

Job rotation The periodic shifting of a worker from one task to another.

Job satisfaction A general attitude toward one's job; the difference between the amount of rewards workers receive and the amount they believe they should receive.

Job sharing The practice of having two or more people split a 40-hours-a-week job.

Job specification States the minimum acceptable qualifications that an employee must possess to perform a given job successfully.

Justice view of ethics Requires individuals to improve and enforce rules fairly and impartially so there is an equitable distribution of benefits and costs.

Kinesics The study of body motions.

Knowledge power   The ability to control unique and valuable information.

KOIS   The Kuder Occupational Interest Survey. This is an interest test that is used for the purposes of vocational counseling and placement. Like other interest tests, it is more useful for predicting job satisfaction, persistence, and choice than job success.

Labor union   An organization, made up of employees, that acts collectively to protect and promote employee interests.

Laboratory experiment   In an artificial environment, the researcher manipulates an independent variable under controlled conditions, and then concludes that any change in the dependent variable is due to the manipulation or change imposed on the independent variable.

Leader-member-exchange theory   In-groups and out-groups that are created by leaders. Subordinates with in-group status will have higher performance ratings, less turnover, and greater satisfaction with their superior.

Leader-member relations   The degree of confidence, trust, and respect subordinates have in their leader.

Leader-participation model   A leadership theory that provides a set of rules to determine the form and amount of participative decision making in different situations.

Leadership   The ability to influence a group toward the achievement of goals.

Leadership styles   The research on leadership styles has either distinguished between two key dimensions (consideration and initiating structure) or three different styles (autocratic, democratic, and laissez-faire). Each dimension and style is associated with different outcomes (e.g., the autocratic style is associated with greater productivity, while the democratic style is linked with higher satisfaction, at least in some situations).

Leading   Includes motivating subordinates, directing others, selecting the most effective communication channels, and resolving conflicts.

Learning   Any relatively permanent change in behavior that occurs as a result of experience.

Legitimate political behavior   Normal everyday politics.

Leniency error   The tendency to evaluate a set of employees too high (positive) or too low (negative).

Leniency/Structure bias   Rater bias in which all ratees are assigned ratings that are predominantly positive (leniency) or negative (strictness).

Line authority   Authority to direct the work of a subordinate.

Locus of control   The degree to which people believe they are masters of their own fate.

Long-linked technology   Tasks or operations that are sequentially interdependent.

Lower-order needs   Needs that are satisfied externally; physiological and safety needs.

Loyalty   Dissatisfaction expressed by passively waiting for conditions to improve.

LPC   Least preferred coworker questionnaire that measures task or relationship-oriented leadership style.

Machiavellianism   Degree to which an individual is pragmatic, maintains emotional distance, and believes that ends can justify means.

Machine bureaucracy   A structure that rates high in complexity, formalization, and centralization.

McClelland's theory of needs   Achievement, power, and affiliation are three important needs that help to understand motivation.

Management by objectives (MBO)   A program that encompasses specific goals, participatively set, for an explicit time period, with feedback on goal progress.

Managerial grid   A nine-by-nine matrix outlining eighty-one different leadership styles.

Managers   Individuals who achieve goals through other people.

Maquiladoras   Domestic Mexican firms that manufacture or assemble products for a company of another nation, which are then sent back to the foreign company for sale and distribution.

Mass production   Large-batch manufacturing.

Matrix structure   A structure that creates dual lines of authority; combines functional and product departmentalization.

Maturity   The ability and willingness of people to take responsibility for directing their own behavior.

Mechanistic structure   A structure characterized by high complexity, high formalization, and centralization.

Mediating technology   Linking of independent units.

Mediator   A neutral third party who facilitates a negotiated solution by using reasoning, persuasion, and suggestions for alternatives.

Mental health consultation   One of the three major types of consultation. It attempts to focus on the "psychological" well-being of all the parties involved in consultation. Its ultimate goal is to create a mentally healthier society.

Message   What is communicated.

Meta-analysis   A statistical technique that quantitatively integrates and synthesizes a number of independent studies to determine if they consistently produced similar results.

Metamorphosis stage   The stage in the socialization process in which a new employee adjusts to his or her work group's values and norms.

Middle line   Managers who connect the operating core to the strategic apex.

Model   Abstraction of reality; simplified representation of some real-world phenomenon.

Moderating variable   Abates the effect of the independent variable on the dependent variable; also known as *contingency variable.*

Motivating potential score   A predictive index suggesting the motivation potential in a job.

Motivation   The willingness to exert high levels of effort toward organizational goals, conditioned by the effort's ability to satisfy some individual need.

Motivation-hygiene theory   A reference to intrinsic factors, which are related to job satisfaction, and extrinsic factors, which are associated with dissatisfaction.

Multiple cutoff   A method for combining test scores that involves establishing minimum cutoff scores for each test. If an examinee falls below the cutoff for even one test, the person is rejected. Examinees who reach or exceed the minimum cutoff scores on all tests are accepted.

Multiple regression   A method for combining test scores that involves the use of a statistically derived equation to yield a predictor score for each examinee on the basis of performance on each test in a test battery. Multiple regression equations assign weights to each test score, based on the test's correlation with the criterion and with other tests in the battery.

Multiple (Successive) hurdles   A method of administering multiple predictors that involves ordering the predictors and then administering each predictor only after the previous one has been successfully passed or completed.

nAch   Need to achieve or strive continually to do things better.

National culture   The primary values and practices that characterize a particular country.

Need   Some internal state that makes certain outcomes appear attractive.

Need for achievement   One of the needs proposed by McClelland as a primary motivator of behavior. A person with a high need for achievement sets moderately difficult self-goals, engages in activities that have a moderate degree of risk, desires feedback about performance, and prefers to be personally responsible for his or her activities.

Need hierarchy theory   Maslow's theory of motivation proposing that five basic needs are arranged in a hierarchical order such that a need higher in the hierarchy doesn't serve as a source of motivation until all lower needs have been fulfilled.

Needs assessment (analysis)   Systematic process of determining job performance requirements and employee performance deficits to identify training needs and the content of training programs.

Neglect   Dissatisfaction expressed through allowing conditions to worsen.

Negotiation   A process in which two or more parties exchange goods or services and attempt to agree on the exchange rate for them.

Noise   A potential cause of learning and performance failures when present in the environment. In general, noise is most likely to have adverse effects when it is intermittent, uncontrollable, and unpredictable.

Nominal group technique   A group decision-making method in which individual members meet face-to-face to pool their judgments in a systematic but independent fashion.

Nonverbal communications   Messages conveyed through body movements, the intonations or emphasis we give to words, facial expressions, and the physical distance between the sender and receiver.

Norming   The third stage in group development, characterized by close relationships and cohesiveness.

Norms   Acceptable standards of behavior within a group that are shared by the group's members.

OB Mod   A program where managers identify performance-related employee behaviors and then implement an intervention strategy to strengthen desirable performance behaviors and weaken undesirable behaviors.

Objective measures   Measures of job performance that directly assess productivity (e.g., number of units produced, number of errors) or other job-related behaviors (absenteeism, tardiness, etc.)

Older employees   Employees who may require special consideration in selection and training due to changes in intellectual functioning. Most research suggests that deficits in performance among older employees are more often due to declines in psychomotor skills than cognitive failures.

Operant conditioning   A type of conditioning in which desired voluntary behavior leads to a reward or prevents a punishment.

Operating core   Employees who perform the basic work related to the production of products and services.

Opportunity power   Influence obtained as a result of being in the right place at the right time.

Opportunity to perform   High level of performance is partially a function of an absence of obstacles that constrain the employee.

Optimizing model   A decision-making model that describes how individuals should behave to maximize some outcome.

Organic structure   A structure characterized by low complexity, low formalization, and decentralization.

Organization   (1) A consciously coordinated social unit, composed of two or more people, that functions on a relatively continuous basis to achieve a common goal or set of goals. (2) A group of people put together for a common purpose. Almost all consultation, regardless of the type, occurs within some type of organization. It is one of the factors that influence the process and outcomes of consultation. Throughout this book (*Consultation Skills*) this term is used synonymously with the term *agency*.

Organization size   The number of people employed in an organization.

Organization structure   The degree of complexity, formalization, and centralization in the organization.

Organizational behavior (OB)   A field of study that investigates the impact that individuals, groups, and structure have on behavior within organizations, for the purpose of applying such knowledge toward improving an organization's effectiveness.

Organizational commitment   An individual's orientation toward the organization in terms of loyalty, identification, and involvement.

Organization consultation   One of the three major types of consultation. Its primary goal is the enhancement of an organization's effectiveness. The organization is the client system, and the members of the organization involved in consultation are the consultees. Consultants frequently work together in teams when performing organizational consultation.

Organizational culture   A common perception held by the organization's members; a system of shared meaning.

Organizational development   (1) A collection of planned-change interventions, built on humanistic-democratic values, that seek to improve organizational effectiveness and employee well-being. (2) A term referring to a broad range of techniques designed to increase overall organizational effectiveness. Most techniques share in common a systems approach, top management commitment, the use of a change agent, and an emphasis on people and their relationships. Includes the managerial grid, QWL (quality of work life) interventions, process consultation, and the sociotechnical approach.

Organizing   Determining what tasks are to be done, who is to do them, how the tasks are to be grouped, who reports to whom, and where decisions are to be made.

Overlearning   Learning and practice past the point of mastery; helps ensure that information and skills will be remembered.

Paired comparison   (1) An evaluation method that compares each employee with every other employee and assigns a summary ranking based on the number of superior scores that the employee achieves. (2) A relative method of performance appraisal involving comparing an employee with every other employee on all dimensions of job behavior.

Paraphrasing   Restating what the speaker has said in one's own words.

Parochialism   A narrow view of the world; an inability to recognize differences between people.

Participative management   A process where subordinates share a significant degree of decision-making power with their immediate superiors.

Parties-at-interest   Those people (who usually belong to the organization in which consultation is occurring) who are not directly involved in consultation but are affected by the consultation process in some way. Parties-at-interest typically include contact persons and administrators. If the consultant belongs to an organization (e.g., a mental health center), then those members of the consultant's organization indirectly affected by the consultation are also parties-at-interest.

Path-goal theory   (1) The theory that a leader's behavior is acceptable to subordinates insofar as they view it as a source of either immediate or future satisfaction. (2) A theory of leadership that proposes an effective leader is one who helps employees identify and achieve personal goals through the achievement of organizational goals.

Perceived conflict   Awareness by one or more parties of the existence of conditions that create opportunities for conflict to arise.

Perception   A process by which individuals organize and interpret their sensory impressions to give meaning to their environment.

Performance-based compensation   Paying employees on the basis of some performance measure.

Performing   The fourth stage in group development, when the group is fully functional.

Permanent part-time employment   Increasingly popular method of scheduling work. Includes job sharing and job pairing in which two (or more) employees share a job. Associated with greater productivity and satisfaction.

Person-machine system   The target of most human factors interventions. From the human factors perspective, any failure in performance is due to a person-machine mismatch.

Personal power   Influence attributed to one's personal characteristics.

Personality   The sum total of ways in which an individual reacts and interacts with others.

Personality traits   Enduring characteristics that describe an individual's behavior.

Persuasive power   The ability to allocate and manipulate symbolic rewards.

Physical ability   That required to do tasks demanding stamina, dexterity, strength, and similar skills.

Physiological symptoms of stress   Changes in an individual's health as a result of stress.

Piece-rate pay plans   Workers are paid a fixed sum for each unit of production completed.

Placid-clustered environment   An environment in which change occurs slowly, but threats occur in clusters.

Placid-randomized environment   An environment in which demands are randomly distributed and change occurs slowly.

Planned change   Change activities that are intentional and goal oriented.

Planning   Includes defining goals, establishing strategy, and developing plans to coordinate activities.

Political behavior   Those activities that are not required as part of one's formal role in the organization, but that influence, or attempt to influence, the distribution of advantages and disadvantages within the organization.

Pooled interdependence   Where two groups function with relative independence but their combined output contributes to the organization's overall goals.

Position power   Influence derived from one's formal structural position in the organization; includes power to hire, fire, discipline, promote, and give salary increases.

Power   A capacity that A has to influence the behavior of B so that B does things he or she would not otherwise do.

Power-control view of structure   An organization's structure is the result of a power struggle by internal constituencies who are seeking to further their interests.

Power distance   A national culture attribute describing the extent to which a society accepts that power in institutions and organizations is distributed unequally.

Power need   The desire to make others behave in a way that they would not otherwise have behaved.

Power tactics   Identifies how individuals manipulate the power bases.

Prearrival stage   The period of learning in the socialization process that occurs before a new employee joins the organization.

Predictor   Any test or measuring device used to predict performance on some other variable. In organizations, selection tests are used as predictors of future job performance to assist in selection decisions.

Problem analyzability   The type of search procedure employees follow in responding to exceptions.

Process consultation   (1) Insights that a consultant gives a client into what is going on around the client, within the client, and between the client and other people; identifies processes that need improvement. (2) An organizational development in which a consultant helps the client (members of the organization) perceive, understand, and change the processes that are undermining their interactions and the organization's effectiveness.

Process departmentalization   Grouping activities on the basis of product or customer flow.

Process production   Continuous-process production.

Product departmentalization   Grouping activities by product line.

Production-oriented leader   One who emphasizes technical or task aspects of the job.

Productivity   A performance measure including effectiveness and efficiency.

Professional bureaucracy   A structure that rates high in complexity and formalization, and low in centralization.

Projection   Attributing one's own characteristics to other people.

Psychological contract   An unwritten agreement that sets out what management expects from the employee, and vice versa.

Psychological symptoms of stress   Changes in an individual's attitudes and disposition due to stress.

Psychomotor tests   Tests requiring a coordination of sensory processes and motor activities. Unlike intelligence, psychomotor skill seems to represent independent abilities that do not have an underlying "g" factor.

Quality circle   (1) A work group of employees who meet regularly to discuss their quality problems, investigate causes, recommend solutions, and take corrective actions. (2) An organizational development strategy involving work groups that meet periodically to discuss ways to improve productivity.

Quality of life   A national culture attribute that emphasizes relationships and concern for others.

Quantity of life   A national culture attribute describing the extent to which societal values are characterized by assertiveness and materialism.

Rationality   Choices that are consistent and value-maximizing.

Reciprocal interdependence   Where groups exchange inputs and outputs.

Referent power   Influence held by A based on B's admiration and desire to model himself or herself after A.

Refreezing   Stabilizing a change intervention by balancing driving and restraining forces.

Reinforcement theory   The theory that behavior is a function of its consequences.

Reliability   (1) Consistency of measurement. (2) The degree to which a predictor, criterion, or other measuring device provides consistent results across, different forms of the test, different raters, and so on. Usually measured with a correlation (reliability) coefficient. Reliability is a necessary, but not sufficient, condition for validity.

Research   The systematic gathering of information.

Responsibility   An obligation to perform.

Rest breaks   Brief periods of rest from work that help reduce fatigue. It is best if rest break schedules are empirically determined but, in general, should be provided at least twice: at the beginning of the fourth and eighth hours of work.

Restraining forces   Forces that hinder movement away from the status quo.

Rights view of ethics   Decisions concerned with respecting and protecting the basic rights of individuals.

Risky shift phenomenon   The proposal that group decisions tend to be "riskier" than decisions made by individuals.

Rituals   Repetitive sequences of activities that express and reinforce the key values of the organization, what goals are most important, which people are important, and which are expendable.

Role   A set of expected behavior patterns attributed to someone occupying a given position in a social unit.

Role conflict   A situation in which an individual is confronted by divergent role expectations.

Role expectations   How others believe a person should act in a given situation.

Role identity   Certain attitudes and behaviors consistent with a role.

Role perception   An individual's view of how he or she is supposed to act in a given situation.

Satisfaction and performance   The relationship between satisfaction and performance. Contrary to what might be expected, the research has found only a weak relationship between job satisfaction and performance, with the average correlation being around .14.

Satisficing model   A decision-making model where a decision maker chooses the first solution that is "good enough"; that is, satisfactory and sufficient.

Scientific management   Management theory that advocates the use of scientific methods to achieve improved worker efficiency and productivity. Emphasized having each worker perform a simple, standardized component of the entire job and using pay as the primary motivator.

SCII   The Strong-Campbell Interest Inventory, a widely used interest test. Research has shown that the SCII and its predecessors are better predictors of job choice, persistence, and satisfaction than job success.

Selection ratio   The ratio of the number of applicants hired to the total number of applicants. Utility of a predictor is maximized when the selection ratio is low (e.g., $1:100$ is better than $1:10$).

Selective perception   The tendency of people to selectively interpret what they see based on their interests, background, experience, and attitudes.

Self-actualization   The drive to become what one is capable of becoming.

Self-efficacy   The individual's belief that he or she is capable of performing a task.

Self-esteem   Individuals' degree of liking or disliking for themselves.

Self-managed work teams   Groups that are free to determine how the goals assigned to them are to be accomplished and how tasks are to be allocated.

Self-management   Learning techniques that allow individuals to manage their own behavior so that less external management control is necessary.

Self-monitoring   A personality trait that measures an individual's ability to adjust his or her behavior to external, situational factors.

Self-perception theory   Attitudes that are used after the fact to make sense out of an action that has already occurred.

Self-serving bias   The tendency for individuals to attribute their own successes to internal factors while putting the blame for failures on external factors.

Sensitivity training   Training groups that seek to change behavior through unstructured group interaction.

Sequential interdependence   The situation where one group depends on another for its input but the dependency is only one way.

Shaping behavior   Systematically reinforcing each successive step that moves an individual closer to the desired response.

Similarity error   Giving special consideration when rating others to those qualities that the evaluator perceives in himself or herself.

Simple structure   A structure characterized by low complexity, low formalization, and authority centralized in a single person.

Situational leadership theory   (1) A contingency theory that focuses on followers' maturity. (2) Hersey and Blanchard's model of leadership, which proposes that the best leadership style depends on the maturity of the workers. As a worker's job maturity changes, so, too, should the leader's style.

Skill variety   The degree to which the job requires a variety of different activities.

Socialization   The process that adapts employees to the organization's culture.

Social information-processing model   Attitudes and behaviors that employees adopt in response to the social cues provided by others with whom they have contact.

Social-learning theory   The theory that people can learn through observation and direct experience.

Social facilitation   The increase in learning and performance that occurs in the presence of others. Most likely to occur when the task is simple or well learned.

Social inhibition   The decrease in learning and performance that occurs in the presence of others. Most likely to occur when the task is new or complex.

Social loafing   The tendency of group members to do less than they are capable of individually, resulting in an inverse relationship between group size and individual performance.

Sociotechnical approach   An organizational development approach that simultaneously focuses on both the social and technical aspects of the organization. Views the organization as basically a social system rather than a technical system for providing goods and services.

Source of power   How power holders come to control the bases of power.

Span of control   The number of subordinates a manager can efficiently and effectively direct.

Spatial differentiation   The degree to which the location of an organization's offices, plants, and personnel are geographically dispersed.

Staff authority   Positions that support, assist, and advise line managers.

Status   A socially defined position or rank given to groups or group members by others.

Stereotyping   Judging someone on the basis of one's perception of the group to which that person belongs.

Storming   The second stage in group development, characterized by intragroup conflict.

Strategic apex   Top-level managers.

Stress   (1) A dynamic condition in which an individual is confronted with an opportunity, constraint, or demand related to what he or she desires and for which the outcome is perceived to be both uncertain and important. (2) The physiological response of the body to a stressor. While work-related factors can serve as sources of stress, Holmes and Rahe (1967) found that certain factors related to marriage are most likely to lead to stress-related illness.

Strong cultures   Cultures where the core values are intensely held and widely shared.

Structured interview   Interview format involving the use of predetermined questions designed to obtain information that has been found to be related to job performance. Associated with higher levels of validity than nonstructured interviews.

Subcultures   Minicultures within an organization, typically defined by department designations and geographical separation.

Subjective measures   Measures of performance or other behavior that reflect the opinion or judgment of the rater. The major problem with subjective measures is that they are susceptible to rater biases.

Support staff   People in an organization who fill the staff units.

Survey feedback   The use of questionnaires to identify discrepancies among member perceptions; discussion follows and remedies are suggested.

Synergy   An action of two or more substances that results in an effect that is different from the individual summation of the substances.

Systematic study   Looking at relationships, attempting to attribute causes and effects, and drawing a conclusion based on scientific evidence.

Task characteristic theories   Theories that seek to identify task characteristics of jobs, how these characteristics are combined to form different jobs, and their relationship to employee motivation, satisfaction, and performance.

Task group   Those working together to complete a job task.

Task identity   The degree to which the job requires completion of a whole and identifiable piece of work.

Task significance   The degree to which the job has a substantial impact on the lives or work of other people.

Task structure   The degree to which job assignments are procedurized.

Task uncertainty   The greater the uncertainty in a task, the more custom the response. Conversely, low uncertainty encompasses routine tasks with standardized activities.

Task variability   The number of exceptions individuals encounter in their work.

Team building   High interaction among group members to increase trust and openness.

Technical skills   The ability to apply specialized knowledge or expertise.

Technology   How an organization transfers its inputs into outputs.

Technostructure   Analysts in the organization.

Telecommuting   A work arrangement where employees do their work at home on a computer that is linked to their office.

Terminal values   Desirable end-states of existence; the goals that a person would like to achieve during his or her lifetime.

Theory   A set of systematically interrelated concepts or hypotheses that purport to explain and predict phenomena.

Theory X   (1) The assumption that employees dislike work, are lazy, dislike responsibility, and must be coerced to perform. (2) Management approach that assumes that employees are inherently lazy, incapable of self-discipline, and seek to avoid work and, therefore, must be externally controlled and motivated. Similar to the traditional scientific management approach.

Theory Y   (1) The assumption that employees like work, are creative, seek responsibility, and can exercise self-direction. (2) Management approach that assumes that employees are capable of autonomy, are primarily self-motivated, and will naturally integrate personal goals with those of the organization. Similar to the human relations approach.

Traditional view of conflict   The belief that all conflict is harmful and must be avoided.

Trait theories of leadership   Theories that sought personality, social, physical, or intellectual traits that differentiated leaders from nonleaders.

Transactional leaders   Leaders who guide or motivate their followers in the direction of established goals by clarifying role and task requirements.

Transformational leaders   Leaders who provide individualized consideration and intellectual stimulation, and who possess charisma.

Tripartite   Composed of three parts. With respect to consultation, it refers to the three parties involved: consultant, consultee, and client system.

Turbulent-field environment   An environment that changes constantly and that contains interrelated elements.

Turnover   Voluntary and involuntary permanent withdrawal from the organization.

Type A behavior   Aggressive involvement in a chronic, incessant struggle to achieve more and more in less and less time and, if necessary, against the opposing efforts of other things or other people.

Type B behavior   Rarely harried by the desire to obtain a wildly increasing number of things or to participate in an endlessly growing series of events in an ever-decreasing amount of time.

Uncertainty avoidance   A national culture attribute describing the extent to which a society feels threatened by uncertain and ambiguous situations and tries to avoid them.

Unfairness   Unfair hiring, placement, or related discrimination against a minority group that occurs when members of the minority group consistently score lower on a predictor but perform approximately the same on the criterion as members of the majority group. A cause of adverse impact.

Unfreezing   Change efforts to overcome the pressures of both individual resistance and group conformity.

Unit production   The production of items in units or small batches.

Unity of command   The belief that a subordinate should have only one superior to whom he or she is directly responsible.

Utilitarian view of ethics   A view in which decisions are made solely on the basis of their outcome or consequences.

Validity   (1) The degree to which a research study is actually measuring what it claims to be measuring. (2) The extent to which a predictor, criterion, or other measure actually assesses what it is intended to measure. Types of validity include content, construct, and criterion-related.

Validity generalization studies   Reviews of validity studies using meta-analytic techniques that have found that criterion-related validity coefficients are usually higher than what is found in a single organization or study, that validity coefficients generalize across different organizations and jobs, and that differential validity is actually rare and, when reported, is often due to methodological flaws in the validation studies.

Values   Basic convictions that a specific mode of conduct or end-state of existence is personally or socially preferable to an opposite or converse mode of conduct or end-state of existence.

Variable   Any general characteristic that can be measured and that changes in either amplitude, intensity, or both.

Variable-interval schedule   Rewards that are distributed in time so that reinforcements are unpredictable.

Variable-ratio schedule   A reward distribution that varies relative to the behavior of the individual.

Vertical differentiation   The number of hierarchical levels in the organization.

Vestibule training   A method of off-the-job training that involves the use of simulated equipment or a simulated job environment. Useful when on-the-job training would be too dangerous or too costly.

Voice   Dissatisfaction expressed through active and constructive attempts to improve conditions.

Weighted application blanks   A type of empirically-derived application blank in which items are assigned weights depending on their correlation with a criterion. Item weights are used to calculate a total score for the applicant.

Wellness programs   Organizationally supported programs that focus on the employee's total physical and mental condition.

Wonderlic personnel test   A 12-minute test of intelligence often used in industry as a selection technique.

Workforce diversity   The increasing heterogeneity of organizations with the inclusion of different groups.

Work (Job) samples   Tests that require the individual (e.g., job applicant) to perform a task or operation actually required by the job.

Work sampling   Creating a miniature replica of a job to evaluate the performance abilities of job candidates.

Work-related problem   The kind of problem considered to be suitable for the primary focus in consultation. In the case of consultation with people such as parents, the term *caretaking-related* is sometimes used instead. This term is often contrasted with *personal problem,* a type of problem not dealt with in consultation.

References

Abrahams, J. (1995). *The mission statement book*. Berkeley, CA: Ten Speed Press.

Abrams, R. (2003). *The successful business plan: Secrets and strategies* (4th ed.). Palo Alto, CA: Planning Shop.

Academy of Psychosomatic Medicine. (1992). *Proposal for the designation of consultation-liaison psychiatry as a subspecialty: Internal report*. Chicago: Author.

Academy of Psychosomatic Medicine. (1998). Practice guidelines for psychiatric consultation in the general medical setting. *Psychosomatics, 39*(4), S8–S30.

Adams, B. (2002). *Streetwise complete business plan*. Avon, MA: Adams Media Corporation.

Adams, G. P. (1963). The making of economic society. *American Economic Review, 53*(1), 185–187.

Advisor on the Web. (2003). Career development. Available from Thomson/West Publishing at https://advisor.west.thomson.com.

Akin, G., & Palmer, I. (2000). Putting metaphors to work for change in organizations. *Organizational Dynamics, 28*(3), 67–79.

Aldana, S. G., & Pronk, N. P. (2001). Health promotion programs, modifiable health risks, and employee absenteeism. *Journal of Occupational and Environmental Medicine, 43*(1), 36–46.

Allen, A. (1994, May 29). Black unlike me: Confessions of a White man confused by racial etiquette. *Washington Post,* pp. C1, C2.

Alinsky, S. (1969). *Reveille for radicals*. New York: Vintage Books.

Alinsky, S. (1971). *Rules for radicals: A practical primer for realistic radicals*. New York: Vintage Books.

Allport, G. W., & Odbert, H. S. (1936). Trait-names: A psycholexical study. *Psychological Monographs, 47*(211), 1–171.

Althen, G. (2002). *American ways: A guide for foreigners in the United States* (2nd ed.). Yarmouth, ME: Intercultural Press.

American Institute of Stress. (2005). *Job stress*. Available from www.stress.org/job.htm.

American Marketing Association. (2005). Marketing definitions. Available from http://www.marketingpower.com/content4620.php.

American Psychological Association. (1972). *Ethical standards of psychologists*. Washington, DC: Author.

American Psychological Association. (1981). Specialty guidelines for the delivery of services by industrial/organizational psychologists. *American Psychologist, 36,* 664–669.

American Psychological Association. (2002). Ethical principles of psychologists and code of conduct. *American Psychologist, 57*(12), 1060–1073.

American Psychological Association. (2005). *Psychologically Healthy Workplace Award*. Available from www.helping.apa.org.

American Psychological Association, Division 13, Education and Training Committee. (2002). Principles for education and training at the doctoral and post-doctoral level in consulting psychology/organizational. In R. L. Lowman (Ed.), *Handbook of organizational consulting psychology* (pp. 773–785). San Francisco: Jossey-Bass.

Angelica, E., & Hyman, V. (1997). *Coping with cutbacks: The nonprofit guide to success when times are tight.* New York: Amerherst H. Wilder Foundation.

Angerer, J. M. (2003). Job burnout. *Journal of Employment Counseling, 40,* 98–107.

Anglin, T. M. (2003). Mental health in schools: Programs of the federal government. In M. D. Weist, S. W. Evans, & N. A. Lever (Eds.), *Handbook of school mental health: Advancing practice and research* (pp. 89–106). New York: Kluwer Academic/Plenum Press.

Applegate, L. M., Austin, R. D., & McFarlan, F. W. (2003). *Corporate information strategy and management: Text and cases* (6th ed.). Boston: McGraw-Hill/Irwin.

Aronson, E. (1999). *The social animal* (8th ed.). New York: Worth.

Association of Psychology Postdoctoral and Internship Centers. (2005). The APPIC Directory. Available from http://www.appic.org/directory/index.html.

Autry, J. A. (1991). *Love and profit: The art of caring leadership.* New York: Morrow.

Baker, S., & Baker, K. (1998). *The complete idiot's guide to project management.* New York: Macmillan.

Bandura, A. (1986). The explanatory and predictive scope of self-efficacy theory. *Journal of Social and Clinical Psychology, 4*(3), 359–373.

Bardwick, J. (1991). Stemming the entitlement tide in American business. *Management Review, 80*(10), 54–59.

Barling, J., & Frone, M. R. (2004). *The psychology of workplace safety.* Washington, DC: American Psychological Association.

Baron, R. (1998). *What type am I? Discover who you really are.* New York: Penguin Putnam.

Baron, R. (2002). *Bar-On Emotional Quotient Inventory.* North Tonawanda, NY: Multi-Health Systems.

Baron, R. A., & Byrne, D. (1991). *Social psychology: Understanding human interaction* (6th ed.). Boston: Allyn & Bacon.

Barrick, M. R., & Mount, M. K. (1993, February). Autonomy as a moderator of the relationship between the Big Five personality dimensions and job performance. *Journal of Applied Psychology,* 111–118.

Bass, B. M. (1992). From transactional to transformational leadership: Learning to share the vision. In R. R. Sims, D. D. White, & D. A. Bednar (Eds.), *Readings in organizational behavior* (pp. 208–221). Boston: Allyn & Bacon.

Bass, B. M., & Avolio, B. J. (1990). Developing transformational leadership: 1992 and beyond. *Journal of European Industrial Training, 14*(5), 21–27.

Batchelor, S. (1983). *Alone with others.* New York: Grove Press.

Beatty, J. F., & Samuelson, S. S. (2001). *Business law for a new century* (2nd ed.). Cincinnati, OH: West Legal Studies in Business.

Bellah, R. N., Madsen, R., Sullivan, W. M., Swidler, A., & Tipton, S. M. (1996). *Habits of the heart.* Berkeley, CA: University of California Press.

Bellman, G. (1990). *The consultant's calling: Bringing who you are to what you do.* San Francisco: Jossey-Bass.

Benne, K. D. (1969). Some ethical problems in group and organizational consultation. In W. G. Bennis, K. D. Benne, & R. Chin (Eds.), *The planning of change* (pp. 595–604). New York: Holt, Rinehart and Winston.

Bennett, J. B., & Lehman, W. E. K. (2003). *Preventing workplace substance abuse: Beyond drug testing to wellness.* Washington, DC: American Psychological Association.

Bennis, W. G., Benne, K. D., Chin, R., & Corey, K. E. (1976). *The planning of change* (3rd ed.). Oxford, England: Holt, Rinehart and Winston.

Bennis, W., & Goldsmith, J. (1997). *Learning to lead: A workbook on becoming a leader.* Cambridge, MA: Perseus Publishing.

Bent, R. (1992). The professional core competency areas. In R. L. Peterson, J. D. McHolland, R. J. Bent, E. Davis-Russell, G. E. Edwall, K. Polite, et al. (Eds.), *The core curriculum in professional psychology* (pp. 77–81). Washington, DC: American Psychological Association.

Benton, D. A. (1999). *Secrets of a CEO coach: Your personal training guide to thinking like a leader and acting like a CEO.* New York: McGraw-Hill.

Bergan, J. R. (1977). *Behavioral consultation.* Columbus, OH: Charles E. Merrill.

Bergan, J. R., & Kratochwill, T. R. (1990). *Behavioral consultation and therapy.* New York: Plenum.

Bergan, J. R., & Tombari, M. L. (1975). The analysis of verbal interactions occurring during consultation. *Journal of School Psychology, 13,* 209–226.

Bergan, J. R., & Tombari, M. L. (1976). Consultant skill and efficiency and the implementation of outcomes of consultation. *Journal of School Psychology, 14,* 3–14.

Berger, C. J., Olson, C. A., & Boudreau, J. W. (1983, December). Effects of unions on job satisfaction: The role of work-related values and perceived rewards. *Organizational Behavior and Human Performance,* 289–324.

Bhatia, N., & Murrell, K. F. (1969). An industrial experiment in organized rest pauses. *Human Factors, 11,* 167–174.

Blais, M. R., Briere, N. M., Lachance, L., Riddle, A. S., & Vallerand, R. J. (1993). L'inventaire des motivation au travail de Blais [The Blais Work Motivation Inventory]. *Revue Quebecoise de Psychologie, 14,* 185–215.

Blake, R. R., & Mouton, J. S. (1964). *The managerial grid.* Houston, TX: Gulf.

Blake, R. R., & Mouton, J. S. (1983). *Consultation* (2nd ed.). Reading, MA: Addison-Wesley.

Blauner, B. (1993). "But things are much worse for the Negro people": Race and radicalism in my life and work. In J. H. Stanfield II (Ed.), *A history of race relations research: First generation recollections* (pp. 1–36). Newbury Park, CA: Sage.

Bledsoe, B. E. (2003). Critical Incident Stress Management (CISM): Benefit or risk for emergency services. *Prehospital Emergency Care, 7*(2), 272–279.

Blevins, W. (1993). *Your family yourself.* Oakland, CA: New Harbinger Publications.

Block, P. (2000). *Flawless consulting: A guide to getting your expertise used* (2nd ed.). San Francisco: Jossey-Bass/Pfeiffer.

Block, P., & Markowitz, A. (2001). *The flawless consulting fieldbook and companion: A guide understanding your expertise.* San Francisco: Jossey-Bass.

Blythe, B. (2002). *Blindsided: A manager's guide to catastrophic incidents in the workplace.* New York: Penguin Books.

Boekaerts, M., & Roeder, I. (1999). Stress, coping, and adjustment in children with a chronic disease: A review of the literature. *Disability and Rehabilitation: An International Multidisciplinary Journal, 21,* 311–337.

Boldt, L. G. (1999). *Zen and the art of making a living.* New York: Viking Penguin.

Bolles, R. N., & Bolles, M. E. (2005). *What color is your parachute? 2005: A practical manual for job-hunters and career-changers.* Berkeley, CA: Ten Speed Press.

Bolman, L., & Deal, T. (2003). *Reframing organizations: Artistry, choice, and leadership* (3rd ed.). San Francisco: Jossey-Bass.

Bond, C. F. (1982). Social facilitation: A self-presentational view. *Journal of Personality and Social Psychology, 42,* 1042–1050.

Bond, F. W., & Bunce, D. (2003). The role of acceptance and job control in mental health, job satisfaction, and work performance. *Journal of Applied Psychology, 88*(6), 1057–1068.

Borman, W. C., White, L. A., Pulakos, E. D., & Oppler, S. H. (1991). Models of supervisory job performance ratings. *Journal of Applied Psychology, 76,* 863–872.

Brake, T., Walker, D., & Walker, T. (1995). *Doing business internationally.* New York: McGraw-Hill.

Brannon, L., & Feist, J. (1997). *Health psychology: An introduction to behavior and health* (3rd ed.). Pacific Grove, CA: Brooks/Cole.

Bray, R. M., & Sugarman, R. (1980). Social facilitation among interaction groups: Evidence for the evaluation apprehension hypothesis. *Personality and Social Psychology Bulletin, 6,* 137–142.

Bridges, W. (1980). *Transitions: Making sense of life's changes* (2nd ed.). New York: Perseus Books.

Bridges, W. (1991). *Managing transitions: Making the most of change.* New York: Perseus Books.

Brigham, E. F., & Ehrhardt, M. C. (2002). *Financial management: Theory and practice* (10th ed.). New York: South-Western/Thomson Learning.

Brockner, J., & Grover, S. (1994). Layoff and surviving employees: The relationship between job insecurity and work effort. *Stores Magazine, 76*(1), RR10–RR12.

Brounstein, M. (1993). *Handling the difficult employee: Solving performance problems.* Menlo Park, CA: Crisp Learning.

Brown, D., Pryzwansky, W. B., & Schulte, A. C. (2001). *Psychological consultation: Introduction to theory and practice* (5th ed.). Boston: Allyn & Bacon.

Brown, R. T., Freeman, W. S., Brown, R. A., Belar, C., Hersch, L., Hornyak, L. M., et al. (2002). The role of psychology in health care delivery. *Professional Psychology: Research and Practice, 33,* 536–545.

Brumback, G. B., Romashko, T., Hahn, C. P., & Fleishman, E. A. (1974). *Model procedures for job analysis, test development and validation.* Washington, DC: American Institutes for Research.

Bugental, J. (1965). *The search for authenticity.* New York: Holt, Rinehart and Winston.

Bugental, J. (1987). *The art of the psychotherapist.* New York: Norton.

Burns, B. J., Costello, E. J., Angold, A., Tweed, D., Stangl, D., Farmer, E., et al. (1995). Children's mental health service use across serviced sectors. *Health Affairs, 14,* 147–159.

Butler, D., & Geis, F. L. (1990). Nonverbal affect responses to male and female leaders: Implications for leadership evaluations. *Journal of Personality and Social Psychology, 58,* 48–59.

Callahan, D. (1998). Crisis intervention model for teachers. *Journal of Instructional Psychology, 25,* 226–234.

Callahan, J. (1996). Negative effects of a school suicide postvention program: A case example. *Crisis, 17*(3), 108–115.

Campbell, D., Draper, R., & Huffington, C. (1991). *A systemic approach to consultation.* New York: Brunner/Mazel.

Campbell, D. P., Hyne, S. A., & Nilsen, D. L. (1992). *Manual for the Campbell Interest and Skill Survey.* Minneapolis, MN: National Computer Systems.

Cannon-Bowers, J. A., & Salas, E. (1998). *Making decisions under stress: Implications for individual and team training.* Washington, DC: American Psychological Association.

Caplan, G. (1963). Types of mental health consultation. *American Journal of Orthopsychiatry, 3,* 470–481.

Caplan, G. (1970). *The theory and practice of mental health consultation.* New York: Basic Books.

Caplan, G., & Caplan, R. B. (1993). *Mental health consultation and collaboration.* San Francisco: Jossey-Bass.

Cardy, R. L., & Dobbins, G. H. (1994). *Performance appraisal: Alternative perspectives.* Cincinnati, OH: South-Western Publishing.

Carpenter, S. L., & Kennedy, W. J. D. (1988). *Managing public disputes.* San Francisco: Jossey-Bass.

Carr-Ruffino, N. (2002). *Managing diversity: People skills for a multicultural workplace* (4th ed.). Boston: Pearson Custom Publishing.

Carver, C. S., & Scheier, M. F. (1981). *Attention and self-regulation: A control-theory approach to human behavior.* New York: Springer-Verlag.

Carver, J., & Carver, M. M. (1997). *Reinventing your board: A step-by-step guide to implementing policy governance.* San Francisco: Jossey-Bass.

Casas, J. M., & Pytluk, S. D. (1995). Hispanic identity development: Implications for research and practice. In J. M. Pontoretto, J. Casas, L. A. Suzuki, & C. M. Alexander (Eds.), *Handbook of multicultural counseling* (pp. 155–180). Thousand Oaks, CA: Sage.

Cascio, W. F. (1991). *Costing human resources: The financial impact of behavior in organizations* (3rd ed.). Boston: PWS-KENT Publishing.

Cass, V. C. (1979). Homosexual identity formation: A theoretical model. *Journal of Homosexuality, 4,* 219–235.

Cattell, H. B. (1989). *The 16PF: Personality in depth.* Champaign, IL: Institute for Personality and Ability Testing.

Cattell, R. B. (1943). The description of personality: Basic traits resolved into clusters. *Journal of Abnormal and Social Psychology, 38,* 476–506.

Cattell, R. B., Eber, H. W., & Tatsuoka, M. M. (1970). *Handbook for the Sixteen Personality Factor Questionnaire (16PF).* Champaign, IL: Institute for Personality and Ability Testing.

Charlop, M. H., Parrish, J. M., Fenton, L. R., & Cataldo, M. J. (1987). Evaluation of hospital-based pediatric psychology services. *Journal of Pediatric Psychology, 12,* 485–503.

Chase, R. B., Aquilano, N. J., & Jacobs, F. R. (2001). *Operations management for competitive advantage* (9th ed.). New York: McGraw-Hill/Irwin.

Cherniss, C., & Goleman, D. (Eds.). (2001). *The emotionally intelligent workplace: How to select for, measure, and improve emotional intelligence in individuals, groups, and organizations.* New York: Wiley.

Chin, R., & K. D. Benne. (1976). General strategies for effecting changes in human systems. In W. G. Bennis, K. D. Benne, R. Chin, & K. E. Corey (Eds.), *The planning of change* (pp. 22–45). New York: Holt, Rinehart and Winston.

Christensen, A., Jacobson, N. S., & Babcock, J. C. (1995). Integrative behavioral couple therapy. In N. S. Jacobson & A. S. Gurman (Eds.), *Clinical handbook of couple therapy* (pp. 31–64). New York: Guilford Press.

CoachVille.com. (2003). *The coaching starter kit: Everything you need to launch and expand your coaching practice.* New York: Norton.

Coch, L., & French, J. R. P. (1948). Overcoming resistance to change. *Human Relations, 1,* 512–532.

Cohen, W. A. (2001). *How to make it big as a consultant.* New York: AMACOM, American Management Association.

Conger, J. A., & Kanungo, R. N. (1988). *Charismatic leadership.* San Francisco: Jossey-Bass.

Connell, J. B. (2002). Organizational consulting to virtual teams. In R. L. Lowman (Ed.), *Handbook of organizational consulting psychology* (pp. 285–311). San Francisco: Jossey-Bass.

Conner, D. (1992). *Managing at the speed of change.* New York: Villard Books.

Conoley, J. C., & Conoley, C. W. (1992). *School consultation: Practice and training* (2nd ed.). Needham Heights, MA: Allyn & Bacon.

Constenbader, V., Swartz, J., & Petrix, L. (1992). Consultation in the schools: The relationship between preservice training, perception of consultative skills, and actual time spent in consultation. *School Psychology Review, 21,* 95–108.

Cooper, R., & Foster, M. (1971). Sociotechnical systems. *American Psychologist, 26*(5), 467–474.

Corey, G. (1991). *Theory and practice of counseling and psychotherapy* (4th ed.). Pacific Grove, CA: Brooks/Cole Publishing.

Corey, G. (2000). *Theory and practice of group counseling* (5th ed.). Belmont, CA: Wadsworth/Thomson Learning.

Cormier, S., & Cormier, B. (1998). *Interviewing strategies for helpers: Fundamental skills and cognitive behavioral interventions* (4th ed.). Pacific Grove, CA: Brooks/Cole Publishing.

Corrigan, P. W., & Kleinlein, P. (2005). The impact of mental illness stigma. In P. W. Corrigan (Ed.), *On the stigma of mental illness: Practical strategies for research and social change* (pp. 11–44). Washington, DC: American Psychological Association.

Costa, P., & McCrae, R. (1992). *Revised NEO Personality Inventory (NEO-PI-R) and NEO Five-Factor Inventory (NEO-FFI) professional manual.* Odessa, FL: Psychological Assessment Resources.

Costa, P., & Widiger, T. (2002). *Personality disorders and the five-factor model of personality* (2nd ed.). Washington, DC: American Psychological Association.

Covey, S. (1996). *What is empowerment?* Available from http://www.qualitydigest.com/jan/covey.html.

Cox, P. H., Qi, Y., & Liu, Z. (1993). Overview of sport psychology. In R. N. Singer, M. Murphy, & L. K. Tennant (Eds.), *Handbook of research on sport psychology* (pp. 3–311). Old Tappan, NY: Macmillan.

Crisp, A. H., Gelder, M. G., Rix, S., Meltzer, H. I., & Rowlands, O. J. (2000). Stigmatisation of people with mental illnesses. *British Journal of Psychiatry, 177,* 4–7.

Crum, T. F. (1987). *The magic of conflict.* New York: Touchstone Books.

Csikszentmihalyi, M. (2003). *Good business: Leadership, flow, and the making of meaning.* New York: Penguin Putnam.

Cummings, T. G., & Worley, C. G. (1993). *Organization development and change* (7th ed.). Cincinnati, OH: South-Western College Publishing.

Cunningham, C. E., Woodward, C. A., Shannon, H. S., MacIntosh, J., Lendrum, B., & Howe, M. A. (1989). Using imagery to facilitate organizational development and change. *Group and Organization Studies, 14*(1), 70–82.

Danna, K., & Griffin, R. (1999). Health and well-being in the workplace: A review and synthesis of the literature. *Journal of Management, 25*(3), 357–385.

David, F. (2001). *Strategic management* (8th ed.). Upper Saddle River, NJ: Prentice-Hall.

David, G., & Watson, G. (1982). *Black life in corporate America: Swimming in the mainstream.* New York: Anchor Press/Doubleday.

David, M. H. (1980). A multidimensional approach to individual differences in empathy. *JSAS Catalog of Selected Documents in Psychology, 10,* 85.

David, M. H., Luce, C., & Kraus, S. J. (1994). The heritability of characteristics associated with dispositional empathy. *Journal of Personality, 62*(3), 369–391.

Davidson, E. J. (2002). Organizational evaluation: Issues and methods. In R. L. Lowman (Ed.), *Handbook of organizational consulting psychology* (pp. 344–369). San Francisco: Jossey-Bass.

Davis, D. L., Skube, C. J., Hellervik, L. W., Gebelein, S. H., & Sheard, J. L. (1996). *Successful manager's handbook: Development suggestions for today's managers.* Minneapolis, MN: Personnel Decisions International.

Davis, M. H. (1983). Measuring individual differences in empathy: Evidence for a multidimensional approach. *Journal of Personality and Social Psychology, 44,* 113–126.

De Jonge, J., Dormann, C., Jannssen, P. P. M., Dollard, M. F., Landerweerd, J. A., & Nijhuis, F. J. N. (2001). Testing reciprocal relationships between job characteristics and psychological well-being. *Journal of Occupational and Organizational Psychology, 71,* 29–46.

Deming, W. E. (1982a, Winter). Improvement of quality and productivity through action by management. *Productivity Review.*

Deming, W. E. (1982b). *Quality, productivity and competitive position.* Cambridge, MA: MIT Center for Advanced Engineering.

De Raad, B., & Perugini, M. (2002). *Big Five Assessment.* Seattle, WA: Hogrefe & Huber.

Dessler, G. (1999). How to earn your employees' commitment. *Academy of Management Executive, 13*(2), 58–67.

Diamond, M. A., & Allcorn, S. (1987). The psychodynamics of regression in work groups. *Human Relations, 40*(8), 525–544.

Dienesch, R. M., & Liden, R. C. (1986). Leader-member exchange model of leadership: A critique and further development. *Academy of Management Review, 11,* 618–634.

Dilts, R. (1996). *Visionary leadership.* Capitola, CA: Meta Publications.

Dilts, R., & Bonissone, G. (1993). *Skills for the future: Managing for creativity and innovation.* Cupertino, CA: Mata Publications.

Dilts, R., Epstein, T., & Dilts, R. (1991). *Tools for dreamers: Strategies for creativity and innovation.* Capitola, CA: Meta Publications.

Dinkmeyer, D., & Carlson, J. (2001). *Consultation: Creating school based interventions.* Philadelphia: Brunner-Routledge.

Division of Managerial Consultation. (1978). *Standards of professional conduct for academic/management consultants.* New York: Academy of Management.

Dolbier, C. L., Soderstrom, M., & Steinhardt, M. A. (2001). The relationships between self-leadership and enhanced psychological, health, and work outcomes. *Journal of Psychology, 135*(5), 469–486.

Dorgan, W. J., III. (2002). Mental illness in the workplace. *Modern Machine Shop, 75*(5), 106.

Dougherty, A. M. (1995). *Consultation: Practice and perspectives in school and community settings* (2nd ed.). Pacific Grove, CA: Brooks/Cole.

Dresang, J. (2005, February 3). Milwaukee area adds 18,300 jobs over year: Green Bay also does well in U.S. survey. *Milwaukee Journal Sentinel,* p. D1.

Drotar, D. (1995). *Consulting with pediatricians: Psychological perspectives for research and practice.* New York: Plenum Press.

Drotar, D, Spirito, A., & Stancin, T. (2003). Professional roles and practice patterns. In Michael C. Roberts (Ed.), *Handbook of pediatric psychology* (3rd. ed., pp. 50–66). New York: Guilford Press.

Drucker, P. F. (1990). *Managing the nonprofit organization, practices and principles.* New York: HarperBusiness.

DuBrin, A. (2000). *Essentials of management* (5th ed.). Cincinnati, OH: South-Western College Publishing.

Dyer, W. G. (1987). *Team building: Issues and alternatives* (2nd ed.). Reading, MA: Addison-Wesley.

Eagly, A., & Karau, S. (2002). Role congruity theory of prejudice toward female leaders. *Psychological Review, 109*(3), 573–598.

Eagly, A. H., Johannesen-Schmidt, M. C., & Van Engen, M. L. (2003). Transformational, transactional, and laissez-faire leadership styles: A meta-analysis comparing women and men. *Psychological Bulletin, 129*(4), 569–592.

Education and Training Committee of the Society for Industrial and Organizational Psychology. (2005). *An instructor's guide for introducing industrial-organizational psychology.* Available from http://www.siop.org/Instruct/inGuide.htm.

Ellis, A., & Harper, R. (1961). *A guide to rational living.* New York: Institute for Rational Living.

Emery, F. E., & Trist, E. L. (1978). Analytical model for sociotechnical systems. In W. A. Pasmore & J. J. Sherwood (Eds.), *Sociotechnical systems: A sourcebook* (pp. 120–131). San Diego, CA: Pfeiffer.

Erchul, W. P., & Martens, B. K. (2002). *School consultation: Conceptual and empirical bases of practice* (2nd ed.). New York: Kluwer Academic/Plenum Press.

Erez, M., Earley, P. C., & Hulin, C. L. (1985, March). The impact of participation on goal acceptance and performance. *Academy of Management Review, 56.*

Evans, M. G., & Ondrack, D. A. (1990, May). The role of job outcomes and values in understanding the union's impact on job satisfaction: A replication. *Human Relations,* 401–418.

Everly, G. S., & Flynn, B. (in press). *Principles and practice of psychological first aid.* Baltimore: Johns Hopkins University Bloomberg School of Public Health.

Everly, G. S., Lating, J. M., & Mitchell, J. T. (2000). Innovations in group crisis intervention: Critical Incident Stress Debriefing (CISD) and Critical Incident Stress Management (CISM). In A. R. Roberts (Ed.), *Crisis intervention handbook: Assessment, treatment, and research* (2nd ed., pp. 77–97). New York: Oxford University Press.

Eysenck, H. J. (1952). The effects of psychotherapy: An evaluation. *Journal of Consulting Psychology, 16,* 319–324.

Fagan, T. K., & Wise, P. S. (2000). *School psychology: Past, present, and future* (2nd ed.). Bethesda, MD: National Association of School Psychologists.

Fairhurst, G. T. (1993). Leader-member exchange patterns of women leaders in industry: A discourse analysis. *Communication Monographs, 60,* 321–351.

Fairhurst, G. T., & Sarr, R. (1996). *The art of framing: Managing the language of leadership.* San Francisco: Jossey Bass.

Feinstein, C., & Reiss, A. (1996). Psychiatric disorder in mentally retarded children and adolescents: The challenges of meaningful diagnosis. *Child and Adolescent Psychiatric Clinics of North America, 5,* 827–852.

Fiedler, F. E. (1967). *A theory of leadership effectiveness.* New York: McGraw-Hill.

Fiedler, F. E., & Chemers, M. M. (1974). *Leadership and effective management.* Glenview, IL: Scott, Foresman.

Fiedler, F. E., & Chemers, M. M. (1984). *The leader match concept.* New York: Wiley.

Fiedler, F. E., Chemers, M., & Mahar, L. (1976). *Improving leadership effectiveness: The leader match concept.* New York: Wiley.

Fiske, S. T., Beroff, D. N., Borgida, E., Deaux, K., & Heilman, M. E. (1991). Social science research on trial: Use of sex stereotyping research in. *Price Waterhouse v. Hopkins. American Psychologist, 46,* 1049–1060.

Fitzgerald, C., & Berger, J. (2002). *Executive coaching: Practices and perspectives.* Palo Alto, CA: Davies-Black Publishing.

Fitzgerald, L. F., Drasgow, F., Hulin, C. L., Gelfand, J. J., & Magley, V. J. (1997). Antecedents and consequences of sexual harassment in organizations: A test of an integrated model. *Journal of Applied Psychology, 83,* 578–589.

Fitzgerald, L. F., Hulin, C. L., & Drasgow, F. (1995). The antecedents and consequences of sexual harassment in organizations: An integrated model. In G. Keita & J. Hurrell Jr. (Eds.), *Job stress in a changing workforce: Investigating gender, diversity, and family issues* (pp. 55–73). Washington, DC: American Psychological Association.

Flaherty, J. (1999). *Coaching: Provoking excellence in others.* Boston: Butterworth-Heinemann.

Flynn, B., & Schultz, J. (2004, December). *Behavioral Health and Awareness Training for Terrorism and Disasters Workshop* [Handout]. Columbus, IN.

Forrester, R., & Drexler, A. B. (1998). A model for team-based organization performance. *Academy of Management Executive, 13*(3), 36–49.

Frankl, V. (1963). *Man's search for meaning.* Boston: Beacon Press.

Frankl, V. (1969). *The will to meaning.* Cleveland, OH: New American Library.

Fraser, J. S. (1989). The strategic rapid intervention approach. In C. Figley (Ed.), *Treating stress: In the family* (pp. 122–157). New York: Brunner/Mazel.

Fraser, J. S. (1995). Strategic rapid intervention: Constructing the process of rapid change. In J. Weakland & W. Ray (Eds.), *Propagations: Thirty years of influence of the Mental Research Institute* (pp. 211–235). New York: Haworth Press.

Fraser, J. S. (2001). Crisis, chaos, and brief therapy: Constructive interventions in high-risk situations. In L. VandeCreek & T. L. Jackson (Eds.), *Innovations in clinical practice: A source book* (Vol. 19, pp. 95–111). Sarasota, FL: Professional Resource Press.

Frease, M., & Zawaki, R. A. (1979). Job sharing: An answer to productivity problems? *Personnel Adminstrator, 100,* 35–38.

Freeman, A., & Fusco, G. (2000). Treating high-arousal patients: Differentiating between patients in crisis and crisis-prone patients. In F. M. Dattilio & A. Freeman (Eds.), *Cognitive-behavioral strategies in crisis intervention* (2nd ed., pp. 27–58). New York: Guilford Press.

French, J. R. P., Jr., & Raven, B. (1959). The bases of social power. In D. Cartwright (Ed.), *Studies in social power* (pp. 150–167). Ann Arbor: University of Michigan, Institute for Social Research.

Freudenberger, H. J., & Richelson, G. (1980). *Burnout: The high cost of high achievement.* New York: Doubleday.

Fried, Y., & Ferris, G. R. (1987, Summer). The validity of the job characteristics model: A review meta-analysis. *Personnel Psychology,* 287–322.

Friedman, T. L. (2000). *The Lexus and the olive tree.* New York: Random House.

Fuchs, D., & Fuchs, L. S. (1989). Exploring effective and efficient prereferral interventions: A component analysis of behavioral consultation. *School Psychology Review, 18*(2), 260–283.

Fuller, G. (1991). *The negotiator's handbook.* Upper Saddle River, NJ: Prentice-Hall.

Galbraith, J. R. (1973). *Designing complex organizations.* Reading, MA: Addison-Wesley.

Gallessich, J. (1982). *The profession and practice of consultation: A handbook for consultants, trainers of consultation and consumers of consultation services.* San Francisco: Jossey-Bass.

Gallup, J. (1998). How to gain access to a company as consultant. In S. Klarreich (Ed.), *Handbook of organizational health psychology: Programs to make the workplace healthier* (pp. 43–54). Madison, CT: Psychosocial Press.

Garfield, C. (1989). *Peak performers.* New York: Avon.

Gatewood, R. D., & Feild, H. S. (1998). *Human resource selection* (4th ed.). Orlando, FL: Dryden Press.

Gelder, M., Gath, D., Mayou, R., & Cowen, P. (1996). *Oxford textbook of psychiatry* (3rd ed.). New York: Oxford University Press.

Gersick, K. E., Davis, J. A., McCollom, M. H., & Lansberg, I. (1997). *Generation to generation: Life cycles of the family business.* Boston: Harvard Business School Press.

Gilbert, J. A., Stead, B. A., & Ivancevich, J. M. (1999). Diversity management: A new organizational paradigm. *Journal of Business Ethics, 21,* 61–76.

Gladding, S. T. (2002). *Family therapy: History, theory, and practice* (3rd ed.). Upper Saddle River, NJ: Prentice-Hall.

Gladding, S. T., & Newsome, D. W. (2004). *Community and agency counseling* (2nd ed.). Upper Saddle River, NJ: Pearson Education.

Gleick, J. (1987). *Chaos: Making a new science.* New York: Penguin Viking.

Godleski, L. S. (1997). Tornado disasters and stress responses. *Journal of the Kentucky Medical Association, 95*(4), 145–148.

Goetsch, D. L., & Davis, S. B. (2000). *Quality management: Introduction to total quality management for production, processing, and services.* Upper Saddle River, NJ: Prentice-Hall.

Golden, C. J. (1990). *Clinical interpretation of objective psychological tests* (2nd ed.). Needham Heights, MA: Allyn & Bacon.

Goleman, D. (1995). *Emotional intelligence: Why it can matter more than IQ.* New York: Bantam Books.

Goleman, D. (1997). *Emotional intelligence.* New York: Bantam Books.

Golembiewski, R. T. (1993). *Handbook of organizational consultation.* New York: Marcel Dekker.

Goodspeed, S. W. (1998). *Community stewardship.* Chicago: AHA Press.

Goodstein, L. (1978). *Consulting with human service systems.* Reading, MA: Addison-Wesley.

Gottfredson, G., & Holland, J. (1996). *Dictionary of Holland occupational codes* (3rd ed.). Odessa, FL: Psychological Assessment Resources.

Gottman, J. M. (1981). *Time-series analysis: A comprehensive introduction for social scientists.* New York: Cambridge University Press.

Gottman, J. M. (1994). *What predicts divorce: The relationship between marital processes and marital outcomes.* Hillsdale, NJ: Erlbaum.

Gottman, J. M. (2002). A multidimensional approach to couples. In F. W. Kaslow (Ed.), *A comprehensive handbook of psychotherapy: Cognitive-behavioral approaches* (Vol. 2, pp. 355–372). Hoboken, NJ: Wiley.

Graen, G., & Cashman, J. F. (1975). A role-making model of leadership in formal organizations: A developmental approach. In J. G. Hunt & L. L. Larson (Eds.), *Leadership frontiers* (pp. 143–165). Kent, OH: Kent State University Press.

Graen, G. B., & Uhl-Bien, M. (1995). Relationship-based approach to leadership: Development of Leader-Member Exchange (LMX) theory of leadership over 25 years—Applying a multi-level multi-domain perspective [Special issue: Leadership: The multiple-level approaches]. *Leadership Quarterly, 6*(Pt. 1), 219–247.

Greenly, D., & Carnall, C. (2001). Workshops as a technique for strategic change. *Journal of Change Management, 2*(1), 33–46.

Greenstone, J., & Leviton, S. (1993). *Elements of crisis intervention.* Pacific Grove, CA: Brooks/Cole Publishing.

Greenwood, D. M. (2002). Gaining and sustaining organizational support through a sociotechnical intervention. *Consulting Psychology Journal: Practice and Research, 54*(2), 104–115.

Griggs, L. B., & Louw, L. L. (1999). *Valuing diversity: New tools for a new reality.* New York: McGraw-Hill.

Gutkin, T. B., & Curtis, M. J. (1990). School-based consultation: Theory, techniques, and research. In T. B. Gtukin & C. R. Reynolds (Eds.), *The handbook of school psychology* (2nd ed., pp. 577–611). New York: Wiley.

Haas, L. J., & Fennimore, D. (1983). Ethical and legal issues in professional psychology: Selected works, 1970–1981. *Professional Psychology: Research and Practice, 14*(4), 540–548.

Haas, L. J., & Malouf, J. L. (2002). *Keeping up the good work: A practitioner's guide to mental health ethics* (3rd ed.). Sarasota, FL: Professional Resource Press/Professional Resource Exchange.

Hackett, R. D., & Guion, R. M. (1985, June). A reevaluation of the absenteeism-job satisfaction relationship. *Organizational Behavior and Human Decisions Processes,* 340–381.

Hackman, J. R. (1977). Work design. In J. R. Hackman & J. L. Suttle (Eds.), *Improving life at work* (pp. 132–133). Santa Monica, CA: Goodyear.

Hackman, J. R., & Oldham, G. R. (1980). *Work redesign*. Reading, MA: Addison-Wesley.

Hackman, J. R., Oldham, G. R., Janson, R., & Purdy, K. (1975). A new strategy for job enrichment. *California Management Review, 17,* 57–71.

Hackman, J. R., & Wageman, R. (1995, June). Total quality management: Empirical, conceptual, and practical issues. *Administrative Science Quarterly,* 309–342.

Haines, S. (1998). *The manager's pocket guide to systems thinking*. Amherst, MA: Human Resources Development Press.

Hakstian, A. R., & Cattell, R. B. (1982). *Manual for the Comprehensive Ability Battery (CAB)*. Champaign, IL: Institute for Personality and Ability Testing.

Hall, E. T. (1983). *The dance of life: The other dimensions of time*. New York: Anchor/Doubleday.

Hall, E. T., & Hall, M. R. (1990). *Understanding cultural differences: Germans, French, and Americans*. Yarmouth, ME: Intercultural Press.

Hammer, T. H. (1978, December). Relationship between local union characteristics and worker behavior and attitudes. *Academy of Management Journal,* 560–577.

Hammond, R., & Howard, J. (1988, September 9). Rumors of inferiority: The hidden obstacles to black success. *New Republic,* 17–21.

Hankins, G. G. (2000). *Diversity blues: How to shake 'em*. Cincinnati, OH: Telvic Press.

Hansen, J. C. (2000). Interpretation of the Strong Interest Inventory. In C. E. Watkins & V. L. Campbell (Eds.), *Testing and assessment in counseling practice* (2nd ed., pp. 227–262). Mahwah, NJ: Erlbaum.

Hanson, P. G., & Lubin, B. (1995). *Answers to questions most frequently asked about organization development*. Thousand Oaks, CA: Sage.

Harbert, K. R. (2000). Critical incident stress debriefing. In F. M. Dattilio & A. Freeman (Eds.), *Cognitive-behavioral strategies in crisis intervention* (2nd ed., pp. 385–408). New York: Guilford Press.

Hardiman, R. (1982). *White identity development: A process oriented model for describing the racial consciousness of White Americans*. Unpublished doctoral dissertation, University of Massachusetts, Amherst.

Hargrove, R. (1995). *Masterful coaching*. San Diego, CA: Pfeiffer.

Hargrove, R., & Kaestner, C. (1998). *Masterful coaching field guide*. San Diego, CA: Pfeiffer.

Harmon, L. W., Hansen, J. C., Borgen, F. H., & Hammer, A. L. (1994). *Strong Interest Inventory applications and technical guide*. Palo Alto, CA: Consulting Psychologists Press.

Harrison, T. C. (2004). *Consultation for contemporary helping professionals*. Boston: Allyn & Bacon.

Hatch, M. J., & Ehrlich, S. B. (1993). Spontaneous humour as an indicator of paradox and ambiguity in organizations. *Organization Studies, 14*(4), 505–526.

Hays, K. F., & Brown, C. H. (2004). *You're on! Consulting for peak performance*. Washington, DC: American Psychological Association.

Hedge, J. W., & Borman, W. C. (1995). Changing conceptions and practices in performance appraisal. In A. Howard (Ed.), *The changing nature of work* (pp. 451–482). San Francisco: Jossey-Bass.

Heffron, F. (1988). *Organization theory and public organizations*. New York: Prentice-Hall.

Helms, J. E. (1994a). The conceptualization of racial identity and other "racial" constructs. In E. J. Tricket, R. J. Watts, & D. Birman (Eds.), *Human diversity: Perspectives on people in context* (pp. 285–311). San Francisco: Jossey-Bass.

Helms, J. E. (1994b). How multiculturalism obscures racial factors in the psychotherapy process. *Journal of Consulting Psychology, 41,* 162–165.

Helms, J. E. (1994c). Racial identity and career assessment. *Journal of Career Assessment, 2,* 199–209.

Helms, J. E. (1995). An update of Helms' white and people of color racial identity models. In J. M. Pontoretto, J. Casas, L. A. Suzuki, & C. M. Alexander (Eds.), *Handbook of multicultural counseling* (pp. 181–198). Thousand Oaks, CA: Sage.

Helms, J. E., & Piper, R. E. (1994). Implications of racial identity theory for vocational psychology. *Journal of Vocational Behavior, 44,* 124–136.

Hendricks, J. E., McKean, J., & Hendricks, C. G. (2003). *Crisis intervention: Contemporary issues for on-site interveners.* Springfield, IL: Charles C Thomas.

Heneman, H. G., & Schwab, D. P. (1972, July). Evaluation of research on expectancy theory prediction of employee performance. *Psychological Bulletin,* 1–9.

Herlihy, B., & Corey, G. (1997). *Boundary issues in counseling: Multiple roles and responsibilities.* Alexandria, VA: American Counseling Association.

Herman, N. J., & Smith, C. M. (1989). Mental hospital depopulation in Canada: Patient perspectives. *Canadian Journal of Psychiatry, 34*(5), 386–391.

Hersey, P., & Blanchard, K. (1982). *Management of organizational behavior: Utilizing human resources* (4th ed.). Englewood Cliffs, NJ: Prentice-Hall.

Herzberg, F., Mausner, B., & Snyderman, B. (1959). *The motivation to work.* New York: Wiley.

Hicks, M., & Peterson, D. (1999). Leaders coaching across borders. In W. Mobley, M. Gessner, & V. Arnold (Eds.), *Advances in global leadership* (Vol. 1, pp. 295–314). Stamford, CT: JAI Press.

Higgins, M. C., & Fram, K. E. (2001). Reconceptualizing mentoring at work: A developmental network perspective. *Academy of Management Review, 26,* 264.

Hobbs, N. (1963). Strategies for the development of clinical psychology. *American Psychological Association Division of Clinical Psychology Newsletter, 16,* 3–5.

Hodgson, P., & Crainer, S. (1993). *What do high performance managers really do?* London: Financial Times/Pitman Publishing.

Hoff, K., & Zirkel, P. (1999). The IDEA's final regulations: Our top ten list for school psychologists. *NASP Communique, 28*(4), 6–7.

Hofstede, G. J., Pederson, P., & Hofstede, G. (2002). *Exploring culture: Exercises, stories, and synthetic cultures.* Yarmouth, ME: Intercultural Press.

Holland, J. L. (1966). *The psychology of vocational choice.* Waltham, MA: Blaisdell.

Holland, J. L. (1985). *Vocational Preference Inventory (VPI) manual* Odessa, FL: Psychological Assessment Resources.

Holland, J. L. (1994). *The self-directed search.* Odessa, FL: Psychological Assessment Resources.

Hollander, S. C. (1960). The wheel of marketing. *Journal of Marketing, 25*(1), 37–42.

Holmes, T. H., & Rahe, R. H. (1967). The Social Readjustment Rating Scale. *Journal of Psychosomatic Research, 11,* 213–218.

Holtz, H. (1993). *How to succeed as an independent consultant* (3rd ed.). New York: Wiley.

Houle, C. O. (1997). *Governing boards: Their nature and nurture.* San Francisco: Jossey-Bass.

House, R. J. (1971, September). A path-goal theory of leader effectiveness. *Administrative Science Quarterly,* 321–338.

House, R. J., & Aditya, R. (1997). The social scientific study of leadership: Quo vadis? *Journal of Management, 23,* 409–474.

House, R. J., & Wigdor, L. A. (1967, Winter). Herzberg's dual-factor theory of job satisfaction and motivations: A review of the evidence and criticism. *Personnel Psychology,* 369–389.

Hubble, M., Duncan, B., & Miller, S. (1999). *The heart and soul of change: What works in therapy.* Washington, DC: American Psychological Association.

Hunter, D., Bailey, A., & Taylor, B. (1995). *The art of facilitation, how to create group synergy.* Cambridge, MA: Fisher Books.

Iaffaldano, M. T., & Muchinsky, P. M. (1985, March). Job satisfaction and job performance: A meta-analysis. *Psychological Bulletin, 251*–273.

Ilgen, D. R., & Hulin, C. L. (2000). *Computational modeling of behavior in organizations.* Washington, DC: American Psychological Association.

Institute of Medicine. (2003). *Preparing for the psychological consequences of terrorism: A public health strategy.* Washington, DC: National Academies Press.

International Society for Performance Improvement. (2005). *ISPI diversity policy.* Available from www.ispi.org.

Jackson, S. E. (Ed.). (1992). *Diversity in the workplace: Human Resource initiatives.* New York: Guilford Press.

Jackson, S. E., & Ruderman, M. N. (Eds.). (1995). *Diversity in work teams: Research paradigms for a changing workplace.* Washington, DC: American Psychological Association.

Janis, I. (1982). *Groupthink* (2nd ed.). Boston: Houghton Mifflin.

Jewell, L. M. (1998). *Contemporary industrial/organizational psychology* (3rd ed.). Pacific Grove, CA: Brooks/Cole.

Johansson, C. B. (2002). *The Career Assessment Inventory.* Minneapolis, MN: Pearson Assessments.

Johnson, D. A., Beyerlein, M. M., Huff, J. W., Halfhill, T. R., & Ballentine, R. D. (2002). Successfully implementing teams in organizations. In R. L. Lowman (Ed.), *Handbook of organizational consulting psychology* (pp. 235–259). San Francisco: Jossey-Bass.

Jones, L. (1994, May). Mama's White. *Essence Magazine,* pp. 78, 80, 148.

Journal of Accountancy. (2000). How to succeed in business by really trying. *Journal of Accountancy, 190*(1), 12.

Judge, T. A., Bono, J. E., Ilies, R., & Gerhardt, M. W. (2002). Personality and leadership: A qualitative and quantitative review. *Journal of Applied Psychology, 87*(4), 765–780.

Jurgensen, C. E. (1978). Job preferences: What makes a job good or bad? *Journal of Applied Psychology, 63*(3), 267–277.

Kagan, J. (1965). The new marriage: Pediatrics and psychology. *American Journal of Diseases of Children, 110,* 272–278.

Kahn, R. L. (1972). The meaning of work: Interpretation and proposals of measurement. In A. Campbell & P. E. Converse (Eds.), *The human meaning of social change* (pp. 159–203). New York: Sage.

Kahn, R. L., & Katz, D. (1960). Leadership practices in relation to productivity and morale. In D. Cartwright & A. Zander (Eds.), *Group dynamics: Research and theory* (2nd ed., pp. 554–570). Elmsford, NY: Row/Paterson.

Kampwirth, T. J. (1999). *Collaborative consultation in the schools: Effective practices for students with learning and behavior problems.* Upper Saddle River, NJ: Prentice-Hall.

Kaplan, R. E. (1997). *Skillscope for managers.* Greensboro, NC: Center for Creative Leadership.

Kaplan, R. E., & Kaiser, R. B. (2003). Developing versatile leadership. *MIT Sloan Management Review, 44*(4), 19–26.

Kaplan, R. S., & Norton, D. P. (1996, January/February). Using the balanced scorecard as a strategic management system. *Harvard Business Review,* 75–77.

Karr, A. R. (2000, April 18). The checkoff. *Wall Street Journal,* p. A1.

Karson, M., Karson, S., & O'Dell J. (1997). *16PF interpretation in clinical practice: A guide to the fifth edition.* Champaign, IL: Institute for Personality and Ability Testing.

Karson, S., & O'Dell, J. W. (1976). *A guide to the clinical use of the 16PF.* Champaign, IL: Institute for Personality and Ability Testing.

Katz, N. H., & Lawyer, J. W. (1985). *Communication and conflict resolution skills.* Dubuque, IA: Kendall/Hunt Publishing.

Katzenbach, J. R., & Smith, D. K. (1999). *The wisdom of teams: Creating the high-performance organization.* New York: HarperCollins.

Kazdin, A. E., Bass, D., Ayers, W. A., & Rodgers, A. (1990). Empirical and clinical focus of child and adolescent psychotherapy research. *Journal of Consulting and Clinical Psychology, 58,* 729–740.

Keller, H. R. (1981). Behavioral consultation. In J. C. Conoley (Ed.), *Consultation in schools: Theory, research, and procedures* (pp. 59–99). New York: Academic Press.

Kelly, L. (1994). *The ASTD technical and skills training handbook.* Alexandria, VA: American Society for Training and Development.

Kesselman, G. A., Hagen, E. L., & Wherry, R. J. (1974). A factor analytic test of the Porter-Lawler expectancy model of work motivation. *Personnel Psychology, 27,* 569–579.

Kilburg, R. R. (2000). *Executive coaching: Developing managerial wisdom in a world of chaos.* Washington, DC: American Psychological Association.

Kilburg, R. R. (2002). Failure and negative outcomes: The taboo topic in executive coaching. In C. Fitzgerald & J. Garvey Berger (Eds.), *Executive coaching, practices and perspectives* (pp. 283–301). Palo Alto, CA: Davies-Black Publishing.

Kirkpatrick, S. A., & Locke, E. A. (1991). Leadership: Do traits matter? *Executive, 5*(2), 48–60.

Klarreich, S. (1998). *Handbook of organizational health psychology.* Madison, CT: Psychosocial Press.

Klaus, M., & Heinz, S. (2004). Is involvement a suppressor on the job satisfaction: Life satisfaction relationship? *Journal of Applied Psychology, 34*(11), 2377–2389.

Klein, J. K., & Kim, J. S. (1998). A field study of the influence of situational constraints, leader-member exchange, and goal commitment on performance. *Academy of Management, 41*(1), 86–95.

Knaus, N. H. (1998). A cognitive perspective on absenteeism. In S. Klarreich (Ed.), *Handbook of organizational health psychology: Programs to make the workplace healthier* (pp. 125–138). Madison, CT: Psychosocial Press.

Knitzer, J. (1996). The role of education in systems of care. In B. A. Stroul & R. M. Friedman (Eds.), *Children's mental health: Creating systems of care in a changing society* (pp. 197–213). Baltimore: Paul H. Brookes.

Kochman, T. (1981). *Black and white styles in conflict.* Chicago: University of Chicago Press.

Kolb, D., Rubin, I., & Osland, J. (1995). *The organizational behavior reader* (6th ed.). Englewood Cliffs, NJ: Prentice-Hall.

Koocher, G. P., Soisson, E. L., VandeCreek, L., Knapp, S., Appelbaum, P. S., & Newman, R. (1995). The business of psychology. In D. N. Bersoff (Ed.), *Ethical conflicts in psychology* (pp. 477–511). Washington, DC: American Psychological Association.

Koortzen, P., & Cilliers, F. (2002). The psychoanalytic approach to team development. In R. L. Lowman (Ed.), *Handbook of organizational consulting psychology* (pp. 260–284). San Francisco: Jossey-Bass.

Kossek, E. E., & Ozeki, C. (1998). Work-family conflict, policies, and the job-life satisfaction relationship: A review and directions for organizational behavior: Human resources research. *Journal of Applied Psychology, 83*(2), 139–150.

Kotter, J. P. (1996a, August 5). Kill complacency . . . before it kills you. *Fortune,* 168–170.

Kotter, J. P. (1996b). *Leading change.* Cambridge, MA: Harvard Business School Press.

Kraiger, K. (Ed.). (2002). *Creating, implementing, and managing effective training and development: State-of-the-art lessons for practice.* San Francisco: Jossey-Bass.

Kroeger, O., & Thuesen, J. M. (1992). *Type talk at work: How the 16 personality types determine your success on the job.* New York: Bantam Doubleday Dell Publishing Group.

Krug, S. E. (Ed.). (1977). *Psychological assessment in medicine.* Champaign, IL: Institute for Personality and Ability Testing.

Kurpius, D. (1978). Consultation theory and practice: An integrated model. *Personnel and Guidance Journal, 56*(6), 335–338.

Kurpius, D., & Robinson, S. E. (1978). An overview of consultation. *Personnel and Guidance Journal, 56*(6), 321–323.

Lamb, C., Hair, J., & McDaniel, C. (2003). *Essentials of marketing* (3rd ed.). Mason, OH: South-Western Publishing.

Lambert, M. J. (1992). Implications of outcome research for psychotherapy integration. In J. C. Norcross & M. R. Goldfried (Eds.), *Handbook of psychotherapy integration* (pp. 94–129). New York: Basic Books.

Lambert, S. (1990). Processes linking work and family. *Human Relations, 43,* 239–257.

Latane, B., Williams, K., & Harkins, S. (1979). Many hands make light the work: The causes and consequents of social loafing. *Journal of Personality and Social Psychology, 37,* 822–832.

Lavigne, J. V., & Faier-Routman, J. (1992). Psychological adjustment to pediatric physical disorders: A meta-analytic review. *Journal of Pediatrics, 17,* 133–158.

Lavigne, J. V., Gibbons, R. D., Arend, R., Rosenbaum, D., Binns, H., & Christoffel, K. K. (1999). Rational service planning in pediatric primary care: Continuity and change in psychopathology among children enrolled in pediatric practices. *Journal of Pediatric Psychology, 24,* 393–403.

Levant, R. F. (2003). *The road to resilience.* Available from www.helping.apa.org.

Levinson, H. (2002a). Assessing organizations. In R. L. Lowman (Ed.), *Handbook of organizational consulting psychology* (pp. 315–343). San Francisco: Jossey-Bass.

Levinson, H. (2002b). *Organizational assessment: A step-by-step guide to effective consulting.* Washington, DC: American Psychological Association.

Lewin, K. (1951). *Field theory in social science.* New York: Harper & Row.

Lewin, K., Lippitt, R., & White, R. K. (1939). Patterns of aggressive behavior in experimentally created social climates. *Journal of Social Psychology, 10,* 271–299.

Lewis, J. A., Lewis, M. D., Daniels, J. A., & D'Andrea, M. J. (1998). *Community counseling: Empowerment strategies for a diverse society* (2nd ed.). Pacific Grove, CA: Brooks/Cole.

Lewis, R., & Walker, B. S. (1997). *Why should white guys have all the fun? How Reginald Lewis created a billion-dollar business empire.* New York: Wiley.

Liccione, W. J. (1997). Effective goal setting: A prerequisite for compensation plans with incentive value. *Compensation and Benefits Management, 13*(1), 19–25.

Likert, R. (1976). *New ways of managing conflict.* New York: McGraw-Hill.

Lippitt, G., & Lippitt, R. (1978). *The consulting process in action.* San Diego, CA: University Associates.

Lippitt, G., & Lippitt, R. (1986). *Consulting process in action* (2nd ed.). San Diego, CA: Pfeiffer.

Lippitt, R., & Lippitt, G. (1975a). Consulting process in action. *Training and Development Journal, 29*(5), 48–54.

Lippitt, R., & Lippitt, G. (1975b). Consulting process in action. *Training and Development Journal, 29*(6), 38–41.

Livers, A., & Carver, K. (2002). *Leading in black and white: Working across the racial divide in corporate America.* San Francisco: Jossey-Bass and the Center for Creative Leadership.

Locke, E. A. (1968). Toward a theory of task motivation and incentives. *Organizational Behavior and Human Performance, 3*(2), 157–190.

Locke, E. A. (1976). The nature and causes of job satisfaction. In M. D. Dunnette (Ed.), *Handbook of industrial and organizational psychology* (pp. 1297–1350). Chicago: Rand McNally.

Loden, M., & Rosener, J. B. (1991). *Workforce America! Managing employee diversity as a vital resource.* New York: McGraw-Hill.

Lombardo, M. M., & Eichinger, R. W. (1989). *Preventing derailment: What to do before it's too late.* Greensboro, NC: Center for Creative Leadership.

London, M. (1997). *Job feedback: Giving, seeking, and using feedback for performance improvement.* Mahwah, NJ: Erlbaum.

Lord, R. G., DeVader, C. L., & Alliger, G. M. (1986, August). A meta-analysis of the relation between personality traits and leadership perceptions: An application of validity generalization procedures. *Journal of Applied Psychology,* 402–410.

Lord, R. G., & Maher, K. J. (1991). *Leadership and information processing: Linking perceptions and performance.* Boston: Unwin Hyman.

Losada, M. (1999). The complex dynamics of high performance teams. *Mathematics and Computer Modeling, 30,* 179–192.

Losada, M., & Heaphy, E. (2004). The role of positivity and connectivity in the performance of business teams: A nonlinear dynamics model. *American Behavioral Scientist, 47*(6), 740–765.

Lowe, K. B., Kroeck, K. G., & Sivasubramaniam, N. (1996, Fall). Effectiveness correlates of transformational and transactional leadership. *Leadership Quarterly, 7,* 385–425.

Lowman, R. L. (1989). *Pre-employment screening for psychopathology: A guide to professional practice.* Sarasota, FL: Professional Resource Exchange.

Lowman, R. L. (1991). *The clinical practice of career assessment: Interests, abilities, and personality.* Washington, DC: American Psychological Association.

Lowman, R. L. (1993). *Counseling and psychotherapy of work dysfunctions.* Washington, DC: American Psychological Association.

Lowman, R. L. (2002a). *The ethical practice of psychology in organizations.* Washington, DC: American Psychological Association.

Lowman, R. L. (Ed.). (2002b). *Handbook of organizational consulting psychology.* San Francisco: Jossey-Bass.

Lublin, J. S. (1996, February 28). Women at top still are distant from CEO jobs. *Wall Street Journal,* p. B1.

Lussier, R. N. (2002). *Human relations in organizations: Applications and skill building* (5th ed.). Boston: McGraw-Hill/Irwin.

Luthans, F. (1988, May). Successful vs. effective real managers. *Academy of Management Executive,* 127–132.

Luthans, F., Hodgetts, R. M., & Rosenkrantz, S. A. (1988). *Real managers.* Cambridge, MA: Ballinger.

Macnab, A. J., Russel, J. A., Lowe, J. P., & Gagnon F. (1999). Critical incident stress intervention after loss of an air ambulance: Two-year follow-up. *Prehospital Disaster Medicine, 14*(1), 8–12.

Maddux, R. B. (2000). *Effective performance appraisals* (4th ed.). Los Altos, CA: Crisp.

Major, B., & O'Brien, L. T. (2005). The social psychology of stigma. *Annual Review of Psychology, 56,* 393–421.

Manning, G., Curtis, K., & McMillen, S. (1996). *Building community: The human side of work.* Cincinnati, OH: Thompson Executive Press.

Mannino, F. V., Trickett, E. J., Shore, M. F., Kidder, M. G., & Levin, G. (Eds.). (1986). *Handbook of mental health consultation.* Rockville, MD: National Institute for Mental Health.

Marcus, L., Dorn, B., Kritek, P., Miller, V., & Wyatt, J. (1995). *Renegotiating health care: Resolving conflict to build collaboration.* San Francisco: Jossey-Bass.

Marks, M. L., & Mirvis, P. H. (1992). Rebuilding after the merger: Dealing with "survivor sickness." *Organizational Dynamics, 21*(2), 18–32.

Marks, M. L., & Mirvis, P. H. (2000). Managing mergers, acquisitions, and alliances: Creating an effective transition structure. *Organizational Dynamics, 28*(3), 35–47.

Martin, I. (1996). *From couch to corporation: Becoming a successful corporate therapist.* New York: Wiley.

Marvin, R. (1978). *Organizational diagnosis: A workbook of theory and practice.* Reading, MA: Addison-Wesley.

Maslach, C., Jackson, S. L., & Letter, M. P. (1996). *Maslach Burnout Inventory* (3rd ed.). Palo Alto, CA: Consulting Psychologists Press.

Maslach, C., & Leiter, M. P. (1997). *The truth about burnout: How organizations cause personal stress and what to do about it.* San Francisco: Jossey-Bass.

Maslow, A. (1970). *Motivation and personality* (2nd ed.). New York: Harper & Row.

Massarik, F., & Pei-Carpenter, M. (2002). *Organization development and consulting: Perspectives and foundations.* San Francisco: Jossey-Bass/Pfeiffer.

Mathis, R. L., & Jackson, J. H. (2003). *Human resource management* (10th ed.). Mason, OH: South-Western.

Matteson, M., & Ivancevich, J. (1993). *Management and organizational behavior classics* (5th ed.). Homewood, IL: Irwin Press.

May, R. (1953). *Man's search for himself.* New York: Norton.

May, R. (1975). *The courage to create.* New York: Norton.

Mayou, R. A., Ehlers, A., & Hobbs, M. (2000). Psychological debriefing for road traffic accident victims: Three-year follow-up of a randomised controlled trial. *British Journal of Psychiatry, 176,* 589–593.

McAdams, T., Neslund, N., & Neslund, K. (2004). *Law, business and society* (7th ed.). Homewood, IL: Irwin Press.

McCaskey, M. B. (1982). *The executive challenge: Managing change and ambiguity.* Boston: Pitman.

McClelland, D. C. (1965). Achievement motivation can be developed. *Harvard Business Review, 43*(6), 6–17.

McClelland, D. C. (1967). *The achieving society.* New York: Free Press.

McClelland, D. C. (1985). How motives, skills, and values determine what people do. *American Psychologist, 40*(7), 812–825.

McCormick, E. J., & Ilgen, D. R. (1980). *Industrial psychology* (7th ed.). Englewood Cliffs, NJ: Prentice-Hall.

McCormick, E. J., Jeanneret, P. R., & Mecham, R. C. (1969). *Position Analysis Questionnaire.* West Lafayette, IN: Purdue Research Foundation.

McGoldrick, M. (Ed.). (1998). *Re-visioning family therapy: Race, culture, and gender in clinical practice.* New York: Guilford Press.

McGregor, D. (1960). *The human side of enterprise.* New York: McGraw-Hill.

McShane, S. L. (1984, June). Job satisfaction and absenteeism: A meta-analytic re-examination. *Canadian Journal of Administrative Science,* 61–77.

Mentors in the workplace can boost your careers, but few employees get on-the-job coaching, a recent survey finds. (1996, May 7). *Wall Street Journal,* p. A1.

Meredith, J. R., & Mantel, S. J. (2003). *Project management: A managerial approach* (5th ed.). Hoboken, NJ: Wiley.

Meyer, R. G. (1993). *The clinician's handbook* (3rd ed.). Needham Heights, MA: Allyn & Bacon.

Meyerson, D. E. (1990). Uncovering socially undesirable emotions: Experiences of ambiguity in organizations. *American Behavioral Scientist, 33*(3), 296–307.

Milite, G. (1991, October). When an employee's idea is just plain awful. *Supervisory Management, 3.*

Milkovich, G. T., & Newman, J. M. (2002). *Compensation.* Boston: McGraw-Hill.

Miller, J., & Brown, P. (1993). *The corporate coach: How to build a team of loyal customers and happy employees.* New York: HarperBusiness.

Miller, W. R. (1985). Motivation for treatment: A review with special emphasis on alcoholism. *Psychological Bulletin, 98,* 84–107.

Miller, W. R., & Rollnick, S. (1991). *Motivational interviewing: Preparing people to change addictive behavior.* New York: Guilford Press.

Milojkovic, J. (2001). *Executive coaching.* Available from http://www.knowledgepassion.com /KPvisitor/KP_Documents/KP_Coaching.pdf.

Miner, J. B. (1991). Psychological assessment in a developmental context. In C. P. Hansen & K. A. Conrad (Eds.), *A handbook of psychological assessment in business* (pp. 225–236). New York: Quorom Books.

Mintzberg, H. (1973). *The nature of managerial work.* New York: Harper & Row.

Mischel, W. (1973, July). Toward a cognitive social learning reconceptualization of personality. *Psychological Review,* 252–283.

Mitchell, J. T. (1983). When disaster strikes: The critical incident debriefing process. *Journal of Emergency Medical Services, 13*(11), 49–52.

Mitchell, J. T., & Everly, G. S., Jr. (1993). *Critical incident stress debriefing: An operations manual for the prevention of trauma among emergency service and disaster workers.* Baltimore: Chevron.

Mitchell, J. T., & Everly, G. S. (2000). Critical incident stress management and critical incident stress debriefings: Evolutions, effects and outcomes. In B. Raphael & J. P. Wilson (Eds.), *Psychological debriefing: Theory, practice and evidence* (pp. 71–90). New York: Cambridge University Press.

Mitchell, T. R. (1974, November). Expectancy models of job satisfaction, occupational preference and effort: A theoretical, methodological and empirical appraisal. *Psychological Bulletin,* 1053–1057.

Mobley, W. H., Griffeth, R. W., Hand, H. H., & Meglino, B. M. (1979, May). Review and conceptual analysis of the employee turnover process. *Psychological Bulletin,* 493–522.

Moran, J. W., & Brightman, B. K. (2000). Leading organizational change. *Journal of Workplace Learning, 12*(2), 66–74.

Morrison, A. M. (1992). *The new leaders: Guidelines on leadership diversity in America.* San Francisco: Jossey-Bass.

Morrison, A. M., White, R. P., & Van Velsor, E. (1987). *Breaking the glass ceiling: Can women reach the top of America's largest corporations?* Reading, MA: Addison-Wesley.

Murphy, K. R., & Cleveland, J. N. (1995). *Understanding performance appraisal: Social, organizational and goal-based perspectives.* Thousand Oaks, CA: Sage.

Myers, I. B., McCaulley, M. H., Quenk, N. L., & Hammer, A. L. (1998). *MBTI manual: A guide to the development and use of the Myers-Briggs Type Indicator* (3rd ed.). Palo Alto, CA: Consulting Psychologists Press.

Myrick, R. D. (1977). *Consultation as a counselor intervention.* Ann Arbor, MI: ERIC Counseling and Personnel Services Information Center.

Myrick, R. D. (1987). *Developmental guidance and counseling: A practical approach.* Minneapolis, MN: Educational Media.

National Institute of Mental Health. (2002). *Mental Health and Mass Violence: Evidence-Based Early Psychological Intervention for Victims/Survivors of Mass Violence. A Workshop to Reach Consensus on Best Practices* (NIH Publication No. 02-5138). Washington, DC: U.S. Government Printing Office.

Nelson, B., & Economy, P. (1997). *Consulting for dummies.* Foster City, CA: IDG Books Worldwide.

Nelson, D. L., & Burke, R. J. (2003). *Gender, work stress, and health.* Washington, DC: American Psychological Association.

Nelson, J. (1993). *Volunteer slavery: My authentic Negro experience.* Chicago: Noble.

Neumann, J. E., Kellner, K., & Dawson-Shepherd, A. (1997). *Developing organizational consultancy.* New York: Routledge.

Newacheck, P. W., Strickland, B., Shonkoff, J. P., Perrin, J. M., McPherson, M., McManus, M., et al. (1998). An epidemiological profile of children with special healthcare needs. *Pediatrics, 102,* 117–123.

Newgass, S., & Schonfeld, D. J. (2000). School crisis intervention, crisis prevention, and response. In A. Roberts (Ed.), *Crisis intervention handbook: Assessment, treatment, and research* (2nd ed., pp. 209–228). New York: Oxford University Press.

Nierenberg, G. I. (1968). *The art of negotiating.* New York: Simon & Schuster.

Nikandrou, I., Papalexandris, N., & Bourantas, D. (2000). Gaining employee trust after acquisition: Implications for managerial action. *Employee Relations, 22*(4), 334–355.

Northouse, G. (2001). *Leadership, theory and practice* (2nd ed.). Thousand Oaks, CA: Sage.

Norton, J. R., & Fox, R. E. (1997). *The change equation: Capitalizing on diversity for effective organizational change.* Washington, DC: American Psychological Association.

NTL Institute. (1980). *NTL values and ethics statement.* Arlington, VA: Author.

O'Driscoll, M., & Cooper, C. (1996). Sources and management of excessive job stress and burnout. In P. Warr (Ed.), *Psychology at work* (4th ed., pp. 195–216). London: Penquin Books.

O'Reilly, C. A., III, & Caldwell, D. F. (1980). Job choice: The impact of intrinsic and extrinsic factors on subsequent satisfaction and commitment. *Journal of Applied Psychology, 65*(5), 559–565.

O'Reilly, C. A., III, & Roberts, K. H. (1975). Individual differences in personality, position in the organization, and job satisfaction. *Organizational Behavior and Human Performance, 14*(1), 144–151.

Office of Alcoholism and Substance Abuse Services. (2001). *Hope and recovery.* Available from www.oasas.state.ny.us/www/home.cfm.

Ørner, R. J., King, S., Avery, A., Bretherton, R., Stolz, P., & Ormerod, J. (2003). Coping and adjustment strategies used by emergency services staff after traumatic incidents: Implications for psychological debriefing, reconstructed early intervention and psychological first aid. *Australasian Journal of Disaster and Trauma Studies, 1.* Available from www.massey.ac.nz/~trauma.

Orsburn, J. D., Moran, L., Musselwhite, E., Zenger, J., & Perrin, C. (1990). *Self-directed work teams: The new American challenge.* Homewood, IL: Business One Irwin.

Ortega, B. (1995). Wal-Mart stores' James Walton dies at 73 of aneurysm. *Wall Street Journal—Eastern Edition, 225*(56), p. B3.

Ortega, B. (1998). *In Sam we trust: The untold story of Sam Walton and Wal-Mart, the world's most powerful retailer.* New York: Crown Business.

Osborn, A. F. (1957). *Applied imagination: Principles and procedures of creative thinking* (Rev. ed.). New York: Charles Scribner's Sons.

Ouchi, W. G. (1981). *Theory Z: How American business can meet the Japanese challenge.* New York: Avon Books.

Ouchi, W. G., & Jaeger, A. M. (1978, April). Type Z corporation: Stability in the midst of mobility. *Academy of Management Review, 3,* 305–314.

Owens, D. S. (2004, December). *Substance abuse services: Awareness for terrorism events.* Behavioral Health and Awareness Training for Terrorism and Disasters Workshop, Columbus, IN.

Pasmore, W. A. (1988). *Designing effective organizations: The socio-technical systems perspective.* New York: Wiley.

Pearce, J. A., & Robinson, R. B., Jr. (1997). *Formulation, implementation, and control of competitive strategy* (6th ed.). Boston: Irwin/McGraw-Hill.

Pedersen, P. B. (2004). *110 experiences for multicultural learning.* Washington, DC: American Psychological Association.

Peltier, B. (2001). *The psychology of executive coaching: Theory and application.* New York: Brunner-Routledge.

Pennington, G. (2002). *Getting under the skin: Coaching Black executives.* Wood Dale, IL: RHR International.

Persico, J. (1992). Employee motivation: Is it necessary. In R. R. Sims, D. D. White, & D. A. Bednar (Eds.), *Readings in organizational behavior* (pp. 79–81). Boston: Allyn & Bacon.

Peter, L. J., & Hull, R. (1969). *The Peter principle: Why things always go wrong.* New York: Bantam Books.

Peters, T. J., & Austin, N. (1985). *A passion for excellence: The leadership difference.* New York: Warner Books.

Peters, T. J., & Waterman, R. H. (1982). *In search of excellence: Lessons from America's best-run companies.* New York: Warner Books.

Peterson, D. (2002). Management development: Coaching and mentoring programs. In K. Kraiger (Ed.), *Creating, implementing, and managing effective training and development* (pp. 160–191). San Francisco: Jossey-Bass.

Peterson, D., & Hicks, M. (1996). *Leader as coach: Strategies for coaching and developing others.* Minneapolis, MN: Personnel Decisions International.

Peterson, S., & Jaret, P. E. (2001). *Business plans kit for dummies.* New York: Wiley.

Petrick, J. A. (2005). *Business ethics case analytic framework and case example.* Dayton, OH: Institute for Business Integrity. Available from www.wright.edu/business/ibi.

Petrick, J. A., & Quinn, J. F. (1997). *Management ethics: Integrity at work.* Thousand Oaks, CA: Sage.

Petry, E. S., Mujica, A. E., & Vickery, D. M. (1998). Sources and consequences of workplace pressure: Increasing the risk of unethical and illegal business practices. *Business and Society Review, 99,* 25–30.

Pfeiffer, W. J., & Jones, J. E. (1977). Ethical considerations in consulting. In J. E. Jones & W. J. Pfeiffer (Eds.), *The 1977 annual handbook for group facilitators* (pp. 217–224). San Diego, CA: University Associates.

Pfeiffer, W. J., & Jones, J. E. (Eds.). (1978). *The 1978 annual handbook for group facilitators.* La Jolla, CA: University Associates.

Phillips, K., & Shaw, P. (1998). *A consultancy approach for trainers and developers* (2nd ed.). Brookfield, VT: Gower.

Phillips, S. L., & Elledge, R. L. (1989). *The team-building source book.* San Francisco: Jossey-Bass/Pfeiffer.

Piedmont, R. (1998). *The revised NEO personality inventory: Clinical and research applications.* New York: Plenum Press.

Piersel, W. C., & Gutkin, T. B. (1983). Resistance to school-based consultation: A behavioral analysis of the problem. *Psychology in the Schools, 20,* 311–326.

Pines, A., Aronson, E., & Kafry, D. (1981). *Burnout: From tedium to personal growth.* New York: Free Press.

Pinson, L. (2001). *Anatomy of a business plan: A step-by-step guide to building a business and securing your company's future* (5th ed.). Chicago: Dearborn Trade Publishing.

Porras, J. I., & Robertson, P. J. (1987). Organization development theory: A typology and evaluation. *Research in organizational change and development: An annual series featuring advances in theory, methodology and research* (Vol. 1, pp. 1–57). Greenwich, CT: Elsevier Science/JAI Press.

Porras, J. I., & Robertson, P. J. (1992). Organizational development: Theory, practice, and research. In M. D. Dunnette & L. M. Hough (Eds.), *Handbook of industrial and organizational psychology* (2nd ed., Vol. 3, pp. 719–822). Palo Alto, CA: Consulting Psychologists Press.

Porter, L. W., & Lawler, E. E. (1968). *Managerial attitudes and performance.* Homewood, IL: Irwin-Dorsey.

Powers, B., & Ellis, A. (1995). *A manager's guide to sexual orientation in the work place.* New York: Routledge.

Price Waterhouse v. Hopkins, 109 S. Ct. 1775 (1989).

Price, J. (1977). *The study of turnover.* Ames: Iowa State University Press.

Primoff, E. S., Clark, C. L., & Caplan, J. R. (1982). *How to prepare for and conduct job element examinations* (Suppl.). Washington, DC: Office of Personnel Management, Office of Personnel Research and Development.

Prince, J. P., & Heiser, L. J. (2000). *Essentials of career interest assessment.* New York: Wiley.

Prochaska, J. O. (1999). How do people change, and how can we change to help many more people. In M. Hubble, B. Duncan, & S. Miller (Eds.), *The heart and soul of change: What works in therapy* (pp. 227–258). Washington, DC: American Psychological Association.

Prochaska, J. O., & DiClemente, C. C. (1992). The transtheoretical approach. In J. D. Norcross & M. R. Goldfried (Eds.), *Handbook of psychotherapy integration* (pp. 300–334). New York: Basic Books.

Prochaska, J. O., DiClemente, C. C., & Norcross, J. C. (1992). In search of how people change. *American Psychologist, 47,* 1102–1114.

Prochaska, J. O., Norcross, J. C., & DiClemente, C. C. (1994). *Changing for good.* New York: Morrow.

Pryzwansky, W., & White, G. (1983). The influence of consultee characteristics on preferences for consultation approaches. *Professional Psychology, 14,* 457–461.

Quenk, N. L. (2000). *Essentials of Myers-Briggs Type Indicator assessment.* New York: Wiley.

Quick, J. C., & Tetrick, L. E. (2003). *Handbook of occupational health psychology.* Washington, DC: American Psychological Association.

Quick, J. D., Henley, A. B., & Quick, J. C. (2004). The balancing act: At work and at home. *Organizational Dynamics, 33*(4), 426–438.

Raalte, J. L., & Brewer, B. W. (2002). *Exploring sport and exercise psychology.* Washington, DC: American Psychological Association.

Rackham, N., & Ruff, R. (1991). *Managing major sales.* New York: HarperBusiness.

Rain, J. S., Lane, I. M., & Steiner, D. D. (1991). A current look at the job satisfaction/life satisfaction relationship: Review and future considerations. *Human Relations, 44*(3), 287–308.

Rappaport, N., Osher, D., Garrison, E. G., Anderson-Ketchmark, C., & Dwyer, K. (2003). Enhancing collaboration within and across disciplines to advance mental health programs in schools. In M. D. Weist, S. W. Evans, & N. A. Lever (Eds.), *Handbook of school mental health concerns: Advancing practice and research* (pp. 107–118). New York: Kluwer Academic/Plenum Press.

Rayner, S. R. (1997). *Virtual team.* Freeland, WA: Rayner & Associates.

Reddy, W. B. (1994). *Intervention skills: Process consultation for small groups and teams.* San Diego, CA: Pfeiffer.

Rees, F. (1998). *The facilitator excellence handbook: Helping people work creatively and productively together.* San Diego, CA: Pfeiffer.

Reinharth, L., & Wahba, M. A. (1975, September). Expectancy theory as a predictor of work motivation, effort expenditure, and job performance. *Academy of Management Journal,* 502–537.

Renesch, J. (Ed.). (1994). *Leadership in a new era.* San Francisco: New Leaders Press.

Renstch, J. R., & Steel, R. P. (1998, Spring). Testing the durability of job characteristics as predictors of absenteeism over a six-year period. *Personnel Psychology,* 165–190.

Reschly, D. L., Tilly, W. D., & Grimes, J. P. (Eds.). (1999). *Special education in transition: Functional and non-categorical programming.* Longmont, CO: Sopris West.

Ritter, A. (2000). Total absence management: Practical solutions to prevent and minimize employee absence. *Employee Benefits Journal, 25*(4), 5–8.

Robbins, S. P. (1990). *Organization theory: Structure, design, and applications* (3rd ed.). Englewood Cliffs, NJ: Prentice-Hall.

Robbins, S. P. (2001). *Organizational behavior* (9th ed.). Upper Saddle River, NJ: Prentice-Hall.

Robbins, S. P., & Hunsaker, P. L. (1996). *Training in InterPersonal Skills: TIPS for managing people at work* (2nd ed.). Upper Saddle River, NJ: Prentice-Hall.

Roberts, A. R. (1991). Conceptualizing crisis theory and the crisis intervention model. In A. R. Roberts (Ed.), *Contemporary perspectives on crisis intervention and prevention* (pp. 3–17). Englewood Cliffs, NJ: Prentice-Hall.

Roberts, A. R. (2002). An overview of crisis theory and crisis intervention. In A. R. Roberts (Ed.), *Crisis intervention handbook: Assessment, treatment, and research* (2nd ed., pp. 2–30). New York: Oxford University Press.

Roberts, B. W., & Hogan, R. (2001). *Personality psychology in the workplace.* Washington, DC: American Psychological Association.

Roberts, M., & Lyman, R. D. (1990). The Psychologist as a pediatric consultant: Inpatient and outpatient. In A. M. Gross & R. S. Drabman (Eds.), *Handbook of Clinical Behavioral Pediatrics* (pp. 11–27). New York: Plenum Press.

Roberts, M. C., Mitchell, M. C., & McNeal, R. (2003). The evolving field of pediatric psychology: Critical issues and future challenges. In M. C. Roberts (Ed.), *Handbook of pediatric psychology* (3rd ed., pp. 3–18). New York: Guilford Press.

Robinson, J. L. (1995). *Racism or attitude? The ongoing struggle for black liberation and self-esteem.* New York: Insight Books.

Rokeach, M. (1973). *The nature of human values.* New York: Free Press.

Rones, M., & Hoagwood, K. (2000). School-based mental health services: A research review. *Clinical Child and Family Psychology Review, 3,* 223–240.

Rose, S., Brewin, C. R., Andrews, B., & Kirk, M. (1999). A randomised controlled trial of individual psychological debriefing for victims of violent crime. *Psychological Medicine, 29,* 793–799.

Rosinski, P. (2003). *Coaching across cultures: New tools for leveraging national, corporate, and professional differences.* London: Nicholas Brealey Publishing.

Rothwell, W. J., Sullivan, R., & McLean, G. N. (1995). *Practicing organization development: A guide for consultants.* San Francisco: Jossey-Bass.

Rudisill, J. R., & Archambault, D. A. (1988, August). *Corporate charting: Tracking corporate consultation work.* Paper session to the 1998 American Psychological Association Annual Convention, San Francisco.

Rudisill, J. R., & Archambault, D. A. (1999). Recordkeeping in corporate consulting: The corporate chart. *Innovations in Clinical Practice: A Source Book, 17,* 323–327.

Rudisill, J. R., Hempy, P. E., Eddy, M. E., Zimmerman, G. L., & Rudisill, T. (1998). Executive fit rehearsal. *Consulting Psychology Journal: Practice and Research, 50*(1), 36–39.

Rundell, J. R., & Wise, M. G. (1999). *Essentials of consultation-liaison psychiatry.* Washington, DC: American Psychiatric Press.

Russell, M. T., & Karol, D. L. (1994). *The 16PF fifth edition administrator's manual.* Champaign, IL: Institute for Personality and Ability Testing.

Salas, E., & Fiore, S. (2004). *Team cognition: Understanding the factors that drive processes and performance.* Washington, DC: American Psychological Association.

Salovey, P., & Mayer, J. D. (1990). Emotional intelligence. *Imagination, Cognition, and Personality, 9,* 185–211.

Sarason, I. G., & Sarason, B. R. (1996). *Abnormal psychology: The problem of maladaptive behavior* (8th ed.). Upper Saddle River, NJ: Prentice-Hall.

Sashkin, M., & Kiser, K. J. (1993). *Putting total quality management to work.* San Francisco: Berrett-Koehler.

Sauter, S. L., Brightwell, W. S., Colligan, M. J., Hurrell, J. J., Jr., Katz, T. M., LeGrande, D. E., et al. (2002). *The changing organization of work and the safety and health of working people: Knowledge gaps and research directions.* Washington, DC: Department of Health and Human Services, Centers for Disease Control and Prevention, National Institute for Occupational Safety and Health.

Savickas, M. L., & Walsh, W. B. (1996). *Handbook of career counseling theory and practice.* Palo Alto, CA: Davies-Black Publishing.

Schaef, A. W., & Fassel, D. (1988). *The addictive organization.* San Francisco: Harper & Row.

Schein, E. (1969). *Process consultation.* Reading, MA: Addison-Wesley.

Schein, E. (2000). *Process consultation: Its role in organization development.* Reading, MA: Addison-Wesley.

Schein, E. (2001). *Process consultation revisited: Building the helping relationship.* Reading, MA: Addison-Wesley.

Schermerhorn, J., Hunt, J., & Osborn, R. (2000). *Organizational behavior* (7th ed.). New York: Wiley.

Schmitz, J. (2000). *Cultural orientations guide.* Princeton, NJ: Princeton Training Press.

Schneider, B. (1983). Interactional psychology and organizational behavior. In L. L. Cummings & B. M. Staw (Eds.), *Research in organizational behavior* (Vol. 5, pp. 1–31). Greenwich, CT: JAI Press.

Schneider, K. T., Swan, S., & Fitzgerald, L. F. (1997). Job-related and psychological effects of sexual harassment in the workplace: Empirical evidence from two organizations. *Journal of Applied Psychology, 82,* 401–415.

Schonfeld, D. J., Lichtenstein, R., Kline-Pruett, M., & Speese-Linehan, D. (2002). *How to prepare for and respond to a crisis* (2nd ed.). Alexandria, VA: Association for Supervision and Curriculum Development.

Schriesheim, C. A., Cogliser, C. C., & Neider, L. L. (1995). Is it "trustworthy?" A multiple levels of analysis reexamination of an Ohio State leadership study. *Leadership Quarterly, 6,* 111–145.

Schutz, W. (1958). *FIRO: A three-dimensional theory of interpersonal behavior.* New York: Holt, Rinehart and Winston.

Schutz, W. (1977). *FIRO-B.* Palo Alto, CA: Consulting Psychologists Press.

Schutz, W. (1992). Beyond FIRO-B: Three new theory-derived measures: Element B (behavior), Element F (feelings), and Element S (self). *Psychological Reports, 70,* 915–937.

Schwarz, R. M. (1994). *The skilled facilitator: Practical wisdom for developing effective groups.* San Francisco: Jossey-Bass.

Scott, C. D., & Jaffe, D. T. (1991). *Empowerment: A practical guide for success.* Los Altos, CA: Crisp.

Scott, K. D., & Taylor, G. S. (1985, September). An examination of conflicting findings on the relationship between job satisfaction and absenteeism: A meta-analysis. *Academy of Management Journal,* 599–612.

Seligman, M. (2002). *Authentic happiness: Using the new positive psychology to realize your potential for lasting fulfillment.* New York: Free Press.

Sellers, P. (2004). P&G: Teaching an old dog new tricks. *Fortune, 149*(11), 166–173.

Senge, P. M. (1990). *The fifth discipline: The art and practice of the learning organization.* New York: Doubleday.

Shalev, A. Y. (2000). Stress management and debriefing: Historical concepts and present patterns. In B. Raphael & J. P. Wilson (Eds.), *Psychological debriefing: Theory, practice and evidence* (pp. 17–31). New York: Cambridge University Press.

Shalley, C., & Oldham, G. (1985, September). Effects of goal difficulty and expected external evaluation of intrinsic motivation. *Academy of Management Journal,* 56.

Shellenbarger, S. (2001). Employees are seeking fewer hours; Maybe bosses should listen. *Wall Street Journal—Eastern Edition, 237*(36), p. B1.

Shepard, G. (2005). *How to manage problem employees: A step-by-step guide for turning difficult employees into high performers.* Hoboken, NJ: Wiley.

Sheppard, H. L., & Herrick, N. Q. (1972). *Where have all the robots gone? Worker dissatisfaction in the '70s.* New York: Free Press.

Shuler, C. F. (1998). *Is racial reconciliation really working? Winning the race to unity.* Chicago: Moody Press.

Simmons, A. (1998). *Territorial games.* New York: AMACOM, American Management Association.

Simon, H. A. (1955). A behavioral model of rational choice. *Quarterly Journal of Economics, 69*(1), 99–118.

Sindermann, C. J., & Sawyer, T. K. (1997). *The scientist as consultant: Building new career opportunities.* New York: Plenum Press.

Slaikeu, K. A. (1990). *Crisis intervention: A handbook for practice and research.* Needham Heights, MA: Allyn & Bacon.

Smeltzer, L., & Zener, M. (1992). Development of a model for announcing major layoffs. *Group and Organization Management, 17*(4), 446–473.

Smith, D. (2000). *Women at work: Leadership for the next century.* Upper Saddle River, NJ: Prentice-Hall.

Smith, J. A., & Foti, R. J. (1998, Summer). A pattern approach to the study of leader emergence. *Leadership Quarterly,* 147–160.

Sobel, A. B., Roberts, M. C., Rayfield, A. D., Barnard, M. U., & Rapoff, M. D. (2001). Evaluating outpatient pediatric psychology services in a primary care setting. *Journal of Pediatric Psychology, 26,* 395–405.

Sodowsky, G. R., Kwan, K. K., & Pannu, R. (1995). Ethnic identity of Asians in the United States. In J. M. Pontoretto, J. Casas, L. A. Suzuki, & C. M. Alexander (Eds.), *Handbook of multicultural counseling* (pp. 123–154). Thousand Oaks, CA: Sage.

Spector, R. E. (2000). *Cultural diversity in health and illness.* Upper Saddle River, NJ: Prentice-Hall Health.

Sperry, L. (1996). *Corporate therapy and consulting.* New York: Brunner/Mazel.

Spokane, A. R., & Catalano, M. (2000). The self-directed search: A theory-driven array of self-guiding career interventions. In C. E. Watkins & V. L. Campbell (Eds.), *Testing and assessment in counseling practice* (2nd ed., pp. 339–370). Mahwah, NJ: Erlbaum.

Stacey, R. (1996). *Complexity and creativity in organizations.* San Francisco: Berrett-Koehler.

Stack, J. (1994). *The great game of business: Unlocking the power and profitability of open-book management.* Greenwich, CT: Reed Elsevier.

Steers, R. M. (1981). *Introduction to organizational behavior.* Santa Monica, CA: Goodyear.

Stefan, S. (2001). *Unequal rights: Discrimination against people with mental disabilities and the Americans with Disabilities Act.* Washington, DC: American Psychological Association.

Stefan, S. (2002). *Hollow promises: Employment discrimination against people with mental disabilities.* Washington, DC: American Psychological Association.

Steiner, I. D. (1972). *Group processes and productivity.* New York: Academic Press.

Sternberg, R. J. (Ed.). (2004). *Creativity: From potential to realization.* Washington, DC: American Psychological Association.

Stewart, E. C., & Bennett, M. J. (1991). *American cultural patterns: A cross-cultural perspective.* Yarmouth, ME: Intercultural Press.

Stickney, C. P., & Weil, R. L. (2000). *Financial accounting: An introduction to concepts, methods, and uses* (9th ed.). Fort Worth, TX: Dryden Press.

Stockdale, J. S. (1996). *Sexual harassment in the workplace: Perspectives, frontiers, and response strategies.* Thousand Oaks, CA: Sage.

Stogdill, R. M., & Coons, A. E. (Eds.). (1951). *Leader behavior: Its description and measurement* (Research Monograph No. 88). Columbus: Ohio State University, Bureau of Business Research.

Stone, F. M. (1999). *Coaching, counseling and mentoring: How to choose and use the right technique to boost employee performance.* New York: American Marketing Association Publications.

Storti, C. (1999). *Figuring foreigners out.* Yarmouth, ME: Intercultural Press.

Stoudemire, A., & Fogel, B. S. (1993). *Psychiatric care of the medical patient.* New York: Oxford University Press.

Sue, D., & Sue, S. (1999). *Counseling the culturally different* (3rd ed.). New York: Wiley.

Sugai, G., & Tindel, G. (1993). *Effective school consultation: An interactive approach.* Pacific Grove, CA: Brooks/Cole.

Suinn, R. M. (1997). Mental practice in sport psychology: Where we have been, where do we go? *Clinical Psychology: Science and Practice, 4,* 189–207.

Swedo, S. E., Leonard, H. L., Garvey, M., Mittleman, B., Allen, A. J., Perlmutter, S., et al. (2002). Pediatric autoimmune neruopsychiatric disorders associated with streptococcal infections: Clinical description of the first 50 cases. *American Journal of Psychiatry, 159*(2), 320.

Tait, M., Baldwin, T., & Padgett, M. Y. (1989). Job and life satisfaction: A reevaluation of the strength of the relationship and gender effects. *Journal of Applied Psychology, 74*(3), 502–508.

Talbott, J. A., & Hales, R. E. (2001). *Textbook of administrative psychiatry: New concepts for a changing behavioral health system* (2nd ed.). Washington, DC: American Psychiatric Association.

Taylor, F. W. (1911). *The principles of scientific management.* New York: Harper & Brothers.

Taylor, J. C., & Bowers, D. G. (1972). *Survey of organizations.* Ann Arbor: University of Michigan, Institute for Social Research.

Tejada, C. (2000, June 16). Fickle grads. *Wall Street Journal,* p. A1.

Terkel, S. (1972). *Working: People talk about what they do all day and how they feel about what they do.* New York: New Press.

Terry, D. J., & Callan, V. J. (1997). Employee adjustment to large-scale organizational change. *Australian Psychologist, 32*(3), 203–210.

Thomas, D. A., & Gabarro, J. J. (1999). *Breaking through: The making of minority executives in corporate America*. Boston: Harvard Business School Press.

Thomas, R. R., & Woodruff, M. I. (1999). *Building a house for diversity*. New York: AMACOM, American Management Association.

Thompson, R. J., & Gustafson, K. E. (1996). *Adaptation to chronic childhood illness*. Washington, DC: American Psychological Association.

Tobias, L. L. (1990). *Psychological consultation to management: A clinician's perspective*. New York: Brunner/Mazel.

Triandis, H. C. (1994). *Culture and social behavior*. New York: McGraw-Hill.

Trist, E., Higgin, B., Murray, H., & Pollack, A. (1963). *Organizational choice*. London: Tavistock.

Tuckman, B. W., & Jensen, M. C. (1977). Stages of small-group development revisited. *Group and Organizational Studies, 2,* 419–427.

U.S. Department of Education. (2001). About safe and drug-free schools program. Available from http://www.ed.gov/offices/OESE/SDFS/aboutsdf.html.

U.S. Department of Health and Human Services. (1994). *Disaster response and recovery: A handbook for mental health professionals* (Publication No. SMA 94-3010). Washington, DC: Department of Health and Human Services.

U.S. Department of Health and Human Services. (2000). *Training manual for mental health workers in major disasters*. Washington, DC: Department of Health and Human Services.

U.S. Department of Health and Human Services. (2002a). *After a disaster: Self-care tips for dealing with stress*. Washington, DC: Department of Health and Human Services.

U.S. Department of Health and Human Services. (2002b). *Communicating in a crisis: Risk communication guidelines for public officials*. Washington, DC: Department of Health and Human Services.

U.S. Equal Employment Opportunity Commission. (2005). Uniform guidelines on employee selection procedures. Available from www.eeoc.gov.

U.S. Public Health Service. (2000). *Report of the Surgeon General's conference on children's mental health: A national action agenda*. Washington, DC: U.S. Department of Human Services.

Ungson, G. R., & Steers, R. M. (1984). Motivation and politics in executive compensation. *Academy of Management Review, 9*(2), 313–323.

van Emmerik, A. A. P., Kamphuis, J. H., Hulsbosch, A. M., Emmelkamp, P. M. G. (2002). Single-session debriefing after psychological trauma: A meta-analysis. *Lancet, 360,* 766–771.

VandenBos, G. R., DeLeon, P. H., & Belar, C. D. (1991). How many psychologists are needed? It's too early to know! *Professional Psychology: Research and Practice, 22,* 441–448.

Varney, G. H. (1989). *Building productive teams: An action guide and resource book*. San Francisco: Jossey-Bass.

Vernberg, E. M., & Reppucci, N. D. (1986). Behavioral consultation. In F. V. Mannino, E. J. Trickett, M. F. Shore, M. G. Kidder, & G. Levin (Eds.), *Handbook of mental health consultation* (pp. 49–80). Rockville, MD: National Institute for Mental Health.

Von Bertalanffy, L. (1976). *General systems theory: Foundations, development, applications*. New York: George Braziller.

Von Brock, M. B., & Elliott, S. N. (1987). The influence of treatment effectiveness information on the acceptability of classroom interventions. *Journal of School Psychology, 25,* 131–144.

Vroom, V. H. (1964). *Work and motivation*. New York: Wiley.

Walfish, S. (2001, August). *Clinical practice strategies outside the realm of managed care*. Paper presented at the 109th Convention of the American Psychological Association, San Francisco.

Wallace, W. A., & Hall, D. L. (1996). *Psychological consultation: Perspectives and applications.* Pacific Grove, CA: Brooks/Cole.

Walton, S., & Huey, J. (1993). *Sam Walton: Made in America.* New York: Bantam.

Wanberg, C. R., Bunce, L. W., & Gavin, M. B. (1999). Perceived fairness of layoffs among individuals who have been laid off: A longitudinal study. *Personnel Psychology, 52,* 59–84.

Warr, P. (Ed.). (1996). *Psychology at work* (4th ed.). New York: Penguin Books.

Warrick, S. (2005). *Why adopt a diversity program?* Available from www.scottwarrick.com.

Watkins, C. E., & Campbell, V. (Eds.). (2000). *Testing and assessment in counseling practice* (2nd ed.). Mahwah, NJ: Erlbaum.

Watson, T. J. (2003). *A business and its beliefs: The ideas that helped build IBM.* New York: McGraw-Hill.

Watzlawick, P., Weakland, J. H., & Fisch, R. (1974). *Change: Principles of problem formation and problem resolution.* New York: Norton.

Weber, M. (1947). *The theory of social and economic organizations.* New York: Free Press.

Weinberg, R. S., & Gould, D. (1999). *Foundations of sport and exercise psychology* (2nd ed.). Champaign, IL: Human Kinetics.

Weinberger, M., Hiner, S. L., & Tierney, W. M. (1987). In support of hassles as a measure of stress in predicting health outcomes. *Journal of Behavioral Medicine, 10,* 19–31.

Weisbord, M. R. (1976). Diagnosing your organization: Six places to look with or without a theory. *Group and Organizational Studies, 1,* 430–447.

Weisbord, M. R. (1992). *Discovering common ground.* San Francisco: Berrett-Koehler.

Weisbord, M. R., & Janoff, S. (1995). *Future search.* San Francisco: Berrett-Koehler.

Weisinger, H. (1998). *Emotional intelligence at work.* San Francisco: Jossey-Bass.

Weiss, A. (2004). *Getting started in consulting* (2nd ed.). Hoboken, NJ: Wiley.

Weiten, W., Stalling, R. B., & Wasden, R. E. (1998). *Psychology: Themes and variations* (4th ed.). Pacific Grove, CA: Brooks/Cole.

Wellington, S. W. (1998). *Advancing women in business: The catalyst guide.* San Francisco: Jossey-Bass.

Wenger, J. (1993). Just part of the mix. *Focus, 21*(9), 3, 4.

West, C. (2001). *Race matters* (Rev. ed.). Boston: Beacon Press.

Whetten, D. A., & Cameron, K. S. (2002). *Developing management skills* (5th ed.). Upper Saddle River, NJ: Prentice-Hall.

Whitmore, J. (1992). *Coaching for performance: A practical guide to growing your own skills.* London: Nicholas Beasley.

Wickstrom, K. F., & Witt, J. C. (1993). Resistance within school-based consultation. In J. E. Zina, T. R. Kratochwill, & S. N. Elliott (Eds.), *Handbook of consultation services for children: Applications in educational and clinical settings* (pp. 159–178). San Francisco: Jossey-Bass.

Widdis, W. (2005). *Breakthrough change tips.* Available from www.focusedchange.com.

Williams, P., & David, D. (2002). *Therapist as life coach: Transforming your practice.* New York: Norton.

Wing, R. (1988). *The art of strategy.* New York: Doubleday.

Winum, P. C., Nielson, T. M., & Bradford, R. E. (2002). Assessing the impact of organizational consulting. In R. L. Lowman (Ed.), *Handbook of organizational consulting psychology* (pp. 645–667). San Francisco: Jossey-Bass.

Witherspoon, R., & White, R. (1997). *Four essential ways that coaching can help executives.* Greensboro, NC: Center for Creative Leadership.

Wofford, J. C., & Liska, L. Z. (1993). Path-goal theories of leadership: A meta-analysis. *Journal of Management.* Winter, 857–876.

Wordreference.com. (2005). *Definitions of sociology and structural sociology.* Retrieved February 19, 2005, from www.wordreference.com.

World Tourism Organization. (2001). *Average annual vacation days taken.* Available from http://www.world-tourism.org.

Wrege, C. D., & Greenwood, R. G. (1991). *Frederick W. Taylor, the father of scientific management: Myth and reality.* Homewood, IL: Business One Irwin.

Wright, P., Kroll, M. J., & Parnell, J. (1998). *Strategic management: Concepts and cases* (4th ed.). Upper Saddle River, NJ: Prentice-Hall.

Yalom, I. D. (1980). *Existential psychotherapy.* New York: Basic Books.

Yalom, I. D. (1995). *The theory and practice of group psychotherapy* (4th ed.). New York: Basic Books.

Yenney, S. L. (1994). *Business strategies for a caring profession: A practitioner's guidebook.* Washington, DC: American Psychological Association.

Yukl, G. (1998). *Leadership in organizations* (3rd ed.). Upper Saddle River, NJ: Prentice-Hall.

Yukl, G., & Falbe, C. M. (1991, June). Importance of different power sources in downward and lateral relations. *Journal of Applied Psychology, 76,* 416–423.

Zaccaro, S. J. (2001). *The nature of executive leadership: A conceptual and empirical analysis of success.* Washington, DC: American Psychological Association.

Zajonc, R. (1965). Social facilitation. *Science, 149,* 269–275.

Additional Reference Sources ———————————

MAGAZINES AND NEWSPAPERS RELEVANT TO BUSINESS

Wall Street Journal
Fortune magazine
Financial Times
Economist

JOURNAL REFERENCES THAT PUBLISH MATERIAL RELEVANT TO CONSULTING PSYCHOLOGY

Consulting Psychology Journal: Practice and Research (Div.13)
Professional Psychology: Research and Practice
American Journal of Community Psychology
Journal of Consulting and Clinical Psychology
Journal of Educational and Psychological Consulting
Journal of Community Psychology
Community Mental Health Journal
Group and Organization Studies
Consultation: An International Journal
Research in Ethical Issues in Organization
Research in Organizational Behavior
Organizational Behavior and Human Decision Making Processes
Journal of Applied Behavioral Science
Organization Development Journal
Leadership and Organization Development Journal
Organizational Dynamics
Human Performance
Employee Relations Ethics

Journal of Consumer Psychology

Journal of Educational and Psychological Consultation

Basic and Applied Social Psychology

Journal of Vocational Behavior

International Journal of Stress Management

Consultation

Appendix

WHAT TO EVALUATE IN PSYCHOLOGICAL STUDIES

Lester L. Tobias

The following questions are intended to stimulate reflection about the characteristics of an individual with whom a psychological study is done.

Review Questions for Report Writing
  I. Intellectual Characteristics
  1. What is the person's basic intellectual capacity or intellectual level?
  2. How would you rate her ability to think logically, analytically, and comprehensively in both concrete and abstract areas?
  3. Are there any noteworthy differences among specific kinds of intelligence?
  4. Does she have any special strengths or weaknesses in dealing with certain kinds of problems?
  5. How is the individual's vocabulary and capacity for command of language?
  6. How is her nonverbal or quantitative reasoning ability?
  7. Is she particularly well equipped to handle technical problems, interpersonal abstractions, spatial relationships?
  8. Is the individual's intellectual effectiveness markedly influenced by emotional factors?
  9. Can he maintain concentration under pressure?
  10. Is he so afraid of intellectual risk as to become constricted or inhibited intellectually?
  11. Does he work up to his intellectual potentials or does he underachieve relative to his potentials?
  12. If there is underachievement, is it confined to certain types of problems or is it a more pervasive characteristic?
  13. What are the person's characteristic patterns or styles of problem solving?

Source: From *Psychological Consulting to Management: A Clinician's Perspective* (pp. 123–141), by L. L. Tobias, 1990, New York: Brunner/Mazel.

Copyright 1988 by Nordli, Wilson Associates, Inc. Reprinted with permission.

This section is a substantial revision of original unpublished material by Dr. Edward M. Glaser. I am indebted to him for his graciousness in granting me permission for publication and full freedom to revise. I have also borrowed heavily from the unpublished ideas of J. Watson Wilson and Daniel G. Tear. Naturally, I accept full responsibility for any defects herein.

14. Is she chiefly analytical or intuitive, tender-minded or tough-minded?
15. Is her thinking ponderous, methodical, bold, inspirational, conventional, traditional, and so on?
16. Is she an abstract thinker, or does she prefer concrete, tangible problems?
17. Does she work speedily or slowly?
18. Does she tend to guess or work with precision?
19. Does the individual possess sufficient intellectual discipline?
20. Is he able to be systematic, attentive to detail, organized, and careful when necessary?
21. If so, does he tend to be too detail oriented, too narrow, or too cautious, double- and triple-checking each solution before committing to it even when precision is unwarranted?
22. Or does the person exhibit a scattered or random search until a correct solution is found?
23. Does he tend to give up on a problem after initial failure?
24. Can he correct and reorient after a false start?
25. Does he go off on tangents?
26. Does she tend to exercise forethought and good judgment or to ask first and think later?
27. Can she think on her feet?
28. Can she move by inference from problem to solution without having to carefully check every single step in the process?
29. Does she tend to get caught off guard?
30. Can she vary her approach in dealing with different problems?
31. Does the individual have a cultivated sense of discrimination?
32. Can she distinguish between what is necessary and unnecessary, and between what is important and unimportant?
33. Is she able to reduce complicated subjects, proposals, or discussions to their simplest terms?
34. Can she separate major issues from minor issues?
35. Does he plan in practical and concrete terms in order to translate broad visions into attainable goals?
36. Can he structure his ideas and plans or does he require external structure?
37. Does he manifest good judgment and level headedness?
38. Can he apply knowledge in a realistic and practical way?
39. Does he have the facility to move from ideas to decision to appropriate actions and deeds?
40. Is she able to make competent decisions in the face of conflicting pressures?
41. Can she face and deal with problems without excessive putting-off?
42. Does she need extra time to resolve issues?
43. Is she bold enough to proceed before all the data are in?
44. Does she think with efficiency and focus?
45. Does the individual have the ability to work with ideas and the relationships among ideas?
46. Does she have facility in assembling a group of seemingly unrelated facts and finding out how they are connected?
47. Does she have overall grasp and breadth—the ability to see the broad picture, to tie things beyond immediate concerns? Can she grasp problems outside her special field?

48. Does the person have a vigorously probing mind, a reflective and natural intellectual curiosity, and a spectrum of interests and knowledge?
49. Does he stay well informed of developments in his field and other fields?
50. Is he receptive to new ideas?
51. Does he passively respond to problems that come his way, or does he look for and become interested in taking the intellectual initiative?
52. Does the person have a creative imagination?
53. Can she dream and "paint with a big brush"?
54. Can she visualize bigger things than can actually be brought about—and exert constant intellectual effort toward those things?
55. Does she have originality and freshness of thinking?
56. Can she get beyond what is commonly accepted or customary?
57. Will she cross-fertilize her ideas with associates and respond to intellectual give-and-take?
58. Is the person fluid, alert, and resourceful?
59. Can he find his way around intellectual barriers and reframe questions so they can yield answers?
60. Can the person juggle several balls in the air at once or think on his feet when an obstacle is encountered?
61. Is he observant, inquisitive, and oriented toward scanning for new information?
62. Is the individual's thinking generally objective—flexibly open to the weight of evidence and to reality factors, rather than distorted by personal prejudices, intellectual rigidity, stereotyping, opinionatedness, stubbornness, personality defenses, and private fantasies?
63. Can she listen to the alternatives provided by others and weigh them judiciously? Can she keep emotional or personal interests from unduly influencing her judgment?
64. Can she tolerate ambiguity and discriminate among shades of gray, or does she see the world only in black and white terms?
65. Can she appreciate divergent realities?
66. Can she go beyond the immediate facts, or does she tend to oversimplify?
67. Can she see contrasts and make fine distinctions?
68. Is he characterized by intellectual integrity?
69. Is he able to be constructively self-critical?
70. Does he have the intellectual honesty, independence, and the courage to stick to a decision?
71. Is his thinking characterized by firmness of conviction?
72. Does she reasonably recognize and accept her approximate level of intellectual capacity?
73. Does she overreach or underachieve relative to her potential, and is she unduly surprised by the results of her efforts?
74. Does she have the ability to turn experience into an asset, to extract from an experience its full implications?

II. Emotional Characteristics
  1. What are the person's characteristic and pervasive traits?
  2. How does he feel about himself and his world?
  3. Does he tend to be calm and relaxed or nervous and tense?
  4. Is he generally good-humored or dyspeptic?
  5. Is he even-tempered or mercurial?

6. Do his mood swings result from inner stimuli or outer stimuli?
7. Is he optimistic or pessimistic?
8. Is he carefree or taciturn?
9. Is she reasonably free from excessive anxieties, worries, obsessions, illusions, fears, guilt feelings, hostility and neurotic or psychosomatic symptoms?
10. Does she tend to be open and forthright or cautiously reserved?
11. Does she internalize inner feelings and tensions or externalize through spontaneous expression or action?
12. To what degree is he free of personal ego-hunger and defensiveness?
13. Is he undersensitive or hypersensitive?
14. Will he freely admit mistakes?
15. Does he take himself too seriously or not seriously enough?
16. Can he compete without always having to win; is he able to achieve and relax, to work and play?
17. Does he sacrifice means for ends or ends for means?
18. Can he tolerate stress and remain poised under pressure?
19. Can he take criticism, rejection, frustration, delay, boredom, and fatigue in reasonable stride, roll with the punches, and still rally to take the initiative and carry on?
20. Is he conceited, apprehensive, self-conscious, or self-deprecating?
21. What is her level of energy and vitality?
22. Is she active and zestful or sluggish and complacent?
23. Does she have a basic urge to get things done?
24. Is she able to use most of her endowments and to acquire skills that work, or does she tend to fritter away time and energy in emotional self-restriction, poor self-discipline, excessive self-consciousness, or inadequate sense of proportion and perspective?
25. Is she mainly inner-directed or outer-directed, structure-seeking or structure-making?
26. Does she strive toward mastery and seek challenges?
27. To what degree is the person generally objective and reasonably free from personal ego fragility as contrasted with having many touchy areas, blind spots, illogical hatreds, fanciful ideals, or strong prejudices?
28. Is he suspicious or distrustful, skeptical or cynical?
29. Does he evidence the ability to be reasonable without intellectualizing, to think and to do?
30. To what extent is the person mature emotionally?
31. Is she weaned, independent, and secure?
32. Is she in touch with her feelings and able to manage them?
33. To what extent is she free from self-absorption, self-deprecation, and over-concern with self-gratification and, therefore, able to focus constructively on facing the demands and challenges of life?
34. Does she evidence the ability to stand out as well as to stand back, self-scrutinize without being self-absorbed, to be proud and to be humble, to take herself seriously and to laugh at herself, to want to be her best without having to be the best?
35. How strong is the person's sense of self?
36. Does he accept himself, berate himself, or ignore himself?

37. Is he conscious of his inner dialogue, and in what tone of voice does this dialogue take place?
38. How strong is his ego and self-concept?
39. To what degree is she able to demonstrate a persistent willingness to spend time in accomplishing a task, to plod patiently when the load is heavy and the road is steep?
40. Can she attack a problem aggressively?
41. Can she back off?
42. Can she delay gratification?
43. Can she maintain self-discipline?
44. How easy or difficult is it for him to shift his ideational, motor or attitudinal sets from one task to another without losing efficiency?
45. Does he have a well-developed sense of importance of timing?
46. Does he have a sense of perspective, proportion, and priority?
47. Can he adjust rapidly to changing situations; can he cope with the unexpected?
48. Can he handle rejection and loss?
49. Can he leave well enough alone?
50. Is he aware of immediate realities and their implications, and can he grapple with them in a forthright, feet-on-the-ground manner?
51. What are the person's characteristic styles of adjustment in the face of barriers and obstacles?
52. What are her "fears and fires"?
53. How does she handle frustration?
54. Is she characteristically an action-taker who accepts accountability and tries to pave her fate or a passive, avoidant, perpetual victim of circumstance?
55. Does he evidence the ability to control and to accept control, to lead and to follow, to take action and to tolerate inaction, to be both passive and active when appropriate?
56. Does he tend to be cautious and wait for the "safe bets," or does he have a well-developed sense of adventure, and if so, in what ways?
57. Is there a confident readiness to take calculated risks for desired objectives?
58. Does she have the ability to operate within bounds, to expand her horizons, to inhibit and to express?
59. Does she tend to seek an easy life devoid of challenge—a comfortable rut— or does she have a strong will to do and does she seek fulfillment through doing things that require courage, patience, or concentrated effort?
60. What kinds of standards and tolerance does she have for herself and others?
61. Does she set high standards and maintain a strong drive for achievement and accomplishment?
62. Is she active and striving?
63. Does she feel confident with regard to the major areas of living?
64. Does he evidence the ability to balance self-interest and personal ethics, to navigate through waters of moral ambiguity with both consistency and flexibility?
65. Does he appreciate moral complexity?
66. What are the lines along which he has decided or feels impelled to live his life?
67. What does he stand against and for in his life?

68. What does he seek to be, to become, or to do in life?
69. For what will he make a sacrifice?
70. Are her goals in line with her long-term needs?
71. What are the essentials for her?
72. What are her choices and emphases when faced with options?
73. What is her guiding emotional core?
74. Is she guided by an overriding value system, and is there congruence among her feelings, thought, goals, actions, and values?
75. Can she articulate her value system?
76. Does the individual have patience, devotion of interest, and determination?
77. Does the person have the ability to idealize without having to be perfect, to find a use for order and for chaos, to focus in and focus out, to structure without obsession, to wander with purpose?
78. Is there a balance between the person's conscience, intellect, and motives?
79. Does he have personal integrity and ethical intent?
80. Is he of sound character and characterized by a sound personal philosophy of constructive fundamental principles?
81. Does he have a well-developed conscience and sense of obligation?
82. What does he do about the responsibilities with which he is entrusted?
83. How far does he see his responsibilities extending from himself?
84. Is the person emotionally flexible enough to modify her own attitudes in order to meet the needs of others?
85. Does she have true humility?
86. Can she both give and receive?
87. Can she depend on herself as well as on others, to join and to be alone, to stand on her own two feet and to hold hands?
88. Can he accept authority without rebelliousness or resentment?
89. Does he experience feelings of alienation from others, or common roots, purposes and rhythms?
90. Can he forgive and accept forgiveness?
91. Does he have the ability to conform or synchronize in a manner that affirms the self, to nurture his own inner light and those of others, to be frank and to be tactful?
92. Can he be vulnerable with others and give and accept intimacy?
93. Does he feel connected with others and with the world, or does he experience loneliness and alienation?
94. Does she have zest for life, spontaneity, a creative thrust, and a growing edge?
95. Does she have the ability to refresh her mind and spirit, to feel satisfied, to find sources of strength and renewal for her own spirits?
96. Can she keep an eye on the distant star—to lift her gaze toward the larger purposes of life?
97. Can she transcend daily concerns and her own finite boundaries with a leap of faith?
98. Does she possess a will that is good toward herself, toward others, toward life, and toward living?
99. Does she foster this will in others?

III. Motivational Characteristics
1. What is the person's degree of drive?
2. What basic needs seem to move the person?

3. Are these needs external or internal?
4. How does the individual express these needs in behavior?
5. Are there strong peaks and valleys among needs, possibly reflecting greater drive or compulsive insatiability?
6. Or, are the person's needs fairly level, possibly reflecting a blandness of drive or ambivalence characteristics of adolescents?
7. Is the need strong because it reflects conflicts and fantasies of childhood; and if so, has the individual learned to set mature and attainable goals to meet those needs?
8. Are the needs so low as to suggest unconscious rejection of the need; and if so, does the need nevertheless drive the person's actions directly?
9. Does the person evidence a strong need for affectionate and intimate relationships with others and for deep emotional attachment?
10. Is there an unbounded craving for acceptance and an insecurity about rejection?
11. Does he constantly need reassurance or is he able to do some self-prodding?
12. If his need for affection is low, does it mean that he values cooler distance, or is he afraid of emotional entanglements?
13. If it is high, does the need lead to hypersensitivity; and if low, does it lead to insensitivity?
14. To what extent is the individual motivated by the need to operate interdependently, to achieve a sense of belonging, to join, to be a partner, or to follow?
15. If the need is high, is it an indication of healthy mutuality or immature dependency?
16. On the other hand, is there a need not to have to rely on others?
17. If so, does it lead to a healthy capacity to operate independently or to an inability to truly join, to appreciate boundaries, to ask for help when it is necessary, or to work in tandem with others?
18. To what extent does the person seek restriction and boundedness?
19. Does she prefer the calculated risk, security, harmony, balance, stability, and predictability?
20. If so, does this reflect insecurity and lead to rigidity, passivity, immobility, emotional blandness, and a failure to stretch potentials?
21. Is she afraid to "rock the boat"?
22. On the other hand, does she seek expansion and resist boundaries?
23. Does she look for diversity, change, unlimited possibilities, and freedom and spontaneity of action and expression?
24. If so, can she accept reasonable boundaries, work within structures, and tolerate rules and guidelines?
25. Or, is there evidence of impulsivity, constant impatience, and a refusal to be guided by tradition or rules of the game?
26. Will the person create turmoil for its own sake?
27. Is the individual oriented toward power, persuasion, authority, influence, and impact?
28. Does it lead to a willingness to take on authority, to take charge, to make things happen, and to be where the action is?
29. Does it lead her to be prime moving, assertive, forceful, and dominant?

30. Or, does it reflect a desire to make sure that she is not "bossed" by others, a reaction to felt impotence, a fear of vulnerability, or the acting out of fantasies of omnipotence?
31. Does it lead to authoritarian, domineering, overcontrolling, or intimidating approaches to others or to situations?
32. Or, does she prefer not to lead; but, instead, to let others make the decision and take responsibility for actions?
33. Does this reflect a contentment with going with the flow; or does it reflect deeper passivity, a fatalistic attitude, or passive aggressiveness?
34. Does the person gain satisfaction from the use of logic, reasons, theory, or creativity?
35. Are these a means of self-expression and goal-attainment?
36. Does this lead him to be easily stimulated by intellectual challenges and to test his intellectual limits?
37. Does it reflect an inability to accept the value of emotions; and, does it lead to overrationality, to analyzing but not solving, to thinking but not acting, to insisting on facts but denying intuitions?
38. Does he, on the other hand, stress a practical and down-to-earth approach with less emphasis on theoretical or abstract issues?
39. If so, does this reflect insecurity regarding his intellectual expression, or a lack of intellectual discipline?
40. Does the person evidence a need to behave in a determined, tenacious, and persistent fashion, to use willpower as an end as well as a means toward an end?
41. Does this lead her to be highly self-disciplined, dutiful, and steadfast, or does it lead her to wear blinders, to be stubborn or dogmatic, to fail to take perspective, and to anticipate adversity?
42. Does she practice denial or assume that wishing makes it so?
43. On the other hand, is she more prone toward flexibility regarding persistence and duty, more oriented toward shifting gears and finding shortcuts and short-lived enthusiasms?
44. If so, to what degree can she nevertheless muster discipline when necessary, or does she make excuses for not trying or for not "keeping the plow in the ground"?
45. Is she willing to make the effort and the sacrifices that are required to attain life goals?
46. To what extent does the individual have a need to exploit opportunities, to seize the advantage, to partake in the interplay of the marketplace, to react resourcefully to incoming stimuli, to venture, and to risk?
47. If this need is high, can the person resist distraction and keep a focus on long-term goals and ethical congruence?
48. Can he temper self-interest and short-term gain for broader purposes?
49. Does he require stimulation in order to react?
50. On the other hand, is he less inclined to react to opportunity, more selective regarding goals, characterized by greater uniformity of pace?
51. If so, does he fail to notice opportunity and wonder why others "get all the breaks"?
52. Does he fear exploitation and react with characteristic counterexploitiveness?

53. Does the individual evidence a need for social recognition, respect, status, prestige, and a sense of communality with others?
54. Does this lead her to maintain a conforming, poised and diplomatic stature and to exhibit a strong sense of communal obligation and commitment?
55. Or, does it reflect shallowness and social insecurity and lead to superficiality, pretentiousness, stressing appearance over substance, or intolerance for divergence?
56. On the other hand, is she more inclined toward nonconformity, less of a joiner, and less inclined to identify with the majority, and more individualistic?
57. If so, does this reflect a healthy willingness to question tradition and a preference for following her own inner light; or, does it reflect adolescent nonconformity, a fear of being unacceptable to others, a compensatory "I don't care what others think" attitude, an inability to fit in, an insensitivity to social expectations, or a perpetual rebellion against "the establishment," or a task focus without a people focus?
58. Does the individual evidence a strong need to be his "personal best," to engage in activities that reflect well upon him, bring out the best in him, and lead to pride of accomplishment?
59. If so, is he self-scrutinizing, self-demanding, and selective about the goals he chooses?
60. Does he have to be in the spotlight all the time?
61. Is there evidence of narcissistic self-absorption, grandiosity, emphasis on appearances, selfishness, or an inability to sustain momentum when there is no opportunity to shine?
62. Is the preoccupation on looking good rather than accomplishing, on the process rather than the result?
63. Is the person too selective regarding goals?
64. On the other hand, does he prefer to operate behind the scenes, to emphasize characteristics of modesty and humility, to do what needs to be done without concern for issues of pride or grandeur?
65. If so, is there an underlying lack of sense of self or pride in self, a fear of introspection, a denial of selfhood?
66. Does the individual show a strong need for competitive achievement, for winning, for acquiring, and for building?
67. Does it lead her to attempt to climb the ladder of success based on a long-term game plan?
68. Does it lead to workaholism, over-competitiveness, or an inability to accept defeat?
69. On the other hand, does she tend to deemphasize competitiveness and acquisitiveness?
70. Can she, nevertheless, compete when in competition; or, is she inclined to underachieve, to fear competition, or to live only for the day?
71. Does the person evidence a strong need for autonomy and self-sufficiency?
72. Is it important for him to be self-directing and self-stimulating, to work on his own or by himself; and, does this lead him to venture out, to explore his potentials, and to fend for himself?
73. Does it lead him to be insular, to fear intimacy, to have to do everything alone?

74. On the other hand, does he show a need to be around others and not to maintain independence?
75. If so, does it lead him to be harmonizing and conventional?
76. Or does it reflect a deeper fear of being alone or abandoned?
77. Is he paralyzed when called upon to strike out on his own?
78. Does the individual evidence a strong need for order, attention to detail, structure, and accuracy?
79. If so, does it lead to analytical depth, punctuality, and elegance of craftsmanship?
80. Or, does it lead to obsessiveness, narrowness, and picayune excursions?
81. Or does she, instead, stress spontaneity, breadth, and creative chaos?
82. Does she, therefore, welcome ambiguity, play with possibility, and enjoy the unexpected?
83. If so, can the individual keep track of details, stay within bounds, and stay on track?

IV. Insight into One's Self and into Others

1. To what degree is the person aware of the roots and background forces that have shaped his style of life?
2. Is his awareness only at a descriptive level; or does he understand the major dynamic forces that have tended to shape his development?
3. Does his self-concept reflect perspective and objectivity?
4. Is he aware of his own tendencies, characteristics, potentials, limitations, strengths, and shortcomings?
5. Is he more self-critical than self-analytical?
6. Does he have a good grasp of his inner needs, and are the goals he sets to meet those needs typically well chosen?
7. Has he chosen a realistic and appropriate level of aspiration?
8. Is his self-image consistent with the way others would see him, and is he aware of his own impact on others?
9. Does he often get surprised at others' behavior or attitudes?
10. Does he even think about these kinds of things?
11. Does the person practice internal vigilance as a means of self-improvement on a continuing basis?
12. Is she characterized by sufficient self-accountability, flexibility, and psychological mindedness to be able to use experience in the service of constructive change?
13. What are the blind spots or areas of subjectivity that skew or distort her view of reality in particular directions?
14. Is she prone toward self-justification, rationalization, hyperbole, minimization, or extremes of thought?
15. Is there evidence of projection, repression, or other defensive barriers to fluid insight development?
16. Is the individual reasonably in touch with her own feelings?
17. Can she constructively use internal as well as external data, logical as well as nonlogical data, and verbal as well as nonverbal data?
18. Is she capable of exhibiting a sense of humor about her own foibles and shortcomings as well as those of others?
19. To what degree and in what way does the person understand or evaluate other people and their reactions?

20. Does he make the effort?
21. Can he sense unstated attitudes, feelings, and motives?
22. Can he distinguish between sincerity and bluff?
23. Are there consistent biases in his assessment of others?
24. Is he aware of individual differences?
25. Does he attempt to make differentiations; or, does he tend only to see others at a surface level?
26. Does he have the ability to observe and interpret minimal cues in dealing with people?
27. Does he see the people-component in issues?
28. Can he sense the climate or morale of a group?
29. Is he perceptive, penetrating, sensitive, and/or empathic?
30. Is he able to understand the underlying motives of others?
31. Is he tolerant or intolerant of the weaknesses of others?
32. Does he gloss over negatives or overemphasize them?
33. Is he able to see through others' eyes and listen through others' ears and, thus, appreciate why people feel and act as they do?
34. Does he have appreciation and respect for divergent realities, perspectives, world views, and values?
35. How does the individual use the insights she develops?
36. Is she active or passive regarding insights?
37. Does she use insights to accommodate, to adapt, to manipulate, to help, to rescue, to control others?
38. Does she evidence skill in balancing the feelings, needs, and ideas of others with her own?
39. Does she have skill in resolving discrepancies of meaning in the communication process?
40. Can she judge when to react to the "facts," and when to search for hidden agendas?

V. Interpersonal Characteristics
1. Does the person maintain a pleasant, agreeable, and friendly manner when meeting people?
2. Is he interested in people?
3. Is he introverted and solitary or extroverted and gregarious?
4. Is he well-mannered, poised, and reasonably free of annoying mannerisms, ostentatiousness, approval-seeking behavior, or pretentiousness?
5. How would you characterize his general social impact, and how well does he wear over time?
6. To what extent does he exhibit the characteristic of stature or presence with others?
7. Does he tend to blend in or to stand out, to lead or to follow, to participate or to withdraw?
8. Is he relatively consistent in ideas, attitudes, and behavior, or, is there a good deal of variance, depending upon time, circumstances, or moods?
9. Is he articulate and skilled in oral expression?
10. Is he able to carry on a conversation, to put ideas across, to stay on the point, and to convey what he means?
11. Can he dramatize an issue to bring it alive?
12. Does the individual typically exhibit good will toward others and toward life?

13. Does she generally facilitate or hinder group action in accomplishing a group task?
14. Is she characteristically kind and gracious to people when there is no special need?
15. Is there generosity in her assumptions about the intents of others?
16. Does she give others the benefit of the doubt?
17. Does she exhibit a spirit of compromise and acceptance of the habits, tastes, and preferences of others?
18. Does she convey amicability, appreciation, humility, and receptiveness with others?
19. Can she adjust to different types of people as they are, not as she would like them to be?
20. Does she overreact to or withdraw from certain types of people or to people in general?
21. Does she tend to adopt a cordial and affirming attitude toward others, or one that is aloof and hostile?
22. Is she forgiving or vengeful?
23. Is she oriented toward or away from acceptance and a spirit of accommodation?
24. Is she capable of both experiencing and conveying genuine respect toward others?
25. Does she tend to be more cooperative or competitive, warm or cool, straightforward or circumventive, selfish or unselfish, fairminded or biased, passive or active, trusting or suspicious, and, honest or deceptive?
26. Is she considerate, helpful, thoughtful, gracious, and able to restrain her personal impulses and desires out of consideration for others?
27. Is there evidence of arrogance, crudeness, self-righteousness, sarcasm, self-consciousness, obsequiousness, posturing, hostility, stiffness, deviousness, insincerity, or manipulativeness?
28. Does she put a high value on another person's time?
29. Does she give people a sense of being in a hurry, or is she generally relaxed and available to others?
30. Does she readily like people for themselves, or does she use people as an audience or for personal gain?
31. To which kinds of people is she likely to feel closest or least close?
32. Does the person inspire the confidence of others?
33. To what extent is he characterized by directness, aggressiveness, assertiveness, energy, persuasiveness, and a willingness to take the lead or the social initiative?
34. Can he be adequately forceful in dealing with unpleasant situations?
35. Can he balance diplomacy, discretion, and tact with frankness and confrontation?
36. What are the differences, if any, in the way he treats subordinates, associates, and superiors?
37. Can he respect the ideas and performance of people whom he dislikes personally?
38. Can he energize others?
39. Can he understand and elicit the best from people who are of lower social status, educational attainment, or intellectual capacity?

40. Can he facilitate the attainment of group objectives?
41. Does the individual evidence simple sincerity and searching honesty?
42. Is she a good listener?
43. Does she know when to talk and when to listen?
44. Does she listen with a sincere desire to understand and to make the best use of another person's point of view?
45. Does she generally have a good sense of humor, including the ability to laugh at herself?
46. Is she generally good humored or humorless?
47. Does she have a sense of fun, of shared play?
48. Can she truly share and truly join with others?
49. Can she give to others as well as take from others with comfort and naturalness?
50. Has she developed the skill of concomitantly affirming the self and others?
51. Can she forgive past hurts and deal with relationships in the present?
52. To what extent does this individual exhibit the traits, characteristics, and behaviors common to a particular culture, nationality, geographical region, subculture, socioeconomic class, or ethnic, linguistic, or racial group?
53. Does he exhibit these characteristics with comfort and ease or is there some awkwardness in his outward expression of his self-identity?
54. Can he adapt his behavior to those who fall into other groups and accommodate divergent characteristics with grace?
55. Is he comfortable dealing with others across generational lines?
56. Does he have a willingness to explore cross-cultural differences?

VI. Vocational Characteristics
1. How do the characteristics of the person "come together" in his approach to his job?
2. What are his vocational and career interests and ambitions?
3. How does he go about applying the relevant "technology" of his job?
4. If the job is selling, how does he sell?
5. If the job is managing, how does he manage?
6. If the job is basket weaving, how does he weave baskets?
7. What is the person's ability to initiate, plan, organize, and direct action?
8. Does he typically develop and use a plan?
9. If so, is the plan tactical, strategic, or a combination of both?
10. Is he capable of broad planning, or does he just focus on specific issues or details?
11. Is he able to plan a steady work flow?
12. Is he better as a visionary, implementer, or follower?
13. Can he distinguish between small and great matters for decisions and teach others to do the same?
14. Can he shift fluidly from abstract to concrete and back?
15. Can he focus on the target without losing sight of the details of implementation?
16. Does he characteristically seek and envision better ways of doing things; and, is he resourceful enough to find the means of putting these ideas into practice?
17. Does he see and act upon new opportunities?
18. Does he move ahead reactively or according to well-defined principles or concepts?

19. Is he objective in weighing evidence for or against proposed courses of action?
20. How determined is the individual to accomplish personal objectives?
21. To what degree does she summon energy, drive, and perseverance toward the attainment of goals?
22. Can she endure long periods without success?
23. Is she one who makes things happen, who takes charge, who is willing to rock the boat, who can be an effective prime mover?
24. Is she prompt to take hold of a problem?
25. What is her degree of drive and ingenuity in finding means to achieve ends?
26. Will she characteristically work up to her highest potential?
27. Does she put first things first, or tend to "grease the wheel that squeaks the loudest," or to procrastinate in getting to the less enjoyable portions of the work?
28. Is she more effective at following through on a specific job, organizing a system, or supervising complex organizational details?
29. Or, is she more of a promoter or an "idea person," but disinterested or weak on the follow-through?
30. What are her standards of accuracy and thoroughness?
31. Does she have the capacity to run things—to take responsibility—and to manage things in a well-organized way that makes for superior accomplishment or end results?
32. Does she have a good understanding of the operating mechanism of a business?
33. Does she know how to apply management principles at many levels?
34. Can she handle many pressing problems in rapid-fire order?
35. Can she tolerate constant interruption?
36. Can she retain many problems in mind simultaneously and juggle priorities for action?
37. Can the person feel like an integral part of an organization, and if so, under what circumstances?
38. Can he identify with the organization to the degree that a powerful motivation and source of satisfaction stems from organizational success or business development?
39. Does he give time, effort, and devotion to becoming more and more adept at a job, and what are the conditions which best bring out this behavior?
40. Does he possess a comprehensive philosophy of management and a sensitivity to the problems of building a spirited and effective team of people?
41. Is he able to think from an organizational point of view and, yet, be loyal to subordinates—accepting full accountability for their actions—as well as to superiors and to his own conscience?
42. Can he compromise without being or feeling compromised?
43. Does the individual tend to view superiors as a guiding or consulting source, or as an inhibiting force?
44. Are her attitudes toward authority potential sources of organizational conflict?
45. Does she work best under freedom and responsibility for operation in an unstructured or semi-structured pattern; or does she require a structured situation in which standard practice can be followed?
46. Will the stimulus of greater responsibility or of greater demand set by a superior help to motivate her, or is it best to allow her to proceed at her own pace?

47. Does the person set a sound example of effective leadership?
48. Is he able to inspire loyalty and to work cooperatively and respectfully with people at all levels of the organization?
49. Can he motivate others to full effectiveness?
50. Is he a good teacher, coach, and assessor of people?
51. What is his ability to select, train, and develop subordinates, to assign them suitably, and to keep track of their performance?
52. Does he generally maintain an attitude of trust and approval in dealing with subordinates and associates, even though realistically recognizing their characteristics, tendencies, or limitations?
53. Does he expect others to pace themselves at his rate; or, does he evidence sensitivity to and respect for other people's rates, styles, or energy levels?
54. Can he effectively represent and transmit the values and priorities that guide the organization to his subordinates?
55. Is he willing and able to be responsive to the expectations handed down from superiors?
56. Does the individual keep people properly informed of matters which affect them?
57. Can, and will, she generally make clear the reasons behind her actions?
58. Can she effectively delegate responsibilities and commensurate authority, or does she overcontrol or underinvolve others?
59. Does she avoid going around people or over people's heads?
60. Is she willing to encourage participation on the part of subordinates, and is she skillful in tapping the creative ideas of others?
61. Does she solicit new ideas in order to improve methods and procedures?
62. Does she play a catalytic role as a supervisor?
63. Is she vitally interested in the people around her?
64. Does she have a genuine interest in the training and development of subordinates?
65. How does the person try to lead?
66. What is the individual's characteristic management style: easy-going, benevolent, stern, clear, fair, dynamic, inspirational, demanding, firm, visionary, conservative, rigid, risk-avoidant, challenging, systematic, or authoritarian?
67. Will he err on the lenient side?
68. Can he make hard people decisions, and in what time frame, and with what skill?
69. Does he supervise by authority, suggestions, personal enthusiasm, explanation, example, or by invitation to group problem solving?
70. Will he hold people accountable for their actions or overprotect them?
71. In what areas, with what problems or in what environment is he most and least effective?
72. What would he need to remember about his own error tendencies in order to maximize effectiveness over the long-haul?
73. What can his manager do to bring out his best potentials on an ongoing basis, to help him feel empowered to stretch, and to help him avoid the probable pitfalls of his style?
74. What particular issues need to be considered in managing this individual in a manner that will meet her needs, promote her growth, and foster her effectiveness?

75. How easy is she to manage?
76. Does she need structure, challenge, incentives, praise, applause, reassurance, concrete directions, absence of risk, clear feedback, a safe and predictable environment, a close working relationship, intellectual stimulation, freedom and latitude, prodding, redirection from blind alleys, deadlines, time to think, support in dealing with other departments, or something else?
77. How will she react if what is needed is unavailable?
78. How will she react when there are setbacks, crises, temptations, losses, failures, or disappointments?
79. How will she deal with risk, uncertainty, rejection, lack of control, or unfairness in others?

Author Index

Subject Index

About the Authors

Richard W. Sears, PsyD, MBA   Richard Sears received his doctorate in Clinical Psychology from the School of Professional Psychology and his Master of Business Administration from the Raj Soin College of Business at Wright State University in Dayton, Ohio. Dr. Sears performs consultation services for individuals, businesses, and nonprofit agencies on a wide variety of topics, including executive coaching and development, strategic and tactical business planning, training and development workshops, mental health issues in the workplace, stress reduction, change management, and self-defense and security issues. He also teaches at Wright State University School of Professional Psychology.

In addition to his business, consultation, and clinical experience, he is a fourth degree black belt in Ninjutsu, a licensed private pilot, scuba diver, and musician, and has received past certification as an Emergency Medical Technician. He once served as a personal protection agent for the Dalai Lama of Tibet. Richard can be contacted at richard@psych-insights.com or by visiting www.psych-insights.com.

John R. Rudisill, PhD, ABPP   John Rudisill is a professor and the dean of the School of Professional Psychology at Wright State University in Dayton, Ohio. He is a generalist with expertise in both clinical and organizational psychology, and has over 25 years of organizational consulting and clinical private practice experience. His professional experience includes Director of the Division of Applied Psychology at Wright State University School of Medicine, Chief Psychologist and Program Director at Dayton Mental Health Center, and Director of the Air Force Mental Health Clinics at Seymour-Johnson and Clark Air Bases. Dr. Rudisill has consulted with numerous public and private organizations. He has a variety of publications in medical education, organizational and clinical practice, as well supervision and mentoring of students. His current area of research is coping with unemployment. He is a fellow of the Division of Independent Practice and the Society of Consulting Psychologists in the American Psychological Association. He is a former president of the Dayton Area Psychological Association and has been a trustee and committee chair of the Ohio Psychological Association. Dr. Rudisill has been awarded a diplomate in professional psychology (clinical) by the American Board of Professional Psychology. He has received the Academy of Medicine Senior Faculty Award for outstanding contributions to medical education and research. Dr. Rudisill has served in leadership roles for a number of community social service activities. He received his PhD from Indiana University, where he studied under Dr. Kenneth Heller, who was a student of Gerald Caplan, father of mental health consultation.

Carrie Mason-Sears, PhD   Carrie Mason-Sears received her PhD in Clinical Psychology from the University of Cincinnati with a specialization in child clinical psychology and child development. She is a licensed clinical psychologist who provides direct and indirect psychological consultation to community and home-based teams in the development and implementation of educational and behavioral supports for children with developmental disabilities and their families. Dr. Mason-Sears provides individual and family therapy for children and families and assists in clinical program expansion and program development in her role as the Clinical Coordinator for Child and Family Services for the Community Integrated Training and Education (CITE) program of the Resident Home Corporation. Dr. Mason-Sears is well known in the Cincinnati community for her work with children with developmental disabilities, and worked at the Cincinnati Children's Hospital Medical Center, Department of Developmental Disabilities, before joining CITE. She has pediatric consultation liaison experience from the University of North Carolina Chapel Hill and Cincinnati Children's Hospital. She also currently manages a part-time private practice in the Cincinnati area. She may be contacted at carrie@psych-insights.com or www.psych-insights.com.